Current Advances in Breast Cancer Research: A Molecular Approach

Edited by

Shankar Suman

Cancer Comprehensive Centre, The Ohio State University, West 12th Avenue, Columbus-43210, USA

Garima Suman

Department of Radiodiagnosis, Tata Memorial Hospital, Dr. E Borges Road, Parel, Mumbai-400012, (Maharashtra) India

Sanjay Mishra

Department of Pathology, The Ohio State University, Columbus, Ohio, 43210, USA

Current Advances in Breast Cancer Research: A Molecular Approach

Editors:Shankar Suman, Garima Suman , Sanjay Mishra

ISBN (Online): 978-981-14-5144-7

ISBN (Print): 978-981-14-5142-3

ISBN (Paperback): 978-1-68108-771-9

need for a court order if at any point you breach any terms of this License Agreement. In no event will any delay or failure by Bentham Science Publishers in enforcing your compliance with this License Agreement constitute a waiver of any of its rights.

3. You acknowledge that you have read this License Agreement, and agree to be bound by its terms and conditions. To the extent that any other terms and conditions presented on any website of Bentham Science Publishers conflict with, or are inconsistent with, the terms and conditions set out in this License Agreement, you acknowledge that the terms and conditions set out in this License Agreement shall prevail.

Bentham Science Publishers Pte. Ltd.
80 Robinson Road #02-00
Singapore 068898
Singapore
Email: subscriptions@benthamscience.net

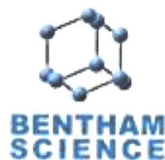

CONTENTS

FOREWORD

Breast cancer is the leading cause of cancer for women both in the developed and the developing world, as per the World Health Organization. Breast cancer also affects men. Over a decade, cancer incidence has declined, but breast cancer incidence in females has increased by 0.4% per year. Although advancements in breast cancer screening, preventive measures, and treatment have resulted in a significant decline in breast cancer mortality, breast cancer still is the second most common cause of cancer-related deaths in females. Unacceptable levels of racial disparity have been consistently reported in breast cancer and offer a challenge in breast cancer prevention, detection, and cure. These disparities are independent of socioeconomic status, access to healthcare or age, or even the stage of breast cancer. Among the major challenges, the heterogeneity in cancer cells makes the disease more complex. Researchers have made significant advancements in studying the heterogenic features in breast cancer, and multiple subsets of breast cancer are discovered. In the molecular biology studies, breast cancer stem-like cells, driver mutations and changes in the tumor microenvironment are investigated as a potential hallmark for the disease progression. The "Omics" approaches in cancer research brought a detailed understanding of breast cancer at a new height. This technology is highly promising in discovering novel biomarkers in different breast cancer subtypes. Genomics, transcriptomics, proteomics, metabolomics, and other omics platforms have opened a new avenue to discover molecular insights in cancer progression. Immunological aspects of breast cancer are considered as cutting-edge science in recent discoveries. This book brings together up-to-date information to address the various challenging aspects of breast cancer. I congratulate the editors for putting together the different pieces of findings of breast cancer research in this book. I hope "Current advances in Breast cancer Research: A molecular approach" will be a good addition to the library of breast cancer literature.

Dr. Smita Misra
School of Graduate Studies and Research,
Centre for Women's Health Research (CWHR),
Meharry Medical College,
Nashville,
TN
USA

PREFACE

Breast cancer is one of the life-threatening diseases in women worldwide, leading to the mortality of millions of people all around the world. The increased prevalence of breast cancer globally in recent years has increased challenges to clinicians and researchers as well. The availability of appropriate detection tools for early detection is the major part of the clinical management of breast cancer patients in the present scenarios. Together with the current imaging techniques, molecular biomarkers based research has gained huge momentum in disease management in recent years. Molecular biomarkers are considered to be the best candidates to evaluate prognosis and therapeutics efficacy. Several biomarkers derived from gene-based technology through invasive approaches have revealed their wide scope in risk assessment of this particular disease. This book, gives details about developments in genomics, transcriptomics, proteomics, and metabolomics for the mining of novel biomarkers for breast cancer early detection. The first four chapters have emphasized to explore the basic understanding of breast cancer and management strategies of breast cancer. The molecular mechanism of carcinogenesis in breast cancer is more concerning to oncologists. The cardinal manifestation of cancer involves gene and protein modification to altering molecular pathways. Chapters 5 to 12 have delineated the basic mechanisms of cancer involved in the progression and metastasis. The role of mitochondrial-mediated energy associate and metabolic pathways has great significance in cancer, and separate chapters have given full emphasis to explore carcinogenic pathways. These chapters also deal with the heterogeneity of breast cancer and new development in diagnosing breast cancer in immunological prospective breast cancer biology. The last two chapters, it have dealt with the current therapeutics and the development of new therapy for breast cancer using natural bioactive compounds and nanotechnology-based approaches. Overall, 14 chapters have been included in this book, which dealwith the current perspectives of breast cancer progression. This book presents a compilation of basic and advanced research on breast cancer biology. This book outlines breast cancer research developments in contemporary years. We hope that the readers will be benefitted by understanding the advances in the biology of breast cancer research through this book.

Shankar Suman
Cancer Comprehensive Centre,
Biomedical Research Tower, The Ohio State University,
West 12th Avenue,
Columbus-43210,
Ohio
USA
Garima Suman
Department of Radiodiagnosis,
Tata Memorial Hospital,
Dr. E Borges Road,
Parel,
Mumbai-400012,
(Maharashtra) India
Sanjay Mishra
Department of Pathology,
The Ohio State University,
Columbus,
Ohio,
43210,
USA

List of Contributors

Akanksha Nigam	Department of Microbiology and Molecular Genetics, The Hebrew University-Hadassah Medical School, Jerusalem, Israel
Anurima Patra	Department of Radiodiagnosis, Tata Memorial Hospital, Mumbai, India
Ajeet Kumar Srivastav	Universal Corporation Limited (LuvLap), 4/1 Middleton Street, Sikkim Commerce House Kolkata, India-700071
Ashna Jha	Chittaranjan National Cancer Institute, Kolkata, India
Bhavana Kushwaha	Endocrinology Division, CSIR-Central Drug Research Institute, Lucknow, India
Brij Nath Tewari	Department of Microbiology, King George University, Lucknow, India
Dinesh Ahirwar	Department of Pathology, The Ohio State University, Columbus, USA
Debangshi Das	Chittaranjan National Cancer Institute, Kolkata, India
Garima Suman	Department of Radiodiagnosis, Tata Memorial Hospital, Mumbai, India
Gatha Thacker	Biochemistry Division, CSIR-Central Drug Research Institute (CSIR-CDRI), Jankipuram Extension, Lucknow, India
Lokesh Baweja	Department of Physics and the Center for Molecular Study of Condensed Soft Matter, Illinois Institute of Technology, Chicago, United States
Manish Charan	Department of Pathology, The Ohio State University, Columbus, USA
Manuraj Pandey	Department of Biotechnology, Unique College, Bhopal, India
Nabanita Chatterjee	Chittaranjan National Cancer Institute, Kolkata, India
Neha Rajoria	Meerut Institute of Engineering and Technology, Meerut, Uttar Pradesh, India
Pradeep K. Sharma	Environmental Carcinogenesis Laboratory, Food Drug and Chemical Toxicology Group, CSIR-Indian Institute of Toxicology Research, Academy of Scientific and Innovative Research, Ghaziabad, India
Pranay Agarwal	Department of Orthopaedic Surgery, Stanford University, Redwood City, California, USA
Rajendra Mehta	Department of Rural Technology and Social Development, Guru Ghasidas Vishwavidhyalaya (Central University), Bilaspur, India
Ramesh K. Ganju	Department of Pathology, The Ohio State University, Columbus, USA
Sanjay Mishra	Department of Pathology, The Ohio State University, Columbus, USA
Saroj Kumar Amar	Department of Forensic Science, School of Bioengineering and Biosciences, Lovely Professional University, Punjab, India Department of Therapeutic Radiology, School of Medicine, Yale University, New Haven, CT, USA
Shankar Suman	Cancer Comprehensive Centre, The Ohio State University, West 12th Avenue, Columbus-43210, USA
Shivam Priya	Institute for Dental Sciences, Faculty of Dental Medicine, Jerusalem, Israel
Sraddhya Roy	Chittaranjan National Cancer Institute, Kolkata, India

Swayam Prakash Srivastava	Department of Pediatrics, Yale University School of Medicine, New Haven, CT, 06511, USA
Swati Misri	Department of Pathology, The Ohio State University, Columbus, USA
Tarjani Agrawal	Projects in Knowledge Inc, Livingston, New Jersey, USA
Vipendra K. Singh	Environmental Carcinogenesis Laboratory, Food Drug and Chemical Toxicology Group, CSIR-Indian Institute of Toxicology Research, India Academy of Scientific and Innovative Research, Ghaziabad, India

CHAPTER 1

Breast Cancer: A Global Burden

Brij Nath Tewari[1,*] and **Sanjay Mishra**[2]

[1]Department of Microbiology, King George's Medical University, Lucknow, 226003, India
[2]Department of Pathology, The Ohio State University, Columbus, OH, USA

Abstract: The burden of breast cancer incidence and related mortality is a major health problem worldwide. In the last few years, the incidence and mortality rate of breast cancer have grown very rapidly in many developing countries and also slowly in developed nations. According to GLOBOCAN 2018 status report, the global cancer burden is estimated to have risen to 18.1 million new cases and 9.6 million deaths in 2018. The etiology of breast cancer depends upon several factors and includes age, genetic, environmental, radiation, breastfeeding, diet, and lifestyle factors, *etc*. The reasons behind the high breast cancer-related mortality are due to the lack of basic knowledge and awareness about breast cancer, less efficient diagnosis, late screening, poor health facilities, and limited access to treatment in developing countries. In this chapter, we summarize key studies on breast cancer epidemiology, types of breast cancer, risk factors, diagnosis, screening tools, predictive marker, surgery, chemotherapy, radiotherapy, hormonal therapy, targeted therapy, and preventative methods on breast cancer over the past years. These integrated findings may help protect and fight against breast cancer.

Keywords: Breast cancer, Carcinoma, ER, Globcan 2018, HER2/neu, Risk factor, PR.

INTRODUCTION

Breast cancer (BC) is among the most widespread invasive cancers and the second-largest major cause of mortality associated with cancer among females. Based on incidence and mortality trends, the incidence rates have increased rapidly in many developing countries and steadily industrialized nations in the past few decades. During their lives, one out of five males and one of every six females globally acquire cancer, and one of every eight males and one in 11 females die from the disease. Cancer incidence and mortality are rapidly growing worldwide. According to GLOBOCAN 2018 status, it is reported that the overall burden of cancer has increased to new instances and a million casualties [1].

---

[*] **Corresponding author Brij Nath Tewari:** Department of Microbiology, King George's Medical University, Lucknow, U.P., 226003, India; Tel: +91-9450664359; India; E-mail: brijnath2008@gmail.com

Globally, the World Health Organization calculated the actual estimate of the population living among five years of cancer diagnosis, known as the 5-year prevalence, which is predicted to be 43.8 million. The global load of breast cancer is progressively drifting from developed to developing countries [2]. The rate of related causes for developing cancer associated with social and economic development is constantly evolving. This is notably true in fast growing-economy countries due to rapid changes in lifestyles more typical of industrialized nations [1]. The progression of the metastatic ability of primary tumor lesions is associated with breast cancer-related mortality [3]. Breast cancer is a complicated, comprehensively inherently heterogeneous disease with distinct morphologies, molecular characteristics and clinical patterns [4]. The metastasis of breast cancer has been a major issue of intense scrutiny of cancer. Probably lung, liver, bones, and brain are the most prevalent sites for cancer metastasis. The brain is one of the most prevalent organs impacted by breast cancer invasion that ultimately leads to the death of breast cancer patients. In women with breast cancer, brain metastasis is increasingly more frequent, and around 15%-30% have brain metastasis [5]. Metastatic breast cancer (MBC) is an incurable disorder. Although the present medical treatments have given adequate palliation unable to eliminate this illness, therefore creating an incurable condition [6]. Being largely incurable, the onset of metastasis is one of the biggest hurdles to the successful treatment of cancer [7]. Once initiated, it can neither be reversed nor stopped, therefore, averting the onset is paramount significance. This essentially requires a better understanding with regards to determinants and biological markers of cancer. Such knowledge may lead to the identification of not only new prognostic markers but also may escort to the development of targeted therapeutic regimen against MBC.

Statistics at a Glance: The Burden of Cancer Worldwide

- In 2015, an estimated 2,4 million cases of incidence and 523,000 deaths were reported as being the most prevalent form of cancer in females worldwide [8]. This Revolution is associated with worldwide economic and socio-demographic outlines, for instance, increasing aging populations [8].
- The major causes of death from cancer worldwide are cancer-related metastasis to distant organs. There have been estimated to be 14.1 million new cases and 8.2 million global death associated with cancer in 2019 [9].
- In less developed areas of the world, along with Central America and parts of Africa and Asia, 57% of instances of fresh disease happened in 2012; and in these areas, 65% of cancer fatalities occurred as well (source: https://www.cancer.gov).
- New cases of cancer are expected to increase annually to 23.6 million by the year 2030(source: https://www.cancer.gov).

A brief History of Breast Cancer

In the present scenario, cancer is one of the major public health issues not only in developed countries but also in developing countries like India. Cancer is basically a group of illnesses characterized by the uncontrolled and abnormal growth of neoplastic cells [10]. It is assumed that the oldest explanation of cancer in Egypt about 3000 BC [11]. In a prehistoric Egyptian textbook on trauma surgery, they described 8 cases of breast tumors abide removed by cauterization with a device called fire drill. The origin of the word 'cancer' is attributed to the Greek physician Hippocrates (460-370 BC), who is known as the "Father of Medicine". Hippocrates used the terms 'carcinos' and 'carcinoma' to illustrate non-ulcer forming and ulcer-forming tumors [11]. In Greek, these phrases mainly refer to a crab, and most likely used before the illness because the finger-like projections from malignant cells describe the shape of a crab [11]. In a while, the Roman physician, Celsius (28-50 BC), converts the Greek word into cancer, the Latin term for crab. Another Greek physician, Galen (130-200 AD), used the term oncos (Greek for swelling) to describe tumors [11]. However, the Hippocrates and Celsus crab analogy still serves to describe malignant lesions.

The female mammary gland is basically comprised of milk-producing glands known as "lobules" and tiny tubes like structures, which allocate the milk from lobules to the nipples, named as "ducts" and finally "stroma" (fatty and connective tissue neighbouring the ducts, lobules, blood vessels, and lymphatic vessels) [12]. Breast cancer is an abnormal development of normal breast cells. The term "breas" attributes to a malignant tumor that is matured cells in the breast [13]. Breast cancer can be categorized into various types based on how breast cancer cells appear beneath the microscope. In most cases, breast cancer starts in the cells that line the ducts of the mammary gland called "ductal breast cancer," and in few cases, cancer occurs in the cells that streak the lobules known as "lobular breast cancer". Alternatively, when breast cancer begins in the epithelial cells that line the mammary gland, then it is termed as "breast carcinomas". In fact, in most cases, breast cancers are frequently rank of carcinoma called "adenocarcinoma", which begins in glandular tissue of mammary gland. Erstwhile of breast cancers can also arise in the mammary gland, such as "breast sarcomas," which start in the cells of connective tissue and muscle. In rare cases, a single breast tumor can also be a mixture of diverse types of *in-situ* and invasive breast cancer. These various kinds of breast cancer are described as following (adapted from the American Cancer Society. Cancer Facts and Figures 2016. Atlanta, Ga: American Cancer Society; 2016).

Types of Breast Cancer

Under the microscope, breast cancer can be divided into distinct kinds depending on how the cancer cells appear. Breast cancers fall into categories:

Ductal Carcinoma In-situ: (DCIS, known as intraductal carcinoma) is a range of abnormal changes in the mammary gland that basically begins in the mammary epithelial cells lining the mammary ducts and also considered as a non-invasive or pre-invasive type of breast cancer. This is the most frequent kind of *in-situ* breast cancer accounting for 83% of *in-situ* cases diagnosed during 2006-2010. About everyone in five new cases of breast cancer will be DCIS, and the majority of females diagnosed at the early stage be cured and treated successfully. The important difference between invasive breast cancer and DCIS is that in DCIS, the breast cancer cells have not invaded through the walls of mammary ducts into the nearby breast tissue. As DCIS can't invade and metastasize the distant organs, it is considered as a pre-cancerous lesion though in rare cases, it can go on to become invasive cancers.

Lobular Carcinoma In-situ: (LCIS, also termed as lobular neoplasia) is not exactly cancer or but a marker of increased risk of having invasive cancer. This type of breast cancer is very rarer than DCIS, and approximately 12% of women *in-situ* breast cancers have been diagnosed from 2006 through 2010.

Infiltrating (Invasive) Ductal Carcinoma: is a very common type of breast cancer. Infiltrating ductal carcinoma (IDC) mainly begins in a milk duct of the mammary gland, and invades through the wall of the mammary duct, which finally grows into the fatty tissue of the mammary gland. From here, it can be metastasized to distant organs throughout the body by the lymphatic organ and bloodstream. Almost eight out of ten invasive breast-cancer cases are IDC.

Inflammatory Breast Cancer (IBC): is a very rare kind of invasive breast cancer, accounting for 1% to 3% of all breast cancer cases. In IBC, the skin of the breast appears red without any single lump or tumor. Other symptoms of IBC include the pitted appearance of the breast, and affected regions may become firmer and itchy also. IBC has a worse prognosis than any other invasive ductal or lobular cancer and tends to have an increased probability of spreading into distant organs.

Phyllodes Tumor: (phyllodes tumor or cystosarcoma phyllodes) is a very uncommon category of breast cancer, whichever occurs in the connective tissue of the mammary gland. This kind of breast tumor is usually benign, and in rare circumstances, it may develop into malignant forms, and the benign tumor can be treated by normal mastectomy. But, when benign phyllodes develop into malignant tumors, then chemotherapy is used as given for soft-tissue sarcomas.

Paget Disease: of the nipple begins in the mammary ducts at first and then spreads in the skin around the nipple and finally to the areola (dark circle in the region of the nipple). It is a very uncommon kind of breast cancer and accounted for 1% of all cases of breast cancer. The symptom of this cancer includes the crusted, reddish, and scaly appearance to the skin of the nipple with areas of bleeding or oozing. This type of breast cancer is more or less linked with either infiltrating ductal carcinoma, or DCIS and treatment of Paget disease often require a mastectomy.

Angiosarcoma: is a very rare kind of breast cancer, and it occurs within the cells lining the blood or lymphatic vessels, and this type of cancer tends to grow and invade other organs very quickly.

There are also some unusual types of breast cancer, which are subtypes of invasive breast carcinoma and include: Low-grade adenosquamous, Adenocystic, Mucinous, Medullary, Papillary, Tubular, Metaplastic, Micropapillary, and mixed carcinoma (which has features of both invasive ductal and lobular carcinoma).

GRADING AND MOLECULAR SUBTYPES OF BREAST CANCER

(It is adopted from American Joint Committee on Cancer. Breast. In: AJCC Cancer Staging Manual, 7th ed. New York: Springer; 2010: 347–369).

Breast Cancer Grading

Breast cancer can also be categorized into different grades based on how the biopsy sample of breast tumors appears to normal breast tissue and how quickly breast cancer cells are multiplying. The breast cancer grading is also helpful in prognosis, and lower grade number indicates the least chance of spreading of cancer cells, while the higher-grade number indicates an increased probability of breast cancer spreading. Tumor grading is also essential to decide whether surgery is required or not after radio or chemotherapies. For invasive breast cancers, the histological grade is sometimes termed as *Richardson grade, Nottingham grade, Scarff-Bloom-Richardson grade*, or *Elston-Ellis grade*. Sometimes, grade expressed with words as a substitute of numbers:

- Grade 1 tumor is similar to well-differentiated.
- Grade 2 tumor is similar to moderately differentiated.
- Grade 3 tumor is similar to poorly differentiated and tends to develop and spread more rapidly.

Breast Cancer Molecular Subtypes

Breast cancer is progressively considered not a single illness, but a combination of diseases, which can be differentiated by different molecular/hormonal subtypes, clinical behaviors, risk factors as well as responses to different clinical treatments [14, 15]. Different hormonal or molecular subtypes of breast cancer have been known using global gene expression profiles. Most suitable for molecular breast cancer subtypes have been recognized with the help of biological markers, which include the existence or nonexistence of estrogen receptors (ER+/ER-), progesterone receptors (PR+/PR-), and human epidermal growth factor receptor 2 also known as (EGFR-2) positive or negative. These molecular subtypes of breast cancer are as following:

Luminal A

Approximately 40% of breast cancer women are found to be luminal A-type, and these breast tumors inclined to be ER(estrogen receptor) positive and/or PR (progesterone receptor) positive and HER2 negative, less aggressive, and slower growing than other molecular subtypes. Luminal-A breast tumors are linked with the most positive short-term prognosis, due to the expression of the hormonal receptor, which is predictive of a positive response to hormonal therapy [16].

Luminal B

It constitutes ~10% - 20% of all breast cancer females and like luminal A-tumor, most of the luminal B-tumors are ER+ and/or PR+. Although, these cases are discriminated by either expression of HER2 or elevated rate of proliferation [16].

Basal-like

It constitutes ~10% - 20% of all breast cancer cases and mass of basal-like breast cancers are termed as "triple-negative breast cancer (TNBC)" since they are ER negative, PR negative, and HER2 negative. These breast cancers are more frequent in African American women, premenopausal females, and those females with *BRCA1* gene alteration. Women with breast cancer diagnosed with TNBC have poorer short-term prognosis than those diagnosed with other molecular subtypes of breast cancer since there are no targeted therapies for these breast cancer cases [16].

HER2 Enriched

This type of molecular subtype comprises ~10% of breast cancer cases and produces excess growth-promoting protein, called HER2, and does not express hormonal receptor-like ER and PR. Just like the basal-like subtype, this subtype inclined to grow and spread much more aggressively than other subtypes of breast cancer and therefore coupled with poorer short-term prognosis. Nevertheless, the use of targeted therapies for this subtype has upturned much of the unfavorable prognostic shock of HER2 overexpression [16].

SIGNS, SYMPTOMS AND RISK FACTORS OF BREAST CANCER

Most of the females recognize a lump or region of thickened tissue in their breast as the first symptom of breast cancer. A newly formed lump or mass is the most prevalent symptom of breast cancer. A relatively painless, hard mass with irregular edges is more likely to be cancerous, but tender, smooth, or rounded. They can often be a pain in the breast.

For this reason, a healthcare professional or a skilled clinician must check any fresh breast mass or a lump or breast alteration in the diagnosis of breast illnesses. American Cancer Society states that the frequent signs and symptoms of breast cancer may include as follows:

- Altered size or shape of the breast.
- Swelling of the entire or part of a breast, nipple, or areola (even if there is no distinct lump).
- Skin irritation or dimpling.
- Pain in breast or nipple.
- Retraction of the nipple (moving inward).
- Redness, scaliness, or thickening of the nipple or breast skin.
- Bloody discharge from the nipple (excluding breast milk).

Risk Factors of Breast Cancer

The risk factor of breast cancer is enormously complex, and its progression is a multi-step process. The consequences are from a series of epigenetic, genetic, endocrine, aging, familial history, lifestyle exposure to the environmental risk factor. To understand the incidence of breast cancer issues, the researcher has identified the 60-70% cases of the known risk factor and the remaining 30-40% of the cases of unknown risk factors. The following factor can raise women's risk of developing breast cancer.

Age

Age is an increasing risk factor for breast cancer, and the incidence of breast cancer is increasing with age, doubling nearly every ten years until menopause, when the pace of growth slows dramatically. In comparison to lung cancer, breast cancer incidence is greater at younger ages [17]. The American Cancer Society reports that in females of under 45 years, approximately 1 in 8 invasive breast cancers grow, whereas in females 55 or older, approximately 2 of 3 invasive breast cancers are detected. Besides sex, aging is one of the most important risk factors for breast cancer because its incidence is strongly linked to growing age. In 2016, females aged 40 and 60, respectively, accounted for around 99.3% and 71.2% of all breast cancer-related fatalities in America [18].

Geographical Variation

There is quite a variation in the incidence and death rate of breast cancer between distinct countries. Age-set incidence and death rates for breast cancer differ by up to five from nation to nation. The biggest variation between far Eastern and Western countries is declining but is at a halt about fivefold [16, 18].

Previous Benign Breast Cancer

Women who experience serious atypical hyperplasia are 4-5 times more susceptible than females who do not experience proliferative breast cancer [20]. Female with this shift and a family history of breast cancer (first-degree relative) are nine times susceptible of having breast cancer than other counterparts. Female with palpable cysts, complex fibroadenomas, duct papillomas, sclerosis adenosis, and moderate or florid epithelial hyperplasia have a relatively higher threat of breast carcinoma (1.53 times). If be female without these alterations, this rise is not clinically significant to warrant any intervention [17].

Age at Menarche and Menopause

A greater risk of breast cancer occurs for women starting their menstrual period early in life or who have late menopause. Women who are under a natural menopause phase after the age of 55 are twice more likely to grow breast cancer than females having menopause before the age of 45. Women who undergo bilateral oophorectomy before the age of 35 have only 40% of females who have natural menopause are under the risk of breast cancer [17].

Oral Contraceptives

The current and latest users of oral contraceptives are 15-25 percent more exposed to breast cancer than those taking exogenous hormones [21]. Further, more than ten years after stopping oral contraceptives, the risk levels off to approach that of never users, independently from the duration of use. This is of meticulous significance since most females who use oral contraceptives are young and have a low baseline incidence of breast cancer. Along these lines, their increased threat during and soon after oral contraceptives employ has little significance [22].

Breast-feeding

Many studies have suggested that a lady's breastfeeding risk of breast cancer is reduced for a year or more slightly. For basal-like breast cancers, the protective influence could be greater [23]. The nonexistence or short duration of breastfeeding that is typical of ladies in developed countries substantially assists in the high incidence of breast cancer. A collaborative analysis estimated that in addition to the reduction of every birth, the risk of the disease was considerably reduced through breastfeeding. An additional protective effect of lactation has been exposed in several populations, most likely attributable to the suppression of the ovulatory function caused by nursing. Breast cancer risk reduced by 4.3% for every year of lactation in a collaborative analysis of 47 studies in 30 nations [24]. Several studies propose that breastfeeding may slightly lower breast cancer risk, especially if it is sustained for 1½ to 2 years. The effect of breastfeeding on the risk of breast cancer has been a subject of debate [25]. However, a growing body of evidence indicates that breastfeeding reduces the risk of developing breast carcinoma [26, 27]. In a current meta-analysis of 27 studies that incorporated 13907 women with breast cancer, the study shows that breastfeeding inversely associated with the risk of breast cancer Zhou *et al.* [26].

Breast Density

A tough, independent risk factor for breast cancer growth was shown to be high-density breast tissue (a mammographic indicator of breast and connective tissue relative to the fatty tissue in the breast) [28]. Several factors that can affect breast density include for example menopause, age, the use of convinced drugs (such as menopausal hormone therapy), pregnancy, and genetics. Breast density predisposes to hereditary genetic factors but decreases with age and further diminishes with menopause and pregnancy [19, 29]. The threat of breast cancer raises with raising breast density; have a 4-6 overlay amplified of breast cancer risk as compared to women with the least density of the breast.

Family History of Breast Cancer

Women with a first-degree relative (mother, sister, daughter, father, or brother) who developed breast cancer have a risk that is approximately double an average woman's risk. If two first-degree relatives developed breast cancer, the risk is five-fold the average risk. The precise risk of breast cancer is unknown, but females with a family history in a father/brother have an enhanced risk of breast cancer. In total, a family with this disease has fewer than 15 percent of females with breast cancer. This means that according to the American Organization of Breast Cancer, most females (more than 85 percent) suffering from breast cancer have no family history.

Personal History of Breast Cancer

A female with cancer in one breast has a three to four-time increased risk for developing new cancer cells in the other breast or another part of the same breast. This is distinct from a cancer recurrence of the primary growth.

Genetic Risk Factors

The genetic risk factors in epidemiology and pathogenesis of both sporadic breast cancer and familial breast cancer are now well established. However, germline mutations of BRCA1 and BRCA2 and other genes account for only 15%–20% of breast cancer that clusters in families and less than 5% of breast cancer overall. Much effort in recent years has been focused on *BRCA1* and *BRCA2*, and the prevalence and penetrance of mutations in these genes have been studied extensively. The genes involved in the hereditary and familial forms of breast cancer include BRCA1, BRCA2, P53, PTEN, ATM, CHEK2 and STK11/LKB1 [30].

The two BRCA genes appear to serve as important regulators of cell-cycle "checkpoint control" mechanisms, involving a cell-cycle arrest, DNA repair, and apoptosis. BRCA1 is a large gene located on chromosome 17, with 24 exons spanning about 100,000 base pairs of genomic DNA, and BRCA2 is located on chromosome 13. Both the BRCA1 and BRCA2 genes are massive, and mutations will occur virtually at any place, making molecular testing to identify mutation for the first time in an affected individual or family technically challenging. Some mutations happen at high frequency in a population. Inherited mutations in two more genes, p53 and PTEN, are related to familial syndromes (Li-Fraumeni and Cowden's respectively) that include a high risk of breast cancer, but both are uncommon [30]. These are almost definitely other genes that increase the risk of disease by only a mild degree but maybe three or four-fold above the overall population. These are unlikely to make florid multi-case families, but they are likely quite prevalent and therefore account for a significant portion of the overall genetic input to breast cancer.

Many families influenced by breast carcinoma demonstrate an overload of ovarian, colon, prostatic, and other cancers due to the same hereditary mutation. Patients with bilateral carcinoma, who acquire a combination of breast cancer and other epithelial cancer, and females who develop the disease at an early age are most probable to create a genetic mutation that makes them susceptible to developing cancer. Most breast cancers are due to a genetic mutation occurring before the age of sixty-five, and a woman with a strong family history of breast cancer of early-onset who is still unaffected at sixty-five has most probably no longer inherited the genetic alteration.

A woman's risk of breast carcinoma is almost more than two times bigger if she has a first-degree relative who developed the disease before the age of 50, and also the younger the relative when she developed breast cancer, the greater the threat of cancer [17]. For instance, a female whose sister developed breast carcinoma aged 30-39 has a cumulative risk of 10% of developing the disease herself through age 65, but that threat is 5% (close to the population risk) if the sister was aged at 50-54. The risk will increase between four to six times if two first degree relatives develop the disease [17].

Radiation

The risk factor of radiation associated between radiation exposure and breast cancer has been confirmed in research of atomic bomb survivors and females who undergone high-dose radiation therapy to the chest, primarily for those who were first exposed at younger ages [31]. This may be because the breast tissue is most prone to carcinogenesis before it is fully distinguished, which occurs with first childbirth [32]. Breast cancer is one of the most prevalent types of a second cancers amongst infancy cancer survivors. Secondary breast cancer is most closely correlated with high-dose radiation therapy to the chest for females treated between 10 and 30 years of age, such as for Hodgkin lymphoma [33]. Breast cancer threat among females with such exposure begins to increase after radiation about eight years and continues to increase for more than 25 years [34]. The risk increases with increased radiation dose. Besides, the risk is higher in female irradiated before age 30, when there is still breast development [35].

Tobacco

Based on 150 studies, the International Cancer Agency found that there was restricted proof that tobacco smoking can cause breast cancer in females [36]. The latest meta-analysis by scientists in the American Cancer Society found that present smokers have a 12% greater risk of breast cancer than the female who never smoked. Researchers also propose that female who starts smoking before their first birth may be at higher risk [37].

Alcohol

A few studies have shown an association between alcohol consumption and breast cancer instances, but the relationship is inconsistent and may be an association with other nutritional factors rather than alcohol [17]. Alcohol drinking is an important breast cancer etiological factor. Consumption of three or more alcoholic drinks per day raises the risk by 30-50%, with daily drink accounting for about 7% higher risk [38].

Diet

Although countless studies have investigated the connection between food consumption (including fat, soy, milk product, meat, and fruits and vegetables) and breast cancer, there is no conclusive confirmation that diet manipulates breast cancer risk [39]. A current meta-analysis of consumption of animal fat and breast cancer, including more than 20,000 instances of breast cancer, found that no connection existed [40]. Similarly, in the Women's Health Initiative, nutritional action, lowering dietary fat in post-menopausal children did not impact breast cancer risk. However, exposure of timing may be essential, as a conclusion from the Nurses' Health Study demonstrated that a high-fat diet during adolescence was linked with a mild increase in premenopausal breast cancer threat [41].

Hormonal Risk Factor

Estrogen Receptor (ER)

The estrogen receptor is a member of the nuclear hormone family of intracellular receptors that are activated by the hormone estrogen (17β-estradiol) [42]. There are two different forms of Estrogen receptor, referred to as ERα and ERβ, each encoded by a separate gene. The ESR1 encodes the ERα isoform and the ERβ isoform is encoded by the ESR2 gene [43]. ESR1 is encoded on chromosome 6 (locus 6q25.1) and ESR2 is encoded on chromosome 14 (locus 14q23-24.1) [44, 45]. The main role of the Estrogen receptor is as a DNA-binding transcription factor that regulates gene expression [46]. ERα and ERβ proteins can be detected in a broad spectrum of tissues. As well, both receptor subtypes may be present in the same tissue but different types of cells. ERα is mainly expressed in uterus, prostate (stroma), ovary (theca cells), testes (Leydig cells), epididymis, bone, breast, various regions of the brain, liver, and white adipose tissue and ERβ is expressed in prostate (epithelium), testis, ovary (granulosa cells), salivary gland, bone marrow, colon, vascular endothelium, and certain regions of the brain [42]. ERα proteins are regarded as being cytoplasmic receptors in their unliganded state, but research has shown that part of ERα resides in the nucleus of ER-negative breast cancer epithelial cells [47]. ERα expression is linked with more differentiated tumors, while evidence that ERβ is involved is controversial [48]. However, recent research proposed that ERβ is associated with proliferation and a poor prognosis [49]. Different descriptions of the ESR1 gene have been identified (with single-nucleotide polymorphisms) and are associated with various risks of developing breast cancer [50]. These two forms of estrogens are co-expressed in various tissues, and they are over-expressed in around 60-70% of breast cancer cases and are ER-positive and estrogen-dependent [51]. Binding of estrogen to ER stimulates the proliferation of mammary cells, with the resulting increase in cell division, DNA replication and increases the mutation rate. This disrupts the cell cycle, apoptosis and DNA repair processes eventually leading to tumor formation [52].

Progesterone Receptor (PR)

The progesterone receptor (PR) is also known as an NR3C3 (nuclear receptor subfamily 3, group C, member 3). In humans, PR is encoded by a single gene located on the long arm of chromosome 11 (11q22) (Law *et al.*, 1987). There are two main nuclear isoforms of PR, A and B that differ in their molecular weight A: 94kD and B: 114kD) [53]. A mutation or change in expression of the co-regulators affects the normal function of the PR and may disrupt the normal growth of the mammary gland, thereby leading to breast cancer [54].

Her2 Neu

The Human Epidermal growth factor Receptor 2 (is also known as HER2/neu or ERBB2) is a protein located at the long arm of chromosome 17 (17q11.2-q12). HER2/neu belongs to a family of four transmembrane receptor tyrosine kinases involved in signal transduction pathways that regulate cell growth and proliferation [55]. HER2/neu is co-localized, and thus most of the time co-amplified, with another proto-oncogene GRB7 [56]. Clinically, HER2/neu is vital because it is the target of the monoclonal antibody trastuzumab (marketed as Herceptin). Trastuzumab is only effective in breast cancer, where the HER2/neu receptor is over-expressed. The mechanism of trastuzumab works after it binds to HER2 is by increasing p27, a protein that detains cell proliferation [57]. Approximately 10% of breast cancers produce excess HER2 (a growth-promoting protein) and do not express ER and PR receptors [58].

TUMOR MARKERS

A tumor marker is described as a substance overexpressed by tumors or the host (associated with the tumor) that can be used to differentiate neoplastic from normal tissue. Body cells, tissues, and body fluids, like cerebrospinal fluid, serum, plasma, and breast milk of women, are the source of tumor markers. The perfect marker would help in diagnosing, staging and forecasting the tumor and serve to detect therapy impacts, detect recurrence, locate tumors, and check the overall populations [59]. Most of the tumor markers do not fit the ideal outline. The reason for this can be the relative lack of sensitivity and specificity of the obtainable analysis. It should be renowned that virtually any protein or chemical has the potential to be a tumor marker. Some substances are increased in tumor tissues and/or leak in bloodstreams or other liquids as tumor cells develop and multiply. Depending upon tumor marker, it can be measured in blood, tissue, urine or stool. Some widely used tumor markers include AFP, Her2/Neu, beta-HCG, CA 19-9, CA 27.29 (CA 15-3), CA 125, CEA, and PSA [60].

Types of Molecular Markers

Molecular Markers address a range of signs. A single marker can serve several purposes and can, therefore, be integrated into several biological markers. Moreover, a single biological marker can be categorized into distinct kinds of the tumor and/or stages of illness. This section describes ordinary terms used to define molecular testing.

Diagnostic Markers

A large group of molecular analyses aid in the diagnosis or sub-classification of a meticulous disease condition. Subclassification of the diagnostic may lead to distinct disease management, but the marker is mainly used to determine the meticulous disease that is present in the sample of a cancer patient. For example, the existence of the Philadelphia chromosome is shown in acute myelogenic leukemia through specific molecular trials, including non-Hodgkin's lymphoma, immunophenotyping, and fluorescence in situ hybridization (FISH) [61, 62].

Prognostic Markers

Prognostic markers are associated with a few clinical upshots. For example, overall survival or recurrence-free survival, independent of the therapy [63]. The existence of p53 mutations is an instance of a prognostic marker subset of patients with more progressive disorder disease for certain cancer [64].

Predictive Markers

Predictive markers estimate the procedure of a specific kind of therapy and are used for further treatment choice. They are used as indications of the probable advantage of precise patient treatment [63]. One instance of a predictive biomarker is a human epidermal growth factor receptor 2 (HER2 (ERBB2). HER2 (ERBB2)-negative tumor cells do not counter with trastuzumab; HER2 positivity, therefore, is predictive of the possible response of trastuzumab in newly diagnosed breast cancer patients [65].

Companion Diagnostic Markers

Companion diagnostic markers may be a diagnostic, prognostic, or predictive diagnostic marker. It can be used to recognize a subgroup of patients who have benefited from therapy. Particularly, prospective data illustrate that patients with positive markers help from the treatment. Consequently, companion diagnostic markers are mainly a subgroup of predictive markers. Evidence may not be adequate to decide whether they have independent prognostic or predictive effectiveness for the disease. One latest example of co-approval of a drug and companion diagnostic is the BRAF V600E mutation test co-approved with the kinase inhibitor vemurafenib. The kinases of activating BRAF V600E mutation are sensitive to vemurafenib, a tiny BRAF molecule inhibitor in 30-60% of melanoma [66, 67].

CURRENT DIAGNOSIS AND TREATMENTS OF BREAST CANCER

Breast cancer is usually diagnosed during any screening test, before any sign has developed, or after when a female feels a lump on her breast [68]. In most cases, lumps can be observed on a mammogram test, and breast lesions turn out to be benign form. But, when breast cancer is suspected based of mammography or breast imaging tools, detailed microscopic investigation of breast tissue is essential for an accurate diagnosis and also to find out the degree of spread of breast cancer cells and finally to decide the types, grades, stages and molecular subtypes of breast cancer. A needle or surgical biopsy can be used to obtain the breast tissue for microscopic assessment. Guidelines for breast cancer detection in the American Cancer Society, which can vary as based on a woman's age and enclose clinical breast examination (CBE) and mammography as well as magnetic resonance imaging (MRI) for a female with elevated at threat.

Screening and Diagnosis of Breast Cancer

Mammography

Mammography is a type of low-dose X-ray machine that permits the visualization of the inside organ of the mammary gland [68, 69]. At present, conventional (film) mammography has been mainly substituted by digital mammography, which emerges to be even more precise for females younger than age 50 and women with dense breast tissue. American Cancer Society also suggested every woman receives an annual mammogram starting at age 40. It is incredibly needed that women are repeatedly screened to raise the probability that breast cancer would be diagnosed at an early stage. Combined outcomes from randomized mammography screening trials recommend that it decrease the risk of dying from breast cancer by 15-20%. Breast cancer early diagnosis by mammography could also show the way to a better range of treatment options; however, mammography screening also has few potential disadvantages.

Overdiagnosis of Breast Cancer

One of the important limitations of mammography is the overdiagnosis of breast cancer patients [70, 71]. Overdiagnosis is the detection of breast cancer cases, which would not have progressed unless a woman underwent screening. Approximate rates of overdiagnosis are extremely variable, which is ranging from 0% to > 30%. False-positive outcomes of mammography are defined as when there is no breast tumor, but it leads to follow-up examinations of breast cancer patients. It is found that on usual, ~10% of women will have reminisced from each screening test for additional testing, but merely 5% of these females will have breast cancer.

Magnetic Resonance Imaging (MRI)

Magnetic resonance imaging, magnetic fields are mainly used to turn out comprehensive and cross-sectional images through the body [69, 72]. MRI examinations for breast imaging employ a contrast material such as gadolinium DTPA that is injected through a vein into the arm to improve the capability to capture detailed images of breast tissues. In 2007, a professional panel of oncologists made by the American Cancer Society published a suggestion on the employ of MRI for screening the women at an increased risk for breast cancer. They suggested yearly MRI testing an additional to regular mammography for women at increased lifetime threat beginning at 30 years of age.

Limitation: According to the panel, MRIs should complement, but not replace mammography-screening test. For females whose lives are below 15% at risk of breast cancer, MRI testing is not suggested.

Breast Ultrasound

Screening or diagnostic mammograms or physical examinations are specially used to evaluate atypical findings of breast ultrasound [73]. Some clinical researchers have also recommended that breast ultrasound may identify female cancer with dense breast tissue more accurately than a mammography test alone.

Limitation: Breast ultrasound also raises the chance of false-positive results, and thus, ultrasound as an alternative to breast mammography is not generally suggested.

PET Scan

For PET scan, patients are being injected with tracer. Then, a device creates 3-D images showing wherever the tracer is gathered. However, these scans demonstrate how tissues and organs function.

X-rays

X-rays are using low doses of radiation in order to generate images within the body of cancer patients.

Biopsy

The removal of cells or tissues from patients, pathologists viewed under a microscope and confirm for signs of disease. If a lump is detected in the breast, a small piece of the lump may have to be removed by the consultant.

There are four types of biopsy used to pathological confirmation of breast cancer:

- **Excision**: The removal of a whole lump of tissue.
- **Incision**: The removal of part of a plump or a sample of tissue.
- **Core**: The removal of tissue employing a wide needle.
- **Fine-Needle Aspiration (FNA)**: The removal of tissue or fluid, using a thin/skinny needle.

Breast Cancer Treatments

The patient and the physician make the decisions regarding the accurate treatment after deliberation of the optimal treatments to be used for the stage and biological features of the breast cancer, the patient's age as well as preference, and the benefits and risks linked with each treatment protocol. Most of the females with breast cancer will have some surgery. Surgery is often used with other treatments for instance, chemotherapy, hormonal, radiation and/or targeted therapy.

Surgery

The main objective of breast cancer surgery is to eradicate the breast tumor mass and to decide the stages of the disease [74 - 77]. This kind of treatment engages breast-conserving surgery (BCS) or mastectomy. In BCS (also known as quadrantectomy or lumpectomy), simply breast tumor mass along with a rim of normal tissue are removed from the body. However, simple mastectomy employs the total removal of the breast. In the recent past, modified radical mastectomy is being used, that employs the removal of the entire breast with axially lymph nodes. Though, this surgical treatment does not involve the removal of the underlying chest wall muscle, along with a simple radical mastectomy. It is reported that 57% of females detected with early-stage breast cancer (stage I or II) have BCS, 36% have a mastectomy, 6% have no surgery, about ~ 1% do not receive any kind of cure. While on the other hand, among females with late-stage breast cancer (III or IV), 13% have BCS, 60% have a mastectomy, 18% have no surgery, and 7% have no therapy.

It is also found that both mastectomy and BCS are performed in combination with the removal of regional lymph nodes near armpit to find out whether cancer has invaded beyond the breast or not. If it is found that breast cancer cells are spread in the lymph nodes, then that information will help decide the need for consequent therapy and the course of treatment. Nowadays, sentinel lymph node biopsy (SLNB) is also commonly used to reduce the need for full axillary lymph node dissections. In this surgery, selected parts of lymph nodes are removed and tested for breast cancer cells spreading before any others are excised. Moreover, recent clinical trials also indicate that axillary lymph node dissection may be prevented for a few breast cancer instances treated with lumpectomy and radiation, even if one or two sentinel lymph nodes have cancer cells.

Limitations

Although removal of axillary lymph nodes with surgery and radiation therapy are effectively used worldwide, this may also cause a serious swelling of the arms, which is caused by the retention of lymph fluids. This type of clinical condition is termed as "lymphedema," and it is also found that breast cancer patients who undergo axillary lymph node removal are ~3 times more possible to develop lymphedema comparatively to those patients who have SLNB [75]. Approximately 5% of breast cancer patients with SLNB and 16%-18% of breast cancer patients were also anticipated. Subsequently, SLNB will create clinically measurable lymphedema undergoing axillary lymph node dissection.

Radiation Therapy

In radiation therapy, high-energy rays or electrons are used in radiation treatment to destroy cells breast cancer [78 - 80]. Behind therapeutic surgery, Radiation therapy can also be used to destroy all surviving breast cells in the breast, chest wall, or underarm region [77, 79]. Radiation therapy is almost suggested for women after BCS, as it has shown to the reduction of ~50% in the incidence of breast cancer recurrence and mortality by ~20%. There are also few clinical studies demonstrate that individuals who have breast tumor greater than 5 cm or who find breast cancer cells are originated in the lymph nodes, also need radiation therapy. This mode of treatment is also needed to cure the signs of an advanced stage of breast cancer. Internal or external radiation therapy may be provided. Few women are treated with both kinds of radiation therapy, and these given therapies are dependent on the stage of breast tumor, form, and location.

Internal Radiation Therapy

Internal radiation therapy is a type of accelerated partial breast irradiation (APBI), in which a radioactive substance is essentially sealed into seeds, wires, nets or catheters, directly located near or into breast tumor. This is also referred to as brachytherapy. Internal radiation therapy also used in the form of intracavitary brachytherapy and is given to breast cancer patients for only five days. While on the other hand, exterior beam radiation is the most common type of radiation treatment used for a female with breast cancer. This sort of treatment focuses on the region impacted by breast cancer from a machine outside the body. This treatment generally involves the entire breast and may also consist of the chest wall and submerged region, based on the size and area of breast cancer. External beam radiation treatment is usually taking place daily for 5-6 weeks; nevertheless, the latest clinical studies have demonstrated just it has been effective to shorten the treatment duration from 6 to 3 weeks (referred to as accelerated breast irradiation).

Limitations

However, there are few limitations associated with radiation therapy and a recent retrospective clinical study reports that patients with breast cancer who received with brachytherapy were more probable than patients with full-breast radiation to experience major problems and to undergo a consequent mastectomy. Further follow-up information is necessary to determine how long-term radiation of the partial breast is enhanced, and to determine which of the finest suitable candidates for breast cancer treatments.

Systemic Therapy

Systemic therapy is a treatment, in which chemotherapeutics drugs travel through the bloodstream of breast cancer patients and affects different parts of the body, not just the breast tumor. These cancer medications are injected into a vein or orally to patients with breast cancer. The main components of systemic therapy mainly include chemotherapy, hormone therapy, and targeted therapy, and all of which will work through the distinct molecular and cell-based methods. For example, chemotherapy drugs, for instance, work by killing unrestricted cells of breast cancer that expand and split. Whereas hormonal therapy works by either diminish the concentration of these women's hormones, which can promote the growth of breast cancer cells or by inhibiting the body's natural hormones system.

But, in individuals with breast cancer before surgery, if any systemic treatment is given it is known as neoadjuvant therapy [81 - 83]. Neo-adjuvant treatment is mainly to shrink breast tumor growth and also sufficient to facilitate and reduce surgical dissection. This type of systemic chemotherapy is as successful as therapy given later than surgery in terms of survival, disease progression, and far-away organ relapse is just as effective as postoperative treatment. While systemic therapy is given after surgical removal of the breast tumor mass, then it is called as adjuvant therapy [84, 85]. This kind of treatment is used to kill those undetected breast cancer cells, which remained after the surgical removal of a breast tumor or had invaded other organs of the female body. The tumor stage, histopathological features decide the use of adjuvant systemic therapy and this is the crucial therapeutic strategy for those breast cancer patients who may not benefit from surgery owing to metastasis.

Chemotherapy

The application and benefits of chemotherapy are dependent on multiple conditions, that include the number of lymph nodes involved, size of breast tumor, the existence of estrogen or progesterone receptors, and also the level of HER2 protein expressed by the breast cancer cells [86, 87]. Chemotherapy is more susceptible to HER2-enriched, basal and breast cancers, while luminal A breast tumors are usually least reactive. In most instances, combinations of medications are more efficient than single therapy; however, over the last few decades, there has still not been any indication that any single combination is best suited to all subtypes of molecular breast cancer. Chemotherapy usually takes 3-6 months based on the combination of medicines used for treatment. Chemotherapy is most helpful when the complete dose and drug cycle have been finished promptly

Hormonal Therapy

In hormonal treatment, tamoxifen and toremifene (Fareston), one of the few well-known drugs are used to eradicate breast cancer cells by inhibiting their proliferation and growth [88, 89]. These drugs inhibit the binding of estrogen to breast cancer cells and hence reduce their unrestricted growth, and these drugs are equally efficient in both pre and post-menopausal females. For the first decades, ER+ therapy for tamoxifen users has demonstrated a 39% reduction in the frequency of breast cancer relapse and a decline in the death rates by around1/3 in the first 15 years. Fulvestrant (Faslodex), letrozole, anastrozole, and exemestane are also a newer class of drugs, which is also being employed to care for the advanced stage of breast cancer patients both pre and post-menopausal women and they work by reducing the estrogen receptors and blocking the binding of estrogen.

Targeted Therapy: Therapy Intended at HER2

In targeted therapy aimed at HER2 protein, Trastuzumab (Herceptin), and

Pertuzumab like monoclonal antibodies, are mainly used to target the HER2 protein [90 - 93] directly. The HER2 protein is very crucial for breast cancer cells to divide rapidly and also grow faster, and generally, breast cancer cells overproducing HER2 protein could cause a relapse of breast cancer. Recent clinical studies show that trastuzumab and pertuzumab, in combination with standard chemotherapy for early-stage HER2-positive breast cancer, decrease the risk of breast cancer recurrence and overall mortality rate by 52% and 33%, correspondingly, as a contrast to standard chemotherapy unaided. In developed instances of HER2-positive breast cancer, these medications are also a standard part of therapy.

Another medicine, ado-trastuzumab emtansine (Kadcyla, formerly called TDM-1), was also recently authorized by the FDA for the use of the same monoclonal antibodies, which is also associated with a chemotherapy medication called DM-1. The drugs are HER2 positive advanced stages of breast cancer and are composed of the same monoclonal antibodies. The drug depending on the antibody is a homing device that carries the chemotherapy drugs to the target directly breast cancer cells. Lapatinib (Tykerb), another important medicinal product that has grown to resist trastuzumab treatment for patients with HER2-positive breast cancer.

Other Targeted Drugs

Everolimus (Afinitor) and bevacizumab (Avastin) are also another class of drugs that target mTOR and vascular endothelial growth factor (VEGF) proteins, respectively, and impede the growth as well as neoangiogenesis of breast tumors [94 - 96]. Everolimus was also recently approved by the FDA to treat metastatic positive hormone receptor, HER2-negative breast cancer cases in the postmenopausal female.

SUMMARY AND CONCLUDING REMARKS

Early detection of cancer can play an important role in the tumbling incidence and burden of breast cancer. Although some threat rebates might be attained with an obstacle, this approach cannot eradicate the majority of breast cancers that build up in low-income and middle-income states. Consequently, early detection may assist in breast cancer diagnosis, and survival remains a vital factor [97]. The effective strategies for diminishing the breast cancer burden globally should be comprehensive approach needed for cancer prevention and public awareness training programme to narrow down the widen gap between advanced evidence-based information of breast cancer control to reduce the established extrinsic and intrinsic risk factors, particularly in less developed countries, which has been convinced to be most potential and indelible control of cancer prevention. In addition to the prevention of breast cancer, we discuss how the implementation of current knowledge, coverage of effective screening, educating, and public awareness programs may ensure breast cancer burden. Owing to lifestyle modification, proper interventions are required to minimize the risk of having breast cancer and thus, ultimately improved the health of breast cancer patients. Identifying modifiable risk variables can contribute to development and prevention policy and reduce breast cancer incidence and mortality rate.

CONSENT FOR PUBLICATION

Not applicable.

CONFLICT OF INTEREST

The authors confirm that the contents of this chapter have no conflict of interest.

ACKNOWLEDGEMENT

Brij Nath Tewari acknowledge to King George's Medical University, Lucknow, India.

REFERENCES

[1] Bray F, Ferlay J, Soerjomataram I, Siegel RL, Torre LA, Jemal A. Global cancer statistics 2018: GLOBOCAN estimates of incidence and mortality worldwide for 36 cancers in 185 countries. CA Cancer J Clin 2018; 68(6): 394-424.http://www.ncbi.nlm.nih.gov/pubmed/30207593 [Internet]. [http://dx.doi.org/10.3322/caac.21492] [PMID: 30207593]

[2] Dey S. Preventing breast cancer in LMICs *via* screening and/or early detection: The real and the surreal. World J Clin Oncol 2014; 5(3): 509-19. [http://dx.doi.org/10.5306/wjco.v5.i3.509] [PMID: 25114864]

[3] Mukherjee D, Zhao J. The Role of chemokine receptor CXCR4 in breast cancer metastasis. Am J Cancer Res 2013; 3(1): 46-57.http://www.pubmedcentral.nih.gov/articlerender. fcgi?artid=3555200&tool=pmcentrez&rendertype=abstract [Internet]. [PMID: 23359227]

[4] Bosch A, Eroles P, Zaragoza R, Viña JR, Lluch A. Triple-negative breast cancer: molecular features, pathogenesis, treatment and current lines of research. Cancer Treat Rev 2010; 36(3): 206-15. [http://dx.doi.org/10.1016/j.ctrv.2009.12.002] [PMID: 20060649]

[5] Mendes O, Kim HT, Stoica G. Expression of MMP2, MMP9 and MMP3 in breast cancer brain metastasis in a rat model. Clin Exp Metastasis 2005; 22(3): 237-46. [http://dx.doi.org/10.1007/s10585-005-8115-6] [PMID: 16158251]

[6] Ellis MHD, Lippman ME, Harris JLM, *et al.* Treatment of metastatic disease. Diseases of the Breast. 2nd edition. Philadelphia: Lippincott-Raven 2000; pp. 749-99.

[7] Lu J, Steeg PS, Price JE, *et al.* Breast cancer metastasis: Challenges and opportunities. Cancer Res 2009; 4951-3.

[8] Fitzmaurice C, Allen C, Barber RM, *et al.* Global, regional, and national cancer incidence, mortality, years of life lost, years lived with disability, and disability-adjusted life-years for 32 cancer groups, 1990 to 2015: A Systematic Analysis for the Global Burden of Disease Study Global Burden. JAMA

Oncol 2017.
[PMID: 27918777]

[9]   Torre LA, Bray F, Siegel RL, Ferlay J, Lortet-Tieulent J, Jemal A. Global cancer statistics, 2012. CA
        Cancer J Clin 2015; 65(2): 87-108.
        [http://dx.doi.org/10.3322/caac.21262] [PMID: 25651787]

[10]   Rosenwald IB. The role of translation in neoplastic transformation from a pathologist's point of view.
        Oncogene 2004.

[11]   Hajdu SI, Vadmal M. A note from history: Landmarks in history of cancer, Part 6. Cancer 2013;
        119(23): 4058-82.http://www.ncbi.nlm.nih.gov/pubmed/24105604 [Internet].
        [http://dx.doi.org/10.1002/cncr.28319] [PMID: 24105604]

[12]   Hassiotou F, Geddes D. Anatomy of the human mammary gland: Current status of knowledge. Clin
        Anat 2013; 26(1): 29-48.
        [http://dx.doi.org/10.1002/ca.22165] [PMID: 22997014]

[13]   Hanahan D, Weinberg RA. Hallmarks of cancer: the next generation. Cell 2011; 144(5):
        646-74.https://linkinghub.elsevier.com/retrieve/pii/S0092867411001279 [Internet].
        [http://dx.doi.org/10.1016/j.cell.2011.02.013] [PMID: 21376230]

[14]   Kapoor A, Vogel VG. Prognostic factors for breast cancer and their use in the clinical setting. Expert
        Rev Anticancer Ther 2005; 5(2): 269-81.
        [http://dx.doi.org/10.1586/14737140.5.2.269] [PMID: 15877524]

[15]   Weigelt B, Reis-Filho JS, Kapoor A, Vogel VG. Histological and molecular types of breast cancer: is
        there a unifying taxonomy? Nat Rev Clin Oncol 2009; 6(12): 718-30.
        [http://dx.doi.org/10.1038/nrclinonc.2009.166] [PMID: 19942925]

[16]   American Cancer Society. Breast Cancer Facts & Figures 2013-2014. Atlanta: American Cancer
        Society 2013.

[17]   McPherson K, Steel CM, Dixon JM. ABC of breast diseases. Breast cancer-epidemiology, risk factors,
        and   genetics.   BMJ   2000;   321(7261):   624-8.http://www.pubmedcentral.nih.gov/
        articlerender.fcgi?artid=1118507&tool=pmcentrez&rendertype=abstract [Internet].
        [http://dx.doi.org/10.1136/bmj.321.7261.624] [PMID: 10977847]

[18]   Siegel RL, Miller KD, Jemal A. Cancer Statistics, 2017. CA Cancer J Clin 2017; 67(1):
        7-30.http://www.ncbi.nlm.nih.gov/pubmed/28055103 [Internet].
        [http://dx.doi.org/10.3322/caac.21387] [PMID: 28055103]

[19]   Boyd NF, Rommens JM, Vogt K, *et al.* Mammographic breast density as an intermediate phenotype
        for breast cancer. Lancet Oncol 2005; 6(10): 798-808.
        [http://dx.doi.org/10.1016/S1470-2045(05)70390-9] [PMID: 16198986]

[20]   Athma P, Rappaport R, Swift M. Molecular genotyping shows that ataxia-telangiectasia heterozygotes
        are predisposed to breast cancer. Cancer Genet Cytogenet 1996; 92(2): 130-4.
        [http://dx.doi.org/10.1016/S0165-4608(96)00328-7] [PMID: 8976369]

[21]   Breast cancer and hormonal contraceptives: collaborative reanalysis of individual data on 53 297
        women with breast cancer and 100 239 women without breast cancer from 54 epidemiological studies.
        Lancet   1996;   347(9017):
        1713-27.
        http://search.ebscohost.com/login.aspx?direct=true&AuthType=shib,cookie,ip,url,uid&db=aph&AN=
        9607177751&site=ehost-live&custid=s2888710 [Internet].
        [http://dx.doi.org/10.1016/S0140-6736(96)90806-5] [PMID: 8656904]

[22]   La Vecchia C, Altieri A, Franceschi S, Tavani A. Oral contraceptives and cancer: an update. Drug Saf
        2001; 24(10): 741-54.
        [http://dx.doi.org/10.2165/00002018-200124100-00003] [PMID: 11676302]

[23]   Faupel-Badger JM, Arcaro KF, Balkam JJ, *et al.* Postpartum remodeling, lactation, and breast cancer

risk: summary of a National Cancer Institute-sponsored workshop. J Natl Cancer Inst 2013; 105(3): 166-74.
[http://dx.doi.org/10.1093/jnci/djs505] [PMID: 23264680]

[24] Breast cancer and breastfeeding: collaborative reanalysis of individual data from 47 epidemiological studies in 30 countries, including 50302 women with breast cancer and 96973 women without the disease. Lancet 2002; 360(9328): 187-95.http://www.ncbi.nlm.nih.gov/pubmed/12133652 [Internet].
[http://dx.doi.org/10.1016/S0140-6736(02)09454-0] [PMID: 12133652]

[25] Key TJ, Verkasalo PK, Banks E. Epidemiology of breast cancer. Lancet Oncol 2001; 2(3): 133-40.http://www.ncbi.nlm.nih.gov/pubmed/11902563 [Internet].
[http://dx.doi.org/10.1016/S1470-2045(00)00254-0] [PMID: 11902563]

[26] Zhou Y, Chen J, Li Q, Huang W, Lan H, Jiang H. Association between breastfeeding and breast cancer risk: evidence from a meta-analysis. Breastfeed Med 2015; 10(3): 175-82.http://www.ncbi.nlm.nih.gov/pubmed/25785349 [Internet].
[http://dx.doi.org/10.1089/bfm.2014.0141] [PMID: 25785349]

[27] Hamajima N, Hirose K, Tajima K, *et al.* Alcohol, tobacco and breast cancer--collaborative reanalysis of individual data from 53 epidemiological studies, including 58,515 women with breast cancer and 95,067 women without the disease. Br J Cancer 2002; 87(11): 1234-45.
[http://dx.doi.org/10.1038/sj.bjc.6600596] [PMID: 12439712]

[28] Tamimi RM, Byrne C, Colditz GA, Hankinson SE. Endogenous hormone levels, mammographic density, and subsequent risk of breast cancer in postmenopausal women. J Natl Cancer Inst 2007; 99(15): 1178-87.
[http://dx.doi.org/10.1093/jnci/djm062] [PMID: 17652278]

[29] Ursin G, Lillie EO, Lee E, *et al.* The relative importance of genetics and environment on mammographic density. Cancer Epidemiol Biomarkers Prev 2009; 18(1): 102-12.
[http://dx.doi.org/10.1158/1055-9965.EPI-07-2857] [PMID: 19124487]

[30] van der Groep P, van der Wall E, van Diest PJ. Pathology of hereditary breast cancer. Cell Oncol (Dordr) 2011; 34(2): 71-88.
[http://dx.doi.org/10.1007/s13402-011-0010-3] [PMID: 21336636]

[31] Preston DL, Mattsson A, Holmberg E, Shore R, Hildreth NG, Boice JD Jr. Radiation effects on breast cancer risk: a pooled analysis of eight cohorts. Radiat Res 2002; 158(2): 220-35.
[http://dx.doi.org/10.1667/0033-7587(2002)158[0220:REOBCR]2.0.CO;2] [PMID: 12105993]

[32] Russo J, Hu YF, Yang X, Russo IH. Developmental, cellular, and molecular basis of human breast cancer. J Natl Cancer Inst Monogr 2000; (27): 17-37.
[http://dx.doi.org/10.1093/oxfordjournals.jncimonographs.a024241] [PMID: 10963618]

[33] Clemons M, Loijens L, Goss P. Breast cancer risk following irradiation for Hodgkin's disease. Cancer Treat Rev 2000; 26(4): 291-302.
[http://dx.doi.org/10.1053/ctrv.2000.0174] [PMID: 10913384]

[34] Travis LB, Hill DA, Dores GM, *et al.* Breast cancer following radiotherapy and chemotherapy among young women with Hodgkin disease. JAMA 2003; 290(4): 465-75.
[http://dx.doi.org/10.1001/jama.290.4.465] [PMID: 12876089]

[35] Mitchell RS, Kumar V, Abbas AK. Robbins Basic Pathology. 8th edition. Philadelphia: Saunders Elsevier 2007; pp. 516-22. ISBN 978-1-4160-2973

[36] Secretan B, Straif K, Baan R, *et al.* A review of human carcinogens--Part E: tobacco, areca nut, alcohol, coal smoke, and salted fish. Lancet Oncol 2009; 10(11): 1033-4.
[http://dx.doi.org/10.1016/S1470-2045(09)70326-2] [PMID: 19891056]

[37] Gaudet MM, Gapstur SM, Sun J, Diver WR, Hannan LM, Thun MJ. Active smoking and breast cancer risk: original cohort data and meta-analysis. J Natl Cancer Inst 2013; 105(8): 515-25.
[http://dx.doi.org/10.1093/jnci/djt023] [PMID: 23449445]

[38]   Hamajima N, Hirose K, Tajima K, *et al.* Alcohol, tobacco and breast cancer--collaborative reanalysis of individual data from 53 epidemiological studies, including 58,515 women with breast cancer and 95,067 women without the disease. Br J Cancer 2002; 87(11): 1234-45.
[http://dx.doi.org/10.1038/sj.bjc.6600596] [PMID: 12439712]

[39]   Vera-Ramirez L, Ramirez-Tortosa MC, Sanchez-Rovira P, *et al.* Impact of diet on breast cancer risk: a review of experimental and observational studies. Crit Rev Food Sci Nutr 2013; 53(1): 49-75.
[http://dx.doi.org/10.1080/10408398.2010.521600] [PMID: 23035920]

[40]   Alexander DD, Morimoto LM, Mink PJ, Lowe KA. Summary and meta-analysis of prospective studies of animal fat intake and breast cancer. Nutr Res Rev 2010; 23(1): 169-79.
[http://dx.doi.org/10.1017/S095442241000003X] [PMID: 20181297]

[41]   Linos E, Willett WC, Cho E, Frazier L. Adolescent diet in relation to breast cancer risk among premenopausal women. Cancer Epidemiol Biomarkers Prev 2010; 19(3): 689-96.
[http://dx.doi.org/10.1158/1055-9965.EPI-09-0802] [PMID: 20200427]

[42]   Dahlman-Wright K, Cavailles V, Fuqua SA, *et al.* International Union of Pharmacology. LXIV. Estrogen receptors. Pharmacol Rev 2006; 58(4): 773-81.
[http://dx.doi.org/10.1124/pr.58.4.8] [PMID: 17132854]

[43]   Cowley SM, Hoare S, Mosselman S, Parker MG. Estrogen receptors alpha and beta form heterodimers on DNA. J Biol Chem 1997; 272(32): 19858-62.
[http://dx.doi.org/10.1074/jbc.272.32.19858] [PMID: 9242648]

[44]   Sluyser M, Rijkers AW, de Goeij CC, Parker M, Hilkens J. Assignment of estradiol receptor gene to mouse chromosome 10. J Steroid Biochem 1988; 31(5): 757-61.
[http://dx.doi.org/10.1016/0022-4731(88)90283-X] [PMID: 3199815]

[45]   Menasce LP, White GR, Harrison CJ, Boyle JM. Localization of the estrogen receptor locus (ESR) to chromosome 6q25.1 by FISH and a simple post-FISH banding technique. Genomics 1993; 17(1): 263-5.
[http://dx.doi.org/10.1006/geno.1993.1320] [PMID: 8406468]

[46]   Levin ER. Integration of the extranuclear and nuclear actions of estrogen. Mol Endocrinol 2005; 19(8): 1951-9.
[http://dx.doi.org/10.1210/me.2004-0390] [PMID: 15705661]

[47]   Htun H, Holth LT, Walker D, Davie JR, Hager GL. Direct visualization of the human estrogen receptor alpha reveals a role for ligand in the nuclear distribution of the receptor. Mol Biol Cell 1999; 10(2): 471-86.
[http://dx.doi.org/10.1091/mbc.10.2.471] [PMID: 9950689]

[48]   Herynk MH, Fuqua SAW. Estrogen receptor mutations in human disease. Endocr Rev 2004; 25(6): 869-98.
[http://dx.doi.org/10.1210/er.2003-0010] [PMID: 15583021]

[49]   Rosa FE, Caldeira JRF, Felipes J, *et al.* Evaluation of estrogen receptor alpha and beta and progesterone receptor expression and correlation with clinicopathologic factors and proliferative marker Ki-67 in breast cancers. Hum Pathol 2008; 39(5): 720-30. http://www.ncbi.nlm.nih.gov/pubmed/18234277 [Internet].
[http://dx.doi.org/10.1016/j.humpath.2007.09.019] [PMID: 18234277]

[50]   Deroo BJ, Korach KS. Estrogen receptors and human disease. J Clin Invest 2006; 116(3): 561-70.
[http://dx.doi.org/10.1172/JCI27987] [PMID: 16511588]

[51]   Masood S, Sim SJ, Lu L. Immunohistochemical differentiation of atypical hyperplasia *vs.* carcinoma in situ of the breast. Cancer Detect Prev 1992; 16(4): 225-35.
[PMID: 1281040]

[52]   Cortez V, Mann M, Brann DW, Vadlamudi RK. Extranuclear signaling by estrogen: role in breast cancer progression and metastasis. Minerva Ginecol 2010; 62(6): 573-83.

[PMID: 21079578]

[53]   Horwitz KB, Alexander PS. *In situ* photolinked nuclear progesterone receptors of human breast cancer cells: subunit molecular weights after transformation and translocation. Endocrinology 1983; 113(6): 2195-201.
[http://dx.doi.org/10.1210/endo-113-6-2195] [PMID: 6685620]

[54]   Gao X, Nawaz Z. Progesterone receptors - animal models and cell signaling in breast cancer: Role of steroid receptor coactivators and corepressors of progesterone receptors in breast cancer. Breast Cancer Res 2002; 4(5): 182-6.
[http://dx.doi.org/10.1186/bcr449] [PMID: 12223121]

[55]   Zhou BP, Hung M-C. Dysregulation of cellular signaling by HER2/neu in breast cancer. Semin Oncol 2003; 30(5) (Suppl. 16): 38-48.
[http://dx.doi.org/10.1053/j.seminoncol.2003.08.006] [PMID: 14613025]

[56]   Vinatzer U, Dampier B, Streubel B, *et al.* Expression of HER2 and the coamplified genes GRB7 and MLN64 in human breast cancer: quantitative real-time reverse transcription-PCR as a diagnostic alternative to immunohistochemistry and fluorescence *in situ* hybridization. Clin Cancer Res 2005; 11(23): 8348-57.
[http://dx.doi.org/10.1158/1078-0432.CCR-05-0841] [PMID: 16322295]

[57]   Le XF, Pruefer F, Bast RC Jr. HER2-targeting antibodies modulate the cyclin-dependent kinase inhibitor p27Kip1 *via* multiple signaling pathways. Cell Cycle 2005; 4(1): 87-95.
[http://dx.doi.org/10.4161/cc.4.1.1360] [PMID: 15611642]

[58]   Perou CM, Børresen-Dale AL. Systems biology and genomics of breast cancer. Cold Spring Harb Perspect Biol 2011; 3(2): 1-17.
[http://dx.doi.org/10.1101/cshperspect.a003293] [PMID: 21047916]

[59]   Pamies RJ, Crawford DR. Tumor markers. An update. Med Clin North Am 1996; 80(1): 185-99.
[http://dx.doi.org/10.1016/S0025-7125(05)70435-1] [PMID: 8569297]

[60]   Febbo PG, Ladanyi M, Aldape KD, *et al.* NCCN Task Force report: Evaluating the clinical utility of tumor markers in oncology. J Natl Compr Canc Netw 2011; 9 (Suppl. 5): S1 -32.http://www.ncbi.nlm.nih.gov/pubmed/22138009 [Internet].
[http://dx.doi.org/10.6004/jnccn.2011.0137] [PMID: 22138009]

[61]   Faderl S, Talpaz M, Estrov Z, O'Brien S, Kurzrock R, Kantarjian HM. The biology of chronic myeloid leukemia. N Engl J Med 1999; 341(3): 164-72.
[http://dx.doi.org/10.1056/NEJM199907153410306] [PMID: 10403855]

[62]   Arber DA. Molecular diagnostic approach to non-Hodgkin's lymphoma. J Mol Diagn 2000; 2(4): 178-90. http://www.ncbi.nlm.nih.gov/pubmed/11232108 [Internet].
[http://dx.doi.org/10.1016/S1525-1578(10)60636-8] [PMID: 11232108]

[63]   McShane LM, Altman DG, Sauerbrei W, Taube SE, Gion M, Clark GM. Reporting recommendations for tumor marker prognostic studies. J Clin Oncol 2005; 23(36): 9067-9072 .http://www.ncbi.nlm.nih.gov/pubmed/16172462 [Internet].
[http://dx.doi.org/10.1200/JCO.2004.01.0454] [PMID: 16172462]

[64]   Goldstein I, Marcel V, Olivier M, Oren M, Rotter V, Hainaut P. Understanding wild-type and mutant p53 activities in human cancer: new landmarks on the way to targeted therapies. Cancer Gene Ther 2011; 18(1): 2-11.
[http://dx.doi.org/10.1038/cgt.2010.63] [PMID: 20966976]

[65]   Joensuu H, Kellokumpu-Lehtinen P-L, Bono P, *et al.* Adjuvant docetaxel or vinorelbine with or without trastuzumab for breast cancer. N Engl J Med 2006; 354(8): 809-820 .http://www.ncbi.nlm.nih.gov/pubmed/16495393 [Internet].
[http://dx.doi.org/10.1056/NEJMoa053028] [PMID: 16495393]

[66]   Pollock PM, Meltzer PS. A genome-based strategy uncovers frequent BRAF mutations in melanoma.

Cancer Cell 2002; 2(1): 5-7.
[http://dx.doi.org/10.1016/S1535-6108(02)00089-2] [PMID: 12150818]

[67]   Chapman PB, Hauschild A, Robert C, *et al.* Improved survival with vemurafenib in melanoma with BRAF V600E mutation. N Engl J Med [Internet] 2011; 364(26): 2507-16. http://www.ncbi.nlm.nih.gov/pubmed/21639808
[http://dx.doi.org/10.1056/NEJMoa1103782]

[68]   Olsen O, Gøtzsche PC. Cochrane review on screening for breast cancer with mammography. Lancet 2001; 358(9290): 1340-2.
[http://dx.doi.org/10.1016/S0140-6736(01)06449-2] [PMID: 11684218]

[69]   Saslow D, Boetes C, Burke W, *et al.* American Cancer Society guidelines for breast screening with MRI as an adjunct to mammography. CA Cancer J Clin 2007; 57(2): 75-89.
[http://dx.doi.org/10.3322/canjclin.57.2.75] [PMID: 17392385]

[70]   Jørgensen KJ, Gøtzsche PC. Overdiagnosis in publicly organised mammography screening programmes: systematic review of incidence trends. BMJ 2009; 339: b2587.
[http://dx.doi.org/10.1136/bmj.b2587] [PMID: 19589821]

[71]   Morrell S, Barratt A, Irwig L, Howard K, Biesheuvel C, Armstrong B. Estimates of overdiagnosis of invasive breast cancer associated with screening mammography. Cancer Causes Control 2010; 21(2): 275-82.
[http://dx.doi.org/10.1007/s10552-009-9459-z] [PMID: 19894130]

[72]   Lehman CD, Gatsonis C, Kuhl CK, *et al.* MRI evaluation of the contralateral breast in women with recently diagnosed breast cancer. N Engl J Med 2007; 356(13): 1295-303.
[http://dx.doi.org/10.1056/NEJMoa065447] [PMID: 17392300]

[73]   Sickles EA, Filly RA, Callen PW. Benign breast lesions: ultrasound detection and diagnosis. Radiology 1984; 151(2): 467-70.http://pubs.rsna.org/doi/10.1148/radiology.151.2.6709920 [Internet].
[http://dx.doi.org/10.1148/radiology.151.2.6709920] [PMID: 6709920]

[74]   Kiebert GM, de Haes JCJM, van de Velde CJH. The impact of breast-conserving treatment and mastectomy on the quality of life of early-stage breast cancer patients: a review. J Clin Oncol 1991; 9(6): 1059-70.
[http://dx.doi.org/10.1200/JCO.1991.9.6.1059] [PMID: 2033420]

[75]   Poleshuck EL, Katz J, Andrus CH, *et al.* Risk factors for chronic pain following breast cancer surgery: a prospective study. J Pain 2006; 7(9): 626-34.
[http://dx.doi.org/10.1016/j.jpain.2006.02.007] [PMID: 16942948]

[76]   Veronesi U, Cascinelli N, Mariani L, *et al.* Twenty-year follow-up of a randomized study comparing breast-conserving surgery with radical mastectomy for early breast cancer. N Engl J Med 2002; 347(16): 1227-32.
[http://dx.doi.org/10.1056/NEJMoa020989] [PMID: 12393819]

[77]   Clarke M, Collins R, Darby S, *et al.* EBCTCG. Effects of radiotherapy and of differences in the extent of surgery for early breast cancer on local recurrence and 15-year survival: an overview of the randomised trials. Lancet 2005.

[78]   Early Breast Cancer Trialists', Collaborative Group. Favourable and unfavourable effects on long-term survival of radiotherapy for early breast cancer: an overview of the randomised trials. Early Breast Cancer Trialists' Collaborative Group. Lancet 2000; 355(9217): 1757-70. http://www.ncbi.nlm.nih.gov/pubmed/10832826 [Internet].
[http://dx.doi.org/10.1016/S0140-6736(00)02263-7] [PMID: 10832826]

[79]   Early Breast Cancer Trialists' Collaborative Group. Effects of radiotherapy and surgery in early breast cancer. An overview of the randomized trials. Early Breast Cancer Trialists' Collaborative Group. N Engl J Med 1995; 334(15): 1757-70. http://www.ncbi.nlm.nih.gov/pubmed/10832826

[80]   Noël G, Mazeron JJ. [Favourable and unfavourable effects on long-term survival of radiotherapy for

early breast cancer: an overview of the randomised trials]. Cancer Radiother 2001; 5(1): 92-4.
[http://dx.doi.org/10.1016/S1278-3218(00)00058-5] [PMID: 11236548]

[81]   Loibl S, Denkert C, von Minckwitz G, *et al.* Neoadjuvant treatment of breast cancer: maximizing
        pathologic complete response rates to improve prognosis. Curr Opin Obstet Gynecol 2015; 27(1): 85-
        91.
        [http://dx.doi.org/10.1097/GCO.0000000000000147] [PMID: 25490376]

[82]   Loibl S, Denkert C, von Minckwitz G. Neoadjuvant treatment of breast cancer--Clinical and research
        perspective. Breast 2015; 24 (Suppl. 2): S73-7. https://linkinghub.elsevier.com/retrieve/pii/
        S0960977615001563 [Internet].
        [http://dx.doi.org/10.1016/j.breast.2015.07.018] [PMID: 26387601]

[83]   Liedtke C, Mazouni C, Hess KR, *et al.* Response to neoadjuvant therapy and long-term survival in
        patients with triple-negative breast cancer. J Clin Oncol 2008; 26(8): 1275-81.
        [http://dx.doi.org/10.1200/JCO.2007.14.4147] [PMID: 18250347]

[84]   Ragaz J, Jackson SM, Le N, *et al.* Adjuvant radiotherapy and chemotherapy in node-positive
        premenopausal women with breast cancer. N Engl J Med 1997; 337(14):
        956-62.http://www.nejm.org/doi/abs/10.1056/NEJM199710023371402 [Internet].
        [http://dx.doi.org/10.1056/NEJM199710023371402] [PMID: 9309100]

[85]   Overgaard M, Hansen PS, Overgaard J, *et al.* Postoperative radiotherapy in high-risk premenopausal
        women with breast cancer who receive adjuvant chemotherapy. Danish Breast Cancer Cooperative
        Group 82b Trial. N Engl J Med 1997; 337(14): 949-55.
        [http://dx.doi.org/10.1056/NEJM199710023371401] [PMID: 9395428]

[86]   Byar KL, Berger AM, Bakken SL, Cetak MA. Impact of adjuvant breast cancer chemotherapy on
        fatigue, other symptoms, and quality of life. Oncol Nurs Forum 2006; 33(1):
        E18-26.
        http://onf.ons.org/onf/33/1/impact-adjuvant-breast-cancer-chemotherapy-fatigue-other-symptoms-and-
        quality-life [Internet].
        [http://dx.doi.org/10.1188/06.ONF.E18-E26] [PMID: 16470230]

[87]   Early Breast Cancer Trialists' Collaborative Group (EBCTCG). Effects of chemotherapy and
        hormonal therapy for early breast cancer on recurrence and 15-year survival: an overview of the
        randomised trials. Lancet 2005; 365(9472): 1687-717.
        https://linkinghub.elsevier.com/retrieve/pii/S0140673605665440 [Internet].
        [http://dx.doi.org/10.1016/S0140-6736(05)66544-0] [PMID: 15894097]

[88]   Narod SA. Hormone replacement therapy and the risk of breast cancer. Nat Rev Clin Oncol 2011;
        8(11): 669-76.http://www.nature.com/articles/nrclinonc.2011.110 [Internet].
        [http://dx.doi.org/10.1038/nrclinonc.2011.110] [PMID: 21808267]

[89]   Beral V. Million Women Study Collaborators. Breast cancer and hormone-replacement therapy in the
        Million Women Study. Lancet (London, England) 2003; 362(9382): 419-27.
        http://www.ncbi.nlm.nih.gov/pubmed/12927427
        [http://dx.doi.org/10.1016/S0140-6736(03)14596-5]

[90]   Slamon DJ, Leyland-Jones B, Shak S, *et al.* Use of chemotherapy plus a monoclonal antibody against
        HER2 for metastatic breast cancer that overexpresses HER2. N Engl J Med 2001; 344(11): 783-92.
        http://www.nejm.org/doi/abs/10.1056/NEJM200103153441101 [Internet].
        [http://dx.doi.org/10.1056/NEJM200103153441101] [PMID: 11248153]

[91]   Pal SK, Pegram M. HER2 targeted therapy in breast cancer...beyond Herceptin. Rev Endocr Metab
        Disord 2007; 8(3): 269-77. http://link.springer.com/10.1007/s11154-007-9040-6 [Internet].
        [http://dx.doi.org/10.1007/s11154-007-9040-6] [PMID: 17899385]

[92]   Ahmed S, Sami A, Xiang J. HER2-directed therapy: current treatment options for HER2-positive
        breast cancer. Breast Cancer 2015; 22(2): 101-16.http://www.ncbi.nlm.nih.gov/pubmed/25634227
        [Internet].

[http://dx.doi.org/10.1007/s12282-015-0587-x] [PMID: 25634227]

[93]   Behr TM, Béhé M, Wörmann B. Trastuzumab and breast cancer. N Engl J Med 2001; 345(13): 995-6.
       [http://dx.doi.org/10.1056/NEJM200109273451312] [PMID: 11575295]

[94]   Miller K, Wang M, Gralow J, *et al.* Paclitaxel plus bevacizumab *versus* paclitaxel alone for metastatic
       breast cancer. N Engl J Med 2007; 357(26): 2666-76. http://www.nejm.org/doi/abs/10.1056/
       NEJMoa072113 [Internet].
       [http://dx.doi.org/10.1056/NEJMoa072113] [PMID: 18160686]

[95]   von Minckwitz G, Eidtmann H, Loibl S, *et al.* Integrating bevacizumab, everolimus, and lapatinib into
       current neoadjuvant chemotherapy regimen for primary breast cancer. Safety results of the
       GeparQuinto trial. Ann Oncol 2011; 22(2): 301-6. https://academic.oup.com/
       annonc/article/22/2/301/170087 [Internet].
       [http://dx.doi.org/10.1093/annonc/mdq350] [PMID: 20624784]

[96]   Gnant M, Greil R, Hubalek M, Steger G. Everolimus in postmenopausal, hormone receptor-positive
       advanced breast cancer: summary and results of an austrian expert panel discussion. Breast Care
       (Basel) 2013; 8(4): 293-9.https://www.karger.com/Article/FullText/354121 [Internet].
       [http://dx.doi.org/10.1159/000354121] [PMID: 24415983]

[97]   Andersen BL, Yang H-C, Farrar WB, *et al.* Psychologic intervention improves survival for breast
       cancer patients: a randomized clinical trial. Cancer 2008; 113(12): 3450-8.
       [http://dx.doi.org/10.1002/cncr.23969] [PMID: 19016270]

CHAPTER 2

Current Imaging Techniques in Breast Cancer: An Overview

Garima Suman[*] and **Anurima Patra**

Department of Radiodiagnosis, Tata Memorial Hospital, Dr. E Borges Road, Parel, Mumbai-400012, (Maharashtra) India

Abstract: Tissue diagnosis has been recognized as the gold standard method of diagnosing breast cancer; however, over the last few decades, radiologic imaging has taken the center-stage in pre-operative diagnosis of breast cancer. Radiological imaging tools play a crucial role in not only early detection of breast cancer and staging but also help the surgeons in chalking out the surgical plan and later also in surveillance of the patients. While the advancements in imaging have improved the rate of early detection of breast cancer, 'false alarms' raised due to limitations of existing imaging methods are an important area of concern. The purpose of this chapter is to provide an overview of the capabilities and limitations of the current imaging techniques in breast cancer.

Keywords: BI-RADS, Breast cancer, Magnetic resonance imaging, Mammography, Positron emission tomography, Screening, USG.

INTRODUCTION

Although the mortality from BC has been on a decreasing trend owing to its early detection and better treatment options, it remains to be one of the commonest causes of cancer related deaths in women worldwide [1]. About 85% of BC occur sporadically due to random genetic mutations occurring in women without any family history of BC. A few important risk factors associated with BC include the onset of menarche at an early age, late menopause, nulliparity, and obesity. All these factors cause prolonged exposure to estrogen, which is implicated to be a determinant of BC causality. About 15% of BC results from inherited genetic mutations, and most of these patients have a history of BC diagnosis in first-degree relatives.

[*] **Corresponding Author Garima Suman:** Department of Radiodiagnosis, Tata Memorial Hospital, Dr. E Borges Road, Parel, Mumbai-400012, (Maharashtra) India; Tel: +91 9869133113; E-mail: garimanmc@gmail.com

Breast imaging methods have undergone a huge transition over the last couple of decades due to various technologic advancements. The advancements in non-invasive imaging tools have enabled the clinicians to move away from a poorly reliable screening method like self-examination to a more sensitive tool like mammography (MMG). The practice of direct exposure film mammography is now being replaced by full-field digital MMG and, more recently, digital breast tomosynthesis (DBT). Introduction of BC screening through MMG has arguably played a key role in the early detection of BC. MMG is the 'gold standard' imaging method for pre-operative evaluation of breast lesions. Breast ultrasonography (USG) and magnetic resonance imaging (MRI), serve as adjuncts to MMG and important tools for screening young high-risk subgroups. In current practice, image-guided breast interventional procedures play an integral role in the management of breast lesions, be it pre-operative diagnosis through percutaneous biopsy or lesion localization to guide surgical excision. Introduction of Breast Imaging Reporting and Data System (BI-RADS) by American College of Radiology in 1993 added a new dimension to breast imaging. BI-RADS has been vital in providing a standard for quality control in MMG and bringing uniformity in reporting of breast lesions on imaging. This chapter is focused on current methods in radiological evaluation of BC and discusses the role of each imaging tool in the diagnostic workup. We also briefly touch upon the limitations and drawbacks of the existing imaging tools and ongoing recent advancements to overcome these shortcomings.

Anatomy of Breast

Breast is an in-homogenous organ overlying the anterior chest wall, separated from the underlying chest muscles *viz.* pectoralis minor and major by a fascia. The volume and shape of breasts in each person vary depending on various factors such as age, developmental stage, and degree of endocrine stimulation. Breast is composed of glandular and fibro-adipose tissue. Each breast consists of 15-20 lobes arranged radially around and behind the nipple. Each of these lobes is an independent entity drained by a collecting/lactiferous duct terminating in the nipple. Each collecting duct has multiple branches. The branches of a collecting duct end in a **terminal ductal-lobular unit (TDLU).** A TDLU is formed by a small segment of the terminal part of collecting duct, its branches, and a cluster of ductules and alveoli surrounding it. TLDU is considered to be the basic functional unit of the breast parenchyma. Invasive ductal carcinoma (IDC), which is the most common invasive BC, arises from the epithelial lining of the small ducts. The stroma consisting of fibrous and adipose tissues lies interposed between the lobes. There are also fibrous suspensory bands of connective tissue (a.k.a suspensory ligament of Cooper), which run from under the skin of the breast up to the chest wall. These ligaments divide breasts into lobes and also maintain the structural integrity of the breasts. For radiological imaging, each breast may be divided into three portions: a pre-mammary zone that lies between the skin and the parenchyma, mammary zone consisting of the lobes and lobules, and a retro-mammary zone, located between the gland and pectoralis muscles.

Clinical Diagnosis of BC

The diagnosis of BC is made through either routine screening of the target population or the patient presenting with a symptom. Most commonly, it is the patient who presents with an incidental lump felt in her breast [2]. A recent study suggests that as much as 83% of patients present with breast lump as their only complaint while in rest of the patients, a breast lump is associated with other symptoms such as nipple discharge, pain, a lump in the axilla, weight loss, *etc.* [3]. Most of the BC arises from the upper and outer aspect of the breast believed to be due to the maximum abundance of parenchyma in this region [4]. In about 3-9% of patients, the presenting symptom is nipple discharge [5]. In some cases, the patient first notices a lump in their axilla. On physical examination, the concerning features of a malignant lump include irregular shape, firm to feel, and fixity to skin or chest wall. Advanced BC or inflammatory type of BC can present with swollen, edematous, and enlarged breast with skin dimpling and nipple retraction. Swelling and edema occur due to involvement and blockade of draining lymph channels by the malignant mass. Skin and nipple retraction occurs due to the invasion of the suspensory ligament of cooper by the malignant cells. This gives a typical appearance of the breast known as "Peaud'orange". Rarely, BC may not be detected until it has spread to the skin of the nipple-areolar region and may present as eczematous itchy lesion around the nipple. Further examination reveals malignant cells in the skin lesion with an underlying invasive or *in-situ* ductal carcinoma, an entity called as Paget's disease [6].

Why Imaging?

Imaging plays a central role in screening, diagnosis, and staging of BC as well as post-treatment surveillance. Early BC may present as very small lumps, which can be difficult to palpate. Detection of such small lesions is the goal of screening through low-dose mammography so that malignant lesions are detected at a stage when they are not yet clinically palpable and amenable to curative surgery. Sometimes, BC could present as abnormal nipple discharge with no palpable lump. In such cases, imaging helps in detecting the underlying pathology and helps the surgeon to reach the correct diagnosis. Imaging is used in the staging of BC, which includes, studying the local extent of disease, regional lymph nodal spread, and distant metastases. Several imaging modalities are used in the workup for BC, such as mammography (MMG), ultrasonography (USG), computed tomography (CT), magnetic resonance imaging (MRI), positron imaging tomography (PET), *etc*. Nowadays, PET study is often combined with CT scans and together known as PET-CT. The uses of imaging tools help during the treatment of BC particularly in solving the clinical issue. In addition, awareness of the role of various imaging methods and their limitations is required for their just use.

RADIOLOGICAL MODALITIES USED IN BC DETECTION

Mammography

MMG is a technique that uses an X-ray beam to form a high-resolution radiographic image of the breasts. The two main indications for MMG are screening of BC and evaluation of symptomatic breast lesions like lumps, nipple retraction, nipple discharge, skin changes, *etc*. Breast is predominantly composed of soft tissues. Therefore, it has a relatively narrow range of inherent radio-densities. Special X-ray tubes are used in the MMG machine to produce the low-energy radiation dose necessary to achieve high tissue contrast. The high spatial resolution of MMG enables visualization of fine details and identification of micro-calcifications.

Due to uneven breast thickness from the subcutaneous region to the chest wall, it is important to apply external compression to the breast during MMG. The primary goal of compression is to bring uniformity in the thickness of the breast, so the X-ray beam more evenly penetrates it. Compression is applied on each breast lasting a few seconds at the time of X-ray exposure, employing a compression paddle. The amount of force exerted by the paddle can be controlled by the operator depending on the thickness of the breast and is usually 14 daN, seldom exceeding 20 daN [7]. A uniform breast thickness helps in avoiding overexposure of the relatively thin anterior part towards the nipple and underexposure of the relatively thick posterior part near the chest wall. This allows for shorter exposure times and thus reduced radiation dose. Uniform breast thickness also decreases the scatter radiation. Compression also immobilizes the breast and diminishes the unsharpness of the image caused by patient motion or movement with respiration. Compression separates superimposed breast tissues, which prevent masking of lesions in the background of heterogeneous dense parenchyma.

In routine practice, two standard mammographic projections are used for screening and diagnosis of BC. These views are Mediolateral oblique (MLO) and craniocaudal (CC) views [8, 9]. To obtain the MLO view, the overhead X-ray tube is angled at 30–60° and the X-ray beam is projected in the inferolateral direction (Fig. **1a**). The MLO view is the projection in which almost the entire breast can be seen on a single image. CC view is obtained when the X-ray beam is directed in a perpendicular direction from the overhead X-ray tube while the chest is being compressed from above (Fig. **1b**). Proper positioning for this view is achieved by pulling the breast up and forward, away from the chest wall. There are supplementary views that may be obtained in specific cases to distinguish true lesions from superimposed normal tissues and for better delineation of the margins of the lesion. Some of the commonly used supplementary views are a mediolateral view, spot compression, magnification view, tangential or rolled back view, extended CC view. Magnification view is frequently performed supplementary view for better visualization and characterization of the microcalcifications. On MMG, the breast can be compartmentalized into premammary, mammary, and retromammary zones. The mammary zone is where the bulk of the fibro-glandular parenchyma is located, and most of the cancers arise in this zone. Parenchyma and stromal connective tissue is radiologically dense and appear bright while fat is radiologically lucent and appears dark on a mammogram [10]. The average mean radiation dose for standard two-view MMG of both breasts is approximately 4. 5 mGy [10].

DBT is a new technique in digital MMG where multiple low dose X-ray projections of the breast are acquired at different angles of the X-ray tube. The images obtained are reconstructed into a stack of thin sections of images. The radiologist can scroll through the stack of images and work through the areas of superimposed tissues. This helps in minimizing patient call-backs by alleviating the false-impressions of lesions on standard MMG caused due to tissue overlap. It also serves as an additional tool for the work-up of abnormalities detected on routine views, reducing the requirement of additional views and ultrasound. As a part of the screening study, DBT improves the specificity of the screening mammogram and significantly decreases the patient call-back rates [11]. Computer-aided detection (CAD) is a software tool that can detect and highlight the abnormal areas in the mammogram, which can be reviewed by the radiologist. The objective of using the CAD tool is to reduce the observational errors if the radiologist fails to notice the abnormality. In screening MMG studies, CAD can detect 86–88% of all masses and almost 90% of all malignant lesions. Its sensitivity in spotting micro calcifications is as high as 98% [11]. DBT and CAD have been discussed in detail later in this chapter.

Ultrasonography

USG has several uses at various stages in the diagnosis of BC. Common indications for using USG in breast evaluation are: in combination with MMG for better characterization of a lesion; in cases of palpable lump with equivocal findings ; screening tool in young patients (particularly less than 30 years of age) although MRI is preferred; preoperative localization of a lesion for breast conservation surgery; re-evaluation of a mammographically occult lesion detected on MRI; as a guiding tool to perform tissue sampling *e.g.* USG guided FNAC and biopsy and, intra-operative evaluation of breast lesions.

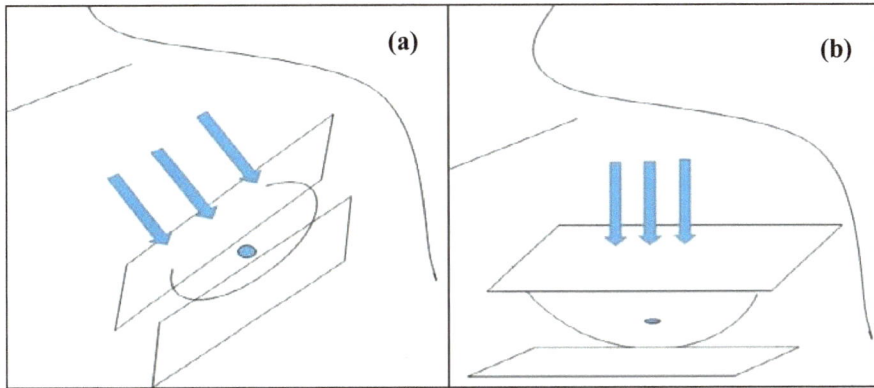

Fig. (1). Projection of X-ray beams (arrows) concerning the breast in MLO view (**a**) and CC view (**b**).

USG is preferred over MMG for breast evaluation in younger women or women with highly dense breast parenchyma on MMG. Besides, USG does not use ionizing radiation as opposed to MMG and is a relatively safe option in young women. Breast density is higher in younger women and decreases with age as the glandular component of parenchyma is replaced by fatty component. In the dense background breast parenchyma on MMG, lesions may get obscured. If the clinical suspicion for a lesion is high, USG is useful in confirming the presence of a lesion and also its characterization. This is especially invaluable for the assessment of palpable abnormalities with negative MMG and dense background parenchyma. In case of a palpable abnormality in the breast, a negative MMG and a negative USG can practically rule out underlying pathology. The negative-predictive value of a combined negative MMG and USG is 99. 8% [7]. Sonographically detected lesions are assessed based on their orientation concerning the chest wall, shape, margin, echogenicity, and acoustic transmission. The classic sonographic characteristics of a lesion concerning for malignancy include nonparallel orientation, "taller than wide" dimensions, irregular shape or margin, hypoechoic internal echogenicity, and posterior acoustic shadowing. Highly aggressive lesions also tend to show increased vascularity. USG can also be used to evaluate the axilla when a suspicious lesion is detected in the breast. Abnormal axillary nodes can be identified pre-operatively and can be sampled through percutaneous ultrasound-guided FNAC/biopsy, thus avoiding sentinel node biopsy and potential risk of lymphedema. Grey-scale USG evaluation of breast is done using high frequencies linear probes with operating frequencies ranging between 7. 5 and 15 MHz Higher the frequency, less the penetrating power. The choice of operating frequency can be adjusted depending upon the thickness of the breast. Currently, available high-frequency linear transducers yield a resolution of approximately 300 μm. Additional option of harmonic imaging can be used to enhance the displayed image quality. Doppler and elastography also contribute to breast lesion characterization. Elastography is a USG technique that can help in the characterization of breast lesions based on tissue stiffness. This technique has the potential to improve the specificity of breast USG to characterize benign *vs.* malignant breast tumors, reducing the intervention rate [12]. An elaborate discussion of elastography follows in the subsequent sections of this chapter.

Magnetic Resonance Imaging

Breast MRI is increasingly being used as an adjunct to MMG and USG due to its good sensitivity. American College of Radiology practice guidelines has laid down the indications for the performance of breast MRI which include screening for high-risk women, equivocal MMG findings, and positive margins after surgery for BC, metastatic axillary adenopathy with unknown primary, response assessment after neo-adjuvant chemotherapy, *etc.* [13]. Breast MRI should be performed on a magnet, which is at least 1.5 T or higher in strength. A dedicated breast coil is used for the scan. The patients are scanned in the prone position using dedicated breast coils, which have in-built compression devices to stabilize the breast. The recommendations for breast MRI include acquiringT1 and T2 weighted images of breasts with and without fat suppression along with early and delayed post-contrast images obtained 4 minutes and 8 minutes respectively after contrast administration. The slice thickness for acquisition should not be more than 3 mm. At 3 Tesla, there is an increase in the signal-to-noise ratio, leading to improvements in image quality. Diffusion-weighted imaging (DWI) and spectroscopy, are being increasingly used to improve the specificity of breast MRI. DWI is a non-contrast echoplanar sequence that measures the rate of diffusion of water molecules within the breast tissue. Malignancy has a higher cellular density and less diffusivity of extracellular water. Thus lower values of apparent diffusion coefficient compared to benign lesions or normal breast tissues. Magnetic resonance spectroscopy (MRS) provides metabolic information about the tumor. The presence of a choline peak on the MR spectra can be used as a way of differentiating malignant from benign lesions. Choline is an important marker of membrane biosynthesis, and its concentration rises when membrane turnover is increased, such as in malignancy. MRS is dependent on the signal-to-noise ratio of the examination, and so the accuracy of spectroscopy is improved when imaging at higher field strengths of 3 teslas. MRS has been further discussed later in the chapter.

A combination of clinical examination, MMG, and MRI are 99% sensitive in preoperative assessment of the local extent of disease in patients with newly diagnosed BC. When used alone, Clinical breast examination has only 50% sensitivity while MMG has 60% sensitivity [13]. The ideal time to perform a breast MRI is in the proliferative phase of a women's menstrual cycle, ideally between days 7 and 13. In this phase, the hormonal influence on the breast is such that the enhancement of background glandular parenchyma is least intense. In newly diagnosed cases of BC, MRI is effective in detecting additional unsuspected tiny lesions in the ipsilateral breast in 15–27% of patients as well as contralateral breast in 3–10% of patients [14, 15]. This may change the management approach, potentially avoiding unnecessary mastectomies; however, there has not been any proven survival benefit in patients with the detection of these additional lesions. There is a considerable overlap in MRI features of benign and malignant breast lesions, which limits the specificity of MRI. The false positivity rate of MRI can range from 9% to as high as 68% [13, 16 - 19]. The small lesions picked up on MRI need to be re-evaluated with MMG or USG and prompt biopsy to be performed to rule out malignancy. Sometimes, these lesions are obscure on MMG and USG [14]. In such cases, an MRI guided biopsy needs to be done. MRI guided biopsy is not available as commonly as USG guided biopsy, especially in the developing countries, and is a costlier affair. Moreover, the interpretation of MRI is difficult and has a long learning curve. Due to these limitations, MRI is not routinely used in all newly diagnosed BC; rather, it is still an adjunctive modality.

In pre-operative local staging, MRI performs better than MMG and USG in the assessment of tumor extent. Lobular carcinoma which is more likely to be multifocal and infiltrative are better evaluated with MRI. It can help in the assessment of response to neoadjuvant chemotherapy in patients with locally advanced primary BC. Neoadjuvant chemotherapy is used to downstage large BC to enable breast-conserving surgery. MRI can recognize responders earlier than other imaging methods such as MMG and USG, by demonstrating a decrease in lesion size, or a change in the enhancement pattern. MRI can help in planning the extent of surgical resection in breast conservative surgery. MRI is used in the postoperative evaluation of breast to differentiate surgical scar from tumor recurrence. MRI has also become an important tool for screening younger women with a high familial risk of BC. The women with known gene mutation carriers have a lifetime risk of developing BC of around 85%. In these younger women, the sensitivity of MMG for detecting malignancy is low due to the presence of mammographically dense breast parenchyma. Screening with MRI is superior to MMG in detecting invasive BC in such women, although MMG remains more sensitive for detecting *in-situ* carcinoma as DCIS most commonly presents as microcalcifications rather than discrete mass [16].

Positron Emission Tomography

PET is a technique of functional imaging which can give information on the metabolic activity of a lesion, unlike CT scan and MRI, which are techniques of anatomical imaging. The principle of PET scan is based on the intravenous injection of a radiopharmaceutical isotope which emits positron. When this positron interacts with an electron, annihilation occurs, resulting in the production of two 511-KeV gamma photons emitted at almost 180° to each other. These photons carry information about the distribution of radioactivity in various tissues. The directionality of annihilation photons is used to localize the origin of these photons [20]. The most common radiopharmaceutical used in practice is 18F-2-deoxy-D-glucose (FDG). Flouride[18] is the radionuclide, and deoxy-glucose acts as the tracer for glucose metabolism. FDG is transported into the cells by glucose transporter proteins. FDG is phosphorylated to form FDG-6-phosphate which cannot cross the cell membrane or undergo further degradation. Since there is increased metabolic requirement of glucose in the cancerous cells, more FDG gets trapped inside malignant cells than normal cells, due to which malignant lesions show much higher uptake (avidity) of FDG in the PET images in comparison to normal tissues. A major advantage of PET imaging over conventional imaging is that the entire body can be screened with just a single study using a single injection of radionuclide. This includes screening for local recurrence, lymph node metastases, and distant organ metastases during a single examination. In practice, PET and CT can be obtained simultaneously in the same sitting in a shorter duration of time and images acquired be co-registered. The combined system allows for simultaneous anatomic as well as functional imaging wherein functional data of PET is added to morphological data of CT which improves the accuracy of lesion localization. Many studies have demonstrated increased diagnostic accuracy of PET-CT compared to PET alone [21].

The three most important roles of PET-CT are the detection of metastasis, monitoring the response to treatment, and early detection of recurrence. Lungs, liver, and bones are the commonest sites of distant metastases in BC. PET has a reported sensitivity of 96% in the detection of locoregional spread and metastasis. PET being a functional imaging modality, is highly sensitive in detecting lesions even before they are seen on anatomical imaging modalities such as MMG, USG, and MRI. PET-CT can accurately differentiate the metastatic and reactive lymph nodes. The sensitivity and specificity of PET imaging in correctly identifying metastatic axillary nodes have been reported as 79-94% and 86-92%, respectively [22].

PET is unique in a way that it can provide qualitative as well as quantitative information on metabolic activity. Standardized uptake value (SUV) can be calculated, which quantifies the metabolic activity. 2. 0–2. 5 SUV is frequently used as the cut-off for discriminating benign lesions from malignant [23]. Serial measurements of SUV throughout follow up during or after therapy helps in assessing response to treatment. Major sites of locoregional recurrence following BC treatment are residual breast, skin, axillary and supraclavicular nodes, and the chest wall. Detecting recurrences early time can significantly improve the long term survival; however, conventional imaging modalities are not as sensitive as PET in differentiating true recurrence from the post-surgical or post-radiation sequel. PET serves as a problem-solving method when conventional imaging findings are equivocal. The recurrent tumor shows significantly higher SUV as compared to post-therapy changes, which may show a similar or minimally increased avidity as the surrounding tissue and tend to become normal over a few weeks. Currently, there is no established role of PET in the primary diagnosis of BC; however, its clinical utility in routine primary detection of BC is under research.

Computed Tomography

CT is not a primary modality for diagnosis or screening of BC. However, it is useful in staging of BC in terms of detecting regional lymphadenopathy and distant metastasis. CT scan is routinely used in the staging of locally advanced BC and advanced cancer. CT often provides the first images of incidentally detected breast abnormality when imaging is performed for unrelated indications. In recent years, technological advancements in the cone-beam CT system have made way for a dedicated CT scan of the breast without unnecessary exposure to the rest of the thorax [24, 25]. In a typical dedicated breast CT, the subject lies in a prone position, and a full 360-degree rotation scan targeted for breasts is performed using cone-beam geometry. Studies in recent years have demonstrated sufficiently good coverage of breast from the chest wall to nipple using this technique and fairly good spatial and contrast resolution [26]. However, its sensitivity in the detection of microcalcifications is not as good as digital MMG.

Screening of BC

Screening aims to detect BC before the appearance of symptoms. The main radiological modality used for screening of BC is MMG. Despite being radiation-free, USG is not used for screening because it is time-consuming, highly operator dependent, and results in more number of false-positive results than MMG [27]. However, targeted USG evaluation of an abnormal mammographic finding can be used along with screening MMG for better evaluation in doubtful cases. As per

American guidelines, women who have a strong family history of BC or a genetic mutation known to increase risk of BC or have had received radiation therapy to the chest before the age of 30; are considered to have a high risk for development of BC. All other women are considered to have a moderate risk of developing BC in their lifetime. For moderate-risk women, annual mammographic screening is recommended starting at 40 years of age. For high-risk women, an MRI and an MMG are recommended every year, typically starting at age 30.

ACR BI-RADS

The American college of radiology has established a standardized system for assessment and reporting of breast imaging called 'Breast imaging reporting and data system' or popularly known as BI-RADS. It lays down standardized descriptors and structured reporting format for MMG, USG, and MRI of the breast. ACR-BI-RADS lays down a standard lexicon based on which a breast lesion should be described. This facilitates clear and consistent communication between radiologists and referring clinician. BI-RADS also allows for an objective way of outcome monitoring and quality assessment, which can be used across the globe. The latest ACR BI-RADS came into existence in 2013 with few modifications in 2017. The standard BI-RADS descriptors used in MMG and USG are summarized in Tables **1** and **2** respectively. These descriptors help in assigning the final BI-RADS category summarized in Table **3**. Readers can refer to the complete BI-RADS atlas on www. acr. org [28].

On MMG, a high grade invasive ductal carcinoma is typically seen as a high-density mass that has an irregular shape, obscured/spiculated margins with or without parenchymal architectural distortion surrounding the lesion. Presence of suspicious-looking calcifications within or outside the increase the likelihood of malignancy. Suspicious calcifications typically are tiny clustered specks of fine, pleomorphic, or fine linear branching pattern. Ductal carcinoma *in-situ* may present as scattered suspicious calcifications without any obvious mass. However, there are certain breast malignancies which lack these characteristics and may be misinterpreted as benign lesions, for example, medullary carcinoma, mucinous carcinoma, and papillary carcinoma tends to be well-defined masses. These masses should be carefully assessed for the presence of any gentle lobulation or irregularity, and if needed, an additional compression view may be used for better evaluation [29]. A typical malignant mass on USG appears as a hypoechoic solid or complex solid-cystic lesion with an irregular shape, non-circumscribed margins, and posterior acoustic shadowing. The orientation of the lesion is usually not parallel to the skin, and there may be increased internal vascularity within the lesion. Calcifications, if present is seen as tiny hyperechoic specs within or outside the lesion. There can be associated dilated duct in direct communication with the lesion, or a part of the lesion may be seen extending within it. On MRI, a malignant mass usually has an irregular shape, non-circumscribed margins, heterogeneous or rim enhancement, and demonstrates a type 3 curve on dynamic contrast kinetics (*i.e.*, rapid initial rise, followed by a washout in the delayed phase. ACR BI-RADS currently does not take into account the elastography features or spectroscopic findings into assigning the final stage.

IMAGE GUIDED BREAST INTERVENTION

Percutaneous image-guided biopsy is a popular, reliable alternative to surgical biopsy. It has many advantages over surgical biopsy; for example, it is minimally invasive, quick to perform, cause minimal post-procedure scarring and has a much lower risk of complications [30].

Pre-operative Localization

Pre-operative localization of the lesion is required when the lesion itself is not palpable. Pre-operative localization helps the surgeon in easily locating the lesion intra-operatively and permits its removal without having to excise a large part of normal breast tissue. Small excision produces a small scar and avoids long term deformity and other cosmetic issues. MMG is the most widely used technique for an image-guided lesion localization [10, 31, 32]. The most common technique uses a combination of needle and hooked wire. The localization procedure is usually performed with the patient in the sitting position. The patient wears a front-open gown, which allows for proper mammographic positioning and minimal disturbance in the needle position while the patient is shifted to the operating room. At the outset, CC and mediolateral (ML) views of the involved breast are performed to confirm the presence of the lesion. A fenestrated compression grid having numbered and alphabetical coordinates are used to determine the location of the lesion. The procedure is performed using aseptic precautions and under local anesthesia. Usually, no premedication is needed. The needle is inserted into the skin parallel to the chest wall at the appropriate location, as determined by the grid co-ordinates. The position is adjusted to be placed within the lesion and confirmed with a mammogram. If properly positioned, the needle is removed while the wire is left in place with a small length extending beyond the skin. The wire hooks itself into the lesion and the length protruding above the skin surface is anchored onto the skin. A final MMG is obtained to check the position after the removal of the needle. It is important to perform this localization procedure on the day of surgery because there is a risk that the position of wire may change if the patient changes posture frequently *e.g.* while sleeping. After the localization is complete, the patient goes to the operating room, and a mammogram is sent to the surgeon to see. There is an alternative way of lesion localization by injecting the methylene blue dye within the lesion. Since this procedure does not involve any hooked wire, there is no risk of mal-positioning, this method can be used to localize the lesion a day before surgery.

Image-guided Breast Lesion Biopsy

The development of percutaneous image-guided breast biopsies has made a significant impact on approach to BC management. Percutaneous image-guided biopsy has become a popular alternative to open surgical biopsies for histopathological diagnosis of breast lesions [30, 33]. As compared to surgical biopsy, a percutaneous biopsy is less invasive, can be performed quickly, causes minimal scarring, and has the fewer risk of complications [34, 35]. There has been remarkable development in the percutaneous biopsy method, from fine-needle aspiration cytology towards vacuum-assisted biopsy [36]. Increasingly sophisticated vacuum-assisted biopsy devices are available to improve the yield of representative tissue during the biopsy. Nowadays, USG guided biopsy has become the most popular technique in practice for performing a percutaneous biopsy for lesions visible on USG [36]. There are several reasons for its popularity, most importantly the real-time nature of USG, which enables the radiologist to have full control over the needle for the entire duration of biopsy, allowing for corrections in the position of needle as and when required. Patient and operator comfort is much better in the USG. USG guided biopsy has a shorter learning curve as compared to MR guided biopsy. There is no risk of ionizing radiation in the USG and has wide acceptance among patients. It is more cost and time effective also as multiple lesions can be sampled in one session.

Table 1. Mammographic descriptors as per ACR BI-RADS.

Breast Composition	a. The breasts are almost entirely fatty b. There are scattered areas of fibroglandular density c. The breasts are heterogeneously dense, which may obscure small masses d. The breasts are extremely dense, which lowers the sensitivity of mammography	
Masses	Shape	Oval
		Round
		Irregular

(Table 1) cont.....

	Margin	Circumscribed
		Obscured
		Microlobulated
		Indistinct
		Spiculated
	Density	High density
		Equal density
		Low density
		Fat-containing
Calcification	Typically benign	Skin
		Vascular
		Coarse or "popcorn-like."
		Large rod-like
		Round
		Rim
		Dystrophic
		Milk of calcium
		Suture
	Suspicious morphology	Amorphous Coarse heterogeneous
		Fine pleomorphic
		Fine linear or fine-linear branching
	Distribution	Diffuse
		Regional
		Grouped
		Linear
		Segmental
Architectural distortion		
Asymmetries	Asymmetry	
	Global asymmetry	
	Focal asymmetry	
	Developing asymmetry	
Intramammary lymph node		
Skin lesion		
Solitary dilated duct		

(Table 1) cont.....

Associated Features	Skin retraction
	Nipple retraction
	Skin thickening
	Trabecular thickening
	Axillary adenopathy
	Architectural distortion
	Calcifications
Location of Lesion	Laterality
	Quadrant and clock face
	Depth
	Distance from the nipple

(Courtesy: Sickles, EA, D'Orsi CJ, Bassett LW, *et al.* ACR BI-RADS® Mammography. In: ACR BI-RADS® Atlas, Breast Imaging Reporting and Data System. Reston, VA, American College of Radiology; 2013.)

All the lesions which are visible on the USG are amenable for biopsy. Indeterminate BI-RADS 3 lesions and suspicious lesions (BI-RADS 4 and 5) are usually targeted for biopsy. USG-guided Biopsy is performed as an outpatient procedure under local anesthesia. High-frequency (10- to 12-MHz) probe is used to assess the lesion and adjustments in dynamic range, greyscale, and the focal point may be needed for the best visualization of the lesion. Status of vascularity within and adjacent to the lesion is assessed using spectral or color Doppler. A wide spectrum of core-needle devices is available having different needle thickness and length. Vacuum-assisted Co-axial needles are being increasingly used as they allow for obtaining multiple samples with single needle-trocar insertion. The biopsy is performed under sterile precautions with a technique called 'Freehand technique' where the radiologists hold the probe in one hand and hold the needle with another hand. The tip of the needle is inserted into the lesion using the shortest path from the skin to the lesion. Multiple tissue samples can be obtained in a single sitting for histopathological assessment as well as immunohistochemistry such as ER, PR, and Erb 2 status. In the same session, fine needle aspiration or core biopsy of suspicious metastatic lesions such as abnormal nodes and liver lesions can also be performed.

MRI guided biopsy is chosen as the method of choice only when a suspicious lesion is visible only on MRI, which guided breast biopsies up to 60% [37 - 41]. The malignancy rate of MRI-guided biopsies is performed, which in common term known as biopsy yield of malignancy [42]. A biopsy is done with the patient in the prone position similar to the breast MRI. All the sequences of breast MRI protocol, as elaborated in the previous section, are obtained. Dynamic Contrast-enhanced images are also obtained following gadolinium administration, and the target lesion is demarcated on the subtracted images. Following lesion localization, local anesthesia is applied, and multiple tissue samples are obtained using an MR-safe vacuum assist biopsy needle similar to that in the USG.

Table 2. USG descriptors as per ACR BI-RADS.

Tissue Composition (screening only)	a. Homogeneous background echotexture – fat b. Homogeneous background echotexture – fibroglandular c. Heterogeneous background echotexture	
Masses	Shape	Oval
		Round
		Irregular
	Orientation	Parallel
		Not Parallel
	Margin	Circumscribed
		Not Circumscribed -Indistinct -Angular -Microbulated -Spiculated
	Echo Pattern	Anechoic
		Hyperechoic
		Complex cystic and solid
		Hypoechoic
		Isochoric
		Heterogeneous
	Posterior features	No Posterior features
		Enhancement
		Shadowing
		Combined pattern
Calcifications	Calcifications in a mass	
	Calcifications outside of a mass	
	Intraductal Calcifications	

(Table 2) cont.....

Associated Features	Architectural distortion	
	Duct changes	
	Skin Changes	Skin thickening
		Skin retraction
	Edema	
	Vascularity	Absent
		Internal Vascularity
		Vessels in rim
	Elasticity assessment	Soft
		Intermediate
		Hard
Special Cases	Simple cyst	
	Clustered microcysts	
	Complicated cyst	
	Mass in or on skin	
	Foreign body including implants	
	Lymph nodes - intramammary	
	Lymph nodes – axillary	
	Vascular abnormalities	AVMs (arteriovenous malformations/ peseudoaneurysms
		Mondor disease
	Postsurgical fluid collection	
	Fat necrosis	

(Courtesy: Mendelson EB, Böhm-Vélez M, Berg WA, *et al.* ACR BI-RADS® Ultrasound. In: ACR BI-RADS® Atlas, Breast Imaging Reporting and Data System. Reston, VA, American College of Radiology; 2013.)

Table 3. Final BI-RADS assessment categories.

Category 0: **Mammography:** Incomplete – Need Additional Imaging Evaluation and/or Prior Mammograms for Comparison **Ultrasound & MRI:** Incomplete – Need Additional Imaging Evaluation		
Category 1: Negative		
Category 2: Benign		
Category 3: Probably Benign		
Category 4: Suspicious	Mammography & Ultrasound:	Category 4A: Low suspicion for malignancy Category 4B: Moderate suspicion for malignancy Category 4C: High suspicion for malignancy

(Table 3) cont.....

Category 5: Highly Suggestive of Malignancy
Category 6: Known Biopsy-Proven Malignancy

(Courtesy: ACR-BI-RADS atlas 5ᵗʰ Edition)

Other Applications

In the postoperative setting, the accumulation of clear serous fluid (a.k.a seroma) in the dead space in the operative bed is fairly common after surgeries. If the fluid volume is large, it can cause pain or pressure symptoms. There is also a risk of secondary infection. USG serves as a non-invasive tool to quantitate the amount of the collection and look for any evidence of secondary infection such as thick internal echoes. If indicated, USG guided fluid aspiration can provide diagnostic as well as therapeutic benefits. USG can also be used to monitor the resolution of a complicated seroma.

RECENT ADVANCES IN BREAST IMAGING

The ongoing technological development has led to advancements in digital MMG and high-resolution USG, which has improved the sensitivity of these modalities in detecting tiny lesions.

Digital Breast Tomosynthesis

The overall sensitivity of traditional diagnostic algorithms using MMG alone or when combined with USG is low, which indicates that there is still plenty of room for improvement in our existing imaging methods [43 - 46]. In addition to that, a major limitation of conventional 2D MMG arises due to potential tissue overlap. This occurs because all the tissue that lies in the path of the X-ray beam contributes to the signal detected by the detector. The tissue overlap may obscure an existing lesion leading to an error in interpretation. Moreover, the overlap of tissues of various densities and texture can create a false impression of a 'pseudo lesion. ' The artifact thus created due to the summation of intervening tissues may lead to false-positive interpretation and increased patient call-back rates. This limitation can be overcome by Digital breast tomosynthesis (DBT). In DBT, the X-ray tube moves in an arc above the compressed breast and generates a series of low-dose exposures each from a different angle at fixed preset intervals. DBT has shown improved sensitivity and specificity compared with digital MMG [47, 48].

Computer reconstruction generates 1-mm slices from the in-plane volumetric dataset. DBT allows three-dimensional (3D) estimation of tissue distribution to help determine the positional status of the lesion, for example, its vertical depth from the skin. Multiple projections create multiple planes in which an object (or lesion) can be seen. When an object is in-plane, its margins can be seen clearly while the objects above or below that specific plane are out of focus, and their margins are blurred out [49]. DBT is becoming increasingly popular in its use due to its benefits. DBT generates a stack of images that can be easily scrolled through. Superimposed tissues can be easily differentiated from true lesions thus decreasing the false-positive callbacks. There is a potential improvement in the detection of conspicuous lesions due to the unmasking of obscured lesions. DBT enables a detailed assessment of lesion margins especially in the areas of the fat-tissue interface. It helps in differentiate actual masses from distortions and focal asymmetry. DBT has been found particularly useful in identifying skin conditions and intramammary lymph nodes with confidence.

The combination of conventional 2D MMG and DBT is also known as "combo-mode" acquisition. Both the images are acquired in a single compression; therefore, there is no chance of misregistration, and patient tolerance is very good. Combo mode acquisition shows better performance than 2D MMG across different breast densities [50]. Food and Drug Administration (FDA) approved the combination of 2D digital MMG and DBT imaging in 2011. The combo-mode may increase the patient's radiation dose by approximately two times when compared to 2D MMG alone [51]. Of course, the dose varies significantly depending on breast size and composition. Still, combo- mode offers the advantage of preventing unnecessary callbacks which otherwise could lead to multiple additional MMG views and a significantly higher radiation dose in the subject [52].

Advances in Breast Ultrasonography

In recent times, improvements in technology have led to the development of novel techniques in USG. Some of these techniques are automated volumetric breast USG, contrast-enhanced breast USG, and breast elastography. Improvement in re-slicing methods has made it possible to display the image in various reconstructed planes for a better depiction of the infiltrative margins.

Two image acquisition techniques that have become the frontrunner in advanced clinical breast imaging are compound imaging and harmonic tissue imaging (THI). In Compound imaging, multiple frames of USG images are obtained to form a single compound image [53, 54]. The method is called frequency compound imaging when multiple different frequencies are used and spatial compound imaging when images are acquired from different angles. Spatial compounding reduces the speckle and improves lateral resolution [54]. Similarly, frequency compounding also decreases speckle and improves contrast resolution and improves penetration [55].

In THI mode, the scanner is configured to receive echoes at multiples (usually double) of the transmitted or fundamental frequency. THI filters out the weak, nonlinear tissue signal and reduces the clutter and side lobes artifacts. It improves the grayscale contrast between the lesion and the background parenchyma and makes the border of the lesion appear well delineated. The overall result is better-contrasted resolution [56]. Spatial compounding and THI are simultaneously used in routine clinical practice [54].

One of the most important improvements in breast USG was brought about by the advent of breast elastography. Elastography is a method of a qualitative and quantitative assessment of the texture or stiffness of a breast lesion. It is based on the concept that malignant lesions are harder or stiffer than surrounding breast tissue as compared to benign lesions. Strain and shear wave elastography are the two main methods in elastography. Strain elastography measures the displacement induced while shear wave elastography measures the velocity of an induced shear wave caused by introducing mechanical excitation within a region of interest [57]. The shear wave technique is commonly used in the newer machines as it is independent of probe compression applied by the operator. The degree of stiffness of tissue is reproduced and displayed as a color-coded map on the screen. The quantitative measurement of tissue elasticity in Kilopascals (kPa) is also displayed. Benign lesions and normal breast parenchyma is easily deformable with the elasticity of <80 kPa and higher values are obtained with malignant lesions, increasing with the grade of the tumor. Breast elastography has also shown to improve the specificity by 20%in distinguishing BI-RADS 3 and 4a lesions and can help in avoiding biopsies in these [12].

Contrast-enhanced ultrasound (CEUS) is an emerging technique in breast imaging. CEUS uses injectable gas microbubbles enclosed in a polymer shell to assess the vascularity of the lesions. Malignant lesions differ from benign lesions in their contrast kinetics, similar to what is seen in MRI. After the injection of microbubbles, the target lesion is evaluated under power Doppler. Insolated microbubbles produce highly nonlinear echoes, which can be selectively filtered to make the lesion appear more prominent in the background of normal parenchyma [58]. The role of CEUS is likely to expand in the near future with the development of tissue-specific and target specific ligands, which can be tagged to the microbubble [59]. Studies have also suggested that THI technique can be used in CEUS to isolate microbubble signals better [60].

A major change in breast imaging has been the development of transducers. Newer transducers allow the generation of electronic volumetric arrays and simultaneous beam steering in all directions. This had made it possible to acquire real-time, high-quality 3D images of the entire breast [61]. Automated 3D whole breast USG systems are being developed as a faster alternative to the usual2D USG while not compromising with the diagnostic accuracy [62 - 64]. It allows us to obtain the image in the desired plane and also allows for better image co-registration with another modality. In 2012, automated breast USG got approved by the FDA as an adjunct screening modality to MMG in asymptomatic women with dense breast tissue with a negative screening mammogram.

Computer-aided Detection

Computer-aided detection (CAD) is an artificial intelligence software tool that identifies and highlights suspicious findings on imaging, which can be later reviewed and interpreted by the radiologist. The main purpose of marking these suspicious findings is to reduce the chances of oversights by interpreting radiologists. CAD system got FDA approval to be used in MMG in 1998. CAD is based on the principle on pattern recognition, where the system is trained with a set of images, and search algorithms are developed. Multiple steps are included in this process. The first step is adjusting the image contrast and reducing the noise in order to train the system to ignore the technique differences. Then the system is trained such that it can separate the lesion from the rest of the normal breast and highlight the abnormalities of interest, for example, clustered micro calcifications in MMG. The sensitivity of CAD for detecting cancer ranges from 60 to 100% [65 - 68], while the sensitivity in detecting calcifications is 80-100% [67 - 70]. Highly dense breast parenchyma poses a challenge in MMG and can obscure small lesions; however, one of the major advantages of CAD is that it is not affected by variations in breast density [67, 69, 71]. The main drawbacks of CAD are an increased number of call back rates, which results in patient anxiety and monetary loss. This occurs due to lesions detected by CAD software, which turn out to be normal parenchyma on further evaluation [72 - 74]. Although there is some data to which suggests that CAD improves cancer detection rate in DCIS and improves the diagnostic accuracy in lobular carcinoma, the overall evidence in support of CAD is equivocal [75, 76].

Recent evidence suggests that CAD software can be used to reduce the reading time of digital breast tomography [77]. Ongoing research in this field indicates that CAD software, when used with DBT, is better at detecting abnormalities that when used with 2D MMG [78 - 80]. The software detects suspicious findings on DBT stack and creates a CAD- enhanced 2D image thus providing both the 2D as well as 3D anatomical location of the lesion. This allows for faster review by the radiologist [77]. The first DBT based CAD system got approved by FDA in 2017 [81].

CAD system was introduced for breast MRI with the idea that it can potentially improve the diagnostic accuracy of breast MRI and aid in the faster interpretation of images. Breast MRI has a long learning curve, and interpretation may significantly vary among radiologists with various levels of experience. CAD can minimize the subjectivity in interpretation in less experienced radiologists [82 - 84]. CAD has shown to have good accuracy in analyzing enhancement kinetics of breast masses; however, its diagnostic utility is limited in lesions presenting as a non-mass-like enhancement [85]. The sensitivity of CAD in the detection of DCIS is also poor [86, 87]. The CAD may be useful in the follow up of lesions post-chemotherapy in the assessment of the changes in contrast enhancement pattern. However, CAD lacks an accurate measurement of the residual lesion and may detect false-negative post-chemotherapy enhancements. The use of CAD in clinical breast MRI is not yet popular, and its main role is complementary at best in the current practice [87].

Magnetic Resonance Spectroscopy

Choline is a constituent of various compounds involved in membrane biosynthesis and degradation. Neoplastic breast tissues have increased cell turnover and thus increased choline levels. Estimation of choline levels forms the basis of MRS in BC. High choline peak in a lesion tends to support a diagnosis of malignancy, although it is not 100% specific nor can be used as a sole criterion to diagnose a malignancy [88]. Its specificity is approximately 88% in BC. However, the accuracy improves when used alongside the DCE sequence [89, 90]. MRS is also useful in response assessment after neoadjuvant chemotherapy in locally advanced BC. A good response to chemotherapy is indicated by a decreasing trend of choline levels [91, 92]. It enables the early identification of non-responders so that appropriate change in the management plan can be brought about at the earliest.

On the other hand, there are some limitations of MRS, such as limited usefulness in minimally invasive (*e.g.*, DCIS), low grade and small (less than 1 cm) lesions in which there are also some shortcomings in terms of poor signal-to-noise ratio and spectral resolution. Moreover, only 1 lesion can be examined at a time with the single-voxel technique and the scan duration gets prolonged if more than 1 lesions are present [93]. In current clinical practice, MRS is used only as an adjunct to the standard breast MRI sequences and as a problem-solving tool in doubtful cases [94].

LIMITATIONS, DRAWBACKS, AND SUMMARY

MMG is the screening method of choice for BC, but it performs poorly in the setting of dense breast parenchyma [95]. In young women, especially those less than 30 years of age, there is a concern about the potential harm that can result from long term exposure to radiation [96]. Due to these demerits, MRI has evolved as the method of choice in young, high-risk women. Moreover, sometimes, the abnormalities detected on screening MMG studies may require additional imaging or even a biopsy and eventually turn out to be benign. Raising false alarms can cause unnecessary anxiety in the patients and also adds to the cost of screening. It has long been debated that older women more than 65 years of age do not benefit from screening MMG. These women in most likelihood would not have known about the disease without screening and these cancers would not have threatened their lives during their individual residual lifespan. In such cases, detection merely causes anxiety and monetary loss. Despite that, the utility of screening with MMG cannot be undermined as it leads to early detection of cancer in a large subgroup of women and thereby a significant decrease in mortality. In short, the advantages of MMG clearly outweigh the disadvantages.

The main drawback of USG in BC assessment is that it is highly operator dependent and can be highly subjective. The interpretation of USG findings is also dependent on the expertise of the radiologist, which makes it highly subjective. ACR BI-RADS aims to remove the subjectivity in interpretation and standardize the reporting of breast lesions. Another issue is a long time taken to perform the exam for which automated USG can be a solution; however, even automated USG requires intensive training in performance and interpretation. These concerns can be addressed by continuing medical education and adequate training.

Some of the drawbacks of breast MRI are high cost, limited availability, and the use of exogenous contrast agents. It can have limited acceptability in claustrophobic patients. Other general absolute contraindications to MRI apply for breast MRI as well, which include patients with pacemakers, defibrillators or other implanted electronic devices. There are certain limitations specific to breast MRI; for example, performing a breast MRI is significantly more time consuming than an MMG. MRI breast takes 40-60 minutes as compared to MMG which takes only 10 minutes. Also, MRI is not very sensitive in the assessment of microcalcifications. MRI findings can often be non-specific, often requiring re-evaluation with USG, and images can be limited by artifacts in the setting of metal implants. To overcome this, abbreviated MRI protocols are being developed that promise to reduce the cost and increase the availability of MRI screening.

A major limitation of PET is its poor sensitivity in detecting tiny lesions with sensitivity as low as 68% for detecting lesions less than 2 cm. Slow-growing tumors that are not very active metabolically and *in-situ* carcinomas (ductal and lobular carcinoma *in situ*) may be overlooked on PET-CT. Its accuracy for detecting in situ carcinomas ranges from 2-25% [97]. Moreover, there are certain non-neoplastic conditions which may be misinterpreted as neoplastic on PET. Body organs having a high basal metabolic activity such as brain, myocardium, urinary bladder, *etc.* show high physiologic FDG uptake and may be misinterpreted to be involved with metastasis. An increase in the glycolytic process in focal inflammation results in high FDG uptake which may be mistaken for malignancies. In the immediate post-surgery period, active granulation tissue may show increased FDG uptake.

Similarly, after recent radiation therapy, the irradiated tissues may show high FDG avidity; however, it usually resolves in a few weeks. These areas of physiologic uptake may be misinterpreted as false positive. Apart from these, FDG PET, which is used for staging of BC, performs poorly in the detection of sclerotic bone metastasis; however, CT scan often done in combination with PET can usually detect these [98, 99].

CONSENT FOR PUBLICATION

Not applicable.

CONFLICT OF INTEREST

The authors confirm that the contents of this chapter have no conflict of interest.

ACKNOWLEDGEMENTS

Declared none.

REFERENCES

[1]   Bray F, Ferlay J, Soerjomataram I, Siegel R L, Torre L A, Jemal A. Global cancer statistics 2018: GLOBOCAN estimates of incidence and mortality worldwide for 36 cancers in 185 countries. CA Cancer J Clin 2018; 68(6): 394-424.
[http://dx.doi.org/10. 3322/caac. 21492] [PMID: 30207593]

[2]   Walker S, Hyde C, Hamilton W. Risk of breast cancer in symptomatic women in primary care: a case-control study using electronic records. Br J Gen Pract 2014; 64(629): e788-93.
[http://dx.doi.org/10. 3399/bjgp14X682873] [PMID: 25452544]

[3]   Koo M M, von Wagner C, Abel GA, McPhail S, Rubin GP, Lyratzopoulos G. Typical and atypical presenting symptoms of breast cancer and their associations with diagnostic intervals: Evidence from a national audit of cancer diagnosis. Cancer Epidemiol 2017; 48: 140-6.
[http://dx.doi.org/10. 1016/j. canep. 2017. 04. 010] [PMID: 28549339]

[4]   Lee A H. Why is carcinoma of the breast more frequent in the upper outer quadrant? A case series based on needle core biopsy diagnoses. Breast 2005; 14(2): 151-2.
[http://dx.doi.org/10. 1016/j. breast. 2004. 07. 002] [PMID: 15767185]

[5]   Seltzer M H. Breast complaints, biopsies, and cancer correlated with age in 10,000 consecutive new surgical referrals. Breast J 2004; 10(2): 111-7.
[http://dx.doi.org/10. 1111/j. 1075-122X. 2004. 21284. x] [PMID: 15009037]

[6]   Trebska-McGowan K, Terracina K P, Takabe K. Update on the surgical management of Paget's disease. Gland Surg 2013; 2(3): 137-42.
[http://dx.doi.org/10.3978/j.issn.2227-684X.2013.08.03] [PMID: 24386631]

[7] de Groot J E, Branderhorst W, Grimbergen C A, den Heeten G J, Broeders M J M. Towards personalized compression in mammography: a comparison study between pressure- and force-standardization. Eur J Radiol 2015; 84(3): 384-91.
[http://dx.doi.org/10. 1016/j. ejrad. 2014. 12. 005] [PMID: 25554008]

[8] Funke M. [Diagnostic imaging of breast cancer : An update]. Radiologe 2016; 56(10): 921-38.
[http://dx.doi.org/10. 1007/s00117-016-0134-6] [PMID: 27600118]

[9] Popli M B, Teotia R, Narang M, Krishna H. Breast positioning during mammography: Mistakes to be avoided. Breast Cancer (Auckl) 2014; 8: 119-24.
[http://dx.doi.org/10. 4137/BCBCR. S17617] [PMID: 25125982]

[10] Liu W H, Teng G J, Jiang J. Mammography and breast localization for the interventionalist. Tech Vasc Interv Radiol 2014; 17(1): 10-5.
[http://dx.doi.org/10. 1053/j. tvir. 2013. 12. 003] [PMID: 24636326]

[11] Wallis M G, Moa E, Zanca F, Leifland K, Danielsson M. Two-view and single-view tomosynthesis *versus* full-field digital mammography: high-resolution X-ray imaging observer study. Radiology 2012; 262(3): 788-96.
[http://dx.doi.org/10. 1148/radiol. 11103514] [PMID: 22274840]

[12] Berg W A, Cosgrove D O, Doré C J, *et al.* BE1 Investigators. Shear-wave elastography improves the specificity of breast US: the BE1 multinational study of 939 masses. Radiology 2012; 262(2): 435-49.
[http://dx.doi.org/10. 1148/radiol. 11110640] [PMID: 22282182]

[13] Saslow D, Boetes C, Burke W, *et al.* American Cancer Society Breast Cancer Advisory Group. American Cancer Society guidelines for breast screening with MRI as an adjunct to mammography. CA Cancer J Clin 2007; 57(2): 75-89.
[http://dx.doi.org/10. 3322/canjclin. 57. 2. 75] [PMID: 17392385]

[14] Berg W A, Gutierrez L, NessAiver M S, *et al.* Diagnostic accuracy of mammography, clinical examination, US, and MR imaging in preoperative assessment of breast cancer. Radiology 2004; 233(3): 830-49.
[http://dx.doi.org/10. 1148/radiol. 2333031484] [PMID: 15486214]

[15] Tsina G, Simon P. Breast magnetic resonance imaging and its impact on the surgical treatment of breast cancer. Obstet Gynecol Int 2014; 2014632074
[http://dx.doi.org/10. 1155/2014/632074] [PMID: 24864145]

[16] Leach M O, Boggis C R, Dixon A K, *et al.* MARIBS study group. Screening with magnetic resonance imaging and mammography of a UK population at high familial risk of breast cancer: a prospective multicentre cohort study (MARIBS). Lancet 2005; 365(9473): 1769-78.
[http://dx.doi.org/10. 1016/S0140-6736(05)66481-1] [PMID: 15910949]

[17] Zhang Y, Fukatsu H, Naganawa S, *et al.* The role of contrast-enhanced MR mammography for determining candidates for breast conservation surgery. Breast Cancer 2002; 9(3): 231-9.
[http://dx.doi.org/10. 1007/BF02967595] [PMID: 12185335]

[18] Schell A M, Rosenkranz K, Lewis P J. Role of breast MRI in the preoperative evaluation of patients with newly diagnosed breast cancer. AJR Am J Roentgenol 2009; 192(5): 1438-44.
[http://dx.doi.org/10. 2214/AJR. 08. 1551] [PMID: 19380574]

[19] Del Frate C, Borghese L, Cedolini C, *et al.* Role of pre-surgical breast MRI in the management of invasive breast carcinoma. Breast 2007; 16(5): 469-81.
[http://dx.doi.org/10. 1016/j. breast. 2007. 02. 004] [PMID: 17433681]

[20] Kapoor V, McCook B M, Torok F S. An introduction to PET-CT imaging. Radiographics 2004; 24(2): 523-43.
[http://dx.doi.org/10. 1148/rg. 242025724] [PMID: 15026598]

[21] Tatsumi M, Cohade C, Mourtzikos K A, Fishman E K, Wahl R L. Initial experience with FDG-PET/CT in the evaluation of breast cancer. Eur J Nucl Med Mol Imaging 2006; 33(3): 254-62.

[http://dx.doi.org/10. 1007/s00259-005-1835-7] [PMID: 16258765]

[22]   Schirrmeister H, Kühn T, Guhlmann A, *et al.* Fluorine-18 2-deoxy-2-fluoro-D-glucose PET in the preoperative staging of breast cancer: comparison with the standard staging procedures. Eur J Nucl Med 2001; 28(3): 351-8.
[http://dx.doi.org/10. 1007/s002590000448] [PMID: 11315604]

[23]   Avril N, Dose J, Jänicke F, *et al.* Metabolic characterization of breast tumors with positron emission tomography using F-18 fluorodeoxyglucose. J Clin Oncol 1996; 14(6): 1848-57.
[http://dx.doi.org/10. 1200/JCO. 1996. 14. 6. 1848] [PMID: 8656253]

[24]   O'Connell A, Conover D L, Zhang Y, *et al.* Cone-beam CT for breast imaging: Radiation dose, breast coverage, and image quality. AJR Am J Roentgenol 2010; 195(2): 496-509.
[http://dx.doi.org/10. 2214/AJR. 08. 1017] [PMID: 20651210]

[25]   Boone J M, Nelson T R, Lindfors K K, Seibert J A. Dedicated breast CT: radiation dose and image quality evaluation. Radiology 2001; 221(3): 657-67.
[http://dx.doi.org/10. 1148/radiol. 2213010334] [PMID: 11719660]

[26]   Lindfors K K, Boone J M, Nelson T R, Yang K, Kwan A L, Miller D F. Dedicated breast CT: initial clinical experience. Radiology 2008; 246(3): 725-33.
[http://dx.doi.org/10. 1148/radiol. 2463070410] [PMID: 18195383]

[27]   Berg W A, Blume J D, Cormack J B, *et al.* ACRIN 6666 Investigators. Combined screening with ultrasound and mammography vs mammography alone in women at elevated risk of breast cancer. JAMA 2008; 299(18): 2151-63.
[http://dx.doi.org/10. 1001/jama. 299. 18. 2151] [PMID: 18477782]

[28]   D'Orsi CJ, Sickles EA, Mendelson EB, *et al.* ACR BI-RADS® Atlas, Breast Imaging Reporting and Data System. Reston, VA, American College of Radiology; 2013.

[29]   Moskowitz M. The predictive value of certain mammographic signs in screening for breast cancer. Cancer 1983; 51(6): 1007-11.
[http://dx.doi.org/10. 1002/1097-0142(19830315)51:6<1007::AID-CNCR2820510607>3. 0. CO;2-P] [PMID: 6821864]

[30]   Apesteguía L, Pina L J. Ultrasound-guided core-needle biopsy of breast lesions. Insights Imaging 2011; 2(4): 493-500.
[http://dx.doi.org/10. 1007/s13244-011-0090-7] [PMID: 22347970]

[31]   Shetty M K. Presurgical localization of breast abnormalities: an overview and analysis of 202 cases. Indian J Surg Oncol 2010; 1(4): 278-83.
[http://dx.doi.org/10. 1007/s13193-010-0016-8] [PMID: 22693379]

[32]   Dimitrovska M J, Mitreska N, Lazareska M, Jovanovska E S, Dodevski A, Stojkoski A. Hook wire localization procedure and early detection of breast cancer - our experience. Open Access Maced J Med Sci 2015; 3(2): 273-7.
[http://dx.doi.org/10. 3889/oamjms. 2015. 055] [PMID: 27275234]

[33]   Mahoney M C, Newell M S. Breast intervention: how I do it. Radiology 2013; 268(1): 12-24.
[http://dx.doi.org/10. 1148/radiol. 13120985] [PMID: 23793589]

[34]   Liberman L. 2000; Centennial dissertation. Percutaneous imaging-guided core breast biopsy: state of the art at the millennium. AJR Am J Roentgenol 2000; 174(5): 1191-9.

[35]   Liberman L. Percutaneous image-guided core breast biopsy. Radiol Clin North Am 2002; 40(3): 483-500, vi.
[http://dx.doi.org/10. 1016/S0033-8389(01)00011-2] [PMID: 12117188]

[36]   AJCC. https://cancerstaging.org/references-tools/deskreferences/Pages/Breast-Cancer-Staging.aspx

[37]   Mahoney M C. Initial clinical experience with a new MRI vacuum-assisted breast biopsy device. J Magn Reson Imaging 2008; 28(4): 900-5.

[http://dx.doi.org/10. 1002/jmri. 21549] [PMID: 18821610]

[38]   Orel S G, Rosen M, Mies C, Schnall M D. MR imaging-guided 9-gauge vacuum-assisted core-needle breast biopsy: initial experience. Radiology 2006; 238(1): 54-61.
[http://dx.doi.org/10. 1148/radiol. 2381050050] [PMID: 16304093]

[39]   Imschweiler T, Haueisen H, Kampmann G, *et al.* MRI-guided vacuum-assisted breast biopsy: comparison with stereotactically guided and ultrasound-guided techniques. Eur Radiol 2014; 24(1): 128-35.
[http://dx.doi.org/10. 1007/s00330-013-2989-5] [PMID: 23979106]

[40]   Malhaire C, El Khoury C, Thibault F, *et al.* Vacuum-assisted biopsies under MR guidance: results of 72 procedures. Eur Radiol 2010; 20(7): 1554-62.
[http://dx.doi.org/10. 1007/s00330-009-1707-9] [PMID: 20119729]

[41]   Rauch G M, Dogan B E, Smith T B, Liu P, Yang W T. Outcome analysis of 9-gauge MRI-guided vacuum-assisted core needle breast biopsies. AJR Am J Roentgenol 2012; 198(2): 292-9.
[http://dx.doi.org/10. 2214/AJR. 11. 7594] [PMID: 22268171]

[42]   Mendelson EB, Böhm-Vélez M, Berg WA, *et al.* ACR BI-RADS Atlas: Breast Imaging Reporting and Data System. Reston: American College of Radiology 2013.

[43]   Lehman C D, Arao R F, Sprague B L, *et al.* National Performance Benchmarks for Modern Screening Digital Mammography: Update from the Breast Cancer Surveillance Consortium. Radiology 2017; 283(1): 49-58.
[http://dx.doi.org/10. 1148/radiol. 2016161174] [PMID: 27918707]

[44]   Sickles E A, Miglioretti D L, Ballard-Barbash R, *et al.* Performance benchmarks for diagnostic mammography. Radiology 2005; 235(3): 775-90.
[http://dx.doi.org/10. 1148/radiol. 2353040738] [PMID: 15914475]

[45]   Sickles E A, Wolverton D E, Dee K E. Performance parameters for screening and diagnostic mammography: specialist and general radiologists. Radiology 2002; 224(3): 861-9.
[http://dx.doi.org/10. 1148/radiol. 2243011482] [PMID: 12202726]

[46]   Barlow W E, Lehman C D, Zheng Y, *et al.* Performance of diagnostic mammography for women with signs or symptoms of breast cancer. J Natl Cancer Inst 2002; 94(15): 1151-9.
[http://dx.doi.org/10. 1093/jnci/94. 15. 1151] [PMID: 12165640]

[47]   Lei J, Yang P, Zhang L, Wang Y, Yang K. Diagnostic accuracy of digital breast tomosynthesis *versus* digital mammography for benign and malignant lesions in breasts: a meta-analysis. Eur Radiol 2014; 24(3): 595-602.
[http://dx.doi.org/10. 1007/s00330-013-3012-x] [PMID: 24121712]

[48]   Andersson I, Ikeda D M, Zackrisson S, *et al.* Breast tomosynthesis and digital mammography: a comparison of breast cancer visibility and BIRADS classification in a population of cancers with subtle mammographic findings. Eur Radiol 2008; 18(12): 2817-25.
[http://dx.doi.org/10. 1007/s00330-008-1076-9] [PMID: 18641998]

[49]   Roth R G, Maidment A D, Weinstein S P, Roth S O, Conant E F. Digital breast tomosynthesis: lessons learned from early clinical implementation. Radiographics 2014; 34(4): E89-E102.
[http://dx.doi.org/10. 1148/rg. 344130087] [PMID: 25019451]

[50]   Bonafede M M, Kalra V B, Miller J D, Fajardo L L. Value analysis of digital breast tomosynthesis for breast cancer screening in a commercially-insured US population. Clinicoecon Outcomes Res 2015; 7: 53-63.
[PMID: 25624767]

[51]   Vedantham S, Karellas A, Vijayaraghavan G R, Kopans D B. Digital breast tomosynthesis: State of the art. Radiology 2015; 277(3): 663-84.
[http://dx.doi.org/10. 1148/radiol. 2015141303] [PMID: 26599926]

[52]   Brandt K R, Craig D A, Hoskins T L, *et al.* Can digital breast tomosynthesis replace conventional

diagnostic mammography views for screening recalls without calcifications? A comparison study in a simulated clinical setting. AJR Am J Roentgenol 2013; 200(2): 291-8.
[http://dx.doi.org/10. 2214/AJR. 12. 8881] [PMID: 23345348]

[53]   Kwak J Y, Kim E K, You J K, Oh K K. Variable breast conditions: comparison of conventional and real-time compound ultrasonography. J Ultrasound Med 2004; 23(1): 85-96.
[http://dx.doi.org/10. 7863/jum. 2004. 23. 1. 85] [PMID: 14756357]

[54]   Hooley R J, Scoutt L M, Philpotts L E. Breast ultrasonography: state of the art. Radiology 2013; 268(3): 642-59.
[http://dx.doi.org/10. 1148/radiol. 13121606] [PMID: 23970509]

[55]   Mesurolle B, Helou T, El-Khoury M, Edwardes M, Sutton E J, Kao E. Tissue harmonic imaging, frequency compound imaging, and conventional imaging: use and benefit in breast sonography. J Ultrasound Med 2007; 26(8): 1041-51.
[http://dx.doi.org/10. 7863/jum. 2007. 26. 8. 1041] [PMID: 17646366]

[56]   Cha J H, Moon W K, Cho N, *et al.* Characterization of benign and malignant solid breast masses: comparison of conventional US and tissue harmonic imaging. Radiology 2007; 242(1): 63-9.
[http://dx.doi.org/10. 1148/radiol. 2421050859] [PMID: 17090709]

[57]   Barr R G. Sonographic breast elastography: a primer. J Ultrasound Med 2012; 31(5): 773-83.
[http://dx.doi.org/10. 7863/jum. 2012. 31. 5. 773] [PMID: 22535725]

[58]   Calliada F, Campani R, Bottinelli O, Bozzini A, Sommaruga M G. Ultrasound contrast agents: basic principles. Eur J Radiol 1998; 27 (Suppl. 2): S157-60.
[http://dx.doi.org/10. 1016/S0720-048X(98)00057-6] [PMID: 9652516]

[59]   Abou-Elkacem L, Bachawal S V, Willmann J K. Ultrasound molecular imaging: Moving toward clinical translation. Eur J Radiol 2015; 84(9): 1685-93.
[http://dx.doi.org/10. 1016/j. ejrad. 2015. 03. 016] [PMID: 25851932]

[60]   Sridharan A, Eisenbrey J R, Machado P, *et al.* Quantitative analysis of vascular heterogeneity in breast lesions using contrast-enhanced 3-D harmonic and subharmonic ultrasound imaging. IEEE Trans Ultrason Ferroelectr Freq Control 2015; 62(3): 502-10.
[http://dx.doi.org/10. 1109/TUFFC. 2014. 006886] [PMID: 25935933]

[61]   Diarra B, Robini M, Tortoli P, Cachard C, Liebgott H. Design of optimal 2-D nongrid sparse arrays for medical ultrasound. IEEE Trans Biomed Eng 2013; 60(11): 3093-102.
[http://dx.doi.org/10. 1109/TBME. 2013. 2267742] [PMID: 23771307]

[62]   Chen L, Chen Y, Diao X H, *et al.* Comparative study of automated breast 3-D ultrasound and handheld B-mode ultrasound for differentiation of benign and malignant breast masses. Ultrasound Med Biol 2013; 39(10): 1735-42.
[http://dx.doi.org/10. 1016/j. ultrasmedbio. 2013. 04. 003] [PMID: 23849390]

[63]   Brem R F, Tabár L, Duffy S W, *et al.* Assessing improvement in detection of breast cancer with three-dimensional automated breast US in women with dense breast tissue: the SomoInsight Study. Radiology 2015; 274(3): 663-73.
[http://dx.doi.org/10. 1148/radiol. 14132832] [PMID: 25329763]

[64]   Jeh S K, Kim S H, Choi J J, *et al.* Comparison of automated breast ultrasonography to handheld ultrasonography in detecting and diagnosing breast lesions. Acta Radiol 2016; 57(2): 162-9.
[http://dx.doi.org/10. 1177/0284185115574872] [PMID: 25766727]

[65]   Cole E B, Zhang Z, Marques H S, Edward Hendrick R, Yaffe M J, Pisano E D. Impact of computer-aided detection systems on radiologist accuracy with digital mammography. AJR Am J Roentgenol 2014; 203(4): 909-16.
[http://dx.doi.org/10. 2214/AJR. 12. 10187] [PMID: 25247960]

[66]   Yang S K, Moon W K, Cho N, *et al.* Screening mammography-detected cancers: sensitivity of a computer-aided detection system applied to full-field digital mammograms. Radiology 2007; 244(1):

104-11.
[http://dx.doi.org/10. 1148/radiol. 2441060756] [PMID: 17507722]

[67] Murakami R, Kumita S, Tani H, *et al.* Detection of breast cancer with a computer-aided detection applied to full-field digital mammography. J Digit Imaging 2013; 26(4): 768-73.
[http://dx.doi.org/10. 1007/s10278-012-9564-5] [PMID: 23319110]

[68] Scaranelo A M, Eiada R, Bukhanov K, Crystal P. Evaluation of breast amorphous calcifications by a computer-aided detection system in full-field digital mammography. Br J Radiol 2012; 85(1013): 517-22.
[http://dx.doi.org/10. 1259/bjr/31850970] [PMID: 22556404]

[69] Sadaf A, Crystal P, Scaranelo A, Helbich T. Performance of computer-aided detection applied to full-field digital mammography in detection of breast cancers. Eur J Radiol 2011; 77(3): 457-61.
[http://dx.doi.org/10. 1016/j. ejrad. 2009. 08. 024] [PMID: 19875260]

[70] The J S, Schilling K J, Hoffmeister J W, Friedmann E, McGinnis R, Holcomb R G. Detection of breast cancer with full-field digital mammography and computer-aided detection. AJR Am J Roentgenol 2009; 192(2): 337-40.
[http://dx.doi.org/10. 2214/AJR. 07. 3884] [PMID: 19155392]

[71] Bolivar A V, Gomez S S, Merino P, *et al.* Computer-aided detection system applied to full-field digital mammograms. Acta Radiol 2010; 51(10): 1086-92.
[http://dx.doi.org/10. 3109/02841851. 2010. 520024] [PMID: 20883182]

[72] Thurfjell E L, Lernevall K A, Taube A A. Benefit of independent double reading in a population-based mammography screening program. Radiology 1994; 191(1): 241-4.
[http://dx.doi.org/10. 1148/radiology. 191. 1. 8134580] [PMID: 8134580]

[73] Posso M, Puig T, Carles M, Rué M, Canelo-Aybar C, Bonfill X. Effectiveness and cost-effectiveness of double reading in digital mammography screening: A systematic review and meta-analysis. Eur J Radiol 2017; 96: 40-9.
[http://dx.doi.org/10. 1016/j. ejrad. 2017. 09. 013] [PMID: 29103474]

[74] Sato M, Kawai M, Nishino Y, Shibuya D, Ohuchi N, Ishibashi T. Cost-effectiveness analysis for breast cancer screening: double reading *versus* single + CAD reading. Breast Cancer 2014; 21(5): 532-41.
[http://dx.doi.org/10. 1007/s12282-012-0423-5] [PMID: 23104393]

[75] Malich A, Sauner D, Marx C, *et al.* Influence of breast lesion size and histologic findings on tumor detection rate of a computer-aided detection system. Radiology 2003; 228(3): 851-6.
[http://dx.doi.org/10. 1148/radiol. 2283011906] [PMID: 12869683]

[76] Evans W P, Warren Burhenne L J, Laurie L, O'Shaughnessy K F, Castellino R A. Invasive lobular carcinoma of the breast: mammographic characteristics and computer-aided detection. Radiology 2002; 225(1): 182-9.
[http://dx.doi.org/10. 1148/radiol. 2251011029] [PMID: 12355003]

[77] Balleyguier C, Arfi-Rouche J, Levy L, *et al.* Improving digital breast tomosynthesis reading time: A pilot multi-reader, multi-case study using concurrent Computer-Aided Detection (CAD). Eur J Radiol 2017; 97: 83-9.
[http://dx.doi.org/10. 1016/j. ejrad. 2017. 10. 014] [PMID: 29153373]

[78] Chan H P, Wei J, Zhang Y, *et al.* Computer-aided detection of masses in digital tomosynthesis mammography: comparison of three approaches. Med Phys 2008; 35(9): 4087-95.
[http://dx.doi.org/10. 1118/1. 2968098] [PMID: 18841861]

[79] Chan H P, Wei J, Sahiner B, *et al.* Computer-aided detection system for breast masses on digital tomosynthesis mammograms: preliminary experience. Radiology 2005; 237(3): 1075-80.
[http://dx.doi.org/10. 1148/radiol. 2373041657] [PMID: 16237141]

[80] Benedikt R A, Boatsman J E, Swann C A, Kirkpatrick A D, Toledano A Y. Concurrent computer-

aided detection improves reading time of digital breast tomosynthesis and maintains interpretation performance in a multireader multicase study. AJR Am J Roentgenol 2018; 210(3): 685-94.
[http://dx.doi.org/10. 2214/AJR. 17. 18185] [PMID: 29064756]

[81]   UFaDA. https://www.accessdata.fda.gov/scripts/cdrh/cfdocs/cfpma/pma.cfm?ID=380594

[82]   Renz D M, Baltzer P A, Kullnig P E, *et al.* [Clinical value of computer-assisted analysis in MR mammography. A comparison between two systems and three observers with different levels of experience]. RoFo Fortschr Geb Rontgenstr Nuklearmed 2008; 180(11): 968-76.
[http://dx.doi.org/10. 1055/s-2008-1027772] [PMID: 18855300]

[83]   Meeuwis C, van de Ven S M, Stapper G, *et al.* Computer-aided detection (CAD) for breast MRI: evaluation of efficacy at 3. 0 T. Eur Radiol 2010; 20(3): 522-8.
[http://dx.doi.org/10. 1007/s00330-009-1573-5] [PMID: 19727750]

[84]   Meinel L A, Stolpen A H, Berbaum K S, Fajardo L L, Reinhardt J M. Breast MRI lesion classification: improved performance of human readers with a backpropagation neural network computer-aided diagnosis (CAD) system. J Magn Reson Imaging 2007; 25(1): 89-95.
[http://dx.doi.org/10. 1002/jmri. 20794] [PMID: 17154399]

[85]   Newell D, Nie K, Chen J H, *et al.* Selection of diagnostic features on breast MRI to differentiate between malignant and benign lesions using computer-aided diagnosis: differences in lesions presenting as mass and non-mass-like enhancement. Eur Radiol 2010; 20(4): 771-81.
[http://dx.doi.org/10. 1007/s00330-009-1616-y] [PMID: 19789878]

[86]   Williams T C, DeMartini W B, Partridge S C, Peacock S, Lehman C D. Breast MR imaging: computer-aided evaluation program for discriminating benign from malignant lesions. Radiology 2007; 244(1): 94-103.
[http://dx.doi.org/10. 1148/radiol. 2441060634] [PMID: 17507720]

[87]   Arazi-Kleinman T, Causer P A, Jong R A, Hill K, Warner E. Can breast MRI computer-aided detection (CAD) improve radiologist accuracy for lesions detected at MRI screening and recommended for biopsy in a high-risk population? Clin Radiol 2009; 64(12): 1166-74.
[http://dx.doi.org/10. 1016/j. crad. 2009. 08. 003] [PMID: 19913125]

[88]   Bartella L, Morris E A, Dershaw D D, *et al.* Proton MR spectroscopy with choline peak as malignancy marker improves positive predictive value for breast cancer diagnosis: preliminary study. Radiology 2006; 239(3): 686-92.
[http://dx.doi.org/10. 1148/radiol. 2393051046] [PMID: 16603660]

[89]   Jacobs M A, Barker P B, Argani P, Ouwerkerk R, Bhujwalla Z M, Bluemke D A. Combined dynamic contrast enhanced breast MR and proton spectroscopic imaging: a feasibility study. J Magn Reson Imaging 2005; 21(1): 23-8.
[http://dx.doi.org/10. 1002/jmri. 20239] [PMID: 15611934]

[90]   Bolan P J, Nelson M T, Yee D, Garwood M. Imaging in breast cancer: Magnetic resonance spectroscopy. Breast Cancer Res 2005; 7(4): 149-52.
[http://dx.doi.org/10. 1186/bcr1202] [PMID: 15987466]

[91]   Jagannathan N R, Kumar M, Seenu V, *et al.* Evaluation of total choline from *in-vivo* volume localized proton MR spectroscopy and its response to neoadjuvant chemotherapy in locally advanced breast cancer. Br J Cancer 2001; 84(8): 1016-22.
[http://dx.doi.org/10. 1054/bjoc. 2000. 1711] [PMID: 11308247]

[92]   Meisamy S, Bolan P J, Baker E H, *et al.* Neoadjuvant chemotherapy of locally advanced breast cancer: predicting response with *in vivo* (1)H MR spectroscopy--a pilot study at 4 T. Radiology 2004; 233(2): 424-31.
[http://dx.doi.org/10. 1148/radiol. 2332031285] [PMID: 15516615]

[93]   Bartella L, Huang W. Proton (1H) MR spectroscopy of the breast. Radiographics 2007; 27 (Suppl. 1): S241-52.
[http://dx.doi.org/10. 1148/rg. 27si075504] [PMID: 18180230]

[94]   Siegmann K C, Krämer B, Claussen C. Current Status and New Developments in Breast MRI. Breast Care (Basel) 2011; 6(2): 87-92.
[http://dx.doi.org/10. 1159/000328273] [PMID: 21673817]

[95]   Lehman C D, Smith R A. The role of MRI in breast cancer screening. J Natl Compr Canc Netw 2009; 7(10): 1109-15.
[http://dx.doi.org/10. 6004/jnccn. 2009. 0072] [PMID: 19930977]

[96]   Heywang-Köbrunner S H, Hacker A, Sedlacek S. Advantages and disadvantages of mammography screening. Breast Care (Basel) 2011; 6(3): 199-207.
[http://dx.doi.org/10. 1159/000329005] [PMID: 21779225]

[97]   Avril N, Rosé C A, Schelling M, *et al.* Breast imaging with positron emission tomography and fluorine-18 fluorodeoxyglucose: use and limitations. J Clin Oncol 2000; 18(20): 3495-502.
[http://dx.doi.org/10. 1200/JCO. 2000. 18. 20. 3495] [PMID: 11032590]

[98]   Bakheet S M, Powe J, Kandil A, Ezzat A, Rostom A, Amartey J. F-18 FDG uptake in breast infection and inflammation. Clin Nucl Med 2000; 25(2): 100-3.
[http://dx.doi.org/10. 1097/00003072-200002000-00003] [PMID: 10656642]

[99]   Gordon B A, Flanagan F L, Dehdashti F. Whole-body positron emission tomography: normal variations, pitfalls, and technical considerations. AJR Am J Roentgenol 1997; 169(6): 1675-80.
[http://dx.doi.org/10. 2214/ajr. 169. 6. 9393189] [PMID: 9393189]

CHAPTER 3

An Overview of Genetic, Proteomic and Metabolomic Biomarkers in Breast Cancer

Tarjani Agrawal[*]

Projects in Knowledge Inc, Livingston, New Jersey, USA

Abstract: The molecular techniques play an important role in the diagnosis and treatment of breast cancer. Recent advances in molecular techniques have contributed significantly to understanding tumor biology, tumor heterogeneity, identification of different biomarkers, and discovery of new therapeutic measures and improvement in overall survival, especially in specific subsets of breast cancer. There are other challenging areas in breast cancer research, such as the development of treatments for the highly aggressive triple-negative breast cancer subtype, chemotherapy-resistant cancer stem cell subpopulation, and male breast cancer. New knowledge emerging from researches in genetics, proteomics, and metabolomics offers a promising opportunity for the identification of new biomarkers, and to find novel targets that could facilitate future therapeutic interventions.

Keywords: Breast cancer, Biomarker, Genetics, Metabolomics, Proteomics.

INTRODUCTION

Breast cancer (BC) is one of the most commonly diagnosed malignancies in females worldwide [1]. Worldwide, approximately one-quarter of all cancers in females are BC, and specifically, in developed countries with a Western lifestyle around 27% of cancers are BC [2]. Among the three most common cancers in women, *i.e.*, breast, lung, and colorectal, BC alone accounts for 30% of all new cancer diagnoses in women [3]. Second, to lung cancer, BC is known to be a common cause of cancer death [4]. Among women 20-59 years of age, the leading cause of cancer death is BC [3]. An estimated 231,840 new invasive BC cases and 40,290 deaths occurred in the United States in 2015 [4]. BC is a complex disease caused by cell proliferation and genetic instability due to increased invasive and resistant character by numerous molecular changes [5].

It contains many different categories of tumors that vary significantly in their res-

---

[*] **Corresponding author Tarjani Agrawal**: Projects in knowledge Inc, Livingston, New Jersey, USA; Tel: 2016998205; E-mail: tarjani.pik@gmail.com

Shankar Suman, Garima Suman and Sanjay Mishra (Eds.)

ponses to treatment, presentation, and biology. For example, histologically similar tumors may response differently to clinical behavior and treatment [6]. Various subgroups at the molecular level are created by this heterogeneity, which would lead to different clinical results and therapeutic responses [5]. Therefore, to be able to make the best prediction of survival, there is a need to evaluate as many clinical and pathological features as possible [7]. Clinical endpoints such as survival define the success of any BC therapy. However, these clinical endpoints require measurements through prolonged follow-up, as well as they cannot be used to guide the treatment very early on in the course of therapy. Therefore, to predict the most efficacious therapies or measure response to therapy early in the course of treatment, there is a need to have biomarkers [8].

In cancer, to gain additional information about classical clinical factors and to enable patients with a more favorable benefit-risk balance in order to receive certain treatments, biomarker analysis is recommended. Especially in BC, it is routine practice to perform biomarker analysis. Originally, it was done by testing for hormone receptor expression for guiding tamoxifen therapy; however, subsequently, targeted treatments against human epidermal growth factor receptor 2 (HER2) were included, which revolutionized the biomarker field [9].

There has been significant progress and a shift to identifying specific mutations associated with breast tumors through a specific genetic screen. This may also lead to improved outcomes through "personalized medicine" [10]. Genetic and genomic biomarkers are more beneficial than clinical methods as they may identify a constitutional basis for an individual's disease. Moreover, either molecular variations in single genes or set of genes or even in entire genomes can also be detected using genomic screening [11]. When applied in the context of appropriate counseling and interpretation, identification of genomic biomarkers of inherited risk for BC may help in prevention through assisted reproduction, as well as can be used as a guide to developing targeted therapy, thus decreasing morbidity and mortality [11].

Our understanding of the molecular fundamentals of BC has been advanced by the genome studies, while the proteomics has helped us understanding cellular functions controlled by the same genome having different proteome outputs [12]. Proteomic analysis studies the biological activities of the proteome which means the ensemble of proteins present in one cell, tissue or organism. The proteomic analysis studies have also shown positive results for early BC diagnosis, follow up and therapeutic predictive markers [5].

The alterations in metabolism that occur after changes in genomics and proteomics of different types of breast tumors were also explored, and only now, their role is gradually being understood [13]. Thus, metabolomics, which analyzes metabolites from biofluids and tissues for new biomarkers, has emerged as a new approach in cancer research [14].

Over the past two decades, there is an improvement in survival and a decline in BC mortality primarily due to advances in early detection and treatment. But the increased survival is difficult to interpret because of changes in detection practice [3], and the 5-year relative survival rates for the metastatic disease remain poor [15]. The rate of local recurrence and distant metastases is also very high [16]. There are also two challenging areas of BC research such as the development of treatments for the highly aggressive triple-negative BC subtype and chemotherapy-resistant cancer stem cell subpopulation [10]. Besides, although there have been many advances in women BC treatment, male BC is still not completely understood, as well as only limited therapies are available for men [10].

It is important to keep developing tests that can predict the risk of recurrence of cancer. And also, these tests should be able to give insights about patients that will respond better to specific therapeutic measures. New knowledge emerging from researches in genetics, proteomics, and metabolomics offers an opportunity to identify new biomarkers and discover new targets for future therapeutic interventions.

BIOMARKERS

According to the National Cancer Institute, a biomarker is a biologic molecule found in blood, other body fluids, or tissues that is a sign of a normal or abnormal process [17]. However, this definition does not include the importance of imaging biomarkers that are currently being used. In a broader scope, biomarkers are recognized as any measurable indicators of biologic processes, obtained from tissue, imaging, or any other source [18].

The definition of biomarker, according to World Health Organization, is "any substance, structure or process that can be measured in the body or its products and influence or predict the incidence or outcome of disease" [19].

Biomarkers are called surrogate end-points when they act as reliable substitutes for clinical end-points. The US National Institutes of Health (NIH) Biomarkers Definitions Working Group has defined biomarkers as "a characteristic that is objectively measured and evaluated as an indicator of normal biological processes, pathogenic processes, or pharmacologic responses to a therapeutic intervention". However, there is a narrower definition that is still commonly used: "disease-associated molecular changes in body tissue and fluids", *i.e.*, a biological marker [20]. Biological molecules produced in the tumor itself or the host system as a result of tumor act as tumor markers, which provide biological material for prediction of cancer occurrence, detection of cancer, classification of cancer, and give an understanding of prognosis and therapeutic responses [21].

Tumor biomarkers include chromosomal alterations that may occur due to rearrangement in chromosomal structure as a result of chromosomal instability, which usually occur at the earliest stages of tumorigenesis and persists throughout tumor development. These chromosomal changes may be changes in cancer-specific gene expression pattern or its mutation or promoter methylation that can also result in variation in protein expression [21, 22]. These altered proteins may act as biomarkers. They may be detected in abundance in circulation as free, shed proteins, or there may be the presence of autoantibodies to these variant proteins. Besides, post-translational modification like glycosylation or phosphorylation of proteins due to tumor-specific biochemical changes can provide a variety of biomarker molecules. These biochemical changes can often result in measurable metabolic changes in a cell, which may act as powerful biomarkers [21].

Biomarkers may be detected in body fluids, including blood, as well as in tissues. They can act as prognostic indicators and diagnostic monitors predicting therapeutic advantage and effectiveness of clinical interventions, thus helping the development of targeted therapies and timely interventions during cancer treatment. These biomarkers also help in a stratification of cancer patients according to the most suitable treatment for individual patients [21].

Biomarkers, by definition, are objective and quantifiable medical signs. Therefore, there measurement with a high degree of accuracy and reproducibility is necessary. They also must be relevant and valid with the capability of reliably characterizing a clinically meaningful endpoint in question. An ideal biomarker would explain the clinical problem at a basic biologic level as well as it will be highly specific to the disease [19].

Tumor biomarkers which appear at the earliest stages of tumor development and those appearing and persisting throughout the tumor serve different purposes such as detection of cancer at the earliest stage, diagnosis of cancer, prediction of prognosis of the disease, and prediction of response to anticancer therapies and recurrence of cancer (Fig. **1**). The tumor markers are produced by the tumor cells that can help in detecting these cells [21].

Various techniques can be used to derive biomarkers from multiple clinical and imaging sources. They can be roughly subdivided by their nature of origin [28] (Table **1**). Depending on the role in research and clinical practice, biomarkers were divided into seven sub-categories by The US Food and Drug Administration

(FDA) - NIH Biomarker Working Group [19] (Table **2**).

Table 1. Types of Biomarkers based on their nature of origin.

category	Source	Biomarker type	Examples
Clinical	Patient history	Environmental exposures Lifestyle factors Age Family history	Mantle chest radiation. High alcohol consumption Older age First-degree relative with BC
Laboratory	Whole blood Serum Plasma Tissue	Genomic Transcriptomic Proteomic Metabolomic	BRCA mutations Long noncoding RNAs PI3K/Akt/mTOR pathway Threonine, glutamine
Imaging	Mammography Ultrasound Dynamic contrast-enhanced MRI MIBI scintigraphy FDG PEM	For-presentation images CAD Radiomics	BI-RADS descriptors Kinetic enhancement curves Energy, homogeneity, entropy, skewness, and kurtosis

PI3K = phosphatidylinositol 3-kinase, RNA = ribonucleic acid, Akt = protein kinase B, mTOR = mammalian target of rapamycin, MIBI = methoxyisobutylisonitrile, PEM = positron emission mammography, CAD = computer-aided detection.

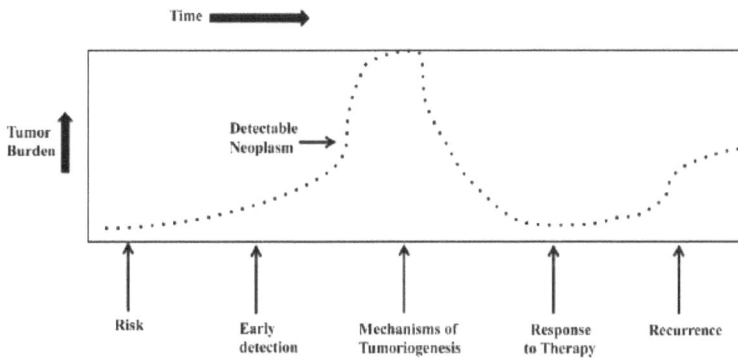

Fig. (1). Application of different biomarkers for different stages of cancer progression.

Detection of BC at an early stage utilizing a biomarker assay is extremely necessary to reduce the burden of disease and to have a better prognosis. BC diagnosed at an early stage is much more treatable than the one detected in the metastatic stage. Thus, the identification of biomarkers having the ability to predict metastasis is also very important [23]. Many potential prognostic and predictive biomarkers for BC have been investigated in the past few decades. With the progression of new techniques for gene expression profiling, it revealed that in comparison to traditional prognostic factors, novel biological factors and molecular markers have more important roles [24]. New technological advances are being made to discover and validate novel biological markers either individually or in series which may help in diagnosis, prognosis, individualized, targeted therapies, and prediction of tumor recurrence [21].

For prognostic and predictive purposes in BC, although many novel biomarkers have been reported, only a few are clinically relevant. Most of these biomarkers could not reach a Level of Evidence I or II due to a lack of sufficient validation, according to the American Society of Clinical Oncology's Tumor Marker Utility Grading System [25, 26]. Nonetheless, the identification of these biomarkers has been very helpful in providing insights for tumor biology and substantiating the relevance of the existing markers [27].

Table 2. Types of biomarkers by use.

Type of biomarker	Function	Example
Diagnostic	Used for the detection or confirmation of a disease or condition and identification of a specific disease subtype	BI-RADS descriptors, ER, PR, and HER2 (also known as ERBB2) status
Monitoring	Serially measured to assess the status of a disease or condition or to find evidence of exposure to, or effects of, a medical product or environmental agent; the focus is on changes in a patient's condition	Tumor size and volume by imaging
Pharmacodynamic response	Used for showing that a medical product, intervention, or environmental exposure results in a biologic response; may not be predictive of whether the intervention will have an effect on the future clinical outcome but rather show that the intervention had an effect	Standardized uptake value at FDG PET to monitor endocrine therapy in BC
Predictive	Used to identify individuals who are more likely to experience a favorable or unfavorable response to an intervention, medical product, or environmental exposure compared with individuals without the biomarker	Possibility that mutations in BRCA genes are predictive of response to PARP inhibitors in patients with advanced breast and ovarian cancer; likelihood that ER- and PR-positive BCs respond to endocrine therapy; possibility that dense breast tissue is a biomarker predictive of the decreased sensitivity of mammography for detecting noncalcified BC
Prognostic	Reflect the likelihood of a clinical event, disease progression, or recurrence irrespective of an intervention	TNM stage, tumor grade, tumor receptor status

(Table 2) cont.....

Type of biomarker	Function	Example
Safety	Indicate the presence of a harmful effect of an intervention if measured before and after the exposure	Serum creatinine and EGFR as safety biomarkers to monitor nephrotoxicity of IV contrast agents
Susceptibility, risk	Used to predict the potential of development of a disease or medical condition in individuals who do not currently have a clinically apparent disease or condition	BRCA gene mutations as indicators of increased lifetime risk of breast and ovarian cancers; mammographically dense breast tissue as an independent risk factor for the development of BC
ER = estrogen receptor, PR = progesterone receptor, PARP = poly (adenosine diphosphate-ribose) polymerase, EGFR = estimated glomerular filtration rate.		

Limitations of Current BC Screening Techniques and the Potential Role of Biomarkers

Screening for BC relies mainly on mammography, which is, in most cases very expensive protocol, as well as detects only 70% of BCs. Mammographic sensitivity is also reported to be as low as less than 50%. Moreover, it is ineffective in younger women. Also, it is constrained by a single patient's characteristics, such as breast density, especially for women who are below the age of 50. Although mammography has shown an increase for the detection of early-stage cancer like stage 0 and 1 cancers, however, it has not been able to show a similar increase in detection of stage II and III cancer incidence, which suggests a bias in the detection of indolent cancers as compared to aggressive cancers [28].

A more powerful approach would be to identify patients for auxiliary imaging based on the use of biomarkers rather than using risk stratification. Theoretically, biomarkers should be able to find the presence of occult cancer in normal mammogram patients, which is a more targeted method than lifetime risk calculations. A typical biomarker-based screening protocol would involve an initial screening using a blood test followed by auxiliary imaging for confirmation and localization of cancer [28].

Integration of Biomarkers into Current Diagnostic Paradigms

A suggested screening protocol incorporating the use of biomarkers is shown in Fig. (**2**) [28].

Commonly Utilized Cancer Biomarkers for BC

Some of the currently utilized cancer biomarkers for BC, and their clinical significance are shown in Table **3** [28, 29].

		MAMMOGRAPHY	
		Normal	Abnormal
BIOMARKER	Normal	Continue annual or biennial screening	Consider 6-month follow up imaging and repeat Biomarker test as alternative to biopsy
	Abnormal	Auxiliary imaging with whole breast ultrasound or magnetic resonance imaging	Diagnostic biopsy

Fig. (2). Suggested standard screening protocol for BC, including at-risk patients who do not qualify for high-risk protocols.

ESTABLISHED BIOMARKERS

Estrogen and Progesterone Receptors

Two prototypical tumor markers that affect the systemic treatment decisions for BC are Progesterone Receptor (PR) and Estrogen Receptor (ER) [6]. Although the oldest, ER, *i.e.*, ER-α, is the most important biomarker for BC because it provides the index for sensitivity to endocrine treatment [30, 31]. The measurement of ER is routinely followed in all cases of BC that are newly diagnosed and also in recurrent/metastatic lesions.

Apart from its use as a prognostic and therapeutic marker, it provides valuable information as a predictive biomarker for endocrine therapy [31]. In ER-positive tumors, ER serves as the direct target for endocrine therapy as such tumors use the steroid hormone estradiol as their main growth stimulus [30]. Thus ER-presence/absence helps in the determination of endocrine therapy, as it is not required in ER-negative tumors. Being a predictive biomarker and a specific target in endocrine therapy, ER is used in most of the diseased settings including the neoadjuvant, adjuvant and advanced [31].

Estrogens play a role in the cell growth in BC by interfering in the regulatory mechanism in the genome. It binds to ER and activates them, which leads to increased transcription of genes such as MYC and Cyclin D (CCND1). Thus the levels of ER correlate with the benefit of antiestrogenic therapy [31].

Table 3. Biomarkers used clinically for BC.

Biomarker or panel	Clinical Utility
ER	ER, positivity indicates better prognosis in BC patients who have better survival than ER-negative BC patients. Predict responsiveness to tamoxifen as when highly expressed; it predicts a better response to tamoxifen therapy particularly in node-negative patients.
PR	A prognostic marker is indicating better survival when positively expressed (PR +ve). High expression of PR predicts beneficial responses to tamoxifen chemotherapy.
HER2/*neu*	Prognostic marker for worse prognosis in patients with HER2/neu-positive tumors as they have more aggressive BCs. Predictor marker for the response to therapy with trastuzumab. Determination of Herceptin sensitivity and prognosis.
BRCA1	Prognostic marker for poor prognosis. High expression of BRCA1 indicates a worse prognosis. If highly expressed, BRCA1 can predict response to chemotherapy in BC patients.
CA27.29	BC monitoring
uPA/PAI-I	Prognosis
MammaPrint™	It is a 70-gene assay, a prognostic indicator in a heterogeneous population for stratification of BC patients into good or poor prognosis.
Oncotype DX®	A 21-gene multiplex prognostic assay used for the determination of the recurrence score.
Isoforms Akt kinase	Akt kinase isoforms and activity are predictive markers to suggest the most likely response to trastuzumab therapy in HER2-neu-positive patients of BC.
Rotterdam Signature	Prognostic for metastasis signature
dtectDx™ Breast	Detection of BC in women under the age of 50 years in conjunction with imaging.
Prosigna	The risk for recurrence, risk category, and subtype
HER2 = human epidermal growth factor receptor; ER = estrogen receptor; PR = progesterone receptor; uPA = urokinase-type plasminogen activator; PAI-I = plasminogen activator inhibitor-1.	

The PR is usually measured concurrently with ER [31]. PR is encoded by gene PGR located on chromosome 11q21.1. This gene is composed of 933 amino acids, and it has three domains: A DNA binding domain, a modulating N-terminal domain, and a ligand-binding C-terminal domain. It is involved in cell-cell signaling, negative regulation of gene expression and transcription initiation from RNA polymerase II promoter. Progesterone has two receptors that are PRA and PRB, which are transcribed by the same gene using an alternative promoter. Both these proteins are identical, but PRB is longer than PRA because it contains extra 164 amino acids on its N-terminal. PRA is a repressor of activity of PRB which is a major activator of transcription factors. During tumorigenesis, there is a change in the ratio between PRA and PRB that is more PRA than PRB [24]. The rationale behind the measurement of PR along with ER is based on the observation that estrogen induces PR, and thus the presence of PR indicates a functional ER [31]. PR-positive tumors are commonly found to be ER-positive as well, whereas tumors positive for PR but negative for ER are very less common and represent only <1% of all BC [32]. On the other hand, PR, in the presence of progesterone, interacts with ER and alters the position of ER binding with chromatin. This ER-chromatin binding alteration leads to switching from regulatory genes associated with cell proliferation to activating the modulating genes involved in cell cycle arrest, cell death and differentiation [31].

In postmenopausal women with low- to intermediate-grade BC, the levels of ER and PR are found to be positive. In such scenarios, both ER and PR are considered weak prognostic markers but very convincing as predictive factors of hormonal therapy response of the tumor (*e.g.*, tamoxifen). PR is also an unconventional predictor of response because ER- and PR-positive patients have shown a good response to treatment than those with have ER-positive and PR-negative patients. Due to wide accessibility and easy usage, immunohistochemistry (IHC) is considered to be the preferred method for ER and PR measurement [6].

Mutation in the ER Gene

Many investigations have been performed to understand the amplification of the ER gene (ESR1) and its effect on BC. An initial report indicated that ESR1 gene amplification in BC could be detected in ~ 20% of all invasive tumors and that there was a correlation between the gene amplification and ER expression levels [30]. Mutation in the ESR1 may lead to the development of resistance to endocrine therapy, which may be less in primary BCs, but 10-40% of recurrent/metastatic lesions present with ESR1 mutations, more commonly after long-term endocrine treatment that includes aromatase inhibitors. These mutations are commonly found in the ER ligand-binding domain, specifically in residues D538G, Y537S, E380Q, Y537C, and Y537N. Multiple prospective, as well as retrospective clinical trials, are conducted to assess the role of ESR1 mutation and its potential clinical significance [31].

HER2

The most heterogeneous group of posttranslational modifications known in proteins is glycoproteins. Many prognostic and predictive biomarkers in cancer are glycoproteins in nature, for example, HER2-neu in the case of BC. The human epidermal growth factor receptor two genes are present on the long arm of chromosome 17 (17q21.1). It encodes a receptor of molecular mass 185 kDa, which is a single-pass transmembrane protein [24].

HER2 was first identified as an initial indicator of the patient's prognosis [30]. It is encoded by oncogene ERBB2 and is a transmembrane glycoprotein member of the HER family. Several normal epithelia such as breast express HER2 at very low levels [6]. In normal cells, the number of HER2 receptors is 20,000, but in the case of a tumor, this number is increased up to 200,000 receptors. It will lead to an aggressive form of BC if left untreated [24]. HER2 amplification and the RNA/protein overexpression correlate strongly, and it occurs in approximately 15% to 20% of BCs [6, 30]. In cases of HER2 overexpression (HER2 positive), BC patients tend to have a shorter overall survival as they are more likely to suffer from relapses. ER-negative tumors are more commonly found to be HER2-positive as compared to ER-positive tumors. Also, around 30% of ER-negative tumors show HER2 gene amplification/overexpression compared to 12% of ER-positive tumors. A significant inverse relationship between both ER/PR and HER2 levels was also seen [31].

The measurement of HER2 is now also compulsory, likewise ER measurement in all new cases of invasive BC as well as in recurrent/metastatic lesions. HER2 overexpression activates the MAPK and PI3K/AKT signaling pathways that, in turn, increases cell growth leading to tumor growth, invasion and metastasis. Another mechanism suggests the deformation of cell membranes and loss of cellular cohesiveness due to HER2 overexpression that enhances the invasive nature of the tumor cells, promotes oncogenesis as well as tumor progression [31].

Overexpression and/or gene amplification of HER2 is considered to be unconventional prognostic markers for clinical outcomes. It also acts as a predictive factor for tumor response to any of the chemotherapeutic agents [6]. In order to determine patients' eligibility for anti-HER2 therapy, the levels of HER2 is typically evaluated. Either used as monotherapy or in combination with other drugs or with chemotherapeutic agents, HER2-targeted drugs show remarkably better response and rates of survival. HER2 gene amplification/overexpression appears to be important for response to all anti-HER2 therapy [31].

To determine the status of HER2, a formalin-fixed or paraffin-embedded (FFPE) tissue is used. Levels are determined by either IHC to assess the amount of protein expressed on the tumor cell membrane or fluorescence in situ hybridization (FISH) or chromatin in situ hybridization (CISH) techniques to measure the number of HER2 copies [6, 33].

Other established markers such as BCRA1/2, p53 are described below.

GENOMIC BIOMARKERS FOR BC

Cancer results from somatic cell genetic damage arising from the dysregulation in the mechanism of recognition and repair of mutations in DNA. Many germline mutations occurring in genes, involved in maintaining the integrity of the genome, predispose individuals to cancer. The proteins, encoded by these genes, are involved in DNA damage recognition or repair. The individuals born with one mutant allele of such genes are at increased risk of acquiring additional DNA damage and genomic instability and therefore accumulate these events leading to the carcinogenic conversion of cells. The remaining wildtype allele of cancer predisposing gene is frequently lost in the tumor cells. Usually, DNA sequencing of candidate genes is used to evaluate the likelihood of forming cancer through the risk of genomic biomarkers [21]. The genomic tests represent clinical "biomarkers" of an individual's susceptibility to developing cancer [11].

A family history of BC indicates the presence of inherited genetic events that predispose to this disease [11]. However, only 5% of BC patients have a strong family history, which implies that most BCs are due to acquired mutations. Of these acquired mutant genes, two genes, which are BRCA1 and BRCA2, show substantial evidence of the early onset of BC. Li-Fraumeni syndrome, ataxia-telangiectasia, and Cowden's disease are also associated with an increased risk of BC [34]. Genetic testing for mutations in BRCA1, BRCA2, and other BC susceptibility genes has served as a model to show that genomics can be integrated into the practice through personalized medicines with increased efficacy required for better screening and prevention strategies, and as biomarkers for targeted therapy [11]. More than one million individuals have been tested for mutations in BRCA1/2. Almost ~ 30% of high-risk BC families and ~ 15% of the BC familial relative risk can be attributed to these pathogenic mutations [11]. Familial risk is defined as the ratio of the risk of disease for an individual who is relative of an affected person as compared to that for the general population. Over the past two decades, the tests for genetic biomarkers of risk have evolved to complement the family history and physical findings. Genomic markers as compared to non-genetic biomarkers show the importance of modifiers of penetrance, allele frequencies related differences in population, and effects of gene-environment interactions [11].

Highly Penetrant BC Genes

BRCA1 and BRCA2

Approximately 5-10% of BCs are hereditary, most of which are due to the mutations in tumor suppressor gene BRCA1 and BRCA2. The BRCA1 and BRCA2 genes are known to be required during in response to DNA damage and homologous recombination. It is a big gene located on chromosome 17q21.31 and has 24 exons, out of which 22 are coding, and two are non-coding. BRCA2 is present on chromosome 13q12.3 [24]. BRCA2 spans more than 70,000 bases and has 27 exons [11]. BRCA1 and BRCA2 are consists of 1863 and 3418 amino acids respectively [36]. Predominant genomic aberrations underlying susceptibility occur due to the formation of premature truncations of the BRCA1 and BRCA2 proteins because of nonsense or frame-shift mutations. More than 2000 distinct rare variants have been shown in BRCA1 and BRCA2. These include intronic changes, missense mutations, and small in-frame insertions and deletions [11].

BRCA1 could function during transcriptional regulation, and the maintenance of chromosomal integrity thus has been implicated in the maintenance of genomic stability [36]. The main domains of BRCA1 located in the RING finger and BRCT domains are critical for DNA repair activity. DNA binding domain of BRCA2 has most of the highly penetrant pathogenic missense mutations. Both BRCA1 and BRCA2 show large genomic rearrangements or structural variations leading to 14% and 2.6% of mutations in respective genes. Population-specific or "founder" mutations have been described in BRCA1/2, *e.g.*, two mutations in BRCA1 (185delG and 5382insC) and one mutation in BRCA2 (6174delT) are commonly encountered, and they are reported in individuals of Ashkenazi (Eastern European) Jewish ancestry [11]. It is highly unlikely that a different mutation will be found, in case if one of these mutations is not present [24]. However, a small portion of the Ashkenazi population, around 5% of all mutations, with BC have non-founder mutations in BRCA1/2, and therefore reflex full gene sequencing is required to find such non-revealing founder mutations [11]. The genomic location of a patient's BRCA1/2 mutation and the risk from modifier genes indicates risk by the gene. BRCA1 and BRCA2 mutation carriers very high-risk category which is 81% or 83% chance of BC by age 80, respectively. However, for better and more precise risk estimates the emerging biomarker data shows that it could add value to the calculations based on other variables modifying risk in BRCA1/2 mutation carriers. A correlation of biomarkers with disease behavior is also possible. In most cases, the tumor of BC patients with BRCA1 mutations show features of more aggressive disease. Therefore genomic biomarkers of risk may also impact the phenotype (*e.g.*, estrogen receptor status) of hereditary disease [11]. A triple assessment of breast surveillance, including self-examination, clinician examination and mammography/magnetic resonance imaging (MRI) should be performed for BRCA mutation carriers [11].

Therapeutic applications have been developed by the identification of mutated genes as biomarkers. As platinum produces interstrand crosslinks that can only be corrected by BRCA1 - and BRCA2 -dependent homologous recombination DNA repair, therefore, many clinical trials either *in-vivo* or *in-vitro* have been able to show that platinum chemotherapy is an effective measure against BRCA1 and, by probably too, BRCA2 mutant tumors [90 - 92]. A new class of drugs that stops the enzyme involved in base excision repair called poly (ADP-ribose) polymerase (PARP) has depicted antitumor activity in the background of BRCA -associated defects in homologous recombination-mediated DNA repair. Clinical trials that have explored the efficacy of molecules that inhibit PARP for the treatment of BRCA1/2 mutant breast cancer have found positive outcomes [93].

Table 4. Biomarkers used clinically for BC indications.

Gene	Location	Familial BC Association	Sporadic BC Association	Other Cancers
BRCA1	17q	High (40%)	High	Ovary (colon, prostate)
BRCA2	13q	High (40%)	High	No ovary, male breast (prostate)
p53	17p	Low	High	Carcinomas, sarcomas, leukemias
RAS (HRAS)	11p	Low in young, higher in old	High in old	Carcinomas, sarcomas, leukemias
Ataxia telangiectasia	11q	Low	Low	Lymphoma, leukemias
hMSH2	2p	Low	Low	Colon, skin, stomach
hMLH1 (lynchII)	3p	Low	Low	Colon, skin, stomach
Neurofibromatosis 1	17q	Very low	Low	Nerve brain
Androgen receptor	Xq	Only males, low	Only males	Male breast

TP53

P53 is one of the most studied biomarkers for BC. It is a transcription factor that regulates the cell cycle, so it acts as a tumor suppressor. The gene TP53 encodes P53. It is present in the short arm of chromosome 17 (17p31.1). Mutation in the TP53 genes leads to the formation of proteins that do not degrade quickly, so accumulates and could be analyzed by immunohistochemistry. The human TP53 gene is a nuclear phosphoprotein composed of 393 amino acids that cause both repression and activation of gene expression by binding at many sites of chromatin. There are two transactivation domains, TAD1 and TAD2, on the N-terminus of p53. Mutation in these domains causes inactivation of p53 completely as a tumor suppressor. At C terminal, there is a tetramerization domain that directly interacts with single-stranded DNA. About 75% of TP53 mutations are missense, 9% are deletions and frameshift insertions, 7% are nonsense mutations, and 5% are silent mutations. These mutations result in a significant loss in transactivation capacity as well as in DNA binding activity. Different mutant forms of p53 protein have different biological and functional effects [24].

Patients that have mutations in the TP53 gene have a high risk of BC [37]. It is reported that, depending upon tumor size and stage of the disease, TP53 mutation can be found in approximately 20-40% of all cases. It seems to be an early event in breast tumorigenesis [24]. However, TP53 mutations are rare as compared to BRCA1/2 mutations. But TP53 testing may be a validated measure in cases with a high family cancer history and showing negative during BRCA1/2 testing. Genomic alteration in the TP53 gene also leads to a multi-cancer predisposing syndrome called Li-Fraumeni syndrome (LFS) [11].

CDH1

People with CDH1 (E-Cadherin) mutations have shown to have around 40-50% risk of lobular BC. There is a 30% chance of having CDH1 mutation in families affected by gastric cancer for multi-generations [94, 95]. Also, almost 70% of carriers of CDH1 mutations have a chance to develop gastric cancer [98]. Although there are no testing recommendations for patients that have CDH1 mutations and BC have been established formally, some researchers propose that patients that have bilateral lobular carcinoma in situ with or without invasive lobular or family history should undergo CDH1 mutation screening [96, 97].

PTEN

Germline mutations in the PTEN gene with a chromosomal locus at 10q23.3 are seen in patients with Cowden syndrome, and they are at increased risk of BC [11, 21].

STK11

Individuals with known STK11 mutations have increased the risk for the development of BC. Aberrant gene function and/or loss of kinase activity could result due to small deletions/insertions of single base substitutions mutations [11]. Individuals with STK11 mutation with a chromosomal locus at 19p13.3 are at increased risk of BC, and it is frequently seen in patients with Peutz-Jeghers Syndrome [21].

Moderate Penetrance BC Genes or Biomarkers

No standardized guidelines have so far been established for the management of risks with other types of cancer or even for the relatives of carriers with moderate penetrance gene mutations; however, screening recommendations should be built based on the patient's personal and family clinical background [11].

CHEK2

CHEK2 serves during DNA damage and suppresses that the entry of cells into mitosis. It functions in DNA damage by phosphorylating BRCA1. The interaction of CHEK2 with BRCA1 is necessary to reinstate the survival after DNA damage. Mutations in CHEK2 predispose individuals to cancer. The truncating mutation CHEK2*1100delC affecting kinase activity may increase the BC risk in females by two-fold and in males by 10-fold. This can be used as a clinical biomarker for pre-symptomatic checks during screening and diagnosis if the harmful mutations in CHEK2 could be detected when a patient has a strong family history of BC [11].

ATM

ATM is a gene that encodes a protein that functions for the proper repair of DNA. ATM, when changed, results in phenotypes from bi-allelic and arguably mono-allelic genomic modifications. Missense mutations in the ATM gene carry the risk of BC [11].

PALB2

PLBA2 is a tumor suppressor gene that functions with the BRCA2 protein to correct and fix DNA breaks. Thus it helps in maintaining the stability of genetic information and controls the rate of cell growth and division. It is reported that germline mutations of PALB2 are associated with hereditary BC. Mutations in PALB2 have been estimated to lead to a two-fold increase in BC risk [11].

RAD51C and RAD51D

Nonsense, frameshift, splice, and non-functional missense mutations have been described in RAD51C, which acts as a DNA repair gene. However, the evidence is limited which holds forth that they are a driver of familial BC. Several authors reported that individuals with mutations in RAD51C, RAD51D carries an increased risk for BC [11].

Low Penetrant Polygenes

Many single nucleotide variations or polymorphisms have been found that result in moderate to low penetrant BC gene biomarkers [11]. Single nucleotide polymorphism (SNP) genotyping will more accurately stratify BC risk and guide disease management. Emerging reports indicate an association between SNPs in certain genes and susceptibility to BC, as well as clinicopathologic status, *e.g.*, an association between FSCN1 single nucleotide polymorphisms (SNPs) and the risk of BC has been reported. FSCN1 overexpression has been reported in BC patients [16].

Other Genetic Biomarkers

PIK3CA Mutation

In all human cancers, PIK3CA is known to be the most frequently mutated oncogene [38]. Next-generation sequencing (NGS) studies have demonstrated that PIK3CA is one of the most frequently mutated genes in BC (31-41%). Concomitant mutations of MAP3K1/PIK3CA, CDH1/PIK3CA are also regularly seen in BC. PIK3CA mutations are reported in 43-57% of Luminal A and in 31-35% of Luminal B carcinomas, respectively [9]. Phosphatidylinositol-4,--biphosphonate 3-kinase (PIK3CA) is part of the PI3K/PTEN/Akt signaling pathway. It acts as a catalytic subunit. It also controls cell growth, proliferation, motility, survival, differentiation and intracellular trafficking [38]. PIK3CA mutations confer the tumor a less treatment-response rate as compared to those seen with the wild-type gene, *e.g.*, and resistance to trastuzumab or lapatinib treatment due to PIK3CA mutations is reported in several studies. The anticancer activity of anti-HER2 therapy also occurs partially through shutting off the PI3K signaling pathway. So mutations in the gene pathways would result in resistance [31].

Mitotic Arrest Deficient Like 1 (MAD1L1)

MAD1L1 is a checkpoint gene known to function in chromosomal instability. Various cancers types such as colon and lung cancers have shown abnormalities in MAD1L1. Nuclear MAD1L1 expression is reported to have an impact on the treatment resistance and the prognosis of BC. Its expression increases the treatment resistance and affects the prognosis of breast cancer thus demonstrating that MAD1L1-positive BC is not susceptible to taxol treatment [39].

Methylation of Paired-like Homeodomain 2 (PITX2P2)

Gene regulatory sites such as C-phosphate-G islands are associated with the gene expression suppression. A common early event, which is methylation of DNA dinucleotides in the PITX2 gene, is associated with subsequent onset of cancer. Methylation patterns are specific to a particular subtype of the tumor and its effect on clinical outcomes. PITX2 DNA methylation has been shown by various reports to be related to high relapse risk in lymph node metastasis-positive and also with hormone receptor-positive BC patients following full-body adjuvant tamoxifen therapy [39].

Lin28

Lin28 is a regulatory stem cell gene that shows high expression levels in undifferentiated cells. It has been shown to have an oncogenic role by promoting cellular proliferation and transformation and, therefore, has been implicated in tumor development. It is reported that Lin28 shows high expression in various tumors including BC. High expression of Lin28 is also reported in recurrent and metastatic BC. Lin28 is an oncoprotein showing posttranscriptional downregulation of microRNA Let-7 and thus affects stem cells. Let-7 is required in normal development and metabolism, and thus it is an important molecule [23].

Cytochrome P450 2D6 Polymorphism

The CYP450 genes result in various phenotypes and are polymorphic. Studies have shown that it could possibly affect the clinical outcomes of BC patients after tamoxifen treatment because some of the genetic variants of CYP450 2D6 (CYP2D6) are shown to be related to even low levels of the active metabolite of Tamoxifen called endoxifen. To predict the patient's response to tamoxifen treatment, it is suggested that the CYP2D6 genotype could be used as a promising biomarker. Also, to further confirm these findings a large-scale, prospective, randomized and well-controlled clinical trial is required [23].

Circulating Tumor Cells and Circulating Free Tumor DNA

A new diagnostic tool known as liquid biopsies, which are done either using tumor nucleic acids (ctDNA, cfmiRNA) or circulating tumor cells (CTCs) of epithelial origin or tumor exosomes in the blood of cancer patients, is becoming very popular [9]. Many circulating tumor cells (CTCs) platforms have been developed in the last decade. Various technologies have been used, such as 1) using specific antibodies, *e.g.* EpCAM (epithelial cell adhesion molecule) alone or combination in immunomagnetic (*e.g.*, CellSearch®) or microfluidics assay; 2) using size-based filtration; 3) using electrical properties. Currently, only CellSearch® is FDA approved for prognosis in metastatic BC [40, 72 - 75]. For BC, an increased CTC count during diagnosis of metastasis is considered to be a negative prognostic factor, and if the CTC count remains high, then the patients are most likely to progress under chemotherapy [30].

Another type of "liquid biopsy" that has been developed to evaluate cancer genetics is called circulating free tumor DNA (cfDNA) [30]. cfDNA could be originally from either nuclear or mitochondria [40]. Outcomes would be affected in cfDNA showing various mutations or posttranslational modifications are seen in the patients. Several cancer types have shown increased levels of cfDNA. Specifically, levels of nuclear cfDNA have also been shown to be associated with malignancy and tumor size [30, 76 - 78].

Gene Expression Profiles and BC Subtypes

Gene expression profiling has become a useful technique in patient care and management to classify tumors and patients according to the stage of the disease and prognosis [21]. The gene expression pattern and threshold of specific gene expression levels can quantify the risk of recurrence more accurately than the traditional method by identifying the tumors with more aggressive biology [41].

Traditional IHC techniques have discovered three subtypes of breast tumors that depict different biologic behaviors: hormone-receptor-positive, triple-negative, and Epidermal Receptor (HER) 2/neu-positive BCs. Human large-scale gene expression profile (GEP) research shown additional subtypes that include luminal BC (LBC) - A, LBC-B, LBC-C, HER2-enriched, claudin-low, triple-negative/basal-like, and normal breast-like. Different management approaches are required as per each specific type depending distinct natural histories of these subtypes [2, 41]. The various subtypes are linked to divergent recurrent genomic modifications. In Western countries, LBC is a highly found subtype that represents more than 60% of all diagnosed BC. These days clinical practices use attributes like estrogen receptor (ER), progesterone receptor (PR), HER2, and Ki67 expression to differentiate between LBC-A (ER+ and/or PR+, HER2-, low Ki67) from LBC-B (ER+ and/or PR+, HER2- or HER2+, high Ki67) and also to determine therapeutic options. LBC-B, as compared to LBC-A, displays a higher rate of early recurrence and worse prognosis. In LBC-B, the biomarkers that can select the most suitable (hormone- with or without chemo-) therapy still have to be confirmed and introduced into the clinic. Thus, it represents a subgroup for which the choice of the optimal therapy still represents a difficult task for the clinician. The triple-negative and HER2+ BC have more vigorous growth. The first stages of BC and *in-situ* lesions have the same molecular characteristics. To identify and aggressively treat (or remove) potentially malignant tumors early diagnosis could be very helpful [2].

Gene expression microarrays such as Affymetrix GeneChip (Affymetrix, Santa Clara, USA) or Illumina (Illumina Inc., San Diego, USA), can be used to define BC subtypes. Even clinical use of gene expression to direct therapeutic decisions: Mammaprint, Oncotype DX (Genomic Health Inc., USA), or PAM50 can describe various BC subtypes. However, at present, due to the high cost and limited availability, such methods are not commonly undertaken. Instead, a clinicopathologic determination of ER, PgR, and HER2 is often used as a simple approximation to determine this classification, and ultimately, this guides the treatment selection in clinical practices [15].

A relatively novel approach of Gene expression profiling is used to identify the genes which can be used as a molecular signature to predict prognosis and guide therapy. To generate molecular signatures, some other techniques like oligonucleotide arrays, cDNA, and multiplex polymerase chain reaction (PCR) or mRNA have been used [41]. Gene expression profiling along with bioinformatics help immensely to identify the culprit gene and the associated cellular pathways involved in cancer development and identify molecular targets for personalized medicine [21]. St Gallen International BC Consensus Conference (2013) has endorsed gene expression profiling for making adjuvant therapy decisions [42].

Nucleic Acid Biomarkers - DNA Sequencing

DNA sequencing is a common method that identifies genetic changes in candidate genes [21].

For many years first-generation sequencing has been in practice to find point mutation, small insertion, and deletions that involve dideoxy-sequencing of every exonic region of interest, which are commonly the mutated exons. But this method has low sensitivity to detect weak signals. There are also chances of contamination with non-cancerous material, and it requires a parallel test of fluorescence *in-situ* hybridization (FISH) for searching for somatic copy number modifications (SCNAS) to be performed. Further limitations are that both the approaches take a lot of time and need a large amount of tissue for testing [31].

The successive generations of DNA sequencing techniques have evolved and come into practice, which is quick, highly efficient, and highly sensitive to analyze many genes and detect multiple "mutational signatures" at a time in a tumor sample. Some of these newer techniques are mass-spectrometric genotyping, real-time PCR, and multiplexed PCR-based parallel "next-generation sequencing". These techniques are advantageous in terms of inspection of a lot of genes at the same time, detection of somatic mutations at low allele frequency, and also with the requirement of a small amount of sample. Though there is a disadvantage with the mass-spectrometric genotyping and real-time PCR that novel and rare mutations cannot be localized by these techniques and therefore need pre-specified mutations to detect properly, this can be overcome by amplification of the regions of interest with PCR followed by parallel sequencing with the next-generation techniques. For the detection of genomic rearrangements and SCNAS, FISH analysis must also be performed in parallel [31].

A small amount of tumor material suffices in next-generation sequencing techniques. They amplify the genomic regions of interest by means of a "hybrid-capture-based enrichment" technique, after which a massive parallel next-generation sequencing is performed, followed by computational analysis [31].

The next-generation sequencing technologies have catapulted revolutionized the process of identification of DNA sequence variants, which may be associated with the cancer process and also may have clinical and therapeutic significance. These Variants in the DNA sequence, small insertions, or deletions in genes may act as diagnostic markers, and they are gradually entering into clinical practice. Advancements in somatic DNA sequence analysis have facilitated studies from single gene to whole-genome analysis to detect DNA sequence variations in tumors [21].

Nucleic Acid Biomarkers - RNA Expression Profiling

Microarray techniques involving a panel of mRNAs that have more effective than the regular methodology of patient stratification based on histopathology biomarkers [21]. These multigene RNA profiling assays are preferred over standard clinical and pathologic markers because they can improve the prediction of outcomes. For example, in patients with ER-positive, HER2-negative early-stage BC who are receiving hormonal therapy with tamoxifen, the risk of distant metastases was quantified by developing a reverse transcriptase-polymerase chain reaction assay of a 21-gene panel, the Oncotype Dx. Based on the high recurrence score on this panel, it was predicted that these patients could benefit from the addition of chemotherapy to their treatment regime [28].

A limitation of these techniques is that it has to be ensured that the RNA preparations are intact with minimal degradation so that the tissue sample, either fresh or archived, can be effectively used to validate the biomarkers. Otherwise, alternative techniques such as gene measurement technologies, which are less sensitive to a slight reduction in the size of RNA, have to be followed [21].

Epigenetics

Epigenetic modifications such as DNA methylation and histone acetylation, which are aberrant chromatin-remodeling mechanisms, have been checked in tumor tissues that lead to a reduction in expression of tumor suppressor gene. A better understanding of these underlying processes might help in the identification of new biomarkers, which may help in therapy decision making as well as predicting the response to cancer chemotherapy. There are no therapeutic interventions that target these epigenetic changes. Clinical trials are being conducted to explore the therapeutic effects of histone deacetylase inhibitors, poly-ADP-ribosylation inhibitors and therapeutic effectiveness of intervening DNA methylation. They may bring novel tools and revolutionize the way cancer is treated with the addition of new options to classical chemotherapies. They may activate tumor suppressor genes or other key checkpoint genes and may help in the development of targeted therapies. Next-generation DNA sequencing provides an opportunity for whole-genome analysis and to find novel epigenetic alterations during DNA methylation. Larger panels of methylation biomarkers are being explored for disease detection and progression by means of higher throughput methods. From such studies, individual as well as panels of biomarkers are also identified which may act as potential tools in early disease detection and prediction of response to chemotherapy [21]. From such studies, for early detection and response to chemotherapy development of panels of biomarkers for individual cancers is being undertaken [21].

MicroRNA

Alterations in gene expression through epigenetic modifications and alterations in protein expression through post-translational changes may also occur due to changes in the expression of microRNAs (miRNAs) [21]. They are small non-coding RNA molecules consisting of 20-25 nucleotides, taking part, at the post-transcriptional level, in the regulation of gene expression associated with various cellular mechanisms including growth, differentiation, angiogenesis, migration, and cell death [43]. A single miRNA can regulate the levels of multiple genes and multiple signaling pathways. They may have different functions ranging from acting as oncogenes, known as oncomirs, tumor suppressor genes, pro-metastatic genes, known as metastasis, metastasis suppressor genes and producing resistance to therapies [44]. Epigenetic alterations repress the expression of miRNAs in cancers [45, 46]. Several studies also report that in cancer as compared to normal tissue, miRNAs are shown to be downregulated [47, 48]. The 6-8 nucleotide sequence at the 5′ end of the miRNA, known as the "seed" sequence, is the basic determinant for miRNA binding to mRNA. miRNAs may significantly influence target mRNA expression, *e.g.*, their expression is significantly reduced if there is any complementary sequence between the loaded miRNA and the seed region, they may be degraded or repressed at translation by miRNAs [49 - 52].

Microarray is an innovative technology that helps in the analysis and profiling of all known miRNAs similar to mRNA profiling [53]. More than 500 miRNAs in humans have been detected so far. They are often found in chromosomal clusters. In different cancers, there is a different expression of different miRNAs [47].

Several studies have shown various miRNA to have high levels in the blood and the tissues of BC patients. It is reported that miR-21, miR-155, miR-210, miR-29c, miR-196a, miR-213, miR-191, miR-203, miR-29b and miR-93 are significantly high in tumors as compared to normal patients, while miR-125b, miR-145, miR-100, miR-10b, Let-7a-2, miR-205, miR-497 and miR-193 are less expressed. Some miRNAs like miR-31 and miR-130b are reported to show both high and low levels [54].

The miRNome is a useful technology for the diagnosis and prediction of prognosis of cancer as it provides a better classification of cancer types than what is achieved with mRNA expression profile [47]. miRNAs are easily quantified in tissue matrix, whether it is normal or cancer tissue or body fluids in spite of their small size. Thus they can act as important biomarkers [55 - 58].

Prognostic miRNAs are important tools to predict the course of the disease and its outcome. Expression patterns of different miRNAs play a role in this, *e.g.*, expression of miR-148 and miR-210 correlates with shorter relapse-free-survival [31].

Predictive miRNAs are useful markers whose expression correlates well with the treatment response, *e.g.*, expression of miR-125b, miR99a, Let-7c is found to have a positive correlation with antiestrogen therapy. These biomarkers, thus help in treatment decision making process and selection of individualized treatment [31].

Microarray-based Multigene Assays

Oncotype DX®

Oncotype DX® (Genomic Health Inc, Redwood City, CA, USA) is a microarray-based multigene assay. It is extensively validated and widely used for outcome prediction in BC [31]. It has an advantage that it can be used in formalin-fixed tissue also [9]. It measures the expression of 21 genes, of which 16 are cancer-related prognostic/predictive, and 5 are reference genes. This measurement is done at the mRNA level utilizing reverse transcriptase PCR [59]. Based on the relative expression of the genes, a score called recurrence score (RS) is calculated. This RS divides the patients into three subgroups based on different risks associated with disease recurrence, *e.g.*, RS <18 indicates low risk, RS 18-30 indicates intermediate risk, and RS ≥30 indicates high risk. Oncotype DX® finds two main uses in BC; it predicts the probability of recurrence, and it identifies those patients who would get advantage from the use of adjuvant therapy [31]. Thus it helps in treatment decisions also [9].

MammaPrint™

MammaPrint™ (or the 70-gene signature) (Agendia, Amsterdam) is a useful tool to predict disease recurrence and guide treatment decisions in patients with BC. This is an extensively validated test that measures the expression of 70 genes by means of the microarray. These 70 genes are implied in all the important signs of cancer. According to the expression levels of these genes, the BC patients are divided into two groups such as low or high-risk for disease recurrence [31]. The clinical utility of MammaPrintTM was recently confirmed in a randomized clinical trial that involved 6692 newly diagnosed BC patients with 0 3 metastatic lymph nodes (MINDACT; EORTC 10041/BIG 3-04, NCT000433589) [59]. The Food and Drug Administration (FDA) first approved it for determining prognosis in patients with node-negative, stage I-II tumors measuring ≤5 cm and are under age 60 years. Later it was also approved for use in patients who are more than 60 years old. MammaPrintTM has been tested for paraffin-embedded material [9].

Prosigna®

The Prosigna® (previously known as PAM50) (NanoString Technologies Inc.) is a test to measure the mRNA level expression of fifty different genes [59]. Initially, RT-qPCR on paraffin-embedded tissue was used to design it. Prosigna® provides data on the intrinsic tumor subtype like Luminal A, Luminal B, HER2-enriched, or basal-like and helps in determining the 10-year risk of distant recurrence. Risk of Recurrence (ROR) are scored on a level of 0-100 and these are categorized as low (ROR score <40, less than 10% risk), intermediate (ROR score 40-60, 10-20% risk), or high (ROR score >60, over 20% risk of recurrence). Several studies have shown that the ROR score gives prognostic data much more than the standard clinical and pathological variables [9].

EndoPredict®

EndoPredict® (Sividon Diagnostics/Myriad) is another second-generation genomic classifier. It uses RT-PCR on paraffin-embedded tissue to test 12 genes: 8 cancer genes, three reference genes used for standardization, and one for genomic DNA level [9, 59]. It generated a comprehensive risk score called EPclin score by combining the expression levels of these 12 genes with lymph node status and tumor size [59]. It uses the scale of 0-15 and defines two classes which are based on the 10-year distant recurrence risk: low risk (score <3.4; overall risk of 6-8%) and high risk (score >3.4; overall risk of 15-22%) [9]. EndoPredict® has been shown to identify a section of patients who have a good long-term prognosis after five years of adjuvant endocrine therapy [59].

BC Index (BCI)

The BCI combines two independent biomarkers, HOXB13: IL17BR and the 5-gene molecular grade index. The distant metastasis risk after ten years of diagnosis is shown by BCI [79, 80]. Among ER-positive lymph node-negative disease, BCI provides novel unrelated prognosis information for both distant-recurrence and free survival (DRFS) [81, 82].

Genomic Grade Index (GGI)

The GGI, a 97 genes micro-array, reclassifies histological grade 2 (HG) patients into two groups: HG1-like or HG2-like. This approach enhances the accuracy and prognostic value of HG in ER-positive invasive breast carcinoma on a heterogeneous cohort [83]. High GGI tumors had a significantly more pathological complete response rate following neoadjuvant chemotherapy for both ER-positive [84] and negative [85], but very less data validating the robustness of GGI is present.

POSTGENOMIC ERA: PROTEOMICS

In the postgenomic era, the enormous amount of data obtained from fully sequenced genomes and co-expression of mRNAs opens a new way to study proteins on a bigger scale, which will greatly enhance our understanding of gene function. The large scale study of proteins is called proteomics, the discipline completely complementary to genomics. To determine links in studying genes and genomes, proteomics can be used. Alteration of the proteins, which are not visible in the DNA sequence, such as isoforms and posttranslational modifications, can be studied only by proteomic techniques. Active molecules in the cells are the main focus of proteomics. For this reason, proteomics directly relates to drug development, which is also of importance in cancer therapy and will eventually become even more important [60].

In BC biology and the other fields proteomics can be categorized into three main areas: (a) protein micro-characterization for large-scale identification and their posttranslational modifications, (b) "differential display" proteomics for comparison of protein levels with potential application in a wide range of diseases, and (c) studies of protein-protein interactions. Indeed, each protein interacts with other molecular partners and as a part of an extended network of these "partners". The area of early diagnostics will be the first application of proteomics that will probably benefit cancer. An ultimate goal in BC research is to develop a relatively easy diagnostic tool which will result in interpretable data in the early stages of pathological mechanism and is based on levels of protein expression to find the proteins that are differentially expressed in BC [60].

Proteomics in BC

Several abnormally regulated proteins and cellular pathways are involved in causing cancer. The proteomics method may be able to find protein-protein interactions, individual proteins, or even driver pathways, leading towards the development of clinical tests based on biomarkers and personalized clinical intervention to increase therapy success rate [61]. There is a high chance that these protein biomarkers can be made into clinical diagnostic tests. These protein biomarkers are often identified in basic science studies of cancer cells as overexpressed proteins. Cancer-specific alterations in proteins may occur at the level of protein abundance or post-translational protein modification such as glycosylation or phosphorylation [21].

For classification of BC, many different body fluids like tissue, serum, plasma, cerebrospinal fluid, urine, saliva, ascites, nipple fluid, and pleural fluid can be used as a matrix. The discovery of protein biomarkers can also be used to predict the patient's response to therapy and for subsequent prognosis. It uses less invasive diagnostic procedures as well as multiple easy sample collection techniques for circulating biomarkers, such as a serum, the blood compartment, enhances the clinical value of possible biomarkers [61]. High-throughput antibody arrays' technique has developed a panel of proteins whose levels are found to be significantly high in malignant breast tissue as compared to normal tissue. Such a panel included p53, MAP kinase 7, and casein kinase Ie and annexin [62].

Significant efforts in clinical proteomics have been made to discover novel BC biomarkers in women, still only a small number of markers such as uPA/PAI-1, circulating tumor cells, estrogen receptor (ER), progesterone receptor (PR), human epidermal growth factor receptor 2 (HER2), cancer antigen (CA)15-3 and CA27.29 have been applied in clinical practice [61].

There are two types of proteomic platforms: antibody-based such as enzyme-linked immunosorbent assay (ELISA), immunohistochemistry (IHC), protein microarray (chip), and western blotting (protein immunoblot) and other are not antibody-based approaches such as mass spectrometric (MS) [61].

The difficulty commonly encountered while establishing a clinical test is often at the level of assaying multiple protein analytes in a body fluid such as the serum, plasma, or urine by sandwich immunoassays and using antibody pairs. If only the post-translational modification of the biomarker protein, which is present in body fluid, is specific to cancer, then there is a considerable challenge associated with the development of antibody pairs to these proteins. Besides, there is also the issue of matrix complexity. There are several direct approaches, such as abundance or post-translational modifications, to identify cancer-specific changes in proteins. A combination of two-dimensional gel electrophoresis for the separation of the proteins alongside any potential methods for their visualization like direct radioactive labeling, fluorescent tags, and silver staining can be used for the identification of proteomic changes in cancer. For the sequence identification of each protein spot, mass spectrometric analysis can be used [21].

Proteomics techniques like nano-techniques are recently emerging to be promising that can beneficial over conventional techniques for the identification of potential biomarkers at the early stages of cancer. Thus, these techniques have to be standardized and applied on a larger scale to validate the potentially valuable biomarkers in cancer patients [63].

Some of the protein biomarkers and assay techniques have been described below.

Ki67

Ki67 is a nuclear nonhistone protein that is expressed during G1, S, and G2 phases of the cell cycle. It showed the highest expression levels during mitosis and no expression during the G0 phase [64]. To understand the proliferative action of BC, the most commonly used technique is the IHC assessment of Ki-67. To distinguish the risk groups in carcinomas positive for ER-alpha and PR, Ki67 can be very important [9].

Initially, the Ki67 antibody was applied only to fresh frozen tissue; however, later, many more antibodies that could be used in paraffin-embedded tissue were developed with MIB-1 (that use the same epitope as the original one) and are being used the most frequently. To determine the Ki67 expression levels, percent of tumor cell nuclei that are stained positive is calculated [30].

In early as well as locally advanced BC, baseline Ki67 can estimate the chemotherapy effect, whereas this is not possible under endocrine treatment. It is also reported that the post-neoadjuvant chemotherapy measurement of Ki67 is a high estimator for recurrence-free and overall survival. However, a high pretreatment score is associated with a high chance to achieve a complete pathological response, and this is a predictor of long-term outcome in these patients. The detection of changes in Ki67 also predicts for treatment benefits as well as Ki67 measurement, early on-treatment, is a superior predictor of long-term outcome than pretreatment expression [30].

Cyclin D

Over 50% of BC cases show overexpression of Cyclin D1 at the mRNA and protein levels. Out of all the cases, gene amplification is observed in around 15% cases. Cyclin D1 is known to regulate the proliferation of estrogen-responsive cells and has a strong positive correlation with ER and PR expression levels. In invasive BC cyclin D1 overexpression acts as a prognostic factor for a better outcome. Particularly among ER-positive patients, early relapse and poor prognosis is associated with amplification of cyclin D1 [30].

Cyclin E

Cyclin E acts as a positive regulator of cell cycle transition, which is similar to cyclin D1 and shows high protein expression levels and forms an enzymatic complex with CDK2 in the G1 phase. Several BC lines have shown expression of Cyclin E gene amplification. The role of cyclin E in tumorigenesis is also supported by strong evidence. Post-translational cleavage results in alteration of full-length protein give rise to hyperactive low molecular weight forms. These are correlated to the increasing stage and grade of BC and are uniquely detectable in tumor cells. The increased levels of cyclin E in the cell cycle are suggestive of alteration of response to chemo and endocrine therapy. It has been reported that altered levels increase the sensitivity of BC cells to cisplatin and paclitaxel effect; however, it also facilitates the resistance to anti-estrogens [30].

Carcinoembryonic Antigen (CEA)

CEA is an oncofetal glycoprotein formed during fetal gut development [21, 65]. CEA is a normal cell product and is highly expressed in adenocarcinomas, mainly of the colon, rectum, breast, pancreas, and lung [65]. CEA-related cell adhesion molecule 6 (CEACAM6) is a multifunctional regulatory protein. It shows overexpression in various cell processes associated with cancer. Atypical ductal hyperplasia's CEACAM6 expression has been suggested to play an important function during breast cancer development. Also, in invasive and treatment-resistant breast cancer CEACAM6 has been shown to play a role [39].

uPA and PAI-1 [PROTEOMICS]

Although not widely used, Urokinase plasminogen activator (uPA) and its inhibitor, PAI-1 is currently among the best validated prognostic biomarkers for BC [59], which uses ELISA to measure the two proteins in fresh tissue extract or freshly frozen BC. Patients reported with high expression of these two proteins are usually found to have a worse outcome than those with low levels [31]. High levels of these two proteins also correlate well with adverse outcomes in patients with newly diagnosed invasive BC. They are also reported to be independent of each other [59].

The measurement of uPA and PAI-1 may prove to be cost-effective to treatment by helping therapy decision making with either elimination or decreasing the administration of adjuvant chemotherapy and determining prognosis. Therefore, their measurement is now widely recommended, particularly in lymph node-negative BC patients [31].

Mammostrat®

The Mammostrat® test is an IHC five-protein assay. Increased Mammostrat scores correlate with lower distant-recurrence free survival (DRFS) and overall survival (OS) for ER-positive early BC despite adjuvant treatment. The impact of Mammostrat on BC outcomes also has been reported in lymph node-positive and ER-negative disease [86, 87]. The recurrence-free-survival (RFS) has also been reported to be improved for Mammostrat® high-risk patients with the addition of chemotherapy to endocrine treatment [88].

IHC4

The IHC4 prognostic score is based on four widely measured IHC markers (ER, progesterone receptor (PgR), HER2, and Ki-67) using formalin-fixed paraffin-embedded tumor samples. ATAC trial cohort of ER-positive early BC was used for the creation and validation of IHC markers as a prognosis factor. This inexpensive biomarker, for which three of four measures are routinely performed, could be as informative as OncotypeDx®. However, these results can only be obtained by standardized procedures because of the lack of reproducibility of IHC [89].

dtectDx™ Breast Serum Biomarker Test

Five serum biomarkers, including IL-8, IL-12, VEGF, CEA, and HGF, were analyzed *via* ELIZA for dtectDx™ Breast (Provista Diagnostics) serum biomarker test. A value of normal or elevated risk is generated by combining the patient characteristics in an algorithm [28].

Mass Spectrometry-based Protein Profiling Studies

The primary aim of mass spectrometry-based protein profiling research in BC is to find new diagnostic biomarkers. Palacios *et al*. confirmed the molecular genotypic classification that is based on BRCA1/2 using a protein-based study with 37 protein biomarkers. A correlation has been found in cell cycle regulators, D-type cyclins (D1, D3), and CDK4 with BRCA2 cancers. However, ER/HER-2 negativity, rapid growth, and ubiquitous basal phenotype are found to be correlated to BRCA1 cancers. The proteins EMP1, DVL1, DDR1, PRKC1, and E-cadherin were identified as biomarkers through the characterization of lobular and ductal cancers [66].

Using cell type and signal pathway protein biomarkers, five molecular subtypes of ER-positive BC have been found. Luminal A, luminal B, basal, HER-2 overexpression, and normal are these four subtypes. Together with the pathological features of BC, 97 biomarker proteins have been found. These include ER, PR, p53, CK5/6, HER-2m CK8/18, Ki-67, BCL2, cyclin D1, cyclin E, E-cadherin and many other markers [66].

The high heterogeneity in cells of full tumor tissue specimens is complicated because of searching for tumor-originating proteins. However, aiding this search with laser capture micro-dissection (LCM) will allow the selective capturing of specific cell subsets [66].

Chaperons

The identification of molecular chaperone 14-3-3σ facilitated the discovery of signaling proteins that are regulated in cancer cells. Seven greatly conserved isoforms form a family of 14-3-3 proteins. These proteins have a molecular weight of around 25-30 kDa. They regulate cell cycle machinery of various important key points. Also, they appear to be linked, directly or indirectly, with signaling proteins, including IGF-1 receptor, Raf, MEK kinases and PI3-kinase. Though, there is a lack of understanding about molecular mechanisms involved in inhibition or activation of these elements. Several studies have shown that the sub-regulation of the 14-3-3σ protein in BC, which suggests that it could be involved in tumor suppression [66].

High expression levels of the α-B-crystallin (Hsp5) and Hsp27 molecules in breast tumor tissues have been reported. Chaperones can reduce accumulated stress, unfolding, and aggregation of the recently formed protein. Their expression has significantly implicated in cell growth. Since high levels of α-B-crystallin proteins were seen in *in-situ* ductal carcinoma, it is suggested that it can be used as a target for altering apoptotic pathways. It is also found that α-B-crystallin could be enough for cancer transformation. It starts EGF and anchorage-independent growth, enhances cell migration and invasion, and constitutively activates the MAPK kinase/ERK (MEK/ERK) pathway. This suggests the role of α---crystallin as a new oncoprotein. Furthermore, these types of chaperones can play a significant role in the process of carcinogenesis as well as act as potential diagnostic markers [66].

Antibody Microarray

Immunoassays such as antibody microarrays resembling highly parallel ELISAs using matrices such as a serum, plasma, urine, liquified extracts of tumor tissue help in multianalyte protein detection, which may in turn help in the testing of prognostic biomarkers or potential therapeutic targets [21].

Cancer Autoantibodies

Overexpressed or mutant tumor proteins lead to production of autoantibodies in the serum of cancer patients. But their sensitivity for cancer diagnosis is very low, *e.g.*, autoantibodies to HER2 protein are detected in only 5-10% of BC patients. These autoantibodies also lack specificity for cancer diagnosis, *e.g.*, autoantibodies to MUC1 have been detected in the sera of women with benign breast disease, invasive BC at an early and advanced stage, as well as in patients with other cancers. Novel technologies such as serologic identification of antigens by recombinant expression (SEREX) technology, higher throughput tumor antigen cloning, *etc.*, assess the autoantigens to discover the autoantibodies [21]. Nonetheless, these autoantibodies and autoantigen detection employing advanced technologies have the potential to play a role in cancer diagnosis, and further research is required on this.

METABOLITES AND METABOLOMICS

The interaction between intracellular pathways and their microenvironment creates metabolites [67]. Metabolomics is the comprehensive analysis of molecules called metabolites, which are produced by various cellular processes. In general, metabolomics uses a variety of analytical tools to understand the chemical profile of metabolites. It employs gas chromatography (GC), high-performance liquid chromatography (HPLC) and capillary electrophoresis for separation of molecules and mass spectroscopy (MS) and nuclear magnetic resonance spectroscopy (NMR) for detection and identification [21]. MS can be coupled with liquid chromatography (LC-MS) or gas chromatography (GC-MS), as well as to NMR [67]. Anyone analytical method does not have the potential to describe the human metabolome. More than 2000 metabolites can be measured using today's technologies. These are only a small number of promising molecular targets as compared to those that are identified by genomics, transcriptomics or proteomics. Tumor staging and stratification can be classified using metabolic patterns and biomarkers that have been developed for BC [21].

The field of metabolomics is still in its infancy and has not yet been applied to clinical practice. It has the potential to provide fast access and easy measure of analytes for the characterization of cancers. This potential can be very beneficial in early recognition and prognostication of BC [99, 100]. The changes in various pathways like glycolysis, apoptotic mechanism, and phosphor-metabolic processes are very well studied and understood. These changes can occur during carcinogenic progression and can also change the metabolic profile of adenine nucleotide and could lead to the discovery of various biomarkers [101, 102]. The integration of other omics with metabolomics technology may provide a more specific classification for alterations that are specific to cancer stage, grade, response to therapy, and prognosis [103 - 106].

Metabolomic analysis can be used for early disease detection, nutritional trials, toxicity analysis, and evaluation of drug action, treatment response, and studying the emergence of resistance to chemotherapy. Metabolomics also enhances the understanding of the detection or drug response of BC. It can be used in the interpretation of molecular measures with the use of computational models that can lead to a clinically relevant result. To understand the biochemical processes that happen at the time of BC diagnosis, metabolite profiling could be very useful [67].

Metabolomics could be targeted and untargeted in their approaches. Targeted metabolomics is based on the identification of a metabolite or a pathway, which is based on an already documented connection between a given metabolite or pathways in the metabolomic composition of a studied sample. However, the untargeted method identifies and quantifies the highest number of metabolites present in a sample [67].

Metabolic Profile of BC

As different factors contribute to clonal evolution, it leads to cancer progression. Also, alongside metabolic reprogramming of cells and adjacent stroma can speed up the process of cancer development. The metabolism of cancer cells can be affected by changes in metabolites of biosynthetic pathway networks. These metabolic changes can be triggered through various processes like tumor growth, tissue remodeling, changes in cell survival, and metastasis. The production of metabolites changes when tumor cells show altered metabolism, which results in a signature capable of characterizing the presence or even the behavior of cancer. The metabolomic profile can also be altered by the surrounding stroma and immune response. It also provides more data about tumor growth and the effect of treatment. The metabolites found in BC cells are different from that of normal epithelial cells of the breast. Moreover, the metabolic profile of drug-sensitive BC cells differs from that of resistant ones. Therefore, for a better understanding of changes in metabolism that could promote carcinogenesis a metabolic pathway analysis is a must [67].

BC cells show increased consumption of glucose, which is linked to activated oncogenes (RAS and MYC) and mutant tumor suppressors (TP53) [67]. But this glucose usage in tumors does not lead to the production of excess NADH for subsequent oxidative phosphorylation in mitochondria for the production of ATP, but instead, lactate accumulates, even when enough oxygen is present for mitochondrial respiration [13]. As lactate mimics physiological mechanisms of the high anaerobic state, it also acts as a source of energy and in molecular signaling of BC cells. Another study reports that lactate levels are inversely correlated with tumor size in patients with early BC. It is difficult to understand the lactate circuit because of the high complexity of a tumor microenvironment and its interconnections between different cell types [67]. In tumor cells, glucose is not used for the production of NADH and ATP. In tumor cells, it is biosynthetic pathways that are activated and lead to the accumulation of building blocks for biopolymers such as glycerol-3-phosphate and, more importantly, NADPH production *via* the pentose phosphate pathway that sustains rapid cell growth. NADPH is required in fatty acid biosynthesis, and with increased biosynthesis of lipids, there is also marked by the accumulation of cholines. However, it is noted that studies in cancer cell lines under normal oxygen levels might lead to false interpretations, and therefore to understand metabolic regulation, a high consideration must be used to mimic *in vivo* tumor microenvironments [13].

A comparative serum analysis study in BC patients and healthy controls showed increased glycolysis, lipogenesis, and the production of volatile organic metabolites compared with healthy women [67].

Studies on different amino acid estimation also elicit useful information. It is suggested that amino acids are consumed during tumor development. Among the amino acids, Glutamine is considered one of the main amino acids involved in tumor development. Patients with early-stage cancer have decreased glutamate levels. However, in women with metastatic cancer, serum glutamine levels are found to be decreased [67]. The glutamic acid/glutamine ratio is significantly correlated with ER status and tumor grade [68]. An *in vivo* study on glutamine and its transporters showed an up-regulated expression of inositol 1, 4, 5-trisphosphate receptors (IP3R) in many BC patients. An increase in lipoprotein content and levels of metabolites such as lactate, lysine, and alanine, and a decrease in serum pyruvate and glucose levels, were also observed in patients who presented with high IP3R levels compared with healthy individuals.

Similarly, Glycine biosynthetic pathway is found to be highly correlated with fast proliferating BC cells. Glycine consumption is required for cancer cell proliferation and is associated with worse prognosis in BC patients. Studies on aspartate show low plasma levels of aspartate and higher levels in lesional tissues in patients with primary BC, which is due to the increased tumor aspartate utilization. Circulating aspartate is a key metabolite characteristic of human BC. Patients with early-stage cancer are found to have increased serum levels of choline, tyrosine, valine, lactate, isoleucine [67]. Variations in plasma concentrations of glucose, lactate, pyruvate, alanine, leucine, isoleucine, glutamate, glutamine, lysine, glycine, proline, N-acetyl cysteine, threonine, tyrosine, phenylalanine, acetate, acetoacetate, β hydroxybutyrate, urea, creatine, and creatinine have also been reported in patients with early or metastatic BC [67, 68].

Studies on lipid profiles in BC showed that tumor grade and ER status affect the lipid profiles most radically, of which highest changes are seen in phospholipids containing major (C16:0 fatty acids, where 16 is the number of carbon atoms and 0 is the number of double bonds) or minor (C14:0 and C18:0 fatty acids) products of the fatty acid synthase (FASN) enzyme. An association between poor survi survival of the patients and increased levels of several related phospholipids has been shown. Both ER status and grade independently affect the same lipids. Also, ER-negative grade 3 tumors have been shown to have the highest levels [13]. Another study on metabolomic analysis of serum lipoproteins in females with newly diagnosed invasive BC at stages I and II showed a positive association between lipoproteins and ER expression, an inverse association between subfractions of high-density lipoprotein and Ki67 and a positive association between low-density lipoproteins with nodal metastasis. So, it may be possible to establish an association between the aggressiveness and prognosis of BC based on subfractions of lipoproteins [67]. Low values of lipids are also reported as a biomarker in metastatic BC [68].

Glycerol-3-phosphate acyltransferase (GPAM) is an enzyme that plays an important role in the biosynthesis of triacylglycerols and phospholipids. Since Expression phospholipids are an important and major component of all cell membranes, the role of GPAM in malignancies is very interesting to the scientist. IHC analysis shows differential expression of GPAM in malignant breast tumors and the levels of its substrate 'sn-glycerol-3-phosphate' are higher in BC than in normal breast tissue. There is also a significant correlation between high cytoplasmic GPAM expression with negative hormone receptor status and better overall patient survival. The metabolomic analysis shows that GPAM expression is associated with increased levels of phospholipids, particularly phosphatidylcholines. In BC, the level of phospholipids is affected more by GPAM as compared to those of triglycerides. The effects of GPAM is independent of those associated with ER status and tumor grade. At least in the context of BC, it implies that the function of GPAM is more involved in phospholipid production rather than in triglyceride synthesis [13, 68].

Taurine and choline-containing compounds are elevated in BC tissue as compared to benign tissue [67]. Various studies have reported alterations in choline metabolism in BC, and these metabolites have been used for classifying tumor types [13]. Increased levels of taurine, glycerophosphocholine, and creatine, and low levels of glycine and phosphocholine were found after five years of surgery in the malignant tissues of healthy patients [67].

Changes in mobile lipid droplets have been observed. It is thought that either the accumulation of lipids in cytosolic vesicles or the formation of microdomains in the cell membrane represents these mobile lipid droplets. However, distinct processes might lead to changes in these mobile lipids.For example, in glioma, selective accumulation of polyunsaturated lipids compared with saturated lipids appears to be distinct to apoptosis rather than necrosis [13].

Urine, as an end product of metabolic processes, is closely linked to clinical phenotypes and has been used in modern metabolomics. Several metabolites have been reported as potential biomarkers for BC, including amino acids such as elevated tryptophan and signs of protein degradation, organic acids, and nucleosides. Biomarkers such as dimethylarginine, tryptophan, phenylalanine, pantothenic acid, succinyladenosine, dimethylguanosine, apronal, threonyl carbamoyl adenosine, kynurenic acid, nicotinuric acid, and indole acetic acid have been identified in the urine samples of BC patients. Several of those are linked to tryptophan (phenylalanine, indoleacetic acid and kynurenic acid). Biomarkers such as s-adenosyl-homocysteine, homovanillate, 4-hydroxy-phenylacetate, five hydroxy indole acetate, 5-hydroxymethyl-2-deoxyuridine and 8-hydroxy-2-deoxyguanosine are also found to have potential value in BC. Urine analysis of early- and late-stage BCs also showed different metabolic profiles about tricarboxylic acid cycle intermediates, metabolites relating to energy metabolism, amino acids and gut microbial metabolites [68].

Metabolomics and BC Chemoresistance

In-vitro cell line (MCF-7) studies demonstrated that glycolysis, as well as the production of lactates and ATP, are associated with resistance to adriamycin. Thus, a therapeutic target for chemoresistant cells may be due to the regulation of sulfur amino acid metabolism [69].

In another *in-vitro* study (with MCF-7 cell line), it was observed that adriamycin deaccelerated several metabolic pathways, including purine, pyrimidine, glutathione, and glycolysis routes. It also was shown to increase oxidative stress. These findings suggest that to evaluate antitumor effects and investigate antitumor candidate agents, it is important to apply cellular metabolomics and the measure metabolic markers quantitatively [70].

In an *in vitro* study with MCF-7 cells exposed to ascididemine, it was observed that there was an increase in citrate, gluconate, and polyunsaturated fatty acids and a decrease in glycerophosphocholine and ethanolamine associated with severe oxidative stress. Thus, central metabolic changes in BC cells might be due to high oxidative stress [71].

SUMMARY AND CONCLUSION

BC is a heterogeneous entity with different subtypes having different molecular profiles, biologic behavior, and risk profiles. Over the years, many prognostic and predictive biomarkers for BC have been discovered, which may help to provide individualized therapies and efficient treatment. Studies on gene expression profile, sequencing, and high-throughput analyses can identify the gene or the pathway involved in each tumor. Currently, researches are focusing on DNA mutation, ctDNA, miRNAs, and CTCs, intending to identify new prognostic and predictive biomarkers. Along with the genetic studies, proteomic studies have also gained pace in recent times and have shown promising results from the point of view of early BC diagnosis, follow up and therapeutic predictive markers. Metabolomic analyses incorporating techniques such as GC-MS, LC-MS and NMR spectroscopy provide valuable information that can be integrated with proteomic and transcriptomic data. These genetic, proteomic and metabolomic studies will provide new insights into the pathogenesis of BC, disease progression, chemoresistance, recurrence, and metastasis. This will lead to better patient management through improved molecular diagnostics and individualized treatment.

CONSENT FOR PUBLICATION

Not applicable.

CONFLICT OF INTEREST

The authors confirm that the contents of this chapter have no conflict of interest.

ACKNOWLEDGEMENTS

I would like to thank Ruchi Jhonsa for help with graphic design.

REFERENCES

[1]   Siegel R, Ma J, Zou Z, Jemal A. Cancer statistics, 2014. CA Cancer J Clin 2014; 64(1): 9-29.
      [http://dx.doi.org/10.3322/caac.21208] [PMID: 24399786]

[2]   Baldassarre G, Belletti B. Molecular biology of breast tumors and prognosis [version 1; referees: 3 approved]. F1000Research 2016; 711.

[3]   Siegel RL, Miller KD, Jemal A. Cancer statistics, 2018. CA Cancer J Clin 2018; 68(1): 7-30.
      [http://dx.doi.org/10.3322/caac.21442] [PMID: 29313949]

[4]   Hagemann IS. Molecular testing in breast cancer a guide to current practices. Arch Pathol Lab Med 2016; 140(8): 815-24.
      [http://dx.doi.org/10.5858/arpa.2016-0051-RA] [PMID: 27472240]

[5]   Baskın Y, Yiğitbaşı T. Clinical proteomics of breast cancer. Curr Genomics 2010; 11(7): 528-36.
        [http://dx.doi.org/10.2174/138920210793175930] [PMID: 21532837]

[6]   Rosa M. Advances in the molecular analysis of breast cancer: pathway toward personalized medicine.
        Cancer Contr 2015; 22(2): 211-9.
        [http://dx.doi.org/10.1177/107327481502200213] [PMID: 26068767]

[7]   Weigelt B, Peterse JL, van 't Veer LJ. Breast cancer metastasis: markers and models. Nat Rev Cancer
        2005; 5(8): 591-602.
        [http://dx.doi.org/10.1038/nrc1670] [PMID: 16056258]

[8]   Ulaner GA, Riedl CC, Dickler MN, Jhaveri K, Pandit-Taskar N, Weber W. Molecular imaging of
        biomarkers in breast cancer. J Nucl Med 2016; 57 (Suppl. 1): 53S-9S.
        [http://dx.doi.org/10.2967/jnumed.115.157909] [PMID: 26834103]

[9]   Colomer R, Aranda-López I, Albanell J, *et al.* Biomarkers in breast cancer: a consensus statement by
        the Spanish Society of Medical Oncology and the Spanish Society of Pathology. Clin Transl Oncol
        2018; 20(7): 815-26.
        [http://dx.doi.org/10.1007/s12094-017-1800-5] [PMID: 29273958]

[10]   de la Mare JA, Contu L, Hunter MC, *et al.* Breast cancer: current developments in molecular
        approaches to diagnosis and treatment. Recent Patents Anticancer Drug Discov 2014; 9(2): 153-75.
        [http://dx.doi.org/10.2174/15748928113086660046] [PMID: 24171821]

[11]   Walsh MF, Nathanson KL, Couch FJ, Offit K. Genomic biomarkers for breast cancer risk. Adv Exp
        Med Biol 2016; 882: 1-32.
        [http://dx.doi.org/10.1007/978-3-319-22909-6_1] [PMID: 26987529]

[12]   Baskin Y. Changes in concepts of the technological progress: personalized medicine. Turk Bull Hyg
        Exp Biol 2007; 64: 41-8.

[13]   Denkert C, Bucher E, Hilvo M, *et al.* Metabolomics of human breast cancer: new approaches for
        tumor typing and biomarker discovery. Genome Med 2012; 4(4): 37.
        [http://dx.doi.org/10.1186/gm336] [PMID: 22546809]

[14]   Lindon JC, Holmes E, Nicholson JK. Metabonomics and its role in drug development and disease
        diagnosis. Expert Rev Mol Diagn 2004; 4(2): 189-99.
        [http://dx.doi.org/10.1586/14737159.4.2.189] [PMID: 14995905]

[15]   Di Leo A, Curigliano G, Diéras V, *et al.* New approaches for improving outcomes in breast cancer in
        Europe. Breast 2015; 24(4): 321-30.
        [http://dx.doi.org/10.1016/j.breast.2015.03.001] [PMID: 25840656]

[16]   Wang D, Xu J, Shi G, Yin G. Molecular markers' progress of breast cancer treatment efficacy. J
        Cancer Res Ther 2015; 11(5) (Suppl. 1): C11-5.
        [http://dx.doi.org/10.4103/0973-1482.191619] [PMID: 26323906]

[17]   Henry NL, Hayes DF. Cancer biomarkers. Mol Oncol 2012; 6(2): 140-6.
        [http://dx.doi.org/10.1016/j.molonc.2012.01.010] [PMID: 22356776]

[18]   Strimbu K, Tavel JA. What are biomarkers? Curr Opin HIV AIDS 2010; 5(6): 463-6.
        [http://dx.doi.org/10.1097/COH.0b013e32833ed177] [PMID: 20978388]

[19]   Weaver O, Leung JWT. Biomarkers and imaging of breast cancer. AJR Am J Roentgenol 2018;
        210(2): 271-8.
        [http://dx.doi.org/10.2214/AJR.17.18708] [PMID: 29166151]

[20]   Cracowski JL. Towards prognostic biomarkers in pulmonary arterial hypertension. Eur Respir J 2012;
        39(4): 799-801.
        [http://dx.doi.org/10.1183/09031936.00155411] [PMID: 22467720]

[21]   Tainsky MA. Genomic and proteomic biomarkers for cancer: a multitude of opportunities. Biochim
        Biophys Acta 2009; 1796(2): 176-93.

[PMID: 19406210]

[22]   Leary RJ, Kinde I, Diehl F, *et al*. Development of personalized tumor biomarkers using massively parallel sequencing. Sci Transl Med 2010; 2(20): 20ra14.
[http://dx.doi.org/10.1126/scitranslmed.3000702] [PMID: 20371490]

[23]   Dos Anjos Pultz B, da Luz FAC, de Faria PR, Oliveira AP, de Araújo RA, Silva MJ. Far beyond the usual biomarkers in breast cancer: a review. J Cancer 2014; 5(7): 559-71.
[http://dx.doi.org/10.7150/jca.8925] [PMID: 25057307]

[24]   Sana M, Malik HJ. Current and emerging breast cancer biomarkers. J Cancer Res Ther 2015; 11(3): 508-13.
[http://dx.doi.org/10.4103/0973-1482.163698] [PMID: 26458575]

[25]   Hayes DF, Bast RC, Desch CE, *et al*. Tumor marker utility grading system: a framework to evaluate clinical utility of tumor markers. J Natl Cancer Inst 1996; 88(20): 1456-66.
[http://dx.doi.org/10.1093/jnci/88.20.1456] [PMID: 8841020]

[26]   Harris L, Fritsche H, Mennel R, *et al*. American Society of Clinical Oncology 2007 update of recommendations for the use of tumor markers in breast cancer. J Clin Oncol 2007; 25(33): 5287-312.
[http://dx.doi.org/10.1200/JCO.2007.14.2364] [PMID: 17954709]

[27]   McShane LM, Altman DG, Sauerbrei W, Taube SE, Gion M, Clark GM. Reporting recommendations for tumor marker prognostic studies. J Clin Oncol 2005; 23(36): 9067-72.
[http://dx.doi.org/10.1200/JCO.2004.01.0454] [PMID: 16172462]

[28]   Hollingsworth AB, Reese DE. Potential use of biomarkers to augment clinical decisions for the early detection of breast cancer. Oncol Hematol Rev 2014; 10(2): 103-9.
[http://dx.doi.org/10.17925/OHR.2014.10.2.103]

[29]   Kamel HFM, Al-Amodi HSB. AbdElmoneim HM Molecular fingerprints and biomarkers of breast cancer. Intechopen 2017; pp. 343-56.

[30]   Weigel MT, Dowsett M. Current and emerging biomarkers in breast cancer: prognosis and prediction. Endocr Relat Cancer 2010; 17(4): R245-62.
[http://dx.doi.org/10.1677/ERC-10-0136] [PMID: 20647302]

[31]   Nicolini A, Ferrari P, Duffy MJ. Prognostic and predictive biomarkers in breast cancer: Past, present and future. Semin Cancer Biol 2018; 52(Pt 1): 56-73.
[http://dx.doi.org/10.1016/j.semcancer.2017.08.010] [PMID: 28882552]

[32]   Viale G, Regan MM, Maiorano E, *et al*. Prognostic and predictive value of centrally reviewed expression of estrogen and progesterone receptors in a randomized trial comparing letrozole and tamoxifen adjuvant therapy for postmenopausal early breast cancer: BIG 1-98. J Clin Oncol 2007; 25(25): 3846-52.
[http://dx.doi.org/10.1200/JCO.2007.11.9453] [PMID: 17679725]

[33]   Wolff AC, Hammond ME, Schwartz JN, *et al*. American Society of Clinical Oncology/College of American Pathologists guideline recommendations for human epidermal growth factor receptor 2 testing in breast cancer. J Clin Oncol 2007; 25(1): 118-45.
[http://dx.doi.org/10.1200/JCO.2006.09.2775] [PMID: 17159189]

[34]   Aloraifi F, Boland MR, Green AJ, Geraghty JG. Gene analysis techniques and susceptibility gene discovery in non-BRCA1/BRCA2 familial breast cancer. Surg Oncol 2015; 24(2): 100-9.
[http://dx.doi.org/10.1016/j.suronc.2015.04.003] [PMID: 25936246]

[35]   Ross JS, Linette GP, Stec J, *et al*. Breast cancer biomarkers and molecular medicine. Expert Rev Mol Diagn 2003; 3(5): 573-85.
[http://dx.doi.org/10.1586/14737159.3.5.573] [PMID: 14510178]

[36]   Pavelić K, Gall-Troselj K. Recent advances in molecular genetics of breast cancer. J Mol Med (Berl) 2001; 79(10): 566-73.
[http://dx.doi.org/10.1007/s001090100256] [PMID: 11692153]

[37]   Hisada M, Garber JE, Fung CY, Fraumeni JF Jr, Li FP. Multiple primary cancers in families with Li-Fraumeni syndrome. J Natl Cancer Inst 1998; 90(8): 606-11.
[http://dx.doi.org/10.1093/jnci/90.8.606] [PMID: 9554443]

[38]   German S, Aslam HM, Saleem S, *et al.* Carcinogenesis of PIK3CA. Hered Cancer Clin Pract 2013; 11(1): 5.
[http://dx.doi.org/10.1186/1897-4287-11-5] [PMID: 23768168]

[39]   Kutomi G, Mizuguchi T, Satomi F, *et al.* Current status of the prognostic molecular biomarkers in breast cancer: A systematic review. Oncol Lett 2017; 13(3): 1491-8. [Review].
[http://dx.doi.org/10.3892/ol.2017.5609] [PMID: 28454281]

[40]   Le Du F, Ueno NT, Gonzalez-Angulo AM. Breast cancer biomarkers: utility in clinical practice. Curr Breast Cancer Rep 2013; 5(4): 1-16.
[http://dx.doi.org/10.1007/s12609-013-0125-9] [PMID: 24416469]

[41]   Kittaneh M, Montero AJ, Glück S. Molecular profiling for breast cancer: a comprehensive review. Biomark Cancer 2013; 5: 61-70.
[http://dx.doi.org/10.4137/BIC.S9455] [PMID: 24250234]

[42]   Goldhirsch A, Winer EP, Coates AS, *et al.* Personalizing the treatment of women with early breast cancer: highlights of the St Gallen International Expert Consensus on the Primary Therapy of Early Breast Cancer 2013. Ann Oncol 2013; 24(9): 2206-23.
[http://dx.doi.org/10.1093/annonc/mdt303] [PMID: 23917950]

[43]   Herranz H, Cohen SM. MicroRNAs and gene regulatory networks: managing the impact of noise in biological systems. Genes Dev 2010; 24(13): 1339-44.
[http://dx.doi.org/10.1101/gad.1937010] [PMID: 20595229]

[44]   van Schooneveld E, Wildiers H, Vergote I, *et al.* Dysregulation of microRNAs in breast cancer and their potential role as prognostic and predictive biomarkers in patient management. Breast Cancer Res 2015; 18: 17.21
[http://dx.doi.org/10.1186/s13058-015-0526-y]

[45]   Lehmann U, Hasemeier B, Christgen M, *et al.* Epigenetic inactivation of microRNA gene hsa-mir-9-1 in human breast cancer. J Pathol 2008; 214(1): 17-24.
[http://dx.doi.org/10.1002/path.2251] [PMID: 17948228]

[46]   Lujambio A, Calin GA, Villanueva A, *et al.* A microRNA DNA methylation signature for human cancer metastasis. Proc Natl Acad Sci USA 2008; 105(36): 13556-61.
[http://dx.doi.org/10.1073/pnas.0803055105] [PMID: 18768788]

[47]   Calin GA, Liu CG, Sevignani C, *et al.* MicroRNA profiling reveals distinct signatures in B cell chronic lymphocytic leukemias. Proc Natl Acad Sci USA 2004; 101(32): 11755-60.
[http://dx.doi.org/10.1073/pnas.0404432101] [PMID: 15284443]

[48]   Porkka KP, Pfeiffer MJ, Waltering KK, Vessella RL, Tammela TL, Visakorpi T. MicroRNA expression profiling in prostate cancer. Cancer Res 2007; 67(13): 6130-5.
[http://dx.doi.org/10.1158/0008-5472.CAN-07-0533] [PMID: 17616669]

[49]   Czech B, Hannon GJ. Small RNA sorting: matchmaking for Argonautes. Nat Rev Genet 2011; 12(1): 19-31.
[http://dx.doi.org/10.1038/nrg2916] [PMID: 21116305]

[50]   Ørom UA, Nielsen FC, Lund AH. MicroRNA-10a binds the 5'UTR of ribosomal protein mRNAs and enhances their translation. Mol Cell 2008; 30(4): 460-71.
[http://dx.doi.org/10.1016/j.molcel.2008.05.001] [PMID: 18498749]

[51]   Qin W, Shi Y, Zhao B, *et al.* miR-24 regulates apoptosis by targeting the open reading frame (ORF) region of FAF1 in cancer cells. PLoS One 2010; 5(2): e9429.
[http://dx.doi.org/10.1371/journal.pone.0009429] [PMID: 20195546]

[52]   Bertoli G, Cava C, Castiglioni I. MicroRNAs: new biomarkers for diagnosis, prognosis, therapy prediction and therapeutic tools for breast cancer. Theranostics 2015; 5(10): 1122-43.
[http://dx.doi.org/10.7150/thno.11543] [PMID: 26199650]

[53]   Borchert GM, Lanier W, Davidson BL. RNA polymerase III transcribes human microRNAs. Nat Struct Mol Biol 2006; 13(12): 1097-101.
[http://dx.doi.org/10.1038/nsmb1167] [PMID: 17099701]

[54]   Andorfer CA, Necela BM, Thompson EA, Perez EA. MicroRNA signatures: clinical biomarkers for the diagnosis and treatment of breast cancer. Trends Mol Med 2011; 17(6): 313-9.
[http://dx.doi.org/10.1016/j.molmed.2011.01.006] [PMID: 21376668]

[55]   Gilad S, Meiri E, Yogev Y, *et al.* Serum microRNAs are promising novel biomarkers. PLoS One 2008; 3(9): e3148.
[http://dx.doi.org/10.1371/journal.pone.0003148] [PMID: 18773077]

[56]   Chen X, Ba Y, Ma L, *et al.* Characterization of microRNAs in serum: a novel class of biomarkers for diagnosis of cancer and other diseases. Cell Res 2008; 18(10): 997-1006.
[http://dx.doi.org/10.1038/cr.2008.282] [PMID: 18766170]

[57]   Mitchell PS, Parkin RK, Kroh EM, *et al.* Circulating microRNAs as stable blood-based markers for cancer detection. Proc Natl Acad Sci USA 2008; 105(30): 10513-8.
[http://dx.doi.org/10.1073/pnas.0804549105] [PMID: 18663219]

[58]   Lawrie CH, Gal S, Dunlop HM, *et al.* Detection of elevated levels of tumour-associated microRNAs in serum of patients with diffuse large B-cell lymphoma. Br J Haematol 2008; 141(5): 672-5.
[http://dx.doi.org/10.1111/j.1365-2141.2008.07077.x] [PMID: 18318758]

[59]   Duffy MJ, Harbeck N, Nap M, *et al.* Clinical use of biomarkers in breast cancer: Updated guidelines from the European Group on Tumor Markers (EGTM). Eur J Cancer 2017; 75: 284-98.
[http://dx.doi.org/10.1016/j.ejca.2017.01.017] [PMID: 28259011]

[60]   Pandey A, Mann M. Proteomics to study genes and genomes. Nature 2000; 405(6788): 837-46.
[http://dx.doi.org/10.1038/35015709] [PMID: 10866210]

[61]   Zografos E, Gazouli M, Tsangaris G, Marinos E. The significance of proteomic biomarkers in male breast cancer. Cancer Genomics Proteomics 2016; 13(3): 183-90.
[PMID: 27107060]

[62]   Hudelist G, Pacher-Zavisin M, Singer CF, *et al.* Use of high-throughput protein array for profiling of differentially expressed proteins in normal and malignant breast tissue. Breast Cancer Res Treat 2004; 86(3): 281-91.
[http://dx.doi.org/10.1023/B:BREA.0000036901.16346.83] [PMID: 15567944]

[63]   Ray S, Reddy PJ, Jain R, Gollapalli K, Moiyadi A, Srivastava S. Proteomic technologies for the identification of disease biomarkers in serum: advances and challenges ahead. Proteomics 2011; 11(11): 2139-61.
[http://dx.doi.org/10.1002/pmic.201000460] [PMID: 21548090]

[64]   Lopez F, Belloc F, Lacombe F, *et al.* Modalities of synthesis of Ki67 antigen during the stimulation of lymphocytes. Cytometry 1991; 12(1): 42-9.
[http://dx.doi.org/10.1002/cyto.990120107] [PMID: 1999122]

[65]   Dbouk HA, Tawil A, Nasr F, Kandakarjian L, Abou-Merhi R. Significance of CEA and VEGF as diagnostic markers of colorectal cancer in lebanese patients. Open Clin Cancer J 2007; 1: 1-5.
[http://dx.doi.org/10.2174/1874189400701010001] [PMID: 18665243]

[66]   Qin XJ, Ling BX. Proteomic studies in breast cancer (Review). Oncol Lett 2012; 3(4): 735-43.
[Review].
[PMID: 22740985]

[67]   Cardoso MR, Santos JC, Ribeiro ML, Talarico MCR, Viana LR, Derchain SFM. A metabolomic

approach to predict breast cancer behavior and chemotherapy response. Int J Mol Sci 2018; 19(2): 1-16.
[http://dx.doi.org/10.3390/ijms19020617] [PMID: 29466297]

[68]   Günther UL. Metabolomics biomarkers for breast cancer. Pathobiology 2015; 82(3-4): 153-65.
[http://dx.doi.org/10.1159/000430844] [PMID: 26330356]

[69]   Ryu CS, Kwak HC, Lee KS, *et al.* Sulfur amino acid metabolism in doxorubicin-resistant breast cancer cells. Toxicol Appl Pharmacol 2011; 255(1): 94-102.
[http://dx.doi.org/10.1016/j.taap.2011.06.004] [PMID: 21703291]

[70]   Cao B, Li M, Zha W, *et al.* Metabolomic approach to evaluating adriamycin pharmacodynamics and resistance in breast cancer cells. Metabolomics 2013; 9(5): 960-73.
[http://dx.doi.org/10.1007/s11306-013-0517-x] [PMID: 24039617]

[71]   Morvan D. Functional metabolomics uncovers metabolic alterations associated to severe oxidative stress in MCF7 breast cancer cells exposed to ascididemin. Mar Drugs 2013; 11(10): 3846-60.
[http://dx.doi.org/10.3390/md11103846] [PMID: 24152560]

[72]   Kling J. Beyond counting tumor cells. Nat Biotechnol 2012; 30(7): 578-80.
[http://dx.doi.org/10.1038/nbt.2295] [PMID: 22781672]

[73]   Cristofanilli M, Budd GT, Ellis MJ, *et al.* Circulating tumor cells, disease progression, and survival in metastatic breast cancer. N Engl J Med 2004; 351(8): 781-91.
[http://dx.doi.org/10.1056/NEJMoa040766] [PMID: 15317891]

[74]   Pierga J-Y, Hajage D, Bachelot T, *et al.* High independent prognostic and predictive value of circulating tumor cells compared with serum tumor markers in a large prospective trial in first-line chemotherapy for metastatic breast cancer patients. Ann Oncol 2012; 23(3): 618-24.
[http://dx.doi.org/10.1093/annonc/mdr263] [PMID: 21642515]

[75]   Zhang L, Riethdorf S, Wu G, *et al.* Meta-analysis of the prognostic value of circulating tumor cells in breast cancer. Clin Cancer Res 2012; 18(20): 5701-10.
[http://dx.doi.org/10.1158/1078-0432.CCR-12-1587] [PMID: 22908097]

[76]   Dawson S-J, Tsui DWY, Murtaza M, *et al.* Analysis of circulating tumor DNA to monitor metastatic breast cancer. N Engl J Med 2013; 368(13): 1199-209.
[http://dx.doi.org/10.1056/NEJMoa1213261] [PMID: 23484797]

[77]   Sorensen BS, Mortensen LS, Andersen J, Nexo E. Circulating HER2 DNA after trastuzumab treatment predicts survival and response in breast cancer. Anticancer Res 2010; 30(6): 2463-8.
[PMID: 20651409]

[78]   Murtaza M, Dawson S-J, Tsui DWY, *et al.* Non-invasive analysis of acquired resistance to cancer therapy by sequencing of plasma DNA. Nature 2013; 497(7447): 108-12.
[http://dx.doi.org/10.1038/nature12065] [PMID: 23563269]

[79]   Jankowitz RC, Cooper K, Erlander MG, *et al.* Prognostic utility of the breast cancer index and comparison to Adjuvant! Online in a clinical case series of early breast cancer. Breast Cancer Res 2011; 13(5): R98.
[http://dx.doi.org/10.1186/bcr3038] [PMID: 21999244]

[80]   Jerevall P-L, Ma X-J, Li H, *et al.* Prognostic utility of HOXB13:IL17BR and molecular grade index in early-stage breast cancer patients from the Stockholm trial. Br J Cancer 2011; 104(11): 1762-9.
[http://dx.doi.org/10.1038/bjc.2011.145] [PMID: 21559019]

[81]   Mathieu MC, Mazouni C, Kesty NC, *et al.* Breast Cancer Index predicts pathological complete response and eligibility for breast conserving surgery in breast cancer patients treated with neoadjuvant chemotherapy. Ann Oncol 2012; 23(8): 2046-52.
[http://dx.doi.org/10.1093/annonc/mdr550] [PMID: 22112967]

[82]   Azim HA Jr, Michiels S, Zagouri F, *et al.* Utility of prognostic genomic tests in breast cancer practice: The IMPAKT 2012 Working Group Consensus Statement. Ann Oncol 2013; 24(3): 647-54.

[http://dx.doi.org/10.1093/annonc/mds645] [PMID: 23337633]

[83] Sotiriou C, Wirapati P, Loi S, *et al.* Gene expression profiling in breast cancer: understanding the molecular basis of histologic grade to improve prognosis. J Natl Cancer Inst 2006; 98(4): 262-72.
[http://dx.doi.org/10.1093/jnci/djj052] [PMID: 16478745]

[84] Naoi Y, Kishi K, Tanei T, *et al.* High genomic grade index associated with poor prognosis for lymph node-negative and estrogen receptor-positive breast cancers and with good response to chemotherapy. Cancer 2011; 117(3): 472-9.
[http://dx.doi.org/10.1002/cncr.25626] [PMID: 20878674]

[85] Liedtke C, Hatzis C, Symmans WF, *et al.* Genomic grade index is associated with response to chemotherapy in patients with breast cancer. J Clin Oncol 2009; 27(19): 3185-91.
[http://dx.doi.org/10.1200/JCO.2008.18.5934] [PMID: 19364972]

[86] Bartlett JM, Thomas J, Ross DT, *et al.* Mammostrat as a tool to stratify breast cancer patients at risk of recurrence during endocrine therapy. Breast Cancer Res 2010; 12(4): R47.
[http://dx.doi.org/10.1186/bcr2604] [PMID: 20615243]

[87] Bartlett JMS, Bloom KJ, Piper T, *et al.* Mammostrat as an immunohistochemical multigene assay for prediction of early relapse risk in the tamoxifen *versus* exemestane adjuvant multicenter trial pathology study. J Clin Oncol 2012; 30(36): 4477-84.
[http://dx.doi.org/10.1200/JCO.2012.42.8896] [PMID: 23045591]

[88] Ross DT, Kim CY, Tang G, *et al.* Chemosensitivity and stratification by a five monoclonal antibody immunohistochemistry test in the NSABP B14 and B20 trials. Clin Cancer Res 2008; 14(20): 6602-9.
[http://dx.doi.org/10.1158/1078-0432.CCR-08-0647] [PMID: 18927301]

[89] Cuzick J, Dowsett M, Pineda S, *et al.* Prognostic value of a combined estrogen receptor, progesterone receptor, Ki-67, and human epidermal growth factor receptor 2 immunohistochemical score and comparison with the Genomic Health recurrence score in early breast cancer. J Clin Oncol 2011; 29(32): 4273-8.
[http://dx.doi.org/10.1200/JCO.2010.31.2835] [PMID: 21990413]

[90] Bahcall OG. iCOGS collection provides a collaborative model. Foreword. Nat Genet 2013; 45(4): 343.
[http://dx.doi.org/10.1038/ng.2592] [PMID: 23535721]

[91] Antoniou AC, Cunningham AP, Peto J, *et al.* The BOADICEA model of genetic susceptibility to breast and ovarian cancers: updates and extensions. Br J Cancer 2008; 98(8): 1457-66.
[http://dx.doi.org/10.1038/sj.bjc.6604305] [PMID: 18349832]

[92] Mavaddat N, Antoniou AC, Easton DF, Garcia-Closas M. Genetic susceptibility to breast cancer. Mol Oncol 2010; 4(3): 174-91.
[http://dx.doi.org/10.1016/j.molonc.2010.04.011] [PMID: 20542480]

[93] Peto J, Collins N, Barfoot R, *et al.* Prevalence of BRCA1 and BRCA2 gene mutations in patients with early-onset breast cancer. J Natl Cancer Inst 1999; 91(11): 943-9.
[http://dx.doi.org/10.1093/jnci/91.11.943] [PMID: 10359546]

[94] Guilford P, Hopkins J, Harraway J, *et al.* E-cadherin germline mutations in familial gastric cancer. Nature 1998; 392(6674): 402-5.
[http://dx.doi.org/10.1038/32918] [PMID: 9537325]

[95] Pharoah PD, Guilford P, Caldas C. Incidence of gastric cancer and breast cancer in CDH1 (E-cadherin) mutation carriers from hereditary diffuse gastric cancer families. Gastroenterology 2001; 121(6): 1348-53. [PubMed: 11729114].
[http://dx.doi.org/10.1053/gast.2001.29611] [PMID: 11729114]

[96] Brooks-Wilson AR, Kaurah P, Suriano G, *et al.* Germline E-cadherin mutations in hereditary diffuse gastric cancer: assessment of 42 new families and review of genetic screening criteria. J Med Genet 2004; 41(7): 508-17.
[http://dx.doi.org/10.1136/jmg.2004.018275] [PMID: 15235021]

[97]   Suriano G, Yew S, Ferreira P, *et al.* Characterization of a recurrent germ line mutation of the E-cadherin gene: implications for genetic testing and clinical management. Clin Cancer Res 2005; 11(15): 5401-9.
[http://dx.doi.org/10.1158/1078-0432.CCR-05-0247] [PMID: 16061854]

[98]   Kaurah P, MacMillan A, Boyd N, *et al.* Founder and recurrent CDH1 mutations in families with hereditary diffuse gastric cancer. JAMA 2007; 297(21): 2360-72.
[http://dx.doi.org/10.1001/jama.297.21.2360] [PMID: 17545690]

[99]   Bathen TF, Jensen LR, Sitter B, *et al.* MR-determined metabolic phenotype of breast cancer in prediction of lymphatic spread, grade, and hormone status. Breast Cancer Res Treat 2007; 104(2): 181-9.
[http://dx.doi.org/10.1007/s10549-006-9400-z] [PMID: 17061040]

[100]   Cheng LL, Burns MA, Taylor JL, *et al.* Metabolic characterization of human prostate cancer with tissue magnetic resonance spectroscopy. Cancer Res 2005; 65(8): 3030-4.
[http://dx.doi.org/10.1158/0008-5472.CAN-04-4106] [PMID: 15833828]

[101]   Mazurek S, Eigenbrodt E. The tumor metabolome. Anticancer Res 2003; 23(2A): 1149-54.
[PMID: 12820363]

[102]   Mazurek S, Grimm H, Boschek CB, Vaupel P, Eigenbrodt E. Pyruvate kinase type M2: a crossroad in the tumor metabolome. Br J Nutr 2002; 87 (Suppl. 1): S23-9.
[http://dx.doi.org/10.1079/BJN2001454] [PMID: 11895152]

[103]   Chung YL, Griffiths JR. Using metabolomics to monitor anticancer drugs. Ernst Schering Found Symp Proc 2007; 4: 55-78.

[104]   Erb G, Elbayed K, Piotto M, *et al.* Toward improved grading of malignancy in oligodendrogliomas using metabolomics. Magn Reson Med 2008; 59(5): 959-65.
[http://dx.doi.org/10.1002/mrm.21486] [PMID: 18429037]

[105]   Kim YS, Maruvada P, Milner JA. Metabolomics in biomarker discovery: future uses for cancer prevention. Future Oncol 2008; 4(1): 93-102.
[http://dx.doi.org/10.2217/14796694.4.1.93] [PMID: 18241004]

[106]   Tomlins SA, Rubin MA, Chinnaiyan AM. Integrative biology of prostate cancer progression. Annu Rev Pathol 2006; 1: 243-71.
[http://dx.doi.org/10.1146/annurev.pathol.1.110304.100047] [PMID: 18039115]

CHAPTER 4

Recent Proteomics Development for Biomarker Detection in Breast Cancer

Gatha Thacker*

Biochemistry Division, CSIR-Central Drug Research Institute (CSIR-CDRI), Jankipuram Extension, Lucknow, 226031, UP, India

Abstract: Breast cancer accounts for a massive and very frequently occurring disease among females throughout the world. In spite of several approaches for the detection of cancer at an early stage and diverse curative strategies that are coming out, the discovery of a potent, efficacious, and unique biomarker is requisite for precise diagnosis at an early stage, as prognostic predictors and as a marker of the development of therapeutic resistance. In the current scenario, the availability of validated breast cancer biomarkers is almost nil. Barely a handful of biomarkers that have a practical advantage in terms of prognosis and diagnosis include estrogen receptor (ER), progesterone receptor (PR), and HER-2 with limitations. Therefore, the urge of precise biomarkers for the detection of breast cancer stands in need. The progress and utilization of proteomic techniques for the discovery of new protein biomarkers have revolutionized the way of understanding the biology and the associated pathways involved in the progression of the disease. With the help of proteomics, now plenty of prospective protein and peptide biomarkers can be identified from the samples using high-throughput analysis. In this chapter, we covered the techniques, which are routinely employed for treatment, diagnosis, and prognosis of breast cancer with all their benefits and drawbacks. It also includes recent advancements in the field of proteomics and their utility in search of new cancer biomarkers.

Keywords: Biomarker, Breast cancer, Differential in-gel electrophoresis, Electrospray ionization, Mammography, Mass spectrometry, Mass-to-charge ratios, Matrix-assisted laser desorption/ionization, Multiple reaction monitoring, Peptide, Proteomics, Surface-enhanced laser desorption/ionization (SALDI).

INTRODUCTION

Breast Cancer (BC) belongs to one of the most formidable diseases and provides major public health risk due to its varied response for prognosis and therapy.

* **Corresponding Author Gatha Thacker:** Biochemistry division, CSIR-Central Drug Research Institute (CSIR-CDRI), Jankipuram Extension, Lucknow, 226031, UP, India; E-mail: gatha.biotech@gmail.com

Shankar Suman, Garima Suman and Sanjay Mishra (Eds.)

Insight from the International Agency for Research on Cancer (IARC) data demonstrate that the cancer occurrence has been raced worldwide with the highest incidence of breast cancer rate found in the United States and Western Europe [1]. The disease is more prevalent and a leading cause of mortality in older age women (more than 50 years) when compared to the younger ones where it is less common. However, younger women are prone to much aggressive type of breast cancer than aged women. Additionally, one-third of patients have experienced recurrence or metastasis of the disease.

The five-year survival rate in the women having breast cancer is found to be approximately 85%, and it is highly correlated with the detection of tumor stage. At very early stages, when cancer is non-metastatic and restricted to the breast, the approximate 5-year survival rate is near about 97%, while it greatly reduces to <25% if it has diagnosed at later stages of metastasis [2]. Therefore, the detection of breast cancer at early-stage while it is yet resectable, makes it easy to diagnose and treat before it metastasizes to other organs, can significantly reduce breast cancer-related mortality. Hence, curtailment in the mortality and morbidity because of breast cancer depends on the identification of a reliable biomarker with innovative approaches for screening, detection at an early stage, prediction of outcome, therapeutic response, and prevention; all that are urgently needed.

At present, mammography is the only contemplate benchmark for the screening and detection of breast cancer. Mammography is the ideal and most suited approach for the diagnosis of breast cancer in women over the age of 50 years; however, the sensitivity of this imaging technique is compromised in younger age women because of the presence of dense breast tissue. Besides, it has other limitations such as tumors smaller than 0.5cm in size remain undetectable by present technology [3]. Above all, the presence of highly invasive metastatic tumors is not being identified by regular mammography imaging. This is why the development of improved diagnostic techniques for breast cancer with the novel approach is required that can lead to increment in the disease-free survival rate of the patients who are diagnosed and suffering from such a deadly disease.

In line, a major focus has given for the search of individuals or a panel of biomarkers, which have clinical applicability in the detection of cancer at an early stage. Biomarkers are proving its utility and efficacy for the detection and monitoring of cancer from a decade. They indicate a difference in the character trait of healthy cell physiology and tumor progression at a given time. According to NIH, biomarkers are designated as "a characteristic that can be objectively measured and evaluated as an indicator of normal biological processes, pathogenic processes, or pharmacologic responses to a therapeutic intervention". Biomarkers are significantly important tools to study a variety of malignancies, and they enabled the process of easy prediction, identification, disease inspection, or drug monitoring and development.

Unlike the conventional methods of clinical detection including biopsy of tissues, MRI imaging, mammogram, and cytology screening, current biomarker discoveries are majorly focussing upon the key approaches like bioinformatics, genomics, metabolomics, and most importantly proteomics. Breast cancer has been studied most intensely through technologies of profiling protein and gene expression. Although genomics has a pivotal role in the discovery biomarker, it only provides information about approximately 35000 corresponding proteins that it encodes. On the other hand, the proteome of a cell is much more potent, effective and comparatively much larger. A total sum of protein that presents in an organism or a certain cell at a given time and in specific conditions which determine and control the expression of various gene expression pattern is called Proteome of that cell or organism. The proteome is responsible for the distinct properties and behaviors of cells and tissues in health and diseased condition.

The occurrence of alternative RNA splicing, single amino acid polymorphisms, and post-translational modifications (PTMs) such as methylation, phosphorylation, acetylation, glycosylation, sumoylation, and ubiquitination result in multiple forms of protein produced from a single gene. Therefore, to study and understand these complex proteo-forms and their role in aggravating cancer biology, the field of proteomics is rapidly emerging. The current chapter provides a comprehensive summary of current proteomic approaches in biomarker identification in breast cancer and expands potential clinical applications for future personalized medicine.

KEY PROTEOMICS TECHNIQUES APPLIED IN BIOMARKER IDENTIFICATION

Proteomics represents a wide-ranging study of proteins and covering many facets to understanding protein structure and protein biology, including identification of new protein, evaluation, and functional analysis, ontology, and to determine persisting interactions among them. Besides that, proteomic approaches found to be very useful in the analysis of thousands of complex biological and clinical samples; commonly studied among them are serum, tissue, plasma, saliva, urine, nipple aspirate fluid (NAF), and cerebrospinal fluid. The core idea of the discovery of novel biomarkers laying in the fact of identifying a crucial protein or peptide is to exhibit varying or distinct expression profiles among healthy and diseased conditions. This feasible yet striking approach makes proteomics an appealing option for biomarker discovery.

There are two basic approaches implied in biomarker identification; one is direct or targets specific while other is global or non-specific. Enzyme-linked immunosorbent assays (ELISA), antibody array, or western blotting to screen specific protein are included in clinically acceptable target specific approaches. However, low-turnout in terms of the number of proteins that can be evaluated or studied in a given time make these techniques unsuitable for biomarker discovery. On the other hand, Mass-spectrometry (MS) based global approaches are well-suited high-throughput screening methods for biomarker discovery, and they are relatively unbiased. Fig. (**1**) outlined various proteomic approaches implied in biomarker discovery in breast cancer;

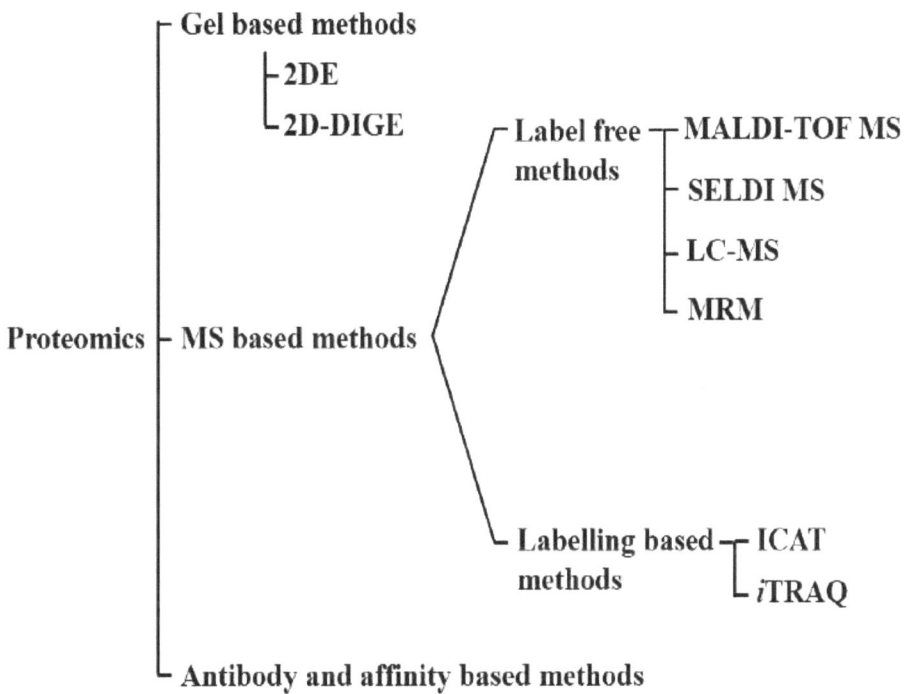

Fig. (1). Schematic of current proteomics technologies utilized for BC biomarker identification.

Gel Based Methods

Complex mixtures of proteins can be separated using electrophoresis, and one of the most routinely employed gel-based techniques is two-dimensional gel electrophoresis (2D-GE), that can be utilized to segregate and visualize a large number of proteins or a complex mixture of proteins in a polyacrylamide gel matrix. Separation of proteins takes place in two dimensions; in the first dimension, migration occurs based on the isoelectric point of the protein. Hence the process called isoelectric focusing (IEF) whereby the proteins are separated in an immobilized pH gradient. Following the migration of proteins in the second dimension based on the differences in their molecular masses, segregated through SDS-PAGE and visualized either by Coomassie Brilliant Blue or silver staining. In biomarker discovery, this technique can be used to detect protein spots, which are altered in abundance between disease and control samples. The differential protein spots detected on a gel can be recovered and further identified by mass spectrometry instruments.

Wulfkuhle, J. D. *et al.* used the traditional 2D-GE approach with the sample of Ductal carcinoma *in situ* (DCIS), an early-stage breast cancer tumor for spotting of new biomarkers [4]. Proteomic profiles of four cases of DCIS were compared with the control of normal epithelial cells of the duct by 2D-GE and confirmed the finding with immunohistochemistry as well. Among the differentially identified proteins, a molecular chaperon HSP27 was found and validated, which is well reported to be upregulated in the early-stage breast cancer tumors, while high levels of actin crosslinking protein transgelin were observed in normal ductal epithelial cells [5]. Fold differences can be evaluated using Image analysis software based on spot volumes by creating a digital reference.

This method is quite handy for the visualization and separation of a large number of proteins ranging from 3,000 to 10,000 approximately. Also, all 2D-GE profiles are already incorporated, and these are compared within existing literature and databases, *i.e.* Expasy, SWISS-2D-PAGE, and UCD-2D-PAGE Database. Although 2D-GE is widely used in proteomic studies, experimental variation in each time running gel, a low range of identification with limited dynamics, repeatability, and standardization are some key problems associated with this technique. Also, proteins having extreme acidic or basic pI, hydrophobic proteins, rare abundant proteins and proteins bound with membranes are comparatively tough to separate with 2DGE. Triplicates of each sample are essential to generate robust results, thus limiting the ability to analyze low volume samples with increased time and labour. Furthermore, it is not an automated process and downstream technologies require the individual attention of each spot of interest.

Differential in-gel electrophoresis (DIGE) provides an advantage over the classical 2D-gel approach in terms of responsiveness, reproducibility, and quantification. In the 2D-DIGE technique, protein extracts of cells or tissues are labeled differentially with a variety of fluorophore-tagged molecules such as Cy2, Cy3, or Cy5 that are eventually mixed and then ultimately separated based on charge and mass in a single 2DE gel. This allows the separation of multiple samples together with internal control and subsequent detection of proteins on one gel. The key to this technique is the normalization within an experiment *via* the inclusion of internal control and the elimination of gel-to-gel variations. This technique was successfully utilized for the identification of a potential circulating biomarker RS/DJ-1 protein, reported to be involved in the regulation of RNA-protein interaction. This protein was spotted from the serum of patients affected by breast cancer using autoantibody [6]. The only drawback of 2D-DIGE is that numerous steps are involved in making it a time-consuming process that requires expertise in processing and handling of samples, good laboratory skills to achieve excellent results.

Mass-Spectrometry (MS) Based Methods

One of the most effective technologies for proteomic studies depends on mass spectrometry (MS) based approaches. Mass spectrometry is not only used to determine the exact molecular weight of peptide using mass-to-charge ratios (m/z). It also predicts the amino acid sequence of a given peptide with a high degree of sensitivity and helps to understand the function and make-up of complex proteome. It allows high-throughput analysis for protein quantification that only requires a small amount of protein sample and provides insight at the molecular level, which is not possible to achieve with conventional gel-based techniques.

In general, ionization followed by separation and detection is the three major and fundamental components that are required for any kind of mass spectrometric techniques. The ionization of the sample molecule by an ion source is a prerequisite in order to accelerate their separation. Subsequently, the sorting of this ionized molecule is carried out by the mass analyzer depending on their mass to charge ratios before detection. The selection of suitable ion sources mainly depends upon the biochemical properties of the sample to be separated. Nowadays, a variety of ion sources have been adopted, out of which electrospray ionization (ESI), matrix-assisted laser desorption/ionization (MALDI) are commonly used and surface-enhanced laser desorption/ionization (SELDI) has been developed with slight modification. Whereas, quadrupole, ion trap, time-o--flight (TOF) and orbitrap are among the top demanding mass analyzers of choice. Different MS instruments utilize a different type of method for the identification and measurement of protein. In general, there are two types of established quantitation methods are utilized in MS: label-free MS quantitation and stable isotope labeling-based MS quantitation.

Label-Free Methods

Label-free MS-based quantitative proteomics techniques are about the detection and measurements of not only changes in the height of digested peptide peak but also the spectral counting of protein that identified. These label-free techniques have many advantages. It can be applied to different sample types, which include urine, blood, tissue, cell culture, and organisms, and there is no cost for labeling reagents though this does increase the length of the MS analysis time.

Matrix-Assisted Laser Desorption/Ionization Time of Flight (MALDI-TOF)

MALDI-TOF is a single step soft-ionization approach. This technique is utilized to understand the biology and physiology of tumors by differentiating and identifying a plethora of previously unidentified proteins. However, the preparation of a sample is a crucial and considerable step of the technique before analysis. Depending on the nature of the sample to be analyzed it is first blended nicely with any one of the following matrices such as; α-cyano-4-hydroxycinnamic acid (CHCA), 3,5-dimethoxy-4-hydroxycinnamic acid, ferulic acid, 2-(4-hydroxyphenylazo)-benzoic acid (HABA), and 2,5-dihydroxybenzoate (DHB), before spotting directly onto sample plates. These matrix substances are usually high energy absorbing in nature, and the choice of appropriate matrix substance is crucial for the identification of specific biomolecules. Besides, a matrix substance also helps in diminishing the shattering and demolition of the sample material during the process of ionization by a direct laser beam.

Charged ions are eventually generated by the ionization step further facing through a vacuum chamber where detectors analyze the time taken by them to cover a fixed distance, which is theoretically directly proportional to their respective masses. Sophisticated predesigned statistical and bioinformatics operations further analyse spectrum generated in this technique. Proteome, Quest, Propek, Bamf, and Biomarker Wizard are some of the popular tools to analyse these data are available commercially.

The main advantages of MALDI are that it is automated, fast, comparatively low cost, and highly sensitive. The technique is multidimensional, requires small sample volumes, and provides accurate measurements of mass even for significantly bigger polypeptides having molecular weight over 30 kDa too. However, it is sensitive to salt contamination, and the reproducibility of data may evoke complexity.

Surface-Enhanced Laser Desorption/Ionization Time of Flight (SELDI-TOF)

At present, SELDI-MS has emerged as a significantly upgraded method for fast and easy identification of specific biomarkers for cancer and also for revealing the specific proteomic pattern. This mass spectrometry technique is an ionization method, recently utilized for high-throughput proteomic screening and footprinting of tumor or cell extracts and biological fluids such as plasma or serum, NAF, ductal fluid, saliva, and urine, *etc*. The sample to be analyzed is spotted onto a chemically modified surface on a protein-binding biochip, to absorb energy and to allow vaporization and ionization by laser for further MS detection.

The binding surface consists of materials having different Physico-chemical properties, *i.e.* a combination of weak cation and strong anion or immobilized metal affinity to provide specific interaction with a particular part of proteins in the given sample. Interaction of specific protein also depends upon certain factors like pH, concentration, amount of salt and existence of lipids, which can significantly interfere within. The chip is then rinsed, and impurities with unbound proteins are removed by washing with buffer, to analyze the sample with a TOF spectrometer. The whole process assists in creating clean mass spectra without any interfering element from extremely complex biological samples. Computer-aided tools are required to read and analyze this finally generated ion spectrum.

SELDI-TOF-MS technology, without any doubts, advantageous over presently used similar kinds of proteomic techniques as it is easy to use and provides high-throughput profiling of complex samples at the same time. Its sensitivity and requirement for only a small amount of sample volumes, when it is compared to conventional approaches, also provide an upper hand to this technique. Small peptides ranging up to 500 Da can also be detected with accuracy through SALDI, and data for large study sets can be generated in minutes or hours.

Also, it has the ability to detect low molecular weight as well as truncated, modified, or fragmented proteins and peptides with high sensitivity and specificity. Because of all these advances, SALDI is now being used majorly for the identification of differential biomarkers present or altered in diseased conditions in various types of cancer. Sauter, E. *et al.* and Paweletz C. P. *et al.* used SALDI-TOF to study nipple aspirate fluid in search of a potential biomarker for breast cancer [7, 8]. At present applicability of this technique is evolving much faster for the detection of tumors at early stages.

Although SELDI-TOF provides a comprehensive way for protein profiling and high-throughput screening, the major drawback of SELDI-TOF-MS is that the results are biased toward peptides and smaller proteins, intricate in detecting larger molecular weight proteins and identification of post-translation modification (PTM). Other limitations of the SELDI-MS approach include the low resolution of MS and it is prone to generate artifacts. A crucial factor of using SELDI-TOF-MS in biomarker research is its low reproducibility and comparability of datasets due to different chip surfaces and analytical conditions.

Therefore, standardization of analytical conditions is critical for accurate data interpretation and comparative purposes.

LC-MS

LC-MS combines chromatographic techniques with MS to enhance the resolving ability and is a widely used approach for the proteomic analysis. In LC-MS, prepared peptide fragments generated either by lysis of protein or by chemical degradation are loaded onto a column called high-performance liquid chromatography (HPLC) column packed with fine chemically modified silica particles for separation. Separation in the HPLC column relies on size, charge, hydrophobicity, and also on binding affinity of the peptide to the stationary phase. After elution, peptides are directed into the mass spectrometer, ionized either by electrospray ionization source or by atmospheric pressure chemical ionization and further separated based on their unique mass to charge ratio. LC-MS is a multidimensional approach utilized to detect large molecular weight molecules upon tryptic digestion. It is one of the most common approaches to identify modified proteins in breast cancer cells [9].

Though this method is a powerful fractionation method that can separate large amounts of peptides with high resolution, however, measurement and identification of peptides that remain in comparatively small proportions still pose a challenge, as detection of the most abundant peptide is common and preferable nature of this technique. Besides, it is time-consuming and not suited for routine clinical analysis.

Multiple Reaction Monitoring (MRM)

Unlike MS-based discovery proteomics where all proteins are detected in an unbiased manner, selected/multiple reaction monitoring (SRM or MRM) is targeted approach to measure only the peptides of interest or selected values of mass to charge ratio (m/z) with great sensitivity, accuracy, and quantification ability. Therefore, the presence of even low abundant peptides in complex biological materials including cell plasma proteins and human tissue, can be detected easily through SRM/MRM. Besides, the MS-based MRM technique exhibits superior multitudinous nature and low-level detection abilities, making it an ideal method for biomarker validation. Besides, it can also facilitate the measurement of post-translational modifications.

SRM is usually operated using a triple quadrupole (Q1, Q2, and Q3) or on a linear ion trap mass spectrometer. In this process, quadrupole one selects unique peptide called parent peptide, which is disintegrated subsequently by collision to generate transition ions in quadrupole 2, and ultimately these sequence-specific products of ionization further analyzed in quadrupole 3. The selection of unique parent peptides depends upon the specificity of the sequence of amino acids in the given protein of interest. Besides, high occurrence, repeated identification in MS runs peptide length, and the absence of missed cleavage sites are some other measures for the selection of candidate peptides. Proteotypic control peptides used and depicted as an intact protein of interest. Furthermore, this technique is acquiescent to multiplex analysis, and a single run of scheduled MRM can analyze approximately hundreds of proteins, wherein MRM transition of each peptide is specifically examined at its expected elution time.

MRM is an excellent label-free technique in terms of reproducibility, sensitivity, and specificity currently used for quantification of targeted protein or peptides. It allows a high level of multiplexing with quantitation of a large number of proteins at the same time in parallel. It is regarded as one among very few effective methods available for quantitative proteomics of clinical samples. However, Different MRM-based quantification results have been reported on the same target proteins by different groups [10 - 12]; a need for suitable fraction preparation is therefore required for analyzing samples having the presence of high abundant proteins. Despite several challenges that are still to be conquered, MRM is coming out as a beneficial approach for the identification of novel biomarkers in clinical proteomics for which antibodies are yet to be discovered.

Labeling-Based MS Quantitation Methods

Stable isotope labelling-based technologies rely on strategy of shifts in mass because of isotope tagging that can be easily determined by a single mass spectrometry experiment. Therefore, quantification of differently expressed proteins between healthy and diseased conditions can be achieved at the same time using differential labeling. The use of isotope labels provides considerable efficacy in protein quantification. However, the high cost of isotope labels and the need for exclusive professional software for statistical calculation are some major drawbacks of this approach. Two important and applicable labeling-based techniques are ICAT (isotope-coded affinity tags) and iTRAQ (isobaric tags for relative and absolute quantitation).

Isotope-Coded Affinity Tags (ICAT)

ICAT reagents are specific for cysteine residues of denatured proteins. In some isotope-labeled proteomics, experiments proteins extracted from the experimental group in question together with the reference groups are labeled either with light or heavy isotope-coded affinity tags utilizing reaction of proteins with cysteinyl thiols. Avidin affinity chromatography is used to retrieve the labeled and LC-MS/MS subsequently analyses unlabelled peptides with the isotopic tags and these peptides. Peak ratio of the isotopic peptide indicates the presence or absence of differential expression of a particular protein in a given sample with control. Profile of potential serological biomarker was reported by Un-Beom Kang *et al.* using ICAT to determine the possibility of breast cancer [13]. Pawlik T. M. *et al.* used ICAT labeling for the identification of BC specific biomarkers from NAF (nipple aspirate fluid) of women who have early-stage breast cancer [14].

Proteins without cysteine residue cannot be analyzed with this technique, which accounts for approximate 10% of the total proteome. Moreover, the number of proteins that can be identified by ICAT ranges between 300 to 400 up to its maximum level, and this is very much lesser than the contemporary methods like 2D-GE. In addition to that, short peptides with large labels make searching for database a more tedious task.

Isobaric Tags for Relative and Absolute Quantitation (iTRAQ)

As the name suggests, iTRAQ is a relative quantitation approach that allows identification of a large number of proteins, approximately up to eight distinct biological samples at the same time in a single run, hence also considered as multiplexing quantitative technique. Because it provides both multiplexing and quantification in a single experiment, it is well suited for biomarker identification studies. Unlike other methods, iTRAQ is unique and generates quality data that is reproducible with definite protein identification due to the incorporation of internal control samples that normalize varying sample sets and combine all the peptide signals. Bouchal, P. *et al.* performed an experimental study using iTRAQ-2DLC-MS/MS for identification of differential protein expression to compare non-invasive early-stage breast cancer tissue samples with the tumors of various metastatic potentials and found 605 unique proteins, demonstrating the sensitivity and capability of this approach [15]. The only pitfall of this technique is that it is of very high cost, time taking, and extremely tedious job to perform.

Antibody and Affinity-Based Methods

Antibodies or affinity based proteomic approaches are applicable in the field of diagnosis and for functional studies. Antibody microarrays, antibody enriched SRM, and affinity mass spectrometry is some routinely used antibody-based proteomic applications that allow profiling and identification of thousands of proteins sensitively and rapidly [16 - 18]. Enrichment of peptides with affinity columns bound with specific antibodies followed by mass spectrometry analysis put forth a great deal to facilitate the characterization of the breast cancer proteome. Although large-scale productions of antibodies are now available, however, batch-to-batch variation and stability of protein epitope can be a complication with such kind of antibody-based assays. Besides, the maintenance of the discrete recognition epitope on the protein to avoid off-target binding provides another challenge.

BIOLOGICAL SAMPLES SUITABLE FOR PROTEOMICS STUDIES

A variety of biological sample sources is available for proteomic investigation, but the selection of a most fitted and worthy biological sample is critical for proteomic profiling studies. Samples of tumor tissue, cell lines, blood, serum, plasma, urine, and biological fluids such as saliva, nipple aspirate fluid [19] are extensively explored for proteomic characterization of the disease. However, breast cancer biomarkers are mostly sourced from tumor tissues and blood samples.

CURRENT BREAST CANCER BIOMARKER PROTEIN PROFILING STUDIES

Breast cancer is one of the fatal diseases causing high worldwide mortality rates; nevertheless, this mortality can be decreased by detection at an early stage. Unfortunately, because of the lack of efficient and easily detectable biomarkers, diagnosis of the disease at its onset is not possible and many patients are diagnosed too late at the metastatic stage. Although the conception of the majority of breast cancer cases is unknown, possible risk factors include gender, age of the patient, family history of having breast cancer, early menarche, late menopause, older maternal age at first live childbirth, and prolonged hormone replacement therapy. The genetic mutation that is frequently associated with the onset of breast cancer involve BRCA1/2 and p53 [20].

The sole idea of utilizing mass spectrometry-based approaches in the study of protein profiling for breast cancer is the identification of unique and efficient biomarkers that have applicability in clinical diagnosis or prognosis. An increased serum level of cancer antigen CA 15-3 is being monitored in patients with breast cancer; however, the presence of this factor is neither beneficial for the diagnosis of patients at an early stage nor helpful in the decision-making for treatment [21, 22]. Traditionally status of the receptor such as Human epithelial growth factor receptor-2, ER, PR, and an upregulated expression of proliferation marker Ki-67 or Mib-1 antigen are used as prognostic markers [23 - 25]. Proteomic studies show that currently, HER2 is the only well-established and routinely used biomarker that is available for the detection of breast cancer in the market [26]. Besides that, Matrix Metallo-Proteinase-2 (MMP-2), Osteopontin, cathepsins B and cathepsins L are also some of the identified prognostic breast cancer biomarkers [27]. However, these markers alone are not efficient enough to differentiate among various conditions and grades of breast cancer.

Studies from mass spectrometry utilizing techniques such as 2DE with MALDI-TOF identified the up-regulation of HSP27 while down-regulation of 14-3-3 σ in the serum of breast cancer patients [28, 29]. 14-3-3 σ is already reported as anti-oncogenic, and it is utilized as a marker of an early-stage breast cancer [30]. Both HSP27 and 14-3-3 σ are closely associated with cell cycle regulation and also intervene, directly or indirectly, with several key proteins of signaling pathways such as receptor IGF-1, Raf, PI3-kinase, and MEK kinases [31]. Similarly, other techniques like SELDI-TOF mass spectrometry has been successfully used to investigate novel and improved biomarkers from serum [32, 33], nipple aspirate fluid (NAF) [33 - 37], tumour tissues [38, 39], tears [40], and cell lines [41] for diagnosis and prognosis of breast cancer. Further, biomarker profiling by such a technique is used to predict lymph node metastasis and relapse-free survival of high-grade breast cancer patients [42, 43] as well as to monitor treatment efficacy for breast cancer metastasis [44].

A variety of 2D-GE based strategies has been employed in the study of preclinical models for breast cancer, including cell lines representing various types and origin of tumor [45 - 47] and animal models [48, 49] although not much data have been generated yet from direct clinical samples. Direct proteomic analysis of breast cancer cells using 2D-GE has identified some interesting protein alterations. 2D-DIGE provides an advancement over 2D-GE technology using a fluorescence detection system. It has been broadly applied for various mechanistic studies and molecular biomarker analysis in BC cell lines and animal models [50 - 52], as well as body fluids of human breast cancer patients such as plasma [53] and saliva [56]. 2D-DIGE analysis of samples from the serum of cancer patients *versus* healthy control identified that apolipoprotein A-I, transferrin, and hemoglobin are upregulated while apolipoprotein A-I, apolipoprotein C-III, and haptoglobin a2 found to be downregulated [54].

Nowadays, iTRAQ is used in preclinical studies and clinical sample analysis. Breast cancer cell lines [55], animal models, human breast cancer serum, and tumor tissues [15, 56] are successfully subjected to iTRAQ to identify biomarkers for diagnosis, metastasis, and drug response. Besides, multiple reaction monitoring (MRM) mass spectrometry technique has been included to identify and validate potential breast cancer biomarkers in an animal model, human blood, and human tissues [57, 58] for diagnosis of metastasis. These results suggest that modern proteomic techniques are very useful and promising in BC biomarker identification.

With the advance of modern proteomic techniques, the identification of novel BC biomarkers has made great progress in the last decade. However, until now, a biomarker that can differentiate between normal subjects or benign breast disease and breast cancer has not been found. Therefore, searching for novel biomarkers from human breast cancer samples holds a great promise for future biomarker studies.

CONCLUDING REMARKS AND FUTURE IMPLICATIONS

In the last ten years of cancer research, the major focus has been given in search of new cancer biomarker identification driven by a strong clinical need to refine the early diagnosis and cure of breast cancer. The majority of mass spectrometry protein profiling studies have emerged and improved tremendously over time, enabled for upgraded cancer diagnosis and treatment. Although it is necessary to have an accurate and deep understanding of the pathophysiological mechanisms associated with the evolution of such quantitative assays, out of which some of these techniques have been satisfactorily validated [59] and created an expansion in proteomic research that has intensified efforts to mine the human proteome.

Although there has been significant progress in breast cancer research, the heterogeneous nature of the disease still causes underlying mechanisms to be poorly understood, and potential candidate protein biomarkers remain to be discovered by proteomics. The use and development of various proteomic techniques have now become greater and grown at a very fast rate. Studies conducted under the guidelines and supervision of the American Society of Clinical Oncology (ASCO) identified several prospective proteins [60] from Serum, needle aspiration fluid (NAF), intercellular fluid, and tumor tissues and seems promising to be developed as a proteomic indicator of clinical value. However, to get a logical conclusion, multiple studies need to be performed with a larger sample size of varying populations and with varying analytical methods. In addition to this, the use of high-throughput methods and analysis of vast numbers of proteins in parallel at the same time enhances the chance of false discovery as well. Moreover, the heterogeneity of biological samples used every time for a different set of experiments causes variation among studies and hamper with the identification of differentially expressed proteins, suggesting the strong need for experimental standardization. Candidate proteins might also be one of the rare occurrence proteins that fall under the detection limits of the applied methods, hence poses the possibility that such tumor-specific secreted proteins remained undetected till now. In such cases, future advancement in the field to study human proteome will depend on the calibration of the applied method, development of well-suited bioinformatics operations, and especially on the collaboration between the scientific groups. Furthermore, the origin of various cancer types including breast cancer, is epithelial so most of the molecular features are commonly shared among these wide varieties of cancers. Thus, the marker identified for breast cancer may not be unique and restricted up to breast cancer and have been found to bear the diagnostic potential for other cancer types too and prove difficult to identify breast cancer-specific biomarker that is expressed solely by these tumor cells.

Although, the search of accurate and efficient biomarker that can be transferred directly into clinical practice is yet at a naive stage, and require integrative and multifaceted approach from experts of these fields. Combined efforts are being done and also sponsored by multiple groups and foundations in the hope that it will accelerate research and output of proteomics-based techniques into the clinical practice to materialize precision medicine or a potential diagnostic/prognostic tool.

CONSENT FOR PUBLICATION

Not applicable.

CONFLICT OF INTEREST

The authors confirm that the contents of this chapter have no conflict of interest.

ACKNOWLEDGEMENTS

Declared none.

REFERENCES

[1]   Dos Anjos Pultz B, da Luz FA, de Faria PR, Oliveira AP, de Araújo RA, Silva MJ. Far beyond the usual biomarkers in breast cancer: a review. J Cancer 2014; 5(7): 559-71.
        [http://dx.doi.org/10.7150/jca.8925] [PMID: 25057307]

[2]   Jemal A, Siegel R, Xu J, Ward E. Cancer statistics, 2010. CA Cancer J Clin 2010; 60(5): 277-300.
        [http://dx.doi.org/10.3322/caac.20073] [PMID: 20610543]

[3]   Ugnat AM, Xie L, Morriss J, Semenciw R, Mao Y. Survival of women with breast cancer in Ottawa, Canada: variation with age, stage, histology, grade and treatment. Br J Cancer 2004; 90(6): 1138-43.
        [http://dx.doi.org/10.1038/sj.bjc.6601662] [PMID: 15026792]

[4]   Wulfkuhle JD, Sgroi DC, Krutzsch H, *et al.* Proteomics of human breast ductal carcinoma *in situ*. Cancer Res 2002; 62(22): 6740-9.
        [PMID: 12438275]

[5]   Storm FK, Gilchrist KW, Warner TF, Mahvi DM. Distribution of Hsp-27 and HER-2/neu in *in situ* and invasive ductal breast carcinomas. Ann Surg Oncol 1995; 2(1): 43-8.
        [http://dx.doi.org/10.1007/BF02303701] [PMID: 7530588]

[6]   Le Naour F, Misek DE, Krause MC, *et al.* Proteomics-based identification of RS/DJ-1 as a novel circulating tumor antigen in breast cancer. Clin Cancer Res 2001; 7(11): 3328-35.
        [PMID: 11705844]

[7]   Paweletz CP, Trock B, Pennanen M, *et al.* Proteomic patterns of nipple aspirate fluids obtained by SELDI-TOF: potential for new biomarkers to aid in the diagnosis of breast cancer. Dis Markers 2001; 17(4): 301-7.
        [http://dx.doi.org/10.1155/2001/674959] [PMID: 11790897]

[8]   Sauter ER, Zhu W, Fan XJ, Wassell RP, Chervoneva I, Du Bois GC. Proteomic analysis of nipple aspirate fluid to detect biologic markers of breast cancer. Br J Cancer 2002; 86(9): 1440-3.
[http://dx.doi.org/10.1038/sj.bjc.6600285] [PMID: 11986778]

[9]   Zhu K, Kim J, Yoo C, Miller FR, Lubman DM. High sequence coverage of proteins isolated from liquid separations of breast cancer cells using capillary electrophoresis-time-of-flight MS and MALDI-TOF MS mapping. Anal Chem 2003; 75(22): 6209-17.
[http://dx.doi.org/10.1021/ac0346454] [PMID: 14616003]

[10]   Fortin T, Salvador A, Charrier JP, *et al.* Multiple reaction monitoring cubed for protein quantification at the low nanogram/milliliter level in nondepleted human serum. Anal Chem 2009; 81(22): 9343-52.
[http://dx.doi.org/10.1021/ac901447h] [PMID: 19839594]

[11]   Keshishian H, Addona T, Burgess M, Kuhn E, Carr SA. Quantitative, multiplexed assays for low abundance proteins in plasma by targeted mass spectrometry and stable isotope dilution. Mol Cell Proteom 2007; 6(12): 2212-29.
[http://dx.doi.org/10.1074/mcp.M700354-MCP200] [PMID: 17939991]

[12]   Kuzyk MA, Smith D, Yang J, *et al.* Multiple reaction monitoring-based, multiplexed, absolute quantitation of 45 proteins in human plasma. Mol Cell Proteom 2009; 8(8): 1860-77.
[http://dx.doi.org/10.1074/mcp.M800540-MCP200] [PMID: 19411661]

[13]   Kang UB, Ahn Y, Lee JW, *et al.* Differential profiling of breast cancer plasma proteome by isotope-coded affinity tagging method reveals biotinidase as a breast cancer biomarker. BMC Cancer 2010; 10: 114.
[http://dx.doi.org/10.1186/1471-2407-10-114] [PMID: 20346108]

[14]   Pawlik TM, Hawke DH, Liu Y, *et al.* Proteomic analysis of nipple aspirate fluid from women with early-stage breast cancer using isotope-coded affinity tags and tandem mass spectrometry reveals differential expression of vitamin D binding protein. BMC Cancer 2006; 6: 68.
[http://dx.doi.org/10.1186/1471-2407-6-68] [PMID: 16542425]

[15]   Bouchal P, Roumeliotis T, Hrstka R, Nenutil R, Vojtesek B, Garbis SD. Biomarker discovery in low-grade breast cancer using isobaric stable isotope tags and two-dimensional liquid chromatography-tandem mass spectrometry (iTRAQ-2DLC-MS/MS) based quantitative proteomic analysis. J Proteom Res 2009; 8(1): 362-73.
[http://dx.doi.org/10.1021/pr800622b] [PMID: 19053527]

[16]   Layton D, Laverty C, Nice EC. Design and operation of an automated high-throughput monoclonal antibody facility. Biophys Rev 2013; 5(1): 47-55.
[http://dx.doi.org/10.1007/s12551-012-0095-6] [PMID: 28510179]

[17]   Voskuil JL. The challenges with the validation of research antibodies. F1000 Res 2017; 6: 161.
[http://dx.doi.org/10.12688/f1000research.10851.1] [PMID: 28357047]

[18]   Wingren C. Antibody-based proteomics. Adv Exp Med Biol 2016; 926: 163-79.
[http://dx.doi.org/10.1007/978-3-319-42316-6_11] [PMID: 27686812]

[19]   Hanash S, Taguchi A. Application of proteomics to cancer early detection. Cancer J 2011; 17(6): 423-8.
[http://dx.doi.org/10.1097/PPO.0b013e3182383cab] [PMID: 22157286]

[20]   Honrado E, Benítez J, Palacios J. Histopathology of BRCA1- and BRCA2-associated breast cancer. Crit Rev Oncol Hematol 2006; 59(1): 27-39.
[http://dx.doi.org/10.1016/j.critrevonc.2006.01.006] [PMID: 16530420]

[21]   Duffy MJ, Duggan C, Keane R, *et al.* High preoperative CA 15-3 concentrations predict adverse outcome in node-negative and node-positive breast cancer: study of 600 patients with histologically confirmed breast cancer. Clin Chem 2004; 50(3): 559-63.
[http://dx.doi.org/10.1373/clinchem.2003.025288] [PMID: 14726467]

[22]   Lumachi F, Basso SM, Brandes AA, Pagano D, Ermani M. Relationship between tumor markers CEA

and CA 15-3, TNM staging, estrogen receptor rate and MIB-1 index in patients with pT1-2 breast cancer. Anticancer Res 2004; 24(5B): 3221-4.
[PMID: 15510614]

[23]   Gutierrez C, Schiff R. HER2: biology, detection, and clinical implications. Arch Pathol Lab Med 2011; 135(1): 55-62.
[PMID: 21204711]

[24]   Millar EK, Graham PH, McNeil CM, *et al.* Prediction of outcome of early ER+ breast cancer is improved using a biomarker panel, which includes Ki-67 and p53. Br J Cancer 2011; 105(2): 272-80.
[http://dx.doi.org/10.1038/bjc.2011.228] [PMID: 21712826]

[25]   O'Toole SA, Selinger CI, Millar EK, Lum T, Beith JM. Molecular assays in breast cancer pathology. Pathology 2011; 43(2): 116-27.
[http://dx.doi.org/10.1097/PAT.0b013e3283430926] [PMID: 21233672]

[26]   Baselga J. Treatment of HER2-overexpressing breast cancer. Ann Oncol 2010; 21 (Suppl. 7): vii36-40.
[http://dx.doi.org/10.1093/annonc/mdq421] [PMID: 20943641]

[27]   Leppä S, Saarto T, Vehmanen L, Blomqvist C, Elomaa I. A high serum matrix metalloproteinase-2 level is associated with an adverse prognosis in node-positive breast carcinoma. Clin Cancer Res 2004; 10(3): 1057-63.
[http://dx.doi.org/10.1158/1078-0432.CCR-03-0047] [PMID: 14871985]

[28]   El Yazidi-Belkoura I, Adriaenssens E, Vercoutter-Edouart AS, Lemoine J, Nurcombe V, Hondermarck H. Proteomics of breast cancer: outcomes and prospects. Technol Cancer Res Treat 2002; 1(4): 287-96.
[http://dx.doi.org/10.1177/153303460200100410] [PMID: 12625788]

[29]   Qin XJ, Ling BX. Proteomic studies in breast cancer (Review). Oncol Lett 2012; 3(4): 735-43. [Review].
[PMID: 22740985]

[30]   Schultz J, Ibrahim SM, Vera J, Kunz M. 14-3-3sigma gene silencing during melanoma progression and its role in cell cycle control and cellular senescence. Mol Cancer 2009; 8: 53.
[http://dx.doi.org/10.1186/1476-4598-8-53] [PMID: 19642975]

[31]   Moreira JM, Ohlsson G, Rank FE, Celis JE. Down-regulation of the tumor suppressor protein 14-3-3 sigma is a sporadic event in cancer of the breast. Mol Cell Proteom 2005; 4(4): 555-69.
[http://dx.doi.org/10.1074/mcp.M400205-MCP200] [PMID: 15644556]

[32]   Hu Y, Zhang S, Yu J, Liu J, Zheng S. SELDI-TOF-MS: the proteomics and bioinformatics approaches in the diagnosis of breast cancer. Breast 2005; 14(4): 250-5.
[http://dx.doi.org/10.1016/j.breast.2005.01.008] [PMID: 16085230]

[33]   Li J, Zhao J, Yu X, *et al.* Identification of biomarkers for breast cancer in nipple aspiration and ductal lavage fluid. Clin Cancer Res 2005; 11(23): 8312-20.
[http://dx.doi.org/10.1158/1078-0432.CCR-05-1538] [PMID: 16322290]

[34]   Pawlik TM, Fritsche H, Coombes KR, *et al.* Significant differences in nipple aspirate fluid protein expression between healthy women and those with breast cancer demonstrated by time-of-flight mass spectrometry. Breast Cancer Res Treat 2005; 89(2): 149-57.
[http://dx.doi.org/10.1007/s10549-004-1710-4] [PMID: 15692757]

[35]   Sauter ER, Shan S, Hewett JE, Speckman P, Du Bois GC. Proteomic analysis of nipple aspirate fluid using SELDI-TOF-MS. Int J Cancer 2005; 114(5): 791-6.
[http://dx.doi.org/10.1002/ijc.20742] [PMID: 15609313]

[36]   Noble JL, Dua RS, Coulton GR, Isacke CM, Gui GP. A comparative proteinomic analysis of nipple aspiration fluid from healthy women and women with breast cancer. Eur J Cancer 2007; 43(16): 2315-20.
[http://dx.doi.org/10.1016/j.ejca.2007.08.009] [PMID: 17904354]

[37]   He J, Gornbein J, Shen D, *et al.* Detection of breast cancer biomarkers in nipple aspirate fluid by SELDI-TOF and their identification by combined liquid chromatography-tandem mass spectrometry. Int J Oncol 2007; 30(1): 145-54.
[http://dx.doi.org/10.3892/ijo.30.1.145] [PMID: 17143523]

[38]   Carter D, Douglass JF, Cornellison CD, *et al.* Purification and characterization of the mammaglobin/lipophilin B complex, a promising diagnostic marker for breast cancer. Biochemistry 2002; 41(21): 6714-22.
[http://dx.doi.org/10.1021/bi0159884] [PMID: 12022875]

[39]   Ricolleau G, Charbonnel C, Lodé L, *et al.* Surface-enhanced laser desorption/ionization time of flight mass spectrometry protein profiling identifies ubiquitin and ferritin light chain as prognostic biomarkers in node-negative breast cancer tumors. Proteom 2006; 6(6): 1963-75.
[http://dx.doi.org/10.1002/pmic.200500283] [PMID: 16470659]

[40]   Lebrecht A, Boehm D, Schmidt M, Koelbl H, Schwirz RL, Grus FH. Diagnosis of breast cancer by tear proteomic pattern. Can Genom Proteom 2009; 6(3): 177-82.
[PMID: 19487546]

[41]   Gonçalves A, Charafe-Jauffret E, Bertucci F, *et al.* Protein profiling of human breast tumor cells identifies novel biomarkers associated with molecular subtypes. Mol Cell Proteom 2008; 7(8): 1420-33.
[http://dx.doi.org/10.1074/mcp.M700487-MCP200] [PMID: 18426791]

[42]   Gast MC, Zapatka M, van Tinteren H, *et al.* Postoperative serum proteomic profiles may predict recurrence-free survival in high-risk primary breast cancer. J Cancer Res Clin Oncol 2011; 137(12): 1773-83.
[http://dx.doi.org/10.1007/s00432-011-1055-4] [PMID: 21913038]

[43]   Nakagawa T, Huang SK, Martinez SR, *et al.* Proteomic profiling of primary breast cancer predicts axillary lymph node metastasis. Cancer Res 2006; 66(24): 11825-30.
[http://dx.doi.org/10.1158/0008-5472.CAN-06-2337] [PMID: 17178879]

[44]   Pusztai L, Gregory BW, Baggerly KA, *et al.* Pharmacoproteomic analysis of prechemotherapy and postchemotherapy plasma samples from patients receiving neoadjuvant or adjuvant chemotherapy for breast carcinoma. Cancer 2004; 100(9): 1814-22.
[http://dx.doi.org/10.1002/cncr.20203] [PMID: 15112261]

[45]   Lee K. Evaluation of an effective sample prefractionation method for the proteome analysis of breast cancer tissue using narrow range two-dimensional gel electrophoresis. Biosci Biotechnol Biochem 2008; 72(6): 1464-74.
[http://dx.doi.org/10.1271/bbb.70777] [PMID: 18540105]

[46]   Smith L, Welham KJ, Watson MB, Drew PJ, Lind MJ, Cawkwell L. The proteomic analysis of cisplatin resistance in breast cancer cells. Oncol Res 2007; 16(11): 497-506.
[http://dx.doi.org/10.3727/096504007783438358] [PMID: 18306929]

[47]   Zhou C, Nitschke AM, Xiong W, *et al.* Proteomic analysis of tumor necrosis factor-alpha resistant human breast cancer cells reveals a MEK5/Erk5-mediated epithelial-mesenchymal transition phenotype. Breast Cancer Res 2008; 10(6): R105.
[http://dx.doi.org/10.1186/bcr2210] [PMID: 19087274]

[48]   Sun B, Zhang S, Zhang D, *et al.* Identification of metastasis-related proteins and their clinical relevance to triple-negative human breast cancer. Clin Cancer Res 2008; 14(21): 7050-9.
[http://dx.doi.org/10.1158/1078-0432.CCR-08-0520] [PMID: 18981002]

[49]   Li DQ, Wang L, Fei F, *et al.* Identification of breast cancer metastasis-associated proteins in an isogenic tumor metastasis model using two-dimensional gel electrophoresis and liquid chromatography-ion trap-mass spectrometry. Proteom 2006; 6(11): 3352-68.
[http://dx.doi.org/10.1002/pmic.200500617] [PMID: 16637015]

[50]   Ambrosino C, Tarallo R, Bamundo A, *et al.* Identification of a hormone-regulated dynamic nuclear actin network associated with estrogen receptor alpha in human breast cancer cell nuclei. Mol Cell Proteom 2010; 9(6): 1352-67.
[http://dx.doi.org/10.1074/mcp.M900519-MCP200] [PMID: 20308691]

[51]   DeAngelis JT, Li Y, Mitchell N, Wilson L, Kim H, Tollefsbol TO. 2D difference gel electrophoresis analysis of different time points during the course of neoplastic transformation of human mammary epithelial cells. J Proteom Res 2011; 10(2): 447-58.
[http://dx.doi.org/10.1021/pr100533k] [PMID: 21105747]

[52]   Lim S, Choong LY, Kuan CP, Yunhao C, Lim YP. Regulation of macrophage inhibitory factor (MIF) by epidermal growth factor receptor (EGFR) in the MCF10AT model of breast cancer progression. J Proteom Res 2009; 8(8): 4062-76.
[http://dx.doi.org/10.1021/pr900430n] [PMID: 19530702]

[53]   Michlmayr A, Bachleitner-Hofmann T, Baumann S, *et al.* Modulation of plasma complement by the initial dose of epirubicin/docetaxel therapy in breast cancer and its predictive value. Br J Cancer 2010; 103(8): 1201-8.
[http://dx.doi.org/10.1038/sj.bjc.6605909] [PMID: 20877360]

[54]   Mathelin C, Cromer A, Wendling C, Tomasetto C, Rio MC. Serum biomarkers for detection of breast cancers: A prospective study. Breast Cancer Res Treat 2006; 96(1): 83-90.
[http://dx.doi.org/10.1007/s10549-005-9046-2] [PMID: 16322896]

[55]   Leong S, Nunez AC, Lin MZ, Crossett B, Christopherson RI, Baxter RC. iTRAQ-based proteomic profiling of breast cancer cell response to doxorubicin and TRAIL. J Proteom Res 2012; 11(7): 3561-72.
[http://dx.doi.org/10.1021/pr2012335] [PMID: 22587632]

[56]   Muraoka S, Kume H, Watanabe S, *et al.* Strategy for SRM-based verification of biomarker candidates discovered by iTRAQ method in limited breast cancer tissue samples. J Proteom Res 2012; 11(8): 4201-10.
[http://dx.doi.org/10.1021/pr300322q] [PMID: 22716024]

[57]   Metodieva G, Greenwood C, Alldridge L, Sauven P, Metodiev M. A peptide-centric approach to breast cancer biomarker discovery utilizing label-free multiple reaction monitoring mass spectrometry. Proteomics Clin Appl 2009; 3(1): 78-82.
[http://dx.doi.org/10.1002/prca.200800072] [PMID: 21136937]

[58]   Sprung RW, Martinez MA, Carpenter KL, *et al.* Precision of multiple reaction monitoring mass spectrometry analysis of formalin-fixed, paraffin-embedded tissue. J Proteom Res 2012; 11(6): 3498-505.
[http://dx.doi.org/10.1021/pr300130t] [PMID: 22530795]

[59]   Goncalves A, Bertucci F. Clinical application of proteomics in breast cancer: state of the art and perspectives. Med Princ Pract 2011; 20(1): 4-18.
[http://dx.doi.org/10.1159/000319544] [PMID: 21160207]

[60]   Harris L, Fritsche H, Mennel R, *et al.* American Society of Clinical Oncology 2007 update of recommendations for the use of tumor markers in breast cancer. J Clin Oncol 2007; 25(33): 5287-312.
[http://dx.doi.org/10.1200/JCO.2007.14.2364] [PMID: 17954709]

CHAPTER 5

Deregulation of Enzymatic Post-Translational Modifications in Breast Cancer

Lokesh Baweja[1,*], Neha Rajoria[2] and Shankar Suman[3]

[1]*Department of Physics and the Center for Molecular Study of Condensed Soft Matter, Illinois Institute of Technology, Chicago, Illinois 60616, USA*
[2]*Meerut Institute of Engineering and Technology, Meerut, Uttar Pradesh250005, India*
[3]*The Ohio State University, Columbus 43210, USA*

Abstract: Post-translational modifications (PTMs) regulate vital cellular processes such as signaling, proteasomal mediated degradation of proteins, and transcription. Deregulation of post-translational modifications (PTMs) has been proven to have a strong association with breast cancer development. Aberrant PTMs can promote carcinogenesis by perturbing normal cellular homeostasis. The current literature review showed that breast cancer cells displayed abnormal ubiquitination, glycosylation, phosphorylation, and SUMOylation patterns. Breast cancer cells also exhibited stable modifications in histone proteins and DNA. These epigenetic modifications can directly affect the expression of cell cycle regulators by disrupting the transcriptional state of the genome. The current chapter summarizes the involvement of PTMs in carcinogenesis and the mechanism by which PTMs promote abnormal cell growth. Enzymes responsible for aberrant PTMs could be targeted to reduce the severity of the disease and may improve the prognosis of breast cancer.

Keywords: Biomarkers, Breast Cancer, Epigenetics, Post-Translational Modifications.

INTRODUCTION

Breast cancer in females is one of the major causes of cancer-related mortalities [1]. Statistical data suggests that around 1 in 8 woman develops breast cancer during her life span [2].

Breast cancer can be described as a cellular anomaly with a high level of heterogeneity and developmental hierarchy [3]. Several studies have reported the deleterious changes at the cellular and molecular levels associated with the development of cancer including aberrant post-translational modifications (PTMs)

* **Corresponding author Lokesh Baweja**: Department of Physics and the Center for Molecular Study of Condensed Soft Matter, Illinois Institute of Technology, Chicago, Illinois 60616, USA; Tel: +15157084065; E-mail: baweja.lokesh@gmail2Ecom

Shankar Suman, Garima Suman and Sanjay Mishra (Eds.)

of the proteome [4]. Association between genomic mutations and breast cancer is very well established through high-throughput next-generation sequencing (NGS) techniques [5, 6]. However, the role of PTMs in breast cancer development is still not well understood. PTMs constitute an additional layer for regulating the structure and activity of proteins. PTMs may affect the function and activity of proteins by modifying their charge, size, and conformations [7, 8]. Moreover, cancer-associated PTMs could be used as a biomarker to develop non-invasive approaches for detecting cancer at an early stage [9]. The majority of the reported PTMs include glycosylation, acetylation, ribosylation, methylation, and SUMOylation are enzymatic [10]. However, non-enzymatic PTMs such as oxidation are also associated with cancer development and metastasis [11, 12]. These modifications may facilitate cancer growth by disturbing cellular homeostasis. Deregulation of histone-modifying enzymes (HME) has been documented in different cell types, which leads to the aberrant modification of histone proteins [13]. Modifications in histones protein and DNA are known as epigenetic changes. Unlike other PTMs, epigenetic changes are reversible and can be corrected *via* therapeutic interventions [14]. For example, drugs targeting HME are in clinical use for hematological malignancies and under clinical trials for treating solid tumors [15]. In this chapter, we discussed the association of PTMs in breast cancer development and their potential as non-invasive early-stage biomarkers and novel therapeutic targets to reduce the severity of the disease.

POST TRANSLATIONAL MODIFICATIONS OF PROTEINS

Glycosylation

Glycosylation is one of the most common PTMs, and the process is catalyzed by enzymes in a specific manner, resulting in the attachment of glycan to proteins. The process that involves the modification of nitrogen of asparagine or arginine amino acid residues is known as N-linked glycosylation, whereas O-linked glycosylation involves the modification of hydroxyl oxygen of serine, threonine, tyrosine, hydroxylysine, and hydroxyproline [16]. Glycans are complex polymers and can be formed by ten monosaccharide sugars, namely glucose, galactose, mannose, glucuronic acid, N-acetlyglucosamine, N-acetlygalactosamine. Glycosylation plays a pivotal role in regulating cell signaling; any alteration in the glycosylation pattern can transform the normal cell into the cancerous cell [17]. In-depth knowledge of mechanisms and consequences of variation in glycosylation patterns is essential in order to understand their contribution to cancer cell development. Significant changes in O-glycans (GalNAc-Ser/Thr) and N-glycans were found to be associated with cellular transformations [18, 19]. Glycosyltransferase regulates the degree of glycan branching, and the expression of this enzyme can modulate the glycosylation patterns [20].

The glycan structure can be further modified to generate unique glycan motifs, such as highly fucosylated glycans and are found in the cell surface of the neoplastic cell. Breast cancer cells showed both O- and N-linked glycosylation modifications [21]. Overexpression of the N-glycosylated HER2 receptor was observed in breast cancer [22]. Recent reports suggested that glycosylation of HER2 directly affected the binding of the Herceptin [22]. In addition to direct binding, glycosylation also affected the sensitivity of doxorubicin towards breast cancer cells [23]. This report potentiates the need for combination therapy, which includes targeting glycosylation patterns in breast cancer along with anti-cancerous drugs for a better prognosis. Breast cancer cells also showed deregulation in O-glycosylation, which resulted in the accumulation of mucin-type tumor-associated antigens [24]. O-glycosylation is regulated by N-acetyl-D-galactosaminyl transferase (GalNAc-Tases) enzymes family and plays a role in the initial steps of mucin O-glycosylation. Altered O-glycosylation is also linked with the proliferation of the cancer cells and the metastasis of breast cancer cells by decreasing cell surface E-cadherin [24]. Yoshinori Ino *et al.,* reported that E-cadherin down-regulation is carried out by Dysadherin, which is a cancer-associated cell membrane glycoprotein and Gu Y *et al.,* explained that E-cadherin downregulation in breast cancer cell due to the glycosylation of p120 and beta-catenin [25, 26]. Immunohistochemistry of breast tumor tissues along with adjacent tissue showed that GlcNAcylation (*i.e.,* a PTM modification that involves the addition of N-acetyl glucosamine residue to serine and threonine residue) is significantly elevated in breast tumor tissues compared to the adjacent tissue [26].

Along with proteins, cancer-specific antigens (CA15.3), which is commonly used for the detection of breast cancer, showed alteration in glycosylation patterns but didn't correlate it with the early stage of breast cancer [27]. CA15-3 is a form of soluble transmembrane protein with variable numbers of glycosylated tandem peptide repeats. The glycosylated form of this protein could be used as an exclusive biomarker for breast cancer cells. However, identifying this PTM in the serum of breast cancer patients is challenging, as suggested by the study of Choi *et al.,* they came up with an antibody-lectin sandwich assay for the detection of glycosylated CA15-3 in patients sera [28]. Autoantibodies against another glycoprotein MUC1 were found in sera of breast cancer patients with stage I and stage II and this modified form of the protein can serve as a useful biomarker for early-stage breast cancer [29]. Glycosylation pattern was also affected by elevated levels of transferase enzymes, such as GCNT2, due to the overexpression of a gene-encoding glucosaminyl (N-acetyl) transferase 2, I-branching in metastatic breast cancer cell lines and basal-like breast tumor samples. GCNT2 has been shown to be involved in epithelial-to-mesenchymal transition and may promote metastasis of cancer cells by modulation their adhesion to endothelial cells [30].

Phosphorylation

Phosphorylation is one of the important PTMs regulated by varieties of kinases, which phosphorylates serine, threonine, and tyrosine residues in proteins [31]. Deregulation of phosphorylation has been associated with breast cancer cell development [32]. Cell migration and invasion are affected by phosphorylation patterns. Authors had reported the involvement of cortactin phosphorylation in actin polymerization, which promoted the breast cell migration and invasion. Integrin signaling induced the phosphorylation of Fos-related antigen (FRA-1) and resulted in enhanced breast cancer invasion [33]. Cell cycle events are controlled by phosphorylation of cell cycle regulatory proteins. Cyclin E is an important cell cycle regulator, which binds and activates cyclin-dependent kinase subunit (CDK2). Mull BB *et al.,* had reported the phosphorylation of threonine 395 in cyclin E and its phosphorylation plays an important role in the proteasome-mediated degradation in tumor cell line [34]. They also reported different phosphorylation sites within the cyclin E generating the larger isoform of each doublet; however, the low molecular weight isoform is stable in both tumor and non-tumor cell lines [34]. Protein Kinase C (PKC) has a diverse role in cellular functions as evident from its multiple forms.

Christoph Borner *et al.* reported the multiple forms of PKC having different molecular weights in human breast cancer cells, which express a specific type of PKC [35]. The study showed that PKC is unphosphorylated when synthesized in membranes as and is later converted into the active 77- and 80-kDa form by post-translational modification events that involves two phosphorylation steps aiding tumor growth and also interferes with the posttranslational processing that converts the 74-kDa PKCs precursor into the 77- and 80-kDa forms of the enzyme [35]. Furthermore, the deregulation of phosphorylation regulating enzymes is also linked with Human Triple-negative breast cancer (TNBC) [36]. This form of breast cancer is poorly understood and refractory to current therapeutic approaches where tumors are negative for ER, PR, and HER2/neu. Specific molecular targets for this subgroup have not been identified, and the directed therapies are unavailable, because of frequent compromisation of PTPN12 tyrosine phosphatase in TNBC [36]. The study also showed the role of the upstream tumor-suppressor network in post-transcriptional controls of PTPN12, which suppressed mammary epithelial cell proliferation and transformation by interacting and inhibiting multiple oncogenic tyrosine kinases, including HER2 and EGFR9. The tumorigenic and metastatic potential of TNBC cells deficient in PTPN12 is weakened upon restoration of PTPN12 function or by the inhibition of PTPN12-regulated tyrosine kinases; this finding suggests that TNBCs are dependent on the tyrosine kinases. Due to tumor suppressor activity of PTPN12 and its regulated kinases are potential targets in TNBC and other cancers [36].

Reports also documented the phosphorylation of small heat shock proteins (sHSPs), which modify their structural and functional properties. Serine 59 phosphorylation of {alpha} B-crystallin impaired its anti-apoptotic function by binding and sequestering Bcl-2 in breast cancer cells [37]. Chronic inflammation is also an important signature, and have a heightened transcriptional factor activity of nuclear factor-κB (NF-κB coupled with the development of many cancers. For example, transcriptional activation of cIAP2 (cellular inhibitor of apoptosis 2) gene is regulated by NF- κB. The phosphorylation of S276 on RelA/p65, a subunit of nuclear factor-κB (NF-κB), acts as a transcriptional repressor by enhancing methylation of the promoter of BRMS1 (breast cancer metastasis suppressor 1) gene through the direct recruitment of DNMT-1 (DNA (cytosine-5--methyltransferase 1). Further, Y. Liu *et al.* highlighted that BRMS1 could be a target for epigenetic onco-pharmaceuticals through NF-κB modification [38].

SUMOylation

SUMO (small ubiquitin-related modifier), a member of ubiquitin-like protein shares high structural similarity with ubiquitin [39, 40]. Despite this similarity, they perform different biological functions. SUMOylation is a three-step process that involves activation, conjugation, and ligation of SUMO moiety. Each of the SUMOlyated pathways requires its own sets of enzymes E2 conjugating enzyme-like Ubc9, it transfers the activated SUMO to protein substrates, and play a critical role in sumoylation-mediated cellular pathways in breast cancer [41]. It is apparent from the studies that SUMO contributes to carcinogenesis by modifying key proteins involved in the cellular process. SUMOylation largely involved in the process for subcellular localization, stabilization of transcriptional cofactors, and chromatin remodeling factors. Several oncogenes and tumor suppressor genes, including Mdm2, p53, p68 and, p72 RNA helicases, undergo SUMOylation [41 - 43]. SUMOylation of p53 decreased its transactivation activity, and it is driven by PIASI (protein inhibitor of activated STAT1), which act as SUMO ligase [44]. Various receptors are targets of SUMO-1 (a small ubiquitin-like modifier). Protein SUMOylation modulates their interaction with binding partners. Progesterone receptor SUMOylation increased its association with steroid receptor coactivator-1 (SRC1), which increase the retention of SRC1 in the nucleus [45]. SUMOylation also modulates the transcriptional activity of glucocorticoid receptors [46]. SUMO-1 can modify the proteins involved in the DNA damage response (DDR). The clinical and biological studies establish the relation between SUMOylation and breast cancer having BRCA1 germline mutations [47]. This PTM not only affects the protein-protein interactions but also plays a role in drug sensitivity towards cells. SUMOylation modulated the forked transcription factor (FORK2) mediated paclitaxel sensitivity in breast cancer [48]. Moreover, there is substantial evidence that SUMOylation is responsible for maintaining breast cancer subtype. The study showed that SUMOylation of TFAP2A is essential for breast cancer cell lines to transform into tumor xenografts. The above evidence suggested that the sumoylation pathway could be targeted to prevent basal breast cancer cell types [49].

Ubiquitination

Ubiquitin is a small protein of 76 amino acid residues, which is ubiquitously present in eukaryotic cells [50]. It not only helps in proteolysis but also modifies the target substrate signals in cellular processes contributing to the mammary tumorigenesis. Approximately 70% of breast cancer cases are estrogen receptor alpha-positive [51]. Ubiquitin can bind covalently and non-covalently with these receptors and which makes it worthy of investigating its role in breast cancer development. Ubiquitination (Ubq) may not serve merely as a target for proteasomal degradation but also implicated in the important cellular process such as cell signaling and DNA repair [52]. Pleiotropic effects of the cognate hormone 17β-estradiol (E2) are mediated by the monoubiquitination of estrogen receptor α (ERα). E2 decreases erα mono-Ubq in breast cancer cells due to inefficient E2 induced ERα phosphorylation at serine residue 118 (S118). Ubiquitylation is responsible for the binding of ERα with the insulin-like growth factor (IGF-1-R), and monoubiquitination impairs E2-induced association ERα to IGF-1-R. The study demonstrated an important role of monoubiquitination in ERα signaling and its role in the regulation of E2-induced cell proliferation [53].

Some studies linked Ubiquitination with carcinogenesis. This PTM modifies the stability of heat shock proteins 90 and its interacting partners. One of the proteins is CHIP (carboxyl-terminus of Hsc70-interacting protein), and it is known to modulate the stability of the estrogen receptor (ESR1) and Her-2/neu (ERBB2). CHIP expression can be used as a prognostic parameter, including tumor grade, as evidenced by its higher expression in normal and benign tumor samples compared to breast cancer tissue. However, no statistical significance can be established [54].

Breast cancer stem cell-like in tumors possess a high resistance towards therapeutic benefit. It has been shown that CHIP E3 ubiquitin ligase is decreased in breast cancer stem cells. CHIP plays an important role in stemness by interacting with OCT4, which is a marker of stem cells. CHIP overexpression can deplete OCT4 through proteasomal degradation [55]. CHIP has a direct effect on the mammosphere formation. Its depletion enhanced the mammosphere formation but reversed by its overexpression [55].

Methylation

Methylation of protein has an important implication in breast cancer progression, and this PTM mostly affects the transcriptional factors activity [56]. Amino acid arginine undergoes methylation in proteins such as H3, Sam68, and H4 [57, 58]. This PTM is catalyzed by protein arginine methyltransferase-1 (PRMT1), and the degree of methylation decides the activating or repressing effects of this PTM. Transcription factors p53, an important tumor suppressor, is mutated in more than 50% of all human cancers [59]. It possesses three methylation sites, such as K370, K372, and K382. p53 methylation at lysine 372 site is correlated with transcription activation by stabilizing p53. However, lysine 382 and lysine 370 methylation inhibited p53 transcriptional activity [60 - 62]. Another important regulator of cell cycle BRCA1 (Tumor Suppressor Protein C) has multifunctional implications in cellular processes such as cell cycle, transcription, DNA damage response, and chromatin remodeling. The methylation BRCA1 influences its transcriptional cofactor function that may lead to affect the tumor suppressor potential of BRCA1 [63].

DNA Methylation and Histone Modifications in Breast Cancer Development

Histone post-translational modifications are epigenetic marks involved in dynamic cellular processes, such as transcription, DNA repair, and maintaining the repressible state of chromatin. Prognosis and the development of cancer are highly correlated with each other [64]. The dynamics of the nucleosome are controlled by covalent modifications of histones, which include acetylation, methylation, phosphorylation, biotinylation, and sumoylation [65]. Among these modifications, acetylation and methylation are stable epigenetic changes and transmitted during cell division [66, 67]. Histone H4 display loss of acetylation and methylation patterns in human cancers [68]. Acetylation of H4K16ac is significantly reduced in 78.9% breast cancer cases. Carcinomas including basal carcinomas, have low levels of lysine acetylation (H3K9ac, H3K18ac, and H4K12ac), lysine (H3K4me2 and H4K20me3), and arginine methylation (H4R3me2) in HER2-positive cells [69]. DNA also showed distinct methylation patterns inside the cell along with histone modifications. CpG island hypermethylation is associated with reduced expression of tumor repressor genes in cancer. Aberrant methylation affects several cellular processes such as cell cycle regulation, DNA repair mechanisms, hormone regulation pathways, invasion and metastasis [70]. A study also reported an exclusive presence of methylated DNA promoter in patients with early invasive and preinvasive breast cancer [71].

Interestingly, methylation was absent in serum samples obtained from normal women suggesting the specificity of this marker in breast cancer [71]. Genes involved in important cellular pathways showed consistent methylation profiles and could differentiate between normal and breast cancer cells. The normal cell also maintains hypermethylated regions, and maintenance of methylation is important for preventing chromosome translocation and gene disruption through reactivation of transposable elements. Tumor characteristics such as size, stage, and histological grade exhibited global DNA hypomethylation in breast cancer [72]. This evidence supports that DNA methylation is an important contributing factor in cancer cell development and may have a high therapeutic value [73].

Lipidation

Isoprenylation and S-acylation modified the membrane proteins, and this process is known as lipidation. Prenylation of proteins is essential for membrane-associated function and important biological activities [74]. It involves the covalent modification of farnesyl (C15) or a geranylgeranyl (C20) moiety to Carboxy terminal cysteine(s) of the target protein by Farnesyltransferase (FT) and geranylgeranyltransferase (GGT) I, respectively. The main target of prenylation is Ras superfamily. Farnesylpyrophosphate and geranylgeranyl pyrophosphate lipids modify Ras and Rho proteins. Prenylated proteins influence cell cycle progression. Philippe Cestac *et al.* showed that prenylation inhibitors modulate the transcriptional activity of the ER by competing with estradiol [75, 76]. In later years they studied that Prenylation inhibitors also modulate the activity of α and β estrogen receptor. They also show that Prenylated Rho proteins have antagonistic effects on estrogen receptor activity. Another inhibitor used for breast cancer is Gliotoxin is a sulfur-containing compound that inhibits both FTase and GGTase and also shows low toxicity and pronounced anti-tumor activity [77].

Acylation

Most of the membrane protein is recognized as post-translationally acylated, which has a high implication of malignant growth of breast cancer. This includes the members of the Src and Ras families of oncoproteins; it works at a leaflet of cellular plasma membranes to control biological signal transduction pathways [78, 79]. The commonly found protein acylations are myristoylation and palmitoylation, which process by myristoyl transferase and palmitoyl acyltransferase (PAT) like enzyme, respectively.

Adenosine Diphosphate (ADP)-ribosylation

Poly (ADP-ribose) polymerase (PARP) is the ubiquitous enzyme of a nucleus, which has an important role in sequence catalysis of the transfer of ADP-ribose to target proteins. The Nuclear proteins, particularly histones and transcription factors, are the primary targets of ribosylation. PARP-1 involved in various cellular apoptosis and survival pathway; meanwhile, it also showed a novel target of breast cancer in the current research scenario. Rojo. *et al.,* observed the higher PARP-1 protein level in higher tumor grade (P = 0.01), estrogen-negative tumors (P <0.001) and triple-negative phenotype (P < 0.001) of breast cancer patients(N=300) [80]. Hence, it is excellent to be targeted PARP inhibitors for breast cancer. PARP1 importantly affects more than ninety genes reported based on the microarray, but their detail mechanism is still unrevealed [81]. Transcriptional factors modification such as AP-2α (activator protein 2α), which regulates an array of genes involved in diverse cellular events, loss of its activity incorporates cancer induction. PARP1 shows dual regulation of AP-2α, where it acts as a co-activator of AP-2α, and it also shows the enzymatic activity as in a temporary shut-off mechanism during unfavorable conditions [82].

OXIDATIVE STRESS MEDIATED REGULATION OF PROTEIN MODIFICATION IN BREAST CANCER

Reactive oxygen species (ROS) generation has important implications in cancer growth. Higher Oxidative Stress is found in nipple aspirated fluid obtained from breast cancer patients [83]. ROS levels were highly correlated with hydroxylation, oxidation, glutathionylation, and S-Nitrosylation. Moreover, ROS scavenger in breast cancer is down-regulated one of the examples is methionine sulfoxide reductase A (Msr A), which is known to protect proteins from oxidation. The level of MsrA can be correlated with advanced tumor grade [84]. Antonella De Luca *et al.* showed that MsrA downregulation involved in tumor suppressor PTEN (phosphatases and tensin homolog deleted on chromosome ten protein) reduction and lead to an activation of PI3K (phosphoinositide-3-kinase) pathway as well as in up-regulation of VEGF which provide additional support for tumor growth.

NO (Nitric acid, an important free radical) encounters many biological significances in cellular metabolism, and it shows an important role in breast cancer progression. NO level in cancer cell expression regulated by some signals like β-estradiol, which induces the expression of endothelial nitric acid synthase and production of NO. NO reversibly target protein in PTM process at certain amino acid residue like tyrosine, cysteine, *via* which tumorigenesis progress. NO often couple with cysteine thiols to form an S-Nitrosothiol, which regulates the enzymatic activities of target proteins specifically c-Src tyrosine kinase that promotes cancer cell invasion and metastasis. c-Src is a non-receptor tyrosine kinase and plays an important role in many cellular processes such as proliferation, migration, and transformation. NO causes S-nitrosylation of c-Src at cysteine 498 (Cys[498]) to stimulate its kinase activity and also important for the

NO-mediated activation of c-Yes [85]. Rahman *et al.* also reported that NO-dependent activation of c-Src favors the enhancement of cell invasion by β-estradiol stimulation and disruption of E-cadherin junctions and hence implicated a role in breast cancer invasion and metastasis.

CONCLUSION AND FUTURE PERSPECTIVES

Several studies reviewed in this chapter have documented the aberrant protein modifications in breast cancer carcinogenesis. Like hereditary mutations, epigenetic modifications can be transmitted during the division of breast cancer cells. Unlike other PTMs, epigenetic modifications are more stable and could help in diagnosing cancer by non-invasive approaches. Histone modifications emerged as new therapeutic targets along with the hormonal therapy. For example, histone-modifying enzymes, histone deacetylases (HDACs class I and class II) are proposed as potential targets for breast cancer. Similarly, several transcription factors that undergo ubiquitination, sumoylation, and methylation can also be targeted. PTMs also generate new epitopes, and autoantibodies against these could be used for early detection of breast cancer. However, the majority of PTMs in breast cancer cells have diverse biological and pathologic consequences influencing growth and survival of the cells and their ability to invade and metastasize. Like other targets, PTMs are present in both the tumor and healthy cells, and their targeting may also lead to undesirable side effects. Current studies also suggested the need for high throughput technologies like NGS to sequence protein for their modifications. Further advances in the field of proteomics may reveal new potential targets and help in generating novel therapeutics for cancer treatments. Therefore, the major concern of PTMs in therapeutic use is the development of most suitable molecular and surrogate markers in breast cancer patients which can be clinically correlated and need also to be transferred it from basic research and technology development for the use of PTMs as tools for early detection, chemoprevention and risk assessment on the basis of their priority.

CONSENT FOR PUBLICATION

Not applicable.

CONFLICT OF INTEREST

The authors confirm that the contents of this chapter have no conflict of interest.

ACKNOWLEDGEMENT

Lokesh Baweja would like to thank Illinois Institute of Technology for providing financial support.

REFERENCES

[1]   Torre LA, Bray F, Siegel RL, Ferlay J, Lortet-Tieulent J, Jemal A. Global cancer statistics, 2012. CA Cancer J Clin 2015; 65(2): 87-108.
[http://dx.doi.org/10.3322/caac.21262] [PMID: 25651787]

[2]   DeSantis CE, Fedewa SA, Goding Sauer A, Kramer JL, Smith RA, Jemal A. Breast cancer statistics, 2015: Convergence of incidence rates between black and white women. CA Cancer J Clin 2016; 66(1): 31-42.
[http://dx.doi.org/10.3322/caac.21320] [PMID: 26513636]

[3]   Polyak K. Heterogeneity in breast cancer. J Clin Invest 2011; 121(10): 3786-8.
[http://dx.doi.org/10.1172/JCI60534] [PMID: 21965334]

[4]   Krueger KE, Srivastava S. Posttranslational protein modifications: current implications for cancer detection, prevention, and therapeutics. Mol Cell Proteom 2006; 5(10): 1799-810.
[http://dx.doi.org/10.1074/mcp.R600009-MCP200] [PMID: 16844681]

[5]   Coles C, Condie A, Chetty U, Steel CM, Evans HJ, Prosser J. p53 mutations in breast cancer. Cancer Res 1992; 52(19): 5291-8.
[PMID: 1394133]

[6]   King MC, Marks JH, Mandell JB. Breast and ovarian cancer risks due to inherited mutations in BRCA1 and BRCA2. Science 2003; 302(5645): 643-6.
[http://dx.doi.org/10.1126/science.1088759] [PMID: 14576434]

[7]   Gavrilov Y, Hagai T, Levy Y. Nonspecific yet decisive: Ubiquitination can affect the native-state dynamics of the modified protein. Protein Sci 2015; 24(10): 1580-92.
[http://dx.doi.org/10.1002/pro.2688] [PMID: 25970168]

[8]   Xin F, Radivojac P. Post-translational modifications induce significant yet not extreme changes to protein structure. Bioinformatics 2012; 28(22): 2905-13.
[http://dx.doi.org/10.1093/bioinformatics/bts541] [PMID: 22947645]

[9]   Hanash SM, Pitteri SJ, Faca VM. Mining the plasma proteome for cancer biomarkers. Nature 2008; 452(7187): 571-9.
[http://dx.doi.org/10.1038/nature06916] [PMID: 18385731]

[10] Jin H, Zangar RC. Protein modifications as potential biomarkers in breast cancer. Biomarker insights 2009; BMI-S2557.
[http://dx.doi.org/10.4137/BMI.S2557]

[11] Karihtala P, Mäntyniemi A, Kang SW, Kinnula VL, Soini Y. Peroxiredoxins in breast carcinoma. Clin Cancer Res 2003; 9(9): 3418-24.
[PMID: 12960131]

[12] Marx J. Cancer research. Inflammation and cancer: the link grows stronger. Science 2004; 306(5698): 966-8.
[http://dx.doi.org/10.1126/science.306.5698.966] [PMID: 15528423]

[13] Noberini R, Osti D, Miccolo C, *et al.* Extensive and systematic rewiring of histone post-translational modifications in cancer model systems. Nucleic Acids Res 2018; 46(8): 3817-32.
[http://dx.doi.org/10.1093/nar/gky224] [PMID: 29618087]

[14] Copeland RA, Olhava EJ, Scott MP. Targeting epigenetic enzymes for drug discovery. Curr Opin Chem Biol 2010; 14(4): 505-10.
[http://dx.doi.org/10.1016/j.cbpa.2010.06.174] [PMID: 20621549]

[15] Mercurio C, Minucci S, Pelicci PG. Histone deacetylases and epigenetic therapies of hematological malignancies. Pharmacol Res 2010; 62(1): 18-34.
[http://dx.doi.org/10.1016/j.phrs.2010.02.010] [PMID: 20219679]

[16] Ohtsubo K, Marth JD. Glycosylation in cellular mechanisms of health and disease. Cell 2006; 126(5):

855-67.
[http://dx.doi.org/10.1016/j.cell.2006.08.019] [PMID: 16959566]

[17]   Dennis JW, Granovsky M, Warren CE. Glycoprotein glycosylation and cancer progression. Biochimica et Biophysica Acta (BBA)-. General Subjects 1999; 1473(1): 21-34.
[http://dx.doi.org/10.1016/S0304-4165(99)00167-1]

[18]   Rodrigues JG, Balmaña M, Macedo JA, *et al.* Glycosylation in cancer: Selected roles in tumour progression, immune modulation and metastasis. Cell Immunol 2018; 333: 46-57.
[http://dx.doi.org/10.1016/j.cellimm.2018.03.007] [PMID: 29576316]

[19]   Kim YJ, Varki A. Perspectives on the significance of altered glycosylation of glycoproteins in cancer. Glycoconj J 1997; 14(5): 569-76.
[http://dx.doi.org/10.1023/A:1018580324971] [PMID: 9298689]

[20]   LaMont JT, Isselbacher KJ. Alterations in glycosyltransferase activity in human colon cancer. J Natl Cancer Inst 1975; 54(1): 53-6.
[http://dx.doi.org/10.1093/jnci/54.1.53] [PMID: 1113312]

[21]   de Leoz ML, Young LJ, An HJ, *et al.* High-mannose glycans are elevated during breast cancer progression. Mol Cell Proteom 2011; 10(1): 002717.
[http://dx.doi.org/10.1074/mcp.M110.002717] [PMID: 21097542]

[22]   Lesniak D, Sabri S, Xu Y, *et al.* Spontaneous epithelial-mesenchymal transition and resistance to HER-2-targeted therapies in HER-2-positive luminal breast cancer. PLoS One 2013; 8(8): e71987.
[http://dx.doi.org/10.1371/journal.pone.0071987] [PMID: 23991019]

[23]   Peiris D, Spector AF, Lomax-Browne H, *et al.* Cellular glycosylation affects Herceptin binding and sensitivity of breast cancer cells to doxorubicin and growth factors. Sci Rep 2017; 7: 43006.
[http://dx.doi.org/10.1038/srep43006] [PMID: 28223691]

[24]   Burchell JM, Mungul A, Taylor-Papadimitriou J. O-linked glycosylation in the mammary gland: changes that occur during malignancy. J Mammary Gland Biol Neoplasia 2001; 6(3): 355-64.
[http://dx.doi.org/10.1023/A:1011331809881] [PMID: 11547903]

[25]   Ino Y, Gotoh M, Sakamoto M, Tsukagoshi K, Hirohashi S. Dysadherin, a cancer-associated cell membrane glycoprotein, down-regulates E-cadherin and promotes metastasis. Proc Natl Acad Sci USA 2002; 99(1): 365-70.
[http://dx.doi.org/10.1073/pnas.012425299] [PMID: 11756660]

[26]   Gu Y, Mi W, Ge Y, *et al.* GlcNAcylation plays an essential role in breast cancer metastasis. Cancer Res 2010; 70(15): 6344-51.
[http://dx.doi.org/10.1158/0008-5472.CAN-09-1887] [PMID: 20610629]

[27]   Kirwan A, Utratna M, O'Dwyer ME, Joshi L, Kilcoyne M. Glycosylation-based serum biomarkers for cancer diagnostics and prognostics. BioMed Res Intern 2015; 2015.
[http://dx.doi.org/10.1155/2015/490531]

[28]   Choi JW, Moon BI, Lee JW, Kim HJ, Jin Y, Kim HJ. Use of CA15-3 for screening breast cancer: An antibody-lectin sandwich assay for detecting glycosylation of CA15-3 in sera. Oncol Rep 2018; 40(1): 145-54.
[http://dx.doi.org/10.3892/or.2018.6433] [PMID: 29749490]

[29]   Blixt O, Bueti D, Burford B, *et al.* Autoantibodies to aberrantly glycosylated MUC1 in early stage breast cancer are associated with a better prognosis. Breast Cancer Res 2011; 13(2): R25.
[http://dx.doi.org/10.1186/bcr2841] [PMID: 21385452]

[30]   Zhang H, Meng F, Wu S, *et al.* Engagement of I-branching β-1, 6-N-acetylglucosaminyltransferase 2 in breast cancer metastasis and TGF-β signaling. Cancer Res 2011; 71(14): 4846-56.
[http://dx.doi.org/10.1158/0008-5472.CAN-11-0414] [PMID: 21750175]

[31]   Rubin CS, Rosen OM. Protein phosphorylation. Annu Rev Biochem 1975; 44(1): 831-87.
[http://dx.doi.org/10.1146/annurev.bi.44.070175.004151] [PMID: 166607]

[32]   Magalhaes MA, Larson DR, Mader CC, *et al.* Cortactin phosphorylation regulates cell invasion through a pH-dependent pathway. J Cell Biol 2011; 195(5): 903-20.
[http://dx.doi.org/10.1083/jcb.201103045] [PMID: 22105349]

[33]   Milde-Langosch K. The Fos family of transcription factors and their role in tumourigenesis. Eur J Cancer 2005; 41(16): 2449-61.
[http://dx.doi.org/10.1016/j.ejca.2005.08.008] [PMID: 16199154]

[34]   Mull BB, Cox J, Bui T, Keyomarsi K. Post-translational modification and stability of low molecular weight cyclin E. Oncogene 2009; 28(35): 3167-76.
[http://dx.doi.org/10.1038/onc.2009.182] [PMID: 19561641]

[35]   Borner C, Filipuzzi I, Wartmann M, Eppenberger U, Fabbro D. Biosynthesis and posttranslational modifications of protein kinase C in human breast cancer cells. J Biol Chem 1989; 264(23): 13902-9.
[PMID: 2474538]

[36]   Sun T, Aceto N, Meerbrey KL, *et al.* Activation of multiple proto-oncogenic tyrosine kinases in breast cancer *via* loss of the PTPN12 phosphatase. Cell 2011; 144(5): 703-18.
[http://dx.doi.org/10.1016/j.cell.2011.02.003] [PMID: 21376233]

[37]   Launay N, Tarze A, Vicart P, Lilienbaum A. Serine 59 phosphorylation of αB-crystallin down-regulates its anti-apoptotic function by binding and sequestering Bcl-2 in breast cancer cells. J Biol Chem 2010; 285(48): 37324-32.
[http://dx.doi.org/10.1074/jbc.M110.124388] [PMID: 20841355]

[38]   Liu Y, Mayo MW, Nagji AS, *et al.* Phosphorylation of RelA/p65 promotes DNMT-1 recruitment to chromatin and represses transcription of the tumor metastasis suppressor gene BRMS1. Oncogene 2012; 31(9): 1143-54.
[http://dx.doi.org/10.1038/onc.2011.308] [PMID: 21765477]

[39]   Wilkinson KA, Henley JM. Mechanisms, regulation and consequences of protein SUMOylation. Biochem J 2010; 428(2): 133-45.
[http://dx.doi.org/10.1042/BJ20100158] [PMID: 20462400]

[40]   Hershko A, Ciechanover A. The ubiquitin system. Annu Rev Biochem 1998; 67: 425-79.
[http://dx.doi.org/10.1146/annurev.biochem.67.1.425] [PMID: 9759494]

[41]   Zhu S, Sachdeva M, Wu F, Lu Z, Mo YY. Ubc9 promotes breast cell invasion and metastasis in a sumoylation-independent manner. Oncogene 2010; 29(12): 1763-72.
[http://dx.doi.org/10.1038/onc.2009.459] [PMID: 20023705]

[42]   Wang L, Banerjee S. Differential PIAS3 expression in human malignancy. Oncol Rep 2004; 11(6): 1319-24.
[PMID: 15138572]

[43]   Meek DW, Knippschild U. Posttranslational modification of MDM2. Mol Cancer Res 2003; 1(14): 1017-26.
[PMID: 14707285]

[44]   Kahyo T, Nishida T, Yasuda H. Involvement of PIAS1 in the sumoylation of tumor suppressor p53. Mol Cell 2001; 8(3): 713-8.
[http://dx.doi.org/10.1016/S1097-2765(01)00349-5] [PMID: 11583632]

[45]   Chauchereau A, Amazit L, Quesne M, Guiochon-Mantel A, Milgrom E. Sumoylation of the progesterone receptor and of the steroid receptor coactivator SRC-1. J Biol Chem 2003; 278(14): 12335-43.
[http://dx.doi.org/10.1074/jbc.M207148200] [PMID: 12529333]

[46]   Le Drean Y, Mincheneau N, Le Goff P, Michel D. Potentiation of glucocorticoid receptor transcriptional activity by sumoylation. Endocrinology 2002; 143(9): 3482-9.
[http://dx.doi.org/10.1210/en.2002-220135] [PMID: 12193561]

[47]   Alshareeda AT, Negm OH, Green AR, *et al.* SUMOylation proteins in breast cancer. Breast Cancer Res Treat 2014; 144(3): 519-30.
[http://dx.doi.org/10.1007/s10549-014-2897-7] [PMID: 24584753]

[48]   Nestal de Moraes G, Ji Z, Fan LY, *et al.* SUMOylation modulates FOXK2-mediated paclitaxel sensitivity in breast cancer cells. Oncogenesis 2018; 7(3): 29.
[http://dx.doi.org/10.1038/s41389-018-0038-6] [PMID: 29540677]

[49]   Bogachek MV, Chen Y, Kulak MV, *et al.* Sumoylation pathway is required to maintain the basal breast cancer subtype. Cancer Cell 2014; 25(6): 748-61.
[http://dx.doi.org/10.1016/j.ccr.2014.04.008] [PMID: 24835590]

[50]   Hershko A, Ciechanover A. The ubiquitin system for protein degradation. Annu Rev Biochem 1992; 61(1): 761-807.
[http://dx.doi.org/10.1146/annurev.bi.61.070192.003553] [PMID: 1323239]

[51]   Murphy LC, Watson P. Steroid receptors in human breast tumorigenesis and breast cancer progression. Biomed Pharmacother 2002; 56(2): 65-77.
[http://dx.doi.org/10.1016/S0753-3322(01)00157-3] [PMID: 12000137]

[52]   Bergink S, Jentsch S. Principles of ubiquitin and SUMO modifications in DNA repair. Nature 2009; 458(7237): 461-7.
[http://dx.doi.org/10.1038/nature07963] [PMID: 19325626]

[53]   La Rosa P, Pesiri V, Marino M, Acconcia F. 17β-Estradiol-induced cell proliferation requires estrogen receptor (ER) α monoubiquitination. Cell Signal 2011; 23(7): 1128-35.
[http://dx.doi.org/10.1016/j.cellsig.2011.02.006] [PMID: 21356307]

[54]   Patani N, Jiang W, Newbold R, Mokbel K. Prognostic implications of carboxyl-terminus of Hsc70 interacting protein and lysyl-oxidase expression in human breast cancer. J Carcinog 2010; 9: 9.
[http://dx.doi.org/10.4103/1477-3163.72505] [PMID: 21139993]

[55]   Cho Y, Kang HG, Kim SJ, *et al.* Post-translational modification of OCT4 in breast cancer tumorigenesis. Cell Death Differ 2018; 25(10): 1781-95.
[http://dx.doi.org/10.1038/s41418-018-0079-6] [PMID: 29511337]

[56]   Yang Y, Bedford MT. Protein arginine methyltransferases and cancer. Nat Rev Cancer 2013; 13(1): 37-50.
[http://dx.doi.org/10.1038/nrc3409] [PMID: 23235912]

[57]   Bauer UM, Daujat S, Nielsen SJ, Nightingale K, Kouzarides T. Methylation at arginine 17 of histone H3 is linked to gene activation. EMBO Rep 2002; 3(1): 39-44.
[http://dx.doi.org/10.1093/embo-reports/kvf013] [PMID: 11751582]

[58]   Côté J, Boisvert FM, Boulanger MC, Bedford MT, Richard S. Sam68 RNA binding protein is an *in vivo* substrate for protein arginine N-methyltransferase 1. Mol Biol Cell 2003; 14(1): 274-87.
[http://dx.doi.org/10.1091/mbc.e02-08-0484] [PMID: 12529443]

[59]   Strahl BD, Briggs SD, Brame CJ, *et al.* Methylation of histone H4 at arginine 3 occurs *in vivo* and is mediated by the nuclear receptor coactivator PRMT1. Curr Biol 2001; 11(12): 996-1000.
[http://dx.doi.org/10.1016/S0960-9822(01)00294-9] [PMID: 11448779]

[60]   Vogelstein B, Lane D, Levine AJ. Surfing the p53 network. Nature 2000; 408(6810): 307-10.
[http://dx.doi.org/10.1038/35042675] [PMID: 11099028]

[61]   Chuikov S, Kurash JK, Wilson JR, *et al.* Regulation of p53 activity through lysine methylation. Nature 2004; 432(7015): 353-60.
[http://dx.doi.org/10.1038/nature03117] [PMID: 15525938]

[62]   Huang J, Perez-Burgos L, Placek BJ, *et al.* Repression of p53 activity by Smyd2-mediated methylation. Nature 2006; 444(7119): 629-32.
[http://dx.doi.org/10.1038/nature05287] [PMID: 17108971]

[63]　Shi X, Kachirskaia I, Yamaguchi H, *et al.* Modulation of p53 function by SET8-mediated methylation at lysine 382. Mol Cell 2007; 27(4): 636-46.
[http://dx.doi.org/10.1016/j.molcel.2007.07.012] [PMID: 17707234]

[64]　Guendel I, Carpio L, Pedati C, *et al.* Methylation of the tumor suppressor protein, BRCA1, influences its transcriptional cofactor function. PLoS One 2010; 5(6): e11379.
[http://dx.doi.org/10.1371/journal.pone.0011379] [PMID: 20614009]

[65]　Widschwendter M, Jones PA. DNA methylation and breast carcinogenesis. Oncogene 2002; 21(35): 5462-82.
[http://dx.doi.org/10.1038/sj.onc.1205606] [PMID: 12154408]

[66]　Bannister AJ, Kouzarides T. Regulation of chromatin by histone modifications. Cell Res 2011; 21(3): 381-95.
[http://dx.doi.org/10.1038/cr.2011.22] [PMID: 21321607]

[67]　Barski A, Cuddapah S, Cui K, *et al.* High-resolution profiling of histone methylations in the human genome. Cell 2007; 129(4): 823-37.
[http://dx.doi.org/10.1016/j.cell.2007.05.009] [PMID: 17512414]

[68]　Wang Z, Zang C, Rosenfeld JA, *et al.* Combinatorial patterns of histone acetylations and methylations in the human genome. Nat Genet 2008; 40(7): 897-903.
[http://dx.doi.org/10.1038/ng.154] [PMID: 18552846]

[69]　Fraga MF, Ballestar E, Villar-Garea A, *et al.* Loss of acetylation at Lys16 and trimethylation at Lys20 of histone H4 is a common hallmark of human cancer. Nat Genet 2005; 37(4): 391-400.
[http://dx.doi.org/10.1038/ng1531] [PMID: 15765097]

[70]　Elsheikh SE, Green AR, Rakha EA, *et al.* Global histone modifications in breast cancer correlate with tumor phenotypes, prognostic factors, and patient outcome. Cancer Res 2009; 69(9): 3802-9.
[http://dx.doi.org/10.1158/0008-5472.CAN-08-3907] [PMID: 19366799]

[71]　Hinshelwood RA, Melki JR, Huschtscha LI, *et al.* Aberrant *de novo* methylation of the p16INK4A CpG island is initiated post gene silencing in association with chromatin remodelling and mimics nucleosome positioning. Hum Mol Genet 2009; 18(16): 3098-109.
[http://dx.doi.org/10.1093/hmg/ddp251] [PMID: 19477956]

[72]　Dulaimi E, Hillinck J, Ibanez de Caceres I, Al-Saleem T, Cairns P. Tumor suppressor gene promoter hypermethylation in serum of breast cancer patients. Clin Cancer Res 2004; 10(18 Pt 1): 6189-93.
[http://dx.doi.org/10.1158/1078-0432.CCR-04-0597] [PMID: 15448006]

[73]　Bernardino J, Roux C, Almeida A, *et al.* DNA hypomethylation in breast cancer: an independent parameter of tumor progression? Cancer Genet Cytogenet 1997; 97(2): 83-9.
[http://dx.doi.org/10.1016/S0165-4608(96)00385-8] [PMID: 9283586]

[74]　Zhang FL, Casey PJ. Protein prenylation: molecular mechanisms and functional consequences. Annu Rev Biochem 1996; 65(1): 241-69.
[http://dx.doi.org/10.1146/annurev.bi.65.070196.001325] [PMID: 8811180]

[75]　Cestac P, Sarrabayrouse G, Médale-Giamarchi C, *et al.* Prenylation inhibitors stimulate both estrogen receptor α transcriptional activity through AF-1 and AF-2 and estrogen receptor β transcriptional activity. Breast Cancer Res 2005; 7(1): R60-70.
[http://dx.doi.org/10.1186/bcr956] [PMID: 15642170]

[76]　Doisneau-Sixou SF, Cestac P, Chouini S, *et al.* Contrasting effects of prenyltransferase inhibitors on estrogen-dependent cell cycle progression and estrogen receptor-mediated transcriptional activity in MCF-7 cells. Endocrinology 2003; 144(3): 989-98.
[http://dx.doi.org/10.1210/en.2002-220726] [PMID: 12586776]

[77]　Vigushin DM, Mirsaidi N, Brooke G, *et al.* Gliotoxin is a dual inhibitor of farnesyltransferase and geranylgeranyltransferase I with antitumor activity against breast cancer *in vivo.* Med Oncol 2004; 21(1): 21-30.

[http://dx.doi.org/10.1385/MO:21:1:21] [PMID: 15034210]

[78]   Völkert M, Wagner M, Peters C, Waldmann H. The chemical biology of Ras lipidation. Biol Chem 2001; 382(8): 1133-45.
[http://dx.doi.org/10.1515/BC.2001.143] [PMID: 11592394]

[79]   Casey PJ. Protein lipidation in cell signaling. Science 1995; 268(5208): 221-5.
[http://dx.doi.org/10.1126/science.7716512] [PMID: 7716512]

[80]   Rojo F, García-Parra J, Zazo S, *et al.* Nuclear PARP-1 protein overexpression is associated with poor overall survival in early breast cancer. Ann Oncol 2012; 23(5): 1156-64.
[http://dx.doi.org/10.1093/annonc/mdr361] [PMID: 21908496]

[81]   Simbulan-Rosenthal CM, Ly DH, Rosenthal DS, *et al.* Misregulation of gene expression in primary fibroblasts lacking poly(ADP-ribose) polymerase. Proc Natl Acad Sci USA 2000; 97(21): 11274-9.
[http://dx.doi.org/10.1073/pnas.200285797] [PMID: 11016956]

[82]   Li M, Naidu P, Yu Y, Berger NA, Kannan P. Dual regulation of AP-2α transcriptional activation by poly(ADP-ribose) polymerase-1. Biochem J 2004; 382(Pt 1): 323-9.
[http://dx.doi.org/10.1042/BJ20040593] [PMID: 15170387]

[83]   Mannello F, Tonti GA, Medda V. Protein oxidation in breast microenvironment: Nipple aspirate fluid collected from breast cancer women contains increased protein carbonyl concentration. Cell Oncol 2009; 31(5): 383-92.
[PMID: 19759418]

[84]   De Luca A, Sanna F, Sallese M, *et al.* Methionine sulfoxide reductase A down-regulation in human breast cancer cells results in a more aggressive phenotype. Proc Natl Acad Sci USA 2010; 107(43): 18628-33.
[http://dx.doi.org/10.1073/pnas.1010171107] [PMID: 20937881]

[85]   Rahman MA, Senga T, Ito S, Hyodo T, Hasegawa H, Hamaguchi M. S-nitrosylation at cysteine 498 of c-Src tyrosine kinase regulates nitric oxide-mediated cell invasion. J Biol Chem 2010; 285(6): 3806-14.
[http://dx.doi.org/10.1074/jbc.M109.059782] [PMID: 19948721]

CHAPTER 6

Genomic Fingerprint of Molecular Mechanisms of Breast Carcinogenesis

Akanksha Nigam[1],* and **Shivam Priya[2]**

[1] *Department of Microbiology and Molecular Genetics, IMRIC, The Hebrew University-Hadassah Medical School, Jerusalem, Israel*

[2] *Institute for Dental Sciences, Faculty of Dental Medicine, The Hebrew University, Jerusalem, Israel*

Abstract: Breast cancer in women is the most frequent cancer with the highest mortality worldwide. The risk factor includes aging, family history, genetic predisposition, and hormone factor. In recent years, many new gene signatures have been identified, which have a profound effect on breast cancer initiation and progression. Extensive research has been done in the past five decades in understanding breast cancer biology through genomics and proteomics. All these comprehensive studies from breast cancer patients elucidate heterogeneity of disease as one of the complex problems in its treatment and management. The outburst of molecular information has led to an understanding of the biological diversity of breast cancer. The involvement of various genes at different steps of cancer progression, such as proliferation, evading apoptosis, migration, immunosuppression, and chemoresistance, have been described in this chapter. With the advent of miRNA and splicing factors, new differential regulators of genes have been identified in breast cancer. The breast cancer therapeutic approach can be accomplished by identifying the oncogene and tumor suppressor genes at an early stage of the disease. Elucidation of novel genes in breast cancer will lead to identifying new molecular pathways that may be targeted for its treatment. For the prognostic and diagnostic treatment of breast cancer it is very important to identify newer genomic fingerprints and to develop novel therapeutic targets against them. Our main goal is to make available inclusive understanding of molecular mechanisms and hallmarks of breast carcinogenesis.

Keywords: BRAC1, Breast Cancer, Chemoresistance, HER2, Metallo-estrogens, mi-RNA, miRNA, Molecular Fingerprinting, TNBC, TME, Treg, Trastuzumab.

INTRODUCTION

Breast cancer (BC) in women is the most common cancer and the leading cause of

---

* **Corresponding author Akanksha Nigam:** Department of Microbiology and Molecular Genetics, IMRIC, the Hebrew University-Hadassah Medical School, Jerusalem, Israel; E-mail: akanksha.nigam@mail.huji.ac.il

Shankar Suman, Garima Suman and Sanjay Mishra (Eds.)

cancer mortality in women; it accounts for 1,300,000 cases and 450,000 deaths each year worldwide [1]. The survival rates of BC patients hugely vary between high and low-income countries. The survival rate is 80% for high-income countries, which reduces to half, *i.e.*, 40%, in low-income countries [2, 3]. In low-income countries, the early detection and treatment of BC is a difficult task [4]. Whereas, in high-income countries like the USA (1975–2000), a continued effort has resulted in a substantial reduction in breast cancer-related deaths [5]. According to the origin of the tumor, BC can be classified as the ductal and lobular tumor. Ductal tumors, which comprise 80% of the tumor, originate in the breast ductal region, and lobular tumors (10-15%) develop from the lobular region [6]. The breast carcinogenesis involves many sequential steps, starting with hyper-proliferation of duct, immunosuppression, leading to invasiveness, and lastly into metastatic status [7]. In this chapter, we will be focusing on risk factors, oncogene, hormone receptors and various hallmarks of BC (proliferation, chemoresistance, TME, mi-RNA, splicing factor). It will be a piece of consolidated information about various molecular fingerprinting genes involved in the induction of breast carcinogenesis (Fig. **1**).

Risk Factors

Normally, there is a balance between negative and positive growth factors in breast tissue, but any imbalance may lead to the development of BC [8]. The following few factors are thought to be related to BC development:

Age

The probability of developing breast cancer increases with the age of women. The lifetime risk for women is very low (1 in 8 women) in the USA. This ratio is even lower (1 in 200 women) for women at an early age (≤39 years), but as the age increases(40-59 years) chances of getting breast cancer also increases (1 in 26 women). This age-related BC incidences further increase in low-income group countries [2, 3]. As women grow older, the chances of having abnormal changes in their cells increase in multi-fold magnitude [1, 3, 4].

Family History

Women with a family history of BC increase the risk for the next generation of women. If a woman is diagnosed with BC at the age of 50 or older, than the chances of her daughter developing BC in the future is relatively high. This comparative risk of BC further increases in daughter, if mother had BC before the age of 50 years [9, 10].

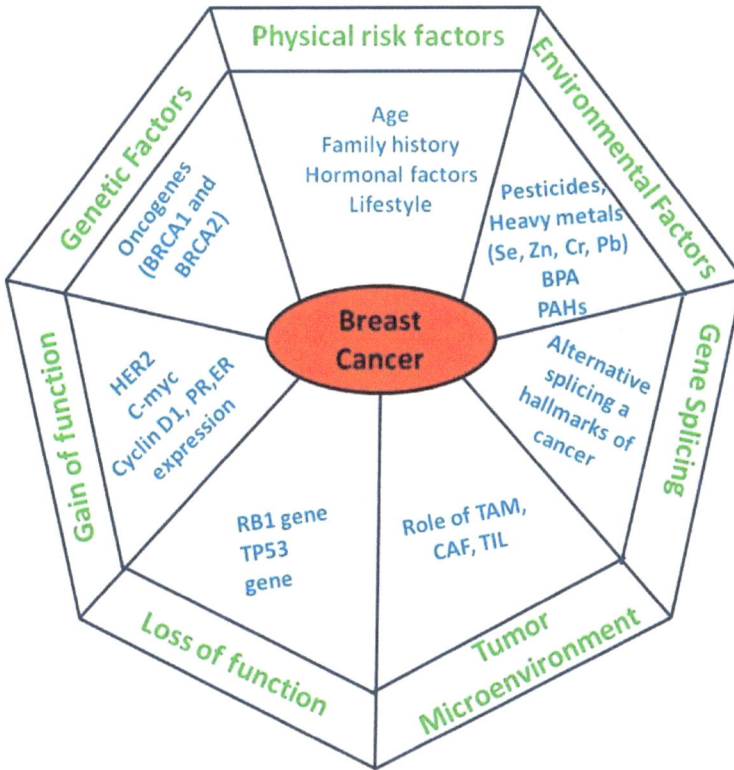

Fig. (1). Diagrammatic representation of different factors responsible for causing breast cancer.

Genetic Predisposition

In BC, there are several inherited genes linked with a genetic predisposition in patients. It is estimated that 25% of patients have a family history of BC, but only 5-10% of cases show the inheritance to next-generation [11, 12]. Genetic predisposition alleles carry 40-85% of lifetime risk, which mainly includes the mutations in BRCA1, BRCA2, TP53, PTEN, STK11, CDH-1 genes. Most mutations in BRCA1 or BRCA2 genes are involved in a high risk of BC. Some other genes are also moderately involved in the occurrence of breast cancer, which include ataxia-telangiectasia (ATM) mutations [13]. The clinical applications of these mutations are still unidentified.

Hormonal Factors

There are so many hormonal dynamics that are directly associated with BC initiation and progression. Early menarche is one of the high-risk factors in women for developing BC. It has been found that women who had early menarche have a higher risk of developing BC at a later stage of life. The initiation of menstruation cycle at an early age increases the risk of BC and is independent of pre or postmenopausal conditions in women. In one of the studies (cancer and nutrition cohort), it has been shown that women with early menstruation (less than 13-year-old) had a two-fold increase in the risk of BC due to hormone receptors. Whereas if menstruation is delayed by two years, then the chances of women having BC are reduced [14]. During the postmenopausal cycle, an increase in testosterone has been correlated with BC development [15]. It has been reported that a 1-year delay in menopause increases the chances of BC by 3%, while every 5-year delay will further increase the risk by 17% [16, 17]. Breastfeeding is one of the protective measures against BC. It is proven that breastfeeding may decrease the endogenous sex hormone level by delaying the return of ovulatory cycles [18]. Hormone replacement therapy (HRT) is also one of the known factors for increasing BC risk. Studies have shown that women having intact uterus after postmenopause have a high risk of BC during HRT [19, 20]. Exposure of exogenous hormone linked with menopause timing further increases the risk of BC in women. BC patients who are treated with combinational HRT for longer time duration have shown a higher rate of recurrence in comparison to those patients who are treated for a much short time frame [21].

Lifestyle

Breast cancer has also been associated with certain lifestyle patterns. These risk factors are mainly associated with obesity, physical fitness, stress, alcohol, and smoking. Physical fitness contributes to the prevention of BC, regular exercise, and a healthy lifestyle help to decrease the stress level. Obesity is also one of the major problems which are correlated to low physical activity. After postmenopausal, if women increase their body weight, the chances of having BC are increased. Alcohol consumption and smoking are some of the other factors which contribute to the risk of BC. These changes in the lifestyle of women contribute to 21% of death worldwide due to BC, which can be averted [22 - 24].

GENETIC FINGERPRINTS OF BREAST CANCER

BRCA1 OR BRCA2 Mutation

In the last few decades, drastic progress has been made towards the treatment of BC. The advancement of treatment techniques and identifying the involvement of novel oncogene have resulted in better management of BC patients. Still, globally, BC is one of the leading causes of death in women. In literature, it is reported that 5 to 10% of mutation is related to BRCA1 or BRCA2 genes. Mutation in these two genes in a woman also signifies that the family has a history of BC [25 - 27].

Mutations in BRCA1 and BRCA2 are also connected to hereditary conditions, *e.g.,* the mutation in Ashkenazi Jews exists at 185delAG and 5382insC in BRCA1 and 6174delT in BRCA2 [28]. Similarly, the mutation in BRCA1(3171ins5) has been commonly found in Swedish family's history (3171ins5) [29]. BRCA1 gene is on chromosome 17 in the human genome which comprises 24 exons and 1863 amino acids. BRCA1 is a well-known tumor suppressor gene that plays an important role in regulating cell cycle and DNA damage repair.BRCA1 causes DNA lesions under the regulation of MDC1 (**M**ediator of **D**NA Damage **C**heckpoint protein **1**) protein. Upon exposure to ionizing radiation ataxia telangiectasia mutated (ATM) phosphorylate BRCA1 [30, 31]. Phosphorylation of BRAC1 facilitates its binding to p53, RAD50-MRE11-NBS1 (R-M-N) complex, and RAD51, which helps in repairing DNA damage.BRCA1 interacts with BARD1 (BRCA1 associated RING domain 1) through its zinc-binding RING-finger domain, and this complex also participates in DNA damage repair [32].

Similar to BRCA1, there is another gene BRCA2, which also has a role in hereditary BC [33]. BRCA2 is found in human chromosome 13, comprising of 70 kb of genomic sequence with 27 exons and encodes 3418 amino acids. BRCA2 gene does not have any homologous similarity with the BRCA1 gene [34]. However, together with BRCA1, BRCA2 binds, and participates in DNA damage repair [35]. BRCA1 and BRCA2 both are associated with hereditary breast cancers. It differs from sporadic breast cancer in their genotypic and phenotypic characteristics. Cancer-related to BRCA1 mutation has the basal-like phenotype, which is a Grade 3 (high grade) cancer [36]. High-grade cancer is characterized by the expression of basal markers like P-cadherin, epidermal growth factor [37 - 40]. BRCA1 associated breast cancer generally shows the overexpression of cell cycle protein, *e.g.,* cyclin A, B1, cyclin E, S-phase proteins, while in BRCA2, carcinoma mostly shows overexpression of cyclin D1 and p27 [37, 40]. The risk of BC is related to mutations in specific genes, the lifestyle of the person and also the environmental factors. BRCA1 and BRCA2 genes mutation can be modified by the expression of RAD51, androgen receptor (AR), H-Ras, and Nuclear receptor coactivator 3 (NCOA3). Surgical removal of both the ovaries in women reduces the risk of ovarian and BC in BRCA1 and BRCA2 mutation-positive patients. Tamoxifen is also known to reduce the risk of BC in BRCA1 and BRCA2 mutation carriers [41, 42].

HER2 Expression in Breast Cancer

Human epidermal growth factor receptor 2 (HER2) is a member of the epidermal growth factor receptor family located on chromosome 17 and encodes 185 kDa protein [43 - 45]. This family of human epidermal growth factor comprises HER-1 or ErbB1, HER-2 or ErbB2, HER-3or or ErbB3, and HER-4 or Erb4 [46]. The

HER2 overexpression and amplification accounts for 30% of tumors and is also associated with the chronic stage of BC patients [47 - 49]. All the HER receptors can assemble into different combinations to form both homodimers and heterodimers for downstream signaling. Except for HER2 receptor, all other receptors undergo dimerization and trans-phosphorylation after the activation by the ligand on their extracellular surface. Activation of HER2 does not take place directly by binding of a ligand; this receptor is activated by heterodimerization of HER1 and HER3. Upon activation of the HER2 cytoplasmic domain results in various downstream signaling, such as MAPK, and PI3K pathways (Fig. **2**). Activation of these pathways results in cell proliferation, differentiation, angiogenesis, and invasion in breast cancer cells [50, 51]. The initiation of BC can be correlated with the amplification status of the HER2 gene. HER2 amplification contributes to different stages of BC progression, such as invasiveness, nodal metastasis, and distant metastasis [52]. HER2 signaling can disrupt cell polarity, cell adhesion and deregulates cell cycle [53, 54]. HER2 deregulation of the cell cycle occurs *via* cyclin D1, cyclin E and cdk6, and degradation of p27 [55]. HER2 also has a role in activating nuclear transcription factors (COX-2, CXCR4, and ETS), resulting in the transformation and proliferation of cancer cells [56 - 61]. HER2 also induces the VEGF expression through HIF-1α dependent [62, 63] and independent mechanism [64]. The increase in VEGF expression assists in tumor growth, metastasis, and angiogenesis [65].

HER2 expression has been used as a prognostic biomarker in breast cancer, and many therapeutic targets have been developed (Table **1**). Determination of HER2 status in breast tumors is of great importance in determining an optimal BC treatment [54].

Trastuzumab, a monoclonal antibody, is the known standard treatment for HER2 positive BC patients. In HER2 positive BC, the use of Trastuzumab along with chemotherapy has shown effective results. The mechanism of action of Trastuzumab is through the immune system (involving both innate and adaptive immunity). Trastuzumab causes a decrease in cyclin D1 expression and an increase in p27 levels, which results in cell cycle arrest and inhibition of angiogenesis [66]. Trastuzumab in combination with other chemotherapy inhibits activation of PI3K/AKT signaling which further inhibits tumor cell survival [67]. Trastuzumab can easily treat women with early stages of BC in combination with other chemotherapy regimens [54]. Treatment with Trastuzumab also results in the development of resistance in cancer cells due to truncated HER2 receptor, which lacks an extracellular domain [68, 69]. Apart from these targets, researchers are also looking to inhibit other signaling pathways (mTOR, PI3K, and AKT), which are overexpressed due to HER2 in BC.

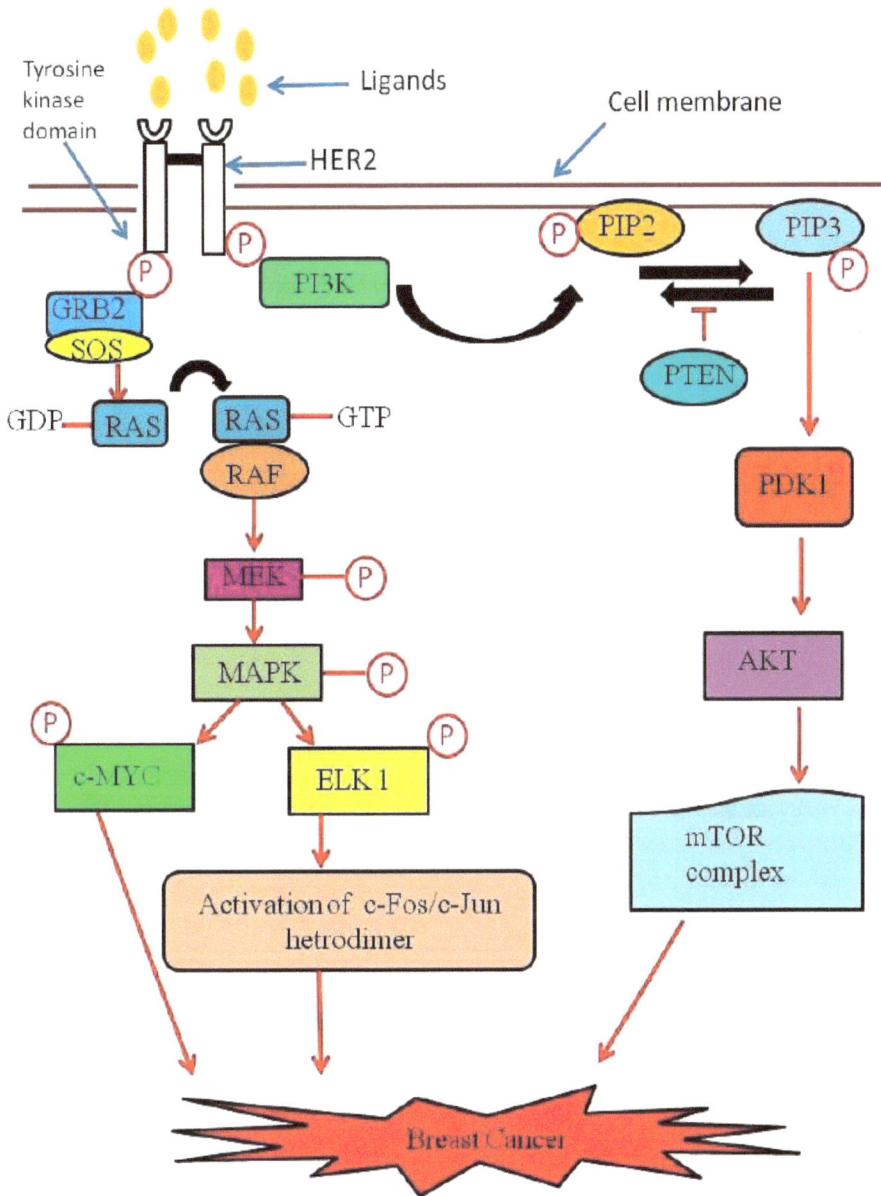

Fig. (2). HER2 signaling pathway: Phosphorylation of tyrosine kinase domain initiates the downstream signaling pathways of MAPK and AKT, which contributes towards the breast cancer progression. Here "P" represents phosphorylation.

Table 1. Use and development combinational drugs against HER2 positive breast cancer patients in different trials and studies; data taken from [54].

Drug	Combined With	Trial/Study Undertaken
Trastuzumab (Herceptin)	Adjuvant therapy	NSABP B31-NCCTG trial
	chemotherapy	BCIRG 006 and FinHer trial
	Epirubicin and Cyclophosphamide	Hercules trial
	Docetaxel	M77001 trial and HERTAX trial
	Paclitaxel or Docetaxel	HRNATA
	Docetaxel or Carboplatin	BCIRG 007 trial
	Anastrozole	TAnDEM study
	Anthracyclines or Taxane	GeparQuattro study
	Neoadjuvant chemotherapy	NOAH clinical trial
Lapatinib (Tykerb)	Chemotherapy or Trastuzumab	-
	Capecitabine	-
Pertuzumab(Perjeta)	Trastuzumab and docetaxel	Cleopatra study
Trastuzumabemtansine (Kadcyla)	Trastuzumab and DM1 moiety	EMILIA study

Estrogen Receptor Expression in Breast Cancer

The steroid hormone (estradiol) has an important role in the initiation, progression, and metastasis of breast cancer. Under the normal homeostasis process, estrogen binds to one of the structurally and functionally distinct estrogen receptors (ER), ER-alpha (ERα, ESR1 gene), and ER-beta (ESR2 gene). As a member of the nuclear receptor family, it has highly conserved DNA and ligand-binding domains [70 - 73]. It has been estimated that approximately 75% of BC patients are ERα positive [74 - 76], suggesting that this receptor is a predominant signaling pathway in estrogen-induced BC [71, 72]. The human ESR1 gene is located on chromosome 6 with 472.9 Kb, translating into 595 amino acids and 66.2 KDa protein [70, 71]. The ESR1 gene comprises two functionally distinct zinc finger motifs helping in receptor dimerization and responsible for specific DNA binding [73, 76]. Molecular characterization of ER revealed that, upon ligand binding, it interacts with co-regulator proteins known as estrogen-responsive elements (EREs) having specific DNA sequences (5'-GGTCAnnnTGACC-3') [72, 77]. Interaction of EREs is assisted by DNA binding protein FOXA1 [78]. Along with this, another member of the forkhead family FOXM1activates forkhead response element at the proximal region of ER promoter which results in overexpression of ERα protein [79]. Transcription factors (AP-1, Sp1, NFκB, RUNX1) helps the ER in binding to DNA directly.

This ER-DNA binding modifies chromatin, making it accessible to other transcriptional factors [80, 81]. These interactions help ER in regulating multiple pathways (DNA replication, cell cycle, apoptosis, and angiogenesis), facilitating the cancer cell survival and metastasis [82, 83].

The engagement of the ER with estrogen through nonnuclear pathways in cytoplasm trigger coregulator growth factor and G-protein coupled signaling (GATA-3) [72, 73]. Mammary gland morphogenesis and luminal cell differentiation are regulated by GATA-3 [84], and its co-expression with ERα is found in BC [85]. Binding of GATA-3 to two *cis*-regulatory elements located within the *ESR1* gene stimulates its overexpression [86]. The ER can be activated through ligand-independent mechanisms, causing crosstalk between ER and growth factors, as well as other protein kinases, resulting in constitutive overexpression of ER. Other co-regulators, which affect ER expression, are insulin-like growth factor-1 receptor, fibroblast growth factor receptor, HER2, kinases (mitogen-activated protein kinases, and receptor tyrosine kinase), PI3K, AKT, mTOR, Src, and CDK [72]. Estrogen is instrumental in facilitating the G_1 to S phase transition utilizing the activation and binding of cyclin D1 and dimerization to CDK4/6 [72, 87]. Dysregulation of the cyclin D1/CDK4/6 pathway is reported to be an early and essential gateway for breast tumorigenesis because the overexpression of cyclin D1 has been implicated in BC and several other solid tumors, as well as hematologic malignancies [72]. Amplification of *CCND1gene* occurs in many human BC tumors [1].

ER[+] BC patients are responsive to endocrine therapies [88], but ER[-] tumors are more aggressive and metastatic [89]. The ERα role in BC is far more complex during its treatment and management [90]. Mutation in the *ESR1* gene results in a gain of function [1] and has been detected in 20% of BC patients with metastatic conditions [75]. Mutations in *ESR1* have also been linked to acquiring HRT resistance, with the most common *ESR1*mutations affecting one of two residues in the ER ligand-binding domain. *ESR1* mutations are rarely found in treatment-naïve patients and are hardly ever the cause of primary resistance [91]. Instead, *ESR1* mutations associated with endocrine resistance are found in patients with metastatic disease who have been treated with aromatase inhibitors (AIs). These *ESR1* mutations confer constitutive or estrogen-independent activation of the ER and resistance to AI therapy. Adjuvant AI therapy appears to select for *ESR1*mutations under the stress of estrogen deprivation, in which there are intratumoral genetic heterogeneity and clonal diversity [72]. Alternative splicing in the ERα mRNA [92] leads to its overexpression and less responsive to tamoxifen treatment. ERα mRNA encodes six different isoforms with the same protein size but the different 5′ untranslated region due to frame-shift mutations or alternative splicing [93, 94]. The role of micro-RNA (miRNA) on ER expression is profounding. In ER⁻ tumors have an expression of miRNA-206, which directly targets ERα expression by base-pairing with the 3′-untranslated region. This overexpression of ERα in ER⁻ tumors further increases the proliferation of BC cells [95, 96].

On the other hand, miR-27a and ZBTB10 inhibit ERα expression [97]. ER expression in ER⁻ tumors can be restored by HDAC inhibitors, inhibition of Src, monoclonal antibodies, and signal transduction inhibitors [98]. Endocrine therapy is generally associated with low toxicity, but it can increase when therapy is combined with certain targeted therapy in BC patients. With the limited success with the HRT in BC, opens the door to understand the estrogen signaling and ligand-ER interaction. The elucidation of the mechanism will help the development of novel therapeutic targets [77].

Progesterone Receptor Expression in Breast Cancer

Progesterone receptors (PRs) are activated by binding of the natural hormone progesterone. PR gene is located on human chromosome 11, and synthesize three PR isoforms from the single gene [99]. The full-length PR-B (116 kDa), N-terminally-truncated PR-A (94 kDa), and PR-C-isoforms (60 kDa) are the protein isoforms from the single gene [100, 101]. All these different types of protein have a very distinctive function like PR-A is required for reproductive function and uterine development [102], PR-B for mammary gland development [103], and PR-C enhances PR activity in BC cell lines [104]. PR isoforms are a member of a large family of steroid hormone receptors (MR, GR ER, and AR) that regulate gene expression by binding directly or indirectly to specific sites in DNA. Concerning BC biology, it's very difficult to study PR in separation from other hormones (EGF and IGF-1) [100, 101]. PR isoforms expression can be ERα dependent as well as independent [101, 105]. During the normal breast development, EGF and IGF-1 promote proliferation in terminal end-buds, whereas ductal outgrowth and side branching are the results of ER and PR [106, 107]. PR is an ER target gene, and it is co-expressed in the same cells, but may also be expressed independently in some conditions [108, 109]. The molecular crosstalk between growth factors and ER causes the downregulation of PR levels [110 - 112]. BC cell lines can be sensitized to growth factor and cytokine signals *via* progesterone [113]. In one of the studies it has been shown that in cultured BC cells after progesterone treatment for the first 18 hrs, cells are proliferative (upregulation of G1/S and G2 cyclins, p21 and CDK2) followed by inhibition(upregulation of p27) in next 24-48 hrs [114 - 116]. Likewise, PR expression decreases by 500-fold due to the overexpression of HER-2 [111]. Many other growth factors (IGF-1, EGF, and Heregulin) and signaling pathways (PI3K–AKT-mTOR) independently cause PR downregulation [111, 112].

Overexpression of PR-A is correlated with an elevated risk for BC [111]. Due to this phenomenon, after HRT treatment, there is a recurrence of BC later in the life of the patients [111]. PR is also associated with the aggressiveness of the tumor; PR⁻ tumors are more aggressive and metastatic. The ER⁺PR⁻ tumors condition also arise in the patients, who are on a high glycaemic index food [100, 117].

RANKL protein is upregulated in PR⁺ cells and acts as mitogen resulting in increased cellular proliferation [102, 118] and pharmacologically inhibiting RANKL delays tumorigenesis [119], due to the PR/RANKL axis, resulting in increases of metastasis of BC. Similarly to RANKL, the Wnt pathway also promotes breast carcinogenesis. Like RANKL, WNT4 (paracrine factor) synthesized in PR⁺ cells can activate both non-canonical and canonical Wnt signaling pathway [120]. Mammary epithelium having hyperplasia, resulting in tumors formation, have an ectopic expression of Wnt1 [121]. MAPK and c-Src are often overexpressed in BC due to the steroid hormone receptor (ER, AR, and PR). This receptor stimulates mitogenic kinases signaling to make breast cells hyper-proliferative. The secretion of active pro-proliferative molecules (Wnts, IGF-II, or stroma-derived HGF) by neighboring cells is due to cross-talk between epithelial and stromal compartments of breast cells [100]. From the epidemiological studies, it has been shown, the risk of BCincreases when an estrogenic compound is combined with progestin. Women who are under oral contraception (comprises of progestin and ethinylestradiol) have a 24% increased risk of getting BC [122]. Molecularly targeted therapies for this type of BC condition will need further exploration. A bridge is needed to build between molecular endocrinology and tumor biology, with much broader knowledge and mechanism of ER and PR signaling.

SUSTAINING PROLIFERATIVE SIGNALING

The fundamental characteristic of cancer cells is to attain unlimited cell division. In our homeostasis process, each cell is designated to define several cell divisions for maintaining organelle architecture. In mammary gland deregulation of these signaling, it makes them take over the control of our body system. Alternation in cellular proliferation and uncontrolled growth is contributed by oncogenes (HER2, c-MYC, RAS, ER), cell cycle (CCND1and cyclin E), tumor suppressor (RB, TP53, PTEN); and susceptibility genes (BRCA1 and BRCA2) [123]. Cellular growth and proliferation contribute to the alteration of genes, which results in metastatic BC (Table **2**) [124]. The progression of the cell to malignant breast cells is not entirely unstated, but it is assumed oncogenes are initially mutated, resulting in unrestrictive cell division [123]. Alteration in oncogenes results in gain-of-function, assisting cell to enter into the cell division phase. The HER2, an oncogene in BC, is overexpressed in 20%–30% of cases. HER2 overexpression is more of lobular origin than ductal origin in BC [125]. Another oncogene c-MYC is usually expressed in cell division. Its gain of function makes the cells to enter into the S phase of the cell cycle, thus increasing the cellular proliferation rate. In the human genome, 15% of the genes are regulated by a nuclear transcription factor, a gene product of c-MYC.

The c-MYC gene has a wide variety of roles in proliferation, apoptosis, differentiation, and metabolism. Cell cycle transition from G1 to S is controlled by c-MYC, is the major mechanism that goes uncontrolled during the progression of BC [126]. This G1 to S transition is further modulated by CCND1 (Cyclin D1), which is under the regulation of the c-MYC gene. CCND1 gene amplification accounts for 13%–20% of BC cases, whereas its protein product (Cyclin D1) is found in 50% of BC [127]. High CCND1 amplification has been associated with poor prognosis in ER-positive BC patients and may require additional chemotherapy later in life [128]. In BC, the mechanism of CCND1 overexpression and the key biomarker such as HER2, ER, and their correlation requires more elucidation. In one of the studies, the tumor showed overexpression of CCND1, resulting in a high risk of BC recurrence in patients' life [129]. CCND1 overexpression, along with cyclin E, has also been found in many of the BC cell lines [123]. Cyclin E overexpression is associated with genomic instability [130], resulting in cell proliferation in the breast cancer genome. Gene (c-MYC) is also involved in the epithelial-to-mesenchymal transition, by repressing E-cadherin expression, a necessary step for cell transformation [131]. The two prototypical tumor suppressors RB (retinoblastoma- associated) and TP53 proteins; have a complex regulatory role in deciding the fate of BC cells. RB and TP53 may facilitate BC cells to undergo cell proliferation, senescence or apoptosis. The RB protein is stimulated by diverse signaling from extracellular and intracellular sources, resulting in cell proliferation *via* changes in the cell cycle. Generally, RB loss occurs *via* chromosomal deletion in BC. Functional inactivation of RB can occur *via* cyclin A or cyclin E overexpression, transcriptional silencing (hypermethylation of promoter), and intragenic mutation [132]. Some of the newly identified genes which are involved in BC cell proliferation have been listed in Table **2**.

Loss of RB1 (gene and protein) is more frequently found in TNBC patients [133]. Alternation in RB along with TP53 is also required for cancer cell initiation and progression. Mutations in TP53 facilitate the cell cycle to continue, even though its DNA is damaged, resulting in breast carcinogenesis. In BC patients, TP53 mutation is found approximately 30% of the population [132]. It has been found that tumors having HER2 expression, show an increased expression of ErbB2 and TP53 mutation [134]. BC cells acquire the capability to sustain proliferative signaling in several alternative ways: The release of excessive growth factor (through ligands), which can bind to receptors available on the cell surface by

ligand-receptor binding results in stimulation of proliferation. This type of autocrine proliferative signaling can also be achieved by cross-talk between tyrosine kinase receptors. The overexpression of ER genes, which also communicates with EGF, IGF-I, and TGFα (growth factors), results in binding to ER and activating mitogenic activity in BC cells [123]. Oncogenic K-RAS mutations are rarer in BC, but genomic studies suggest the participation of the EGFR/HER2/K-RAS pathway [135, 136]. The RAS stimulation leads to activation of P13K/AKT/mTOR pathways resulting in cell proliferation, survival, and metastasis in many types of cancer [135].

Table 2. Identification of genes having a role in cell proliferation can be used as a prognostic biomarker and therapeutic target in breast cancer.

Gene	Therapeutic Targets	Reference
CHP2	CHP2 is overexpressed in breast cancer cells and clinical tumor specimens. Inhibition of the CHP2 blocks cell-cycle.	[137]
GLUL	GLUL expression correlates with the larger tumor size in breast cancer patients. Inhibition of GLUL inhibits p38 and MAPK signaling pathways.	[138]
TUFT1	Induces cell proliferation and evades apoptosis.TUFT1 is overexpressed in many breast cancer cell lines and human specimens.	[139]
E2F1	Involvement in cell proliferation and its expression increases tumor size.	[140]
CARM1	CARM1 inhibits cell proliferation and induces differentiation. It can be used as a therapeutic target.	[141]
RBCK1	RBCK1 mediates proliferation and cell cycle progression in ERα-positive breast cancer cells.	[142]
RRS1	Regulates cell proliferation and its inhibition of increased apoptosis and cell cycle arrest.	[143]

CHEMORESISTANCE

BC heterogeneity is the biggest challenge for its treatment and management. Early detection and treatments have greatly improved the survival of BC patients. Still, there is a paucity of knowledge on its recurrence. The conventional chemotherapy is of limited advantage with chemoresistance being a major hindrance [144, 145]. The **C**yclophosphamide, **M**ethotrexate, and **F**luorouracil (CMF) and/or Anthracyclines- and taxanes are the conventional chemotherapy and have been regularly used in the treatment of TNBC treatment [146, 147]. These therapies give a response to limited patients [148], and in those patients, many would later have reappearance BC due to chemoresistance [149]. These drugs have often resulted in chemoresistance, creating a new challenge to identify the new therapeutic targets. The gene signatures generally associated with chemoresistance comprise of different pathways such as EMT, CDH1 targets, AKT1 signaling, hypoxia, angiogenesis, and ECM degradation [150]. The identification of novel genes and miRNA involved in chemoresistance will provide a better opportunity for BC treatment (Tables **3** and **4**).

Genes Involved in Chemoresistance

Identification of new genes signature, which imparts, chemoresistance is an urgent need for better treatment of BC patients. With recent advances, the use of new drugs that inhibits BC cell line proliferation and invasion are promising but may also lead to chemoresistance later. A set of nine biomarker genes (SYK, LCK, GAB2, PAWR, PPARG, MDFI, ZAP70, CIITA, and ACTA1) for BC have been found, having a role in imparting chemoresistance [151]. Similar study by He *et al.* [152] has identified upregulation of 17 genes (ANPEP, ANTXR1, BTG2, CAV2, MFI2, PSAT1, PVR, AKAP12, DKK3, TUSC3, CLIP4, CAPN2, CRLF1, CYBRD1, PHF10, TRHDE, and ABCC3) in clinical BC samples after the patient underwent chemotherapy. Many of the genes belong to different pathways such as EMT, proliferation, and ATP-binding cassette (ABC) transporters, which promote BC metastasis. In this set of genes, CLIP4, CAPN2, CRLF1, CYBRD1, PHF10, and TRHDE are a group of genes identified for the first time for chemoresistance [153]. With the recent advent of the RNA sequencing and bioinformatics approach, new genes are being identified, which may play an important role in chemoresistance. By using a bioinformatics approach23-genes having chemoresistance signatures have been identified. The chemoresistance in these 23 sets of genes can be overcome by using Decitabine (DAC) drug [152]. These signature chemoresistance genes can be further used for the personalized treatment, and as a prognostic biomarker in BC patients.

Table 3. List of recently identified genes involved in chemoresistance.

Gene	Significance	Reference
LMTK3	LMTK3 provides chemoresistance against doxorubicin and docetaxel	[154]
Transmembrane TNF-α (tmTNF- α)	tmTNF- α is a therapeutic target against doxorubicin-resistant breast cancer cells	[145]
SPP1 and TNC	SPP1 and TNC provides chemoresistance in breast cancer cell line against paclitaxel and doxorubicin	[155]
TCF4	Loss of TCF4 in patient-derived xenografts model leads to chemoresistance	[156]
NRP-1 and TNC	Overexpression of NRP-1 regulates TNC resulting in chemoresistance	[157]

(Table 3) cont.....

Gene	Significance	Reference
WNT10B	Imparts chemoresistance in TNBC patients	[158]
TRIM32	Confer chemoresistance in breast cancer cell line	[159]
EIF-5A2	EIF-5A2 key factor in chemoresistance induced due to doxorubicin in breast cancer cells.	[160]

MicroRNA and Chemo-resistance

MicroRNAs (miRNAs) are small non-coding RNAs (21–25 nucleotides) that negatively regulate gene expression at the post-transcriptional level and are often overexpressed in human cancers [161 - 163]. Recently Wang *et al.* [162] identified a set of miRNAs (miR-196a-5p, miR-4472, miR-16-5p, and miR-489), which can be used as therapeutic targeted in BC treatment. Targeting any single gene or mi-RNA will not be sufficient to reverse chemotherapeutic resistance, suggesting the involvement of multiple molecular pathways that must be considered during the treatment of patients. Considering the involvement of tumor microenvironment, exosomes may also play an important role as delivery cargo between donating and delivering cells in regulating miRNA function [163, 164]. Therefore it is very important to identify the new miRNA which is involved in BC (Table **4**).

Table 4. miRNAs identified in providing the chemoresistance in breast cancer; modified from [163, 164]

Drug and Target Therapy	miRNA
Doxorubicin	miR-451, Let-7a, miR-34a, miR-505, miR-181a, miR-663, miR-25, miR-145, miR-644a, miR-128, miR-30c, miR-326, miR-106b-25 cluster, miR-34a
Doxorubicin plus carboplatin	miR-200c
Paclitaxel	miR-125b, miR-30c, miR-100
Taxol	miR-125b
Gemcitabine	miR-484
Carboplatin	miR-200
MDR	miR-218
Paclitaxel +Carboplatin	miR-621
Cisplatin	miR-383, miR-34a, miR-345, miR-7, miR-302b, miR-24
Adriamycin	miR-489, miR-149
Trastuzumab	miR-200c
PARP1 inhibitor	miR-206
Mitoxantrone	miR-487a

(Table 4) cont.....

Drug and Target Therapy	miRNA
VP-16	miR-326
Docetaxel	miR-129-3p, miR-34a
Tamoxifen	miR-451, miR-451a, miR-320a, miR-15a, miR-16, miR-378-3p, miR-342, miR-574-3p, miR-873, miR-375, miR-214, miR-519a, miR-101, miR-301
Fulvestrant	miR-214, miR-221/222
4-hydroxytamoxifen	miR-221/222
Trastuzumab	miR-21, miR-221, miR-210, miR-205-5p, miR-200c, miR-542-3p, miR-375, miR-7, miR-515, miR-16
Lapatinib	miR-630, miR-16

TUMOR MICROENVIRONMENT (TME)

In recent years, tumors have been recognized as a specialized organ whose homeostatic regulation far differs from normal healthy tissue. When studying BC biology, a tumor can only be understood by studying the specialized (cancer) cells within a closed structure known as the tumor microenvironment. The formation of tumor microenvironment is also a multi-step process like cancer, which is heavily regulated by extracellular matrix (ECM), tumor-associated macrophage (TAM), cancer-associated fibroblast (CAF), mesenchymal stem cells (MSCs), chemokines, endothelial cells, hypoxia, and tumor-infiltrating lymphocytes (TILs) [165, 166]. The BC microenvironment comprises three regions: local (intratumoral), regional (in the breast), and distant (metastatic) site. BC cells secrete various growth factors and cytokines, which leads to an increase in the production of receptor activator nuclear factor κB ligand (RANKL). This activation of RANKL causes activation of osteoclast and increased bone resorption [166]. This phenomenon helps in metastasis of cells in two ways; firstly assisting cell migration from the primary site to bone and secondary from bone to other distant sites. RANKL, along with Treg, has been shown to create an immunosuppressive environment helping metastasis of BC cells to a distant organ such as lung [167]. Tumor stromal cells comprise the extracellular matrix, fibroblast, vascular endothelial cells, and immune-inflammatory cells, which induce cellular proliferation, invasion, and metastasis of BC cells. The growth factors such as IL6, CSF2, CCL5, and VEGF increase the proliferation of BC cells [168]. Some of the prominent players of TME have been elaborated in detail. In recent years, many drugs have been developed against components of TME (Table **5**).

Role of Chemokines in TME

In the context of the tumor, the microenvironment role of chemokine becomes an important functional role in deciding the cancer progression. CCL2 secreted by cancer-associated fibroblasts (CAFs) stimulates cancer stem cell (CSC) type phenotype in TME [169]. Whereas another chemokine CXCL12 recruits CDb11$^+$Gr1$^+$myeloid cells leading to inhibition of apoptosis and increased survival in BC cells [170]. The role of CXCL12 has been found responsible for tumor cell invasion and migration. CXCL12also promotes EMT *via* CXCR4 expression on BC cells [166]. CXCR4 expression is correlated with lymph node metastases and poorer clinical outcomes in BC [171]. CXCR4/CXCL12 complex signaling stimulates the proliferation and migration of stromal cells and secretion of matrix metalloproteinases (MMP) in BC [166]. CCL18 from TAMs in BC inside the tumor microenvironment promotes endothelial cells towards angiogenesis [172]. Chemokines also affect mesenchymal stem cells (MSCs) leading to BC progression. MSCs always migrate to tumor sites and are transformed as tumor-resident MSCs, which results in the production of IL6 and CXCL17. The IL6 and CXCL17 chemokines impart cancer stem cells like phenotype in a tumor, to attain chemoresistance [173]. BC cells and MSCs cross-talk activate Src signaling which itself activates downstream signaling of the PIK3/AKT pathway, giving chemoresistance characteristic to cells [174].

Table 5. Tumor microenvironment components and its therapeutic target; modified from [176]

Molecules involved	Target	Available Drug
CAF	TGF-β secretion	IN-1130
	VEGF secretion	Bevacizumab
	CXCL12 secretion	Byrostatin-5, AMD3100, MSX-11
	Metalloproteinases production (MP)	Metalloproteinase inhibitors
Dendritic cells	M2 polarization	Trabectedin
	ECM remodeling through MP secretion	Doxorubicin
	T$_{reg}$ recruitment	CSFR1 antagonists
^{T}reg	Suppression of immune cells	Anti-CD25 antibodies
	RANKL production	Denosumab
^{T}eff	PD-1/PD-L1 signaling	Anti-PD-L1 antibodies
ECM	ECM remodelling	Magnolol, β-aminopropionitrile

Role of Cancer-associated Fibroblast in TME

The BC stroma is comprised of fibroblasts; these cells in the context of the tumor microenvironment are known as cancer-associated fibroblasts (CAF). This CAF secretes many growth factors and chemokines, which cause changes in tumor stroma lead to tumor growth and invasiveness [175]. CAF also influences by intrinsic genetic variabilities such as SNP in metalloproteinases (MMP3), leading to invasion and metastasis. In BC, metastasis to the brain is being assisted by CAFs [176, 177]. Fibroblast releases many growth factors, such as FGF4, which initiates cancer cells like traits on other normal cells in the tumor microenvironment [178].

Involvement of Immune Compartments in TME

In TME, the immune system comprises basically of macrophages, dendritic cells and tumor-infiltrating lymphocytes (TIL). The tumor-associated macrophage is a major cell type of TME and has a prominent role in promoting tumor growth, immune suppression, and angiogenesis. CCL2 secreted by neoplastic and stromal cells recruits TAM near the site and secrets tumor-promoting factors (VEGF and cytokines). TAM belongs to M2 phenotypes are associated with Th2 cytokines, which also secretes many growth factors (IL-10, CCL2, CCL17, CCL22, TGFB), leading to cancer proliferation and migration [179]. CD68+ TAMs have been shown to interact with IL-6 and promote inflammation in surrounding normal tissue [180]. Dendritic cells (DC) have an important role in attacking neoplastic cells by exerting antitumor responses due to the presence of CD4+ and CD8+ T cells. The maturation of DC is regulated by many factors that may result in the formation of tolerogenic or immunosuppressive DC causing an immunosuppressive condition in BC cells. In the tumor-associated stroma, which favors immature DC, to produce proangiogenic factors and enhance endothelial resulting in invasion and migration of cancer cells [181, 182].

Infiltrated CD4+ lymphocytes and DC produces IL-13, which further assists in BC metastasis [182]. Tumor-infiltrating lymphocytes play a key role in TME and are classified in the following groups CD4+ helper cells, T_{reg} (CD4+, CD25+, FOXP3+), effector cells, and CD8+ T cells. T_{reg} whose primary function is to protect against autoimmune diseases, but in TEM, it works as a blocker against antitumor responses (immunoediting). The BC-specific survival is associated with the infiltration by CD8+ effector T, which is independent of other prognostic factors (tumor grade, tumor size, vascular invasion, lymph node stage, and HER2 status) [183]. There is growing interested in many investigators to study genomic regulation TEM from BC patients. Ma *et al.* [184] have identified the role of TEM even before tumor cells invade into stroma resulting in invasive growth of BC cells in the patients. The heterogeneity of BC also contributes to altered genomic alterations in TEM, which can be used to predict clinical outcomes. Many recent studies have been done that have identified different sets of TEM candidate molecules as a prognostic marker [185, 186].

SPLICING FACTORS AND BREAST CANCER

All eukaryotic genes contain a sequence of introns that are usually not translated to expression sequences for proteins. Exon is responsible for encoding the expression sequence, which finally results in proteins after the translation process. During the expression of a gene, which would be translated into the protein, a splicing event occurs to remove introns. This splicing on the gene occurs differentially, known as alternative splicing, to express different proteins isoform from the same gene. Alternative splicing which accounts for 80% gene variability in the genome, results in more than one isoforms [177]. Splicing is carried with the help of spliceosome and regulatory factors, which facilitates both constitutive and regulated alternative splicing. The regulatory factor includes 300 protein and five small nuclear RNAs (snRNAs). The small nuclear RNAs (U1, U2, U4, U5, and U6) contribute to several key interactions such as RNA–RNA and RNA–protein during spliceosome assembly and splicing catalysis [187, 188]. The alternative splicing has a very key role in cancer initiation and metastasis of BC. This alternative splicing can induce all the hallmarks of BC, such as; proliferation, inhibit apoptosis, invasion, metastasis, and chemoresistance (Table **6**) [189].

ENVIRONMENTAL CONTAMINATES

The factors that are normally involved in the etiology of BC are reproductive, genetic, lifestyle, and environmental (including exogenous estrogen exposures) [198, 199]. Many epidemiological studies have examined BC risks associated with environmental contaminants, such as organochlorine pesticides [200], polychlorinated biphenyls [201], and dioxins [202]. BC could be due to environmental estrogens, which have a tissue and dose dependant estrogenic or antiestrogenic effect [203]. Many of the chemicals to which we are exposed in our daily lifes can have a deleterious effect on our bodies. Some of these chemicals that can change genomic fingerprinting resulting in the initiation of BC have been listed below.

Bisphenol-A and Parabens

BISPHENOL-A (BPA) binds to estrogen receptors, inhibiting the ER-signaling in normal homeostasis process and is classified as an estrogen-disruptor compound (EDC). In one of the studies, mice were exposed to low doses of BPA resulted in mammary tumor formation and metastasis [204]. Exposure of BPA changes the gene expression profile of mammary cells, which has similar genes to metastatic tumors [205]. BPA exposure also alters the expression of LAMP3 [206], EZH2 [207], and long noncoding RNA HOTAIR [208], leading to BC progression in an animal model. Parabens (methylparaben, ethylparaben, n-propylparaben, n-butylparaben, and isobutyl paraben) is a mixture of chemicals that are found in cosmetic products, beverages, pharmaceuticals, and foods are integrated into our daily lifestyle. This mixture of chemicals induces cell growth and proliferation in the human BC cell line (MCF7) [209]. Parabens can also induce migration and invasion of human BC cells [210].

Table 6. Genes involved in alternative splicing in BC; modified from [190].

Gene	Alteration type	Reference
SRSF1	AMP, OE	[190]
SRSF3		
SRSF6		
SRSF5	OE	
TRA2B		
HNRNPA1		
HNRNPK		
RPM		
PTB		
RBM5		
RBM10		
ESPR1,2	OE/KD	
RBFOX2	KD	
ESRP1	OE	[191]
hnRNPA2B1	OE	[192]
LIN28A	OE	[193]
TDP43	OE	[194]
SF3B1	OE	[195]
SF3B3		
KLF6-SV1	OE	[196]
Rac1b	OE	[197]

AMP, Amplification; OE, Overexpression; KD, knockdown.

Polyaromatic Hydrocarbon

PAHs are the most-studied component of air pollution concerning BC. It comprises of hundreds of compounds and their metabolites with different biologic activities. The interaction of PAHs and its effect on the human population has been extensively studied in Long Island Breast Cancer Study Project (LIBCSP) [211]. Treatment of BC cell line MCF-7 with oil samples (containing PAHs) resulted in ROS generation and oxidative stress induction [212]. PAHs exposure can result in p53 mutation and causing BC initiation. On the other hand, PAHs can cause BC through mechanisms independent of p53 mutation [213] PAH activates signaling pathways in MDA-MB-231 (a metastatic human breast cancer cell) resulting in invasion and metastasis process [214]. PAHs halt the DNA mismatch repair system in the human BC cell line [215].

Heavy Metals

Metallo-estrogens are metals (cadmium, calcium, cobalt, copper, nickel, chromium, lead, mercury, and tin) that activate the ER-signaling in the absence of estradiol, leading to initiation of BC [216, 217]. Cadmium, which enters our body through diet or smoke, has been shown to causes cell proliferation and differentiation. Cadmium potentiates the interaction between ERα and c-Jun and enhances the recruitment of transcription factors resulting in overexpression of cyclin D1 and c-myc, thus inducing cell proliferation in BC cells [199]. The presence of Se, Zn, and Cr elements in Sudanese patients has been correlated with the malignant stage of BC status [218]. Lead (Pb) has been shown to initiate mammary tumors development in murine mammary tumor virus-infected female C3H mice through drinking water. The presence of Pb in blood and hair samples of Nigerian women correlates with BC progression [219]. These heavy metals induce breast carcinogenicity *via* interference with cellular redox regulation, dysregulation cellular proliferation, inhibition of DNA repair, and epigenetic inactivation [220].

SUMMARY AND CONCLUDING REMARKS

BC is the most common cancer among women and one of the leading causes women deaths worldwide [221, 222]. Several risk factors associated with cancer include aging, obesity, heavy alcohol consumption, postmenopausal status, adiposity, and physical inactivity [22 - 24]. The surgical treatment of BC was one of the first medical revolutions at the end of the 19th century. The scientific description regarding the history of mastectomy states BC treatment started barely 120 years ago [223]. In the past few decades, significant progress has been made in the field of clinical research, experimental models, and bioinformatics but still, our understanding of BC initiation and metastasis remains limited. The advancement of 'omics' research that includes transcriptomics [224], epigenomics [225], proteomics [226], and metabolomics [227] have provided us with the new candidates of BC. The open-access knowledge-based database such as Cancer Genome Atlas, NCI genomic data commons, and CanSAR have provided with the new insight, but still, there is a paucity of knowledge for better BC treatment.

The BC genome-sequencing data have still not provided adequate information to address challenges in breast carcinogenesis. The comprehensive catalog of mutations in BC is the need of the time. The complexity of BC requires predictive and prognostic biomarkers for the proper management of BC patients. The future challenges of precision medicine research comprise of targeted sequencing, whole-exome sequencing, RNA sequencing, gene expression analysis, phosphoprotein detection, SNP arrays, and ctDNA sequencing. For the early detection of BC and to inhibit its recurrence, we need more research on host-immune interaction and tumor microenvironment.

The identification of a new molecular fingerprinting signature is of utmost importance in the comprehensive treatment of BC patients. The previously known genes BRCA1, BRCA2, and HER2, have been well investigated. Along with this, we have also added new candidate genes from the recent finding. The introduction of a new paradigm in BC, like tumor microenvironment, chemoresistance, and single-cell sequencing, has added a new player to BC genomics. With the advent of the human genome sequence, it has opened a new gateway in understating BC biology. The new molecular fingerprinting signature will be required to identify, especially in TNBCs, of better management of BC. Genomic and genetic studies of tumors by sequencing and understating its molecular fingerprints at the different stages of the disease will help us to assist BC patients in a better way.

ABBREVIATIONS

BPA	Bisphenol-A
CARM1	Coactivator-associated arginine methyltransferase
CCND1	Cyclin D1
CHP2	Calcineurin B homologous protein isoform 2
DC	Dendritic cells
E2F1	Transcription factor E2F1
EGF	Epidermal growth factor
IGF-5A2	eukaryotic initiation factor 5A2
EMT	Epithelial- Mesenchymal Transition
ER	Estrogen Receptor
ERα	Estrogen receptor alpha
GLUL	Glutamate-ammonia ligaseHER2 human epithelial receptor 2 also known as c-neu or c-erbB2
IGF-1	Insulin-like growth factor 1
LATS2	Large tumor suppressor kinase 2
LIBCSP	Long Island Breast Cancer Study Project
LMTK3	Lemur Tyrosine Kinase 3

MMP	Metalloproteinases
MSCs	Mesenchymal stem cell
NRP-1	Neuropilin-1
PAHs	Polycyclic aromatic hydrocarbons
RANKL	Receptor activator nuclear factor κβ ligand
RB	Retinoblastoma
RBCK1	RING finger containing E3 ubiquitin ligases
RRS1	Human regulator of ribosome synthesis 1
SDF-1	Stromal cell-derived factor
SPP1	Secreted Phosphoprotein 1
TAM	Tumor-associated macrophages
TCF4/ITF	2 Transcription factor 4
TGFBR2	Transforming growth factor-beta receptor-2
TIL	Tumor-Infiltrating Lymphocytes
TME	Tumor microenvironment
TNBC; TNC Tenascin C;	Triple-negative breast cancer
TNC	Tenascin C
Treg;	Regulatory T cells
TUFT1	Tuftelin 1

CONSENT FOR PUBLICATION

Not applicable.

CONFLICT OF INTEREST

The authors confirm that the contents of this chapter have no conflict of interest.

ACKNOWLEDGEMENT

We thank editors and publishers of the book for giving us the opportunity.

REFERENCES

[1]   Cancer Genome Atlas Network. Comprehensive molecular portraits of human breast tumours. Nature 2012; 490(7418): 61-70.
[http://dx.doi.org/10.1038/nature11412] [PMID: 23000897]

[2]   Coleman MP, Quaresma M, Berrino F, *et al.* Cancer survival in five continents: a worldwide population-based study (CONCORD). Lancet Oncol 2008; 9(8): 730-56.
[http://dx.doi.org/10.1016/S1470-2045(08)70179-7] [PMID: 18639491]

[3]   Siegel R, Naishadham D, Jemal A. Cancer statistics, 2013. CA Cancer J Clin 2013; 63(1): 11-30.
        [http://dx.doi.org/10.3322/caac.21166] [PMID: 23335087]

[4]   Anderson BO, Yip CH, Smith RA, *et al.* Guideline implementation for breast healthcare in low-income and middle-income countries: overview of the Breast Health Global Initiative Global Summit 2007. Cancer 2008; 113(8) (Suppl.): 2221-43.
        [http://dx.doi.org/10.1002/cncr.23844] [PMID: 18816619]

[5]   Ries LAG, Krapcho M, Stinchcomb DG, *et al.* 2006.https://seer.cancer.gov/csr/1975_2005/

[6]   Vargo-Gogola T, Rosen JM. Modelling breast cancer: one size does not fit all. Nat Rev Cancer 2007; 7(9): 659-72.
        [http://dx.doi.org/10.1038/nrc2193] [PMID: 17721431]

[7]   Polyak K. Breast cancer: origins and evolution. J Clin Invest 2007; 117(11): 3155-63.
        [http://dx.doi.org/10.1172/JCI33295] [PMID: 17975657]

[8]   Maresso KC, Tsai KY, Brown PH, Szabo E, Lippman S, Hawk ET. Molecular cancer prevention: Current status and future directions. CA Cancer J Clin 2015; 65(5): 345-83.
        [http://dx.doi.org/10.3322/caac.21287] [PMID: 26284997]

[9]   Colditz GA, Kaphingst KA, Hankinson SE, Rosner B. Family history and risk of breast cancer: nurses' health study. Breast Cancer Res Treat 2012; 133(3): 1097-104.
        [http://dx.doi.org/10.1007/s10549-012-1985-9] [PMID: 22350789]

[10]   Familial breast cancer: collaborative reanalysis of individual data from 52 epidemiological studies including 58,209 women with breast cancer and 101,986 women without the disease. Lancet 2001; 358(9291): 1389-99.
        [http://dx.doi.org/10.1016/S0140-6736(01)06524-2] [PMID: 11705483]

[11]   Lynch HT, Lynch JF. Breast cancer genetics in an oncology clinic: 328 consecutive patients. Cancer Genet Cytogenet 1986; 22(4): 369-71.
        [http://dx.doi.org/10.1016/0165-4608(86)90032-4] [PMID: 3731052]

[12]   Margolin S, Johansson H, Rutqvist LE, Lindblom A, Fornander T. Family history, and impact on clinical presentation and prognosis, in a population-based breast cancer cohort from the Stockholm County. Fam Cancer 2006; 5(4): 309-21.
        [http://dx.doi.org/10.1007/s10689-006-7851-3] [PMID: 16858627]

[13]   Thompson D, Duedal S, Kirner J, *et al.* Cancer risks and mortality in heterozygous ATM mutation carriers. J Natl Cancer Inst 2005; 97(11): 813-22.
        [http://dx.doi.org/10.1093/jnci/dji141] [PMID: 15928302]

[14]   Ritte R, Lukanova A, Berrino F, *et al.* Adiposity, hormone replacement therapy use and breast cancer risk by age and hormone receptor status: a large prospective cohort study. Breast Cancer Res 2012; 14(3): R76.
        [http://dx.doi.org/10.1186/bcr3186] [PMID: 22583394]

[15]   Sieri S, Krogh V, Bolelli G, *et al.* Sex hormone levels, breast cancer risk, and cancer receptor status in postmenopausal women: the ORDET cohort. Cancer Epidemiol Biomarkers Prev 2009; 18(1): 169-76.
        [http://dx.doi.org/10.1158/1055-9965.EPI-08-0808] [PMID: 19124495]

[16]   Hsieh CC, Trichopoulos D, Katsouyanni K, Yuasa S. Age at menarche, age at menopause, height and obesity as risk factors for breast cancer: associations and interactions in an international case-control study. Int J Cancer 1990; 46(5): 796-800.
        [http://dx.doi.org/10.1002/ijc.2910460508] [PMID: 2228308]

[17]   Kelsey JL, Gammon MD, John EM. Reproductive factors and breast cancer. Epidemiol Rev 1993; 15(1): 36-47.
        [http://dx.doi.org/10.1093/oxfordjournals.epirev.a036115] [PMID: 8405211]

[18]   Breast cancer and breastfeeding: collaborative reanalysis of individual data from 47 epidemiological

studies in 30 countries, including 50302 women with breast cancer and 96973 women without the disease. Lancet 2002; 360(9328): 187-95.
[http://dx.doi.org/10.1016/S0140-6736(02)09454-0] [PMID: 12133652]

[19] Lahmann PH, Hoffmann K, Allen N, *et al.* Body size and breast cancer risk: findings from the European Prospective Investigation into Cancer And Nutrition (EPIC). Int J Cancer 2004; 111(5): 762-71.
[http://dx.doi.org/10.1002/ijc.20315] [PMID: 15252848]

[20] Breast cancer and hormone replacement therapy: collaborative reanalysis of data from 51 epidemiological studies of 52,705 women with breast cancer and 108,411 women without breast cancer. Lancet 1997; 350(9084): 1047-59.
[http://dx.doi.org/10.1016/S0140-6736(97)08233-0] [PMID: 10213546]

[21] Chlebowski RT, Manson JE, Anderson GL, *et al.* Estrogen plus progestin and breast cancer incidence and mortality in the Women's Health Initiative Observational Study. J Natl Cancer Inst 2013; 105(8): 526-35.
[http://dx.doi.org/10.1093/jnci/djt043] [PMID: 23543779]

[22] Danaei G, Vander Hoorn S, Lopez AD, Murray CJ, Ezzati M. Causes of cancer in the world: comparative risk assessment of nine behavioural and environmental risk factors. Lancet 2005; 366(9499): 1784-93.
[http://dx.doi.org/10.1016/S0140-6736(05)67725-2] [PMID: 16298215]

[23] Chen WY, Rosner B, Hankinson SE, Colditz GA, Willett WC. Moderate alcohol consumption during adult life, drinking patterns, and breast cancer risk. JAMA 2011; 306(17): 1884-90.
[http://dx.doi.org/10.1001/jama.2011.1590] [PMID: 22045766]

[24] Wu Y, Zhang D, Kang S. Physical activity and risk of breast cancer: a meta-analysis of prospective studies. Breast Cancer Res Treat 2013; 137(3): 869-82.
[http://dx.doi.org/10.1007/s10549-012-2396-7] [PMID: 23274845]

[25] Claus EB, Schildkraut JM, Thompson WD, Risch NJ. The genetic attributable risk of breast and ovarian cancer. Cancer 1996; 77(11): 2318-24.
[http://dx.doi.org/10.1002/(SICI)1097-0142(19960601)77:11<2318::AID-CNCR21>3.0.CO;2-Z] [PMID: 8635102]

[26] Easton DF, Bishop DT, Ford D, Crockford GP. Genetic linkage analysis in familial breast and ovarian cancer: results from 214 families. Am J Hum Genet 1993; 52(4): 678-701.
[PMID: 8460634]

[27] Struewing JP, Tarone RE, Brody LC, Li FP, Boice JD Jr. BRCA1 mutations in young women with breast cancer. Lancet 1996; 347(9013): 1493.
[http://dx.doi.org/10.1016/S0140-6736(96)91732-8] [PMID: 8676668]

[28] Abeliovich D, Kaduri L, Lerer I, *et al.* The founder mutations 185delAG and 5382insC in BRCA1 and 6174delT in BRCA2 appear in 60% of ovarian cancer and 30% of early-onset breast cancer patients among Ashkenazi women. Am J Hum Genet 1997; 60(3): 505-14.
[PMID: 9042909]

[29] Einbeigi Z, Bergman A, Kindblom LG, *et al.* A founder mutation of the BRCA1 gene in Western Sweden associated with a high incidence of breast and ovarian cancer. Eur J Cancer 2001; 37(15): 1904-9.
[http://dx.doi.org/10.1016/S0959-8049(01)00223-4] [PMID: 11576847]

[30] Cortez D, Wang Y, Qin J, Elledge SJ. Requirement of ATM-dependent phosphorylation of brca1 in the DNA damage response to double-strand breaks. Science 1999; 286(5442): 1162-6.
[http://dx.doi.org/10.1126/science.286.5442.1162] [PMID: 10550055]

[31] Lou Z, Chini CC, Minter-Dykhouse K, Chen J. Mediator of DNA damage checkpoint protein 1 regulates BRCA1 localization and phosphorylation in DNA damage checkpoint control. J Biol Chem 2003; 278(16): 13599-602.

[http://dx.doi.org/10.1074/jbc.C300060200] [PMID: 12611903]

[32]   Hashizume R, Fukuda M, Maeda I, *et al.* The RING heterodimer BRCA1-BARD1 is a ubiquitin ligase inactivated by a breast cancer-derived mutation. J Biol Chem 2001; 276(18): 14537-40.
[http://dx.doi.org/10.1074/jbc.C000881200] [PMID: 11278247]

[33]   Wooster R, Bignell G, Lancaster J, *et al.* Identification of the breast cancer susceptibility gene BRCA2. Nature 1995; 378(6559): 789-92.
[http://dx.doi.org/10.1038/378789a0] [PMID: 8524414]

[34]   Tavtigian SV, Simard J, Rommens J, *et al.* The complete BRCA2 gene and mutations in chromosome 13q-linked kindreds. Nat Genet 1996; 12(3): 333-7.
[http://dx.doi.org/10.1038/ng0396-333] [PMID: 8589730]

[35]   Chen JJ, Silver D, Cantor S, Livingston DM, Scully R. BRCA1, BRCA2, and Rad51 operate in a common DNA damage response pathway. Cancer Res 1999; 59(7) (Suppl.): 1752s-6s.
[PMID: 10197592]

[36]   Perou CM, Sørlie T, Eisen MB, *et al.* Molecular portraits of human breast tumours. Nature 2000; 406(6797): 747-52.
[http://dx.doi.org/10.1038/35021093] [PMID: 10963602]

[37]   Lakhani SR, Jacquemier J, Sloane JP, *et al.* Multifactorial analysis of differences between sporadic breast cancers and cancers involving BRCA1 and BRCA2 mutations. J Natl Cancer Inst 1998; 90(15): 1138-45.
[http://dx.doi.org/10.1093/jnci/90.15.1138] [PMID: 9701363]

[38]   Pathology of familial breast cancer: differences between breast cancers in carriers of BRCA1 or BRCA2 mutations and sporadic cases. Lancet 1997; 349(9064): 1505-10.
[http://dx.doi.org/10.1016/S0140-6736(96)10109-4] [PMID: 9167459]

[39]   Foulkes WD, Stefansson IM, Chappuis PO, *et al.* Germline BRCA1 mutations and a basal epithelial phenotype in breast cancer. J Natl Cancer Inst 2003; 95(19): 1482-5.
[http://dx.doi.org/10.1093/jnci/djg050] [PMID: 14519755]

[40]   Honrado E, Benítez J, Palacios J. The molecular pathology of hereditary breast cancer: genetic testing and therapeutic implications. Mod Pathol 2005; 18(10): 1305-20.
[http://dx.doi.org/10.1038/modpathol.3800453] [PMID: 15933754]

[41]   King MC, Wieand S, Hale K, *et al.* Tamoxifen and breast cancer incidence among women with inherited mutations in BRCA1 and BRCA2: National Surgical Adjuvant Breast and Bowel Project (NSABP-P1) Breast Cancer Prevention Trial. JAMA 2001; 286(18): 2251-6.
[http://dx.doi.org/10.1001/jama.286.18.2251] [PMID: 11710890]

[42]   Narod SA, Brunet JS, Ghadirian P, *et al.* Tamoxifen and risk of contralateral breast cancer in BRCA1 and BRCA2 mutation carriers: a case-control study. Lancet 2000; 356(9245): 1876-81.
[http://dx.doi.org/10.1016/S0140-6736(00)03258-X] [PMID: 11130383]

[43]   Fukushige S, Matsubara K, Yoshida M, *et al.* Localization of a novel v-erbB-related gene, c-erbB-2, on human chromosome 17 and its amplification in a gastric cancer cell line. Mol Cell Biol 1986; 6(3): 955-8.
[http://dx.doi.org/10.1128/MCB.6.3.955] [PMID: 2430175]

[44]   Stern DF, Heffernan PA, Weinberg RA. p185, a product of the neu proto-oncogene, is a receptorlike protein associated with tyrosine kinase activity. Mol Cell Biol 1986; 6(5): 1729-40.
[http://dx.doi.org/10.1128/MCB.6.5.1729] [PMID: 2878363]

[45]   Akiyama T, Sudo C, Ogawara H, Toyoshima K, Yamamoto T. The product of the human c-erbB-2 gene: a 185-kilodalton glycoprotein with tyrosine kinase activity. Science 1986; 232(4758): 1644-6.
[http://dx.doi.org/10.1126/science.3012781] [PMID: 3012781]

[46]   Riese DJ II, Stern DF. Specificity within the EGF family/ErbB receptor family signaling network. BioEssays 1998; 20(1): 41-8.

[http://dx.doi.org/10.1002/(SICI)1521-1878(199801)20:1<41::AID-BIES7>3.0.CO;2-V]   [PMID: 9504046]

[47]   Meric-Bernstam F, Hung MC. Advances in targeting human epidermal growth factor receptor-2 signaling for cancer therapy. Clin Cancer Res 2006; 12(21): 6326-30.
[http://dx.doi.org/10.1158/1078-0432.CCR-06-1732] [PMID: 17085641]

[48]   Slamon DJ, Clark GM, Wong SG, Levin WJ, Ullrich A, McGuire WL. Human breast cancer: correlation of relapse and survival with amplification of the HER-2/neu oncogene. Science 1987; 235(4785): 177-82.
[http://dx.doi.org/10.1126/science.3798106] [PMID: 3798106]

[49]   Slamon DJ, Godolphin W, Jones LA, *et al.* Studies of the HER-2/neu proto-oncogene in human breast and ovarian cancer. Science 1989; 244(4905): 707-12.
[http://dx.doi.org/10.1126/science.2470152] [PMID: 2470152]

[50]   Davoli A, Hocevar BA, Brown TL. Progression and treatment of HER2-positive breast cancer. Cancer Chemother Pharmacol 2010; 65(4): 611-23.
[http://dx.doi.org/10.1007/s00280-009-1208-1] [PMID: 20087739]

[51]   Iqbal N, Iqbal N. Human Epidermal Growth Factor Receptor 2 (HER2) in Cancers: Overexpression and Therapeutic Implications. Mol Biol Int 2014; 2014: 852748.
[http://dx.doi.org/10.1155/2014/852748] [PMID: 25276427]

[52]   Park K, Han S, Kim HJ, Kim J, Shin E. HER2 status in pure ductal carcinoma *in situ* and in the intraductal and invasive components of invasive ductal carcinoma determined by fluorescence *in situ* hybridization and immunohistochemistry. Histopathology 2006; 48(6): 702-7.
[http://dx.doi.org/10.1111/j.1365-2559.2006.02403.x] [PMID: 16681686]

[53]   Moasser MM. The oncogene HER2: its signaling and transforming functions and its role in human cancer pathogenesis. Oncogene 2007; 26(45): 6469-87.
[http://dx.doi.org/10.1038/sj.onc.1210477] [PMID: 17471238]

[54]   Mitri Z, Constantine T, O'Regan R. The HER2 receptor in breast cancer: Pathophysiology, clinical use, and new advances in therapy. Chemother Res Pract 2012; 2012: 743193.
[http://dx.doi.org/10.1155/2012/743193] [PMID: 23320171]

[55]   Timms JF, White SL, O'Hare MJ, Waterfield MD. Effects of ErbB-2 overexpression on mitogenic signalling and cell cycle progression in human breast luminal epithelial cells. Oncogene 2002; 21(43): 6573-86.
[http://dx.doi.org/10.1038/sj.onc.1205847] [PMID: 12242655]

[56]   Subbaramaiah K, Norton L, Gerald W, Dannenberg AJ. Cyclooxygenase-2 is overexpressed in HER-2/neu-positive breast cancer: evidence for involvement of AP-1 and PEA3. J Biol Chem 2002; 277(21): 18649-57.
[http://dx.doi.org/10.1074/jbc.M111415200] [PMID: 11901151]

[57]   Wang SC, Lien HC, Xia W, *et al.* Binding at and transactivation of the COX-2 promoter by nuclear tyrosine kinase receptor ErbB-2. Cancer Cell 2004; 6(3): 251-61.
[http://dx.doi.org/10.1016/j.ccr.2004.07.012] [PMID: 15380516]

[58]   Li YM, Pan Y, Wei Y, *et al.* Upregulation of CXCR4 is essential for HER2-mediated tumor metastasis. Cancer Cell 2004; 6(5): 459-69.
[http://dx.doi.org/10.1016/j.ccr.2004.09.027] [PMID: 15542430]

[59]   Müller A, Homey B, Soto H, *et al.* Involvement of chemokine receptors in breast cancer metastasis. Nature 2001; 410(6824): 50-6.
[http://dx.doi.org/10.1038/35065016] [PMID: 11242036]

[60]   Neve RM, Ylstra B, Chang CH, Albertson DG, Benz CC. ErbB2 activation of ESX gene expression. Oncogene 2002; 21(24): 3934-8.
[http://dx.doi.org/10.1038/sj.onc.1205503] [PMID: 12032832]

[61] Goueli BS, Janknecht R. Upregulation of the catalytic telomerase subunit by the transcription factor ER81 and oncogenic HER2/Neu, Ras, or Raf. Mol Cell Biol 2004; 24(1): 25-35.
[http://dx.doi.org/10.1128/MCB.24.1.25-35.2004] [PMID: 14673140]

[62] Laughner E, Taghavi P, Chiles K, Mahon PC, Semenza GL. HER2 (neu) signaling increases the rate of hypoxia-inducible factor 1alpha (HIF-1alpha) synthesis: novel mechanism for HIF-1-mediated vascular endothelial growth factor expression. Mol Cell Biol 2001; 21(12): 3995-4004.
[http://dx.doi.org/10.1128/MCB.21.12.3995-4004.2001] [PMID: 11359907]

[63] Spangenberg C, Lausch EU, Trost TM, *et al.* ERBB2-mediated transcriptional up-regulation of the alpha5beta1 integrin fibronectin receptor promotes tumor cell survival under adverse conditions. Cancer Res 2006; 66(7): 3715-25.
[http://dx.doi.org/10.1158/0008-5472.CAN-05-2823] [PMID: 16585198]

[64] Loureiro RM, Maharaj AS, Dankort D, Muller WJ, D'Amore PA. ErbB2 overexpression in mammary cells upregulates VEGF through the core promoter. Biochem Biophys Res Commun 2005; 326(2): 455-65.
[http://dx.doi.org/10.1016/j.bbrc.2004.11.053] [PMID: 15582599]

[65] Adams J, Carder PJ, Downey S, *et al.* Vascular endothelial growth factor (VEGF) in breast cancer: comparison of plasma, serum, and tissue VEGF and microvessel density and effects of tamoxifen. Cancer Res 2000; 60(11): 2898-905.
[PMID: 10850435]

[66] Mukohara T. Mechanisms of resistance to anti-human epidermal growth factor receptor 2 agents in breast cancer. Cancer Sci 2011; 102(1): 1-8.
[http://dx.doi.org/10.1111/j.1349-7006.2010.01711.x] [PMID: 20825420]

[67] Pegram MD, Konecny GE, O'Callaghan C, Beryt M, Pietras R, Slamon DJ. Rational combinations of trastuzumab with chemotherapeutic drugs used in the treatment of breast cancer. J Natl Cancer Inst 2004; 96(10): 739-49.
[http://dx.doi.org/10.1093/jnci/djh131] [PMID: 15150302]

[68] Scaltriti M, Rojo F, Ocaña A, *et al.* Expression of p95HER2, a truncated form of the HER2 receptor, and response to anti-HER2 therapies in breast cancer. J Natl Cancer Inst 2007; 99(8): 628-38.
[http://dx.doi.org/10.1093/jnci/djk134] [PMID: 17440164]

[69] Xia W, Liu LH, Ho P, Spector NL. Truncated ErbB2 receptor (p95ErbB2) is regulated by heregulin through heterodimer formation with ErbB3 yet remains sensitive to the dual EGFR/ErbB2 kinase inhibitor GW572016. Oncogene 2004; 23(3): 646-53.
[http://dx.doi.org/10.1038/sj.onc.1207166] [PMID: 14737100]

[70] Saha Roy S, Vadlamudi RK. Role of estrogen receptor signaling in breast cancer metastasis. Int J Breast Cancer 2012; 2012: 654698.
[http://dx.doi.org/10.1155/2012/654698] [PMID: 22295247]

[71] Rondón-Lagos M, Villegas VE, Rangel N, Sánchez MC, Zaphiropoulos PG. Tamoxifen resistance: Emerging molecular targets. Int J Mol Sci 2016; 17(8): E1357.
[http://dx.doi.org/10.3390/ijms17081357] [PMID: 27548161]

[72] Brufsky AM, Dickler MN. Estrogen receptor-positive breast cancer: Exploiting signaling pathways implicated in endocrine resistance. Oncologist 2018; 23(5): 528-39.
[http://dx.doi.org/10.1634/theoncologist.2017-0423] [PMID: 29352052]

[73] Hua H, Zhang H, Kong Q, Jiang Y. Mechanisms for estrogen receptor expression in human cancer. Exp Hematol Oncol 2018; 7: 24.
[http://dx.doi.org/10.1186/s40164-018-0116-7] [PMID: 30250760]

[74] Allred DC, Brown P, Medina D. The origins of estrogen receptor alpha-positive and estrogen receptor alpha-negative human breast cancer. Breast Cancer Res 2004; 6(6): 240-5.
[http://dx.doi.org/10.1186/bcr938] [PMID: 15535853]

[75] Lim E, Tarulli G, Portman N, Hickey TE, Tilley WD, Palmieri C. Pushing estrogen receptor around in breast cancer. Endocr Relat Cancer 2016; 23(12): T227-41.
[http://dx.doi.org/10.1530/ERC-16-0427] [PMID: 27729416]

[76] Hewitt SC, Korach KS. Estrogen receptors: New directions in the new millennium. Endocr Rev 2018; 39(5): 664-75.
[http://dx.doi.org/10.1210/er.2018-00087] [PMID: 29901737]

[77] Williams C, Lin CY. Oestrogen receptors in breast cancer: basic mechanisms and clinical implications. Ecancermedicalscience 2013; 7: 370.
[PMID: 24222786]

[78] Wang L, Nanayakkara G, Yang Q, *et al.* A comprehensive data mining study shows that most nuclear receptors act as newly proposed homeostasis-associated molecular pattern receptors. J Hematol Oncol 2017; 10(1): 168.
[http://dx.doi.org/10.1186/s13045-017-0526-8] [PMID: 29065888]

[79] Madureira PA, Varshochi R, Constantinidou D, *et al.* The Forkhead box M1 protein regulates the transcription of the estrogen receptor alpha in breast cancer cells. J Biol Chem 2006; 281(35): 25167-76.
[http://dx.doi.org/10.1074/jbc.M603906200] [PMID: 16809346]

[80] Shang Y, Hu X, DiRenzo J, Lazar MA, Brown M. Cofactor dynamics and sufficiency in estrogen receptor-regulated transcription. Cell 2000; 103(6): 843-52.
[http://dx.doi.org/10.1016/S0092-8674(00)00188-4] [PMID: 11136970]

[81] Métivier R, Penot G, Hübner MR, *et al.* Estrogen receptor-alpha directs ordered, cyclical, and combinatorial recruitment of cofactors on a natural target promoter. Cell 2003; 115(6): 751-63.
[http://dx.doi.org/10.1016/S0092-8674(03)00934-6] [PMID: 14675539]

[82] Glück S. Consequences of the convergence of multiple alternate pathways on the estrogen receptor in the treatment of metastatic breast cancer. Clin Breast Cancer 2017; 17(2): 79-90.
[http://dx.doi.org/10.1016/j.clbc.2016.08.004] [PMID: 27687476]

[83] Nardone A, De Angelis C, Trivedi MV, Osborne CK, Schiff R. The changing role of ER in endocrine resistance. Breast 2015; 24(24) (Suppl. 2): S60-6.
[http://dx.doi.org/10.1016/j.breast.2015.07.015] [PMID: 26271713]

[84] Asselin-Labat ML, Sutherland KD, Barker H, *et al.* Gata-3 is an essential regulator of mammary-gland morphogenesis and luminal-cell differentiation. Nat Cell Biol 2007; 9(2): 201-9.
[http://dx.doi.org/10.1038/ncb1530] [PMID: 17187062]

[85] Guo Y, Yu P, Liu Z, *et al.* Prognostic and clinicopathological value of GATA binding protein 3 in breast cancer: A systematic review and meta-analysis. PLoS One 2017; 12(4): e0174843.
[http://dx.doi.org/10.1371/journal.pone.0174843] [PMID: 28394898]

[86] Eeckhoute J, Keeton EK, Lupien M, Krum SA, Carroll JS, Brown M. Positive cross-regulatory loop ties GATA-3 to estrogen receptor alpha expression in breast cancer. Cancer Res 2007; 67(13): 6477-83.
[http://dx.doi.org/10.1158/0008-5472.CAN-07-0746] [PMID: 17616709]

[87] Doisneau-Sixou SF, Sergio CM, Carroll JS, Hui R, Musgrove EA, Sutherland RL. Estrogen and antiestrogen regulation of cell cycle progression in breast cancer cells. Endocr Relat Cancer 2003; 10(2): 179-86.
[http://dx.doi.org/10.1677/erc.0.0100179] [PMID: 12790780]

[88] Louie MC, Sevigny MB. Steroid hormone receptors as prognostic markers in breast cancer. Am J Cancer Res 2017; 7(8): 1617-36.
[PMID: 28861319]

[89] Dunnwald LK, Rossing MA, Li CI. Hormone receptor status, tumor characteristics, and prognosis: a prospective cohort of breast cancer patients. Breast Cancer Res 2007; 9(1): R6.

[http://dx.doi.org/10.1186/bcr1639] [PMID: 17239243]

[90]   Johnston SR, Saccani-Jotti G, Smith IE, *et al.* Changes in estrogen receptor, progesterone receptor, and pS2 expression in tamoxifen-resistant human breast cancer. Cancer Res 1995; 55(15): 3331-8.
[PMID: 7614468]

[91]   Murphy CG, Dickler MN. Endocrine resistance in hormone-responsive breast cancer: mechanisms and therapeutic strategies. Endocr Relat Cancer 2016; 23(8): R337-52.
[http://dx.doi.org/10.1530/ERC-16-0121] [PMID: 27406875]

[92]   Hattori Y, Ishii H, Morita A, Sakuma Y, Ozawa H. Characterization of the fundamental properties of the N-terminal truncation (Δ exon 1) variant of estrogen receptor α in the rat. Gene 2015; 571(1): 117-25.
[http://dx.doi.org/10.1016/j.gene.2015.06.086] [PMID: 26151894]

[93]   Green S, Walter P, Kumar V, *et al.* Human oestrogen receptor cDNA: sequence, expression and homology to v-erb-A. Nature 1986; 320(6058): 134-9.
[http://dx.doi.org/10.1038/320134a0] [PMID: 3754034]

[94]   Pfeffer U, Fecarotta E, Arena G, *et al.* Alternative splicing of the estrogen receptor primary transcript normally occurs in estrogen receptor positive tissues and cell lines. J Steroid BiochemMolBiol 1996; 56(1-6 Spec No): 99-105.   [https://doi.org/10.1016/0960-0760(95)00227-8] [PMID: 8603053]

[95]   Iorio MV, Ferracin M, Liu CG, *et al.* MicroRNA gene expression deregulation in human breast cancer. Cancer Res 2005; 65(16): 7065-70.
[http://dx.doi.org/10.1158/0008-5472.CAN-05-1783] [PMID: 16103053]

[96]   Adams BD, Furneaux H, White BA. The micro-ribonucleic acid (miRNA) miR-206 targets the human estrogen receptor-alpha (ERalpha) and represses ERalpha messenger RNA and protein expression in breast cancer cell lines. Mol Endocrinol 2007; 21(5): 1132-47.
[http://dx.doi.org/10.1210/me.2007-0022] [PMID: 17312270]

[97]   Li X, Mertens-Talcott SU, Zhang S, Kim K, Ball J, Safe S. MicroRNA-27a Indirectly Regulates Estrogen Receptor alpha Expression and Hormone Responsiveness in MCF-7 Breast Cancer Cells. Endocrinology 2010; 151(6): 2462-73.
[http://dx.doi.org/10.1210/en.2009-1150] [PMID: 20382698]

[98]   Chu I, Arnaout A, Loiseau S, *et al.* Src promotes estrogen-dependent estrogen receptor alpha proteolysis in human breast cancer. J Clin Invest 2007; 117(8): 2205-15.
[http://dx.doi.org/10.1172/JCI21739] [PMID: 17627304]

[99]   Suzuki R, Orsini N, Saji S, Key TJ, Wolk A. Body weight and incidence of breast cancer defined by estrogen and progesterone receptor status--a meta-analysis. Int J Cancer 2009; 124(3): 698-712.
[http://dx.doi.org/10.1002/ijc.23943] [PMID: 18988226]

[100]   Lange CA, Yee D. Progesterone and breast cancer. Womens Health (Lond) 2008; 4(2): 151-62.
[http://dx.doi.org/10.2217/17455057.4.2.151] [PMID: 19072517]

[101]   Thakkar JP, Mehta DG. A review of an unfavorable subset of breast cancer: estrogen receptor positive progesterone receptor negative. Oncologist 2011; 16(3): 276-85.
[http://dx.doi.org/10.1634/theoncologist.2010-0302] [PMID: 21339261]

[102]   Mulac-Jericevic B, Mullinax RA, DeMayo FJ, Lydon JP, Conneely OM. Subgroup of reproductive functions of progesterone mediated by progesterone receptor-B isoform. Science 2000; 289(5485): 1751-4.
[http://dx.doi.org/10.1126/science.289.5485.1751] [PMID: 10976068]

[103]   Mulac-Jericevic B, Lydon JP, DeMayo FJ, Conneely OM. Defective mammary gland morphogenesis in mice lacking the progesterone receptor B isoform. Proc Natl Acad Sci USA 2003; 100(17): 9744-9.
[http://dx.doi.org/10.1073/pnas.1732707100] [PMID: 12897242]

[104]   Wei LL, Norris BM, Baker CJ. An N-terminally truncated third progesterone receptor protein, PR(C), forms heterodimers with PR(B) but interferes in PR(B)-DNA binding. J Steroid Biochem Mol Biol

1997; 62(4): 287-97.
[http://dx.doi.org/10.1016/S0960-0760(97)00044-7] [PMID: 9408082]

[105] Hewitt SC, Korach KS. Progesterone action and responses in the alphaERKO mouse. Steroids 2000; 65(10-11): 551-7.
[http://dx.doi.org/10.1016/S0039-128X(00)00113-6] [PMID: 11108859]

[106] Haslam SZ, Counterman LJ, Nummy KA. Effects of epidermal growth factor, estrogen, and progestin on DNA synthesis in mammary cells *in vivo* are determined by the developmental state of the gland. J Cell Physiol 1993; 155(1): 72-8.
[http://dx.doi.org/10.1002/jcp.1041550110] [PMID: 8468371]

[107] Ruan W, Monaco ME, Kleinberg DL. Progesterone stimulates mammary gland ductal morphogenesis by synergizing with and enhancing insulin-like growth factor-I action. Endocrinology 2005; 146(3): 1170-8.
[http://dx.doi.org/10.1210/en.2004-1360] [PMID: 15604210]

[108] Hilton HN, Doan TB, Graham JD, *et al.* Acquired convergence of hormone signaling in breast cancer: ER and PR transition from functionally distinct in normal breast to predictors of metastatic disease. Oncotarget 2014; 5(18): 8651-64.
[http://dx.doi.org/10.18632/oncotarget.2354] [PMID: 25261374]

[109] Hilton HN, Santucci N, Silvestri A, *et al.* Progesterone stimulates progenitor cells in normal human breast and breast cancer cells. Breast Cancer Res Treat 2014; 143(3): 423-33.
[http://dx.doi.org/10.1007/s10549-013-2817-2] [PMID: 24395108]

[110] Osborne CK, Shou J, Massarweh S, Schiff R. Crosstalk between estrogen receptor and growth factor receptor pathways as a cause for endocrine therapy resistance in breast cancer. Clin Cancer Res 2005; 11(2 Pt 2): 865s-70s.
[PMID: 15701879]

[111] Cui X, Schiff R, Arpino G, Osborne CK, Lee AV. Biology of progesterone receptor loss in breast cancer and its implications for endocrine therapy. J Clin Oncol 2005; 23(30): 7721-35.
[http://dx.doi.org/10.1200/JCO.2005.09.004] [PMID: 16234531]

[112] Zhang Y, Su H, Rahimi M, Tochihara R, Tang C. EGFRvIII-induced estrogen-independence, tamoxifen-resistance phenotype correlates with PgR expression and modulation of apoptotic molecules in breast cancer. Int J Cancer 2009; 125(9): 2021-8.
[http://dx.doi.org/10.1002/ijc.24540] [PMID: 19588487]

[113] Lange CA. Making sense of cross-talk between steroid hormone receptors and intracellular signaling pathways: who will have the last word? Mol Endocrinol 2004; 18(2): 269-78.
[http://dx.doi.org/10.1210/me.2003-0331] [PMID: 14563938]

[114] Groshong SD, Owen GI, Grimison B, *et al.* Biphasic regulation of breast cancer cell growth by progesterone: role of the cyclin-dependent kinase inhibitors, p21 and p27(Kip1). Mol Endocrinol 1997; 11(11): 1593-607.
[http://dx.doi.org/10.1210/mend.11.11.0006] [PMID: 9328342]

[115] Hissom JR, Moore MR. Progestin effects on growth in the human breast cancer cell line T-47---possible therapeutic implications. Biochem Biophys Res Commun 1987; 145(2): 706-11.
[http://dx.doi.org/10.1016/0006-291X(87)91022-9] [PMID: 3593365]

[116] Musgrove EA, Lee CS, Sutherland RL. Progestins both stimulate and inhibit breast cancer cell cycle progression while increasing expression of transforming growth factor alpha, epidermal growth factor receptor, c-fos, and c-myc genes. Mol Cell Biol 1991; 11(10): 5032-43.
[http://dx.doi.org/10.1128/MCB.11.10.5032] [PMID: 1922031]

[117] Larsson SC, Bergkvist L, Wolk A. Glycemic load, glycemic index and breast cancer risk in a prospective cohort of Swedish women. Int J Cancer 2009; 125(1): 153-7.
[http://dx.doi.org/10.1002/ijc.24310] [PMID: 19319984]

[118] Beleut M, Rajaram RD, Caikovski M, *et al.* Two distinct mechanisms underlie progesterone-induced proliferation in the mammary gland. Proc Natl Acad Sci USA 2010; 107(7): 2989-94.
[http://dx.doi.org/10.1073/pnas.0915148107] [PMID: 20133621]

[119] Schramek D, Leibbrandt A, Sigl V, *et al.* Osteoclast differentiation factor RANKL controls development of progestin-driven mammary cancer. Nature 2010; 468(7320): 98-102.
[http://dx.doi.org/10.1038/nature09387] [PMID: 20881962]

[120] Heinonen KM, Vanegas JR, Lew D, Krosl J, Perreault C. Wnt4 enhances murine hematopoietic progenitor cell expansion through a planar cell polarity-like pathway. PLoS One 2011; 6(4): e19279.
[http://dx.doi.org/10.1371/journal.pone.0019279] [PMID: 21541287]

[121] Tsukamoto AS, Grosschedl R, Guzman RC, Parslow T, Varmus HE. Expression of the int-1 gene in transgenic mice is associated with mammary gland hyperplasia and adenocarcinomas in male and female mice. Cell 1988; 55(4): 619-25.
[http://dx.doi.org/10.1016/0092-8674(88)90220-6] [PMID: 3180222]

[122] Brisken C, Hess K, Jeitziner R. Progesterone and Overlooked Endocrine Pathways in Breast Cancer Pathogenesis. Endocrinology 2015; 156(10): 3442-50.
[http://dx.doi.org/10.1210/en.2015-1392] [PMID: 26241069]

[123] Suter R, Marcum JA. The molecular genetics of breast cancer and targeted therapy. Biologics 2007; 1(3): 241-58.
[PMID: 19707334]

[124] Ingvarsson S. Genetics of breast cancer. Drugs Today (Barc) 2004; 40(12): 991-1002.
[http://dx.doi.org/10.1358/dot.2004.40.12.872574] [PMID: 15645010]

[125] Klapper LN, Kirschbaum MH, Sela M, Yarden Y. Biochemical and clinical implications of the ErbB/HER signaling network of growth factor receptors. Adv Cancer Res 2000; 77: 25-79.
[http://dx.doi.org/10.1016/S0065-230X(08)60784-8] [PMID: 10549355]

[126] Mukherjee S, Conrad SE. c-Myc suppresses p21WAF1/CIP1 expression during estrogen signaling and antiestrogen resistance in human breast cancer cells. J Biol Chem 2005; 280(18): 17617-25.
[http://dx.doi.org/10.1074/jbc.M502278200] [PMID: 15757889]

[127] Roy PG, Thompson AM. Cyclin D1 and breast cancer. Breast 2006; 15(6): 718-27.
[http://dx.doi.org/10.1016/j.breast.2006.02.005] [PMID: 16675218]

[128] Roy PG, Pratt N, Purdie CA, *et al.* High CCND1 amplification identifies a group of poor prognosis women with estrogen receptor positive breast cancer. Int J Cancer 2010; 127(2): 355-60.
[http://dx.doi.org/10.1002/ijc.25034] [PMID: 19904758]

[129] Lundgren K, Brown M, Pineda S, *et al.* Effects of cyclin D1 gene amplification and protein expression on time to recurrence in postmenopausal breast cancer patients treated with anastrozole or tamoxifen: a TransATAC study. Breast Cancer Res 2012; 14(2): R57.
[http://dx.doi.org/10.1186/bcr3161] [PMID: 22475046]

[130] Akli S, Keyomarsi K. Low-molecular-weight cyclin E: the missing link between biology and clinical outcome. Breast Cancer Res 2004; 6(5): 188-91.
[http://dx.doi.org/10.1186/bcr905] [PMID: 15318923]

[131] Cowling VH, Cole MD. E-cadherin repression contributes to c-Myc-induced epithelial cell transformation. Oncogene 2007; 26(24): 3582-6.
[http://dx.doi.org/10.1038/sj.onc.1210132] [PMID: 17146437]

[132] Oliveira AM, Ross JS, Fletcher JA. Tumor suppressor genes in breast cancer: the gatekeepers and the caretakers. Am J Clin Pathol 2005; 124 (Suppl.): S16-28.
[PMID: 16468415]

[133] Stefansson OA, Jonasson JG, Olafsdottir K, *et al.* CpG island hypermethylation of BRCA1 and loss of pRb as co-occurring events in basal/triple-negative breast cancer. Epigenetics 2011; 6(5): 638-49.

[http://dx.doi.org/10.4161/epi.6.5.15667] [PMID: 21593597]

[134] Varna M, Bousquet G, Plassa LF, Bertheau P, Janin A. TP53 status and response to treatment in breast cancers. J Biomed Biotechnol 2011; 2011: 284584.
[http://dx.doi.org/10.1155/2011/284584] [PMID: 21760703]

[135] Siewertsz van Reesema LL, Lee MP, Zheleva V, *et al.* RAS pathway biomarkers for breast cancer prognosis. Clin Lab Int 2016; 40: 18-23.
[PMID: 28579913]

[136] Arteaga CL, Sliwkowski MX, Osborne CK, Perez EA, Puglisi F, Gianni L. Treatment of HER2-positive breast cancer: current status and future perspectives. Nat Rev Clin Oncol 2011; 9(1): 16-32.
[http://dx.doi.org/10.1038/nrclinonc.2011.177] [PMID: 22124364]

[137] Zhao X, Xie T, Dai T, *et al.* CHP2 promotes cell proliferation in breast cancer *via* suppression of FOXO3a. Mol Cancer Res 2018; 16(10): 1512-22.
[http://dx.doi.org/10.1158/1541-7786.MCR-18-0157] [PMID: 29967111]

[138] Wang Y, Fan S, Lu J, *et al.* GLUL promotes cell proliferation in breast cancer. J Cell Biochem 2017; 118(8): 2018-25.
[http://dx.doi.org/10.1002/jcb.25775] [PMID: 27791265]

[139] Liu W, Zhang L, Jin Z, *et al.* TUFT1 is expressed in breast cancer and involved in cancer cell proliferation and survival. Oncotarget 2017; 8(43): 74962-74.
[http://dx.doi.org/10.18632/oncotarget.20472] [PMID: 29088838]

[140] Stender JD, Frasor J, Komm B, Chang KC, Kraus WL, Katzenellenbogen BS. Estrogen-regulated gene networks in human breast cancer cells: involvement of E2F1 in the regulation of cell proliferation. Mol Endocrinol 2007; 21(9): 2112-23.
[http://dx.doi.org/10.1210/me.2006-0474] [PMID: 17550982]

[141] Al-Dhaheri M, Wu J, Skliris GP, *et al.* CARM1 is an important determinant of ERα-dependent breast cancer cell differentiation and proliferation in breast cancer cells. Cancer Res 2011; 71(6): 2118-28.
[http://dx.doi.org/10.1158/0008-5472.CAN-10-2426] [PMID: 21282336]

[142] Gustafsson N, Zhao C, Gustafsson JA, Dahlman-Wright K. RBCK1 drives breast cancer cell proliferation by promoting transcription of estrogen receptor alpha and cyclin B1. Cancer Res 2010; 70(3): 1265-74.
[http://dx.doi.org/10.1158/0008-5472.CAN-09-2674] [PMID: 20103625]

[143] Song J, Ma Z, Hua Y, *et al.* Functional role of RRS1 in breast cancer cell proliferation. J Cell Mol Med 2018; 22(12): 6304-13.
[http://dx.doi.org/10.1111/jcmm.13922] [PMID: 30320499]

[144] O'Driscoll L, Clynes M. Biomarkers and multiple drug resistance in breast cancer. Curr Cancer Drug Targets 2006; 6(5): 365-84.
[http://dx.doi.org/10.2174/156800906777723958] [PMID: 16918307]

[145] Zhang Z, Lin G, Yan Y, *et al.* Transmembrane TNF-alpha promotes chemoresistance in breast cancer cells. Oncogene 2018; 37(25): 3456-70.
[http://dx.doi.org/10.1038/s41388-018-0221-4] [PMID: 29559745]

[146] Coates AS, Winer EP, Goldhirsch A, *et al.* Tailoring therapies--improving the management of early breast cancer: St Gallen International Expert Consensus on the Primary Therapy of Early Breast Cancer 2015. Ann Oncol 2015; 26(8): 1533-46.
[http://dx.doi.org/10.1093/annonc/mdv221] [PMID: 25939896]

[147] Rivera E, Gomez H. Chemotherapy resistance in metastatic breast cancer: the evolving role of ixabepilone. Breast Cancer Res 2010; 12(12) (Suppl. 2): S2.
[http://dx.doi.org/10.1186/bcr2573] [PMID: 21050423]

[148] von Minckwitz G, Untch M, Blohmer JU, *et al.* Definition and impact of pathologic complete response on prognosis after neoadjuvant chemotherapy in various intrinsic breast cancer subtypes. J Clin Oncol

2012; 30(15): 1796-804.
[http://dx.doi.org/10.1200/JCO.2011.38.8595] [PMID: 22508812]

[149] O'Reilly EA, Gubbins L, Sharma S, *et al.* The fate of chemoresistance in triple negative breast cancer (TNBC). BBA Clin 2015; 3: 257-75.
[http://dx.doi.org/10.1016/j.bbacli.2015.03.003] [PMID: 26676166]

[150] Kim C, Gao R, Sei E, *et al.* Chemoresistance evolution in triple-negative breast cancer delineated by single-cell sequencing. Cell 2018; 173(4): 879-893.e13.
[http://dx.doi.org/10.1016/j.cell.2018.03.041] [PMID: 29681456]

[151] Wu T, Wang X, Li J, *et al.* Identification of personalized chemoresistance genes in subtypes of basal-like breast cancer based on functional differences using pathway analysis. PLoS One 2015; 10(6): e0131183.
[http://dx.doi.org/10.1371/journal.pone.0131183] [PMID: 26126114]

[152] He DX, Xia YD, Gu XT, Jin J, Ma X. A transcription/translation-based gene signature predicts resistance to chemotherapy in breast cancer. J Pharm Biomed Anal 2015; 102: 500-8.
[http://dx.doi.org/10.1016/j.jpba.2014.10.018] [PMID: 25459950]

[153] He DX, Gu F, Gao F, *et al.* Genome-wide profiles of methylation, microRNAs, and gene expression in chemoresistant breast cancer. Sci Rep 2016; 6: 24706.
[http://dx.doi.org/10.1038/srep24706] [PMID: 27094684]

[154] Stebbing J, Shah K, Lit LC, *et al.* LMTK3 confers chemo-resistance in breast cancer. Oncogene 2018; 37(23): 3113-30.
[http://dx.doi.org/10.1038/s41388-018-0197-0] [PMID: 29540829]

[155] Insua-Rodríguez J, Pein M, Hongu T, *et al.* Stress signaling in breast cancer cells induces matrix components that promote chemoresistant metastasis. EMBO Mol Med 2018; 10(10): 10.
[http://dx.doi.org/10.15252/emmm.201809003] [PMID: 30190333]

[156] Ruiz de Garibay G, Mateo F, Stradella A, *et al.* Tumor xenograft modeling identifies an association between TCF4 loss and breast cancer chemoresistance. Dis Model Mech 2018; 11(5): 11.
[http://dx.doi.org/10.1242/dmm.032292] [PMID: 29666142]

[157] Naik A, Al-Yahyaee A, Abdullah N, *et al.* Neuropilin-1 promotes the oncogenic Tenascin-C/integrin β3 pathway and modulates chemoresistance in breast cancer cells. BMC Cancer 2018; 18(1): 533.
[http://dx.doi.org/10.1186/s12885-018-4446-y] [PMID: 29728077]

[158] El Ayachi I, Fatima I, Wend P, *et al.* The WNT10B network is associated with survival and metastases in chemoresistant triple-negative breast cancer. Cancer Res 2019; 79(5): 982-93.
[http://dx.doi.org/10.1158/0008-5472.CAN-18-1069] [PMID: 30563890]

[159] Zhao TT, Jin F, Li JG, *et al.* TRIM32 promotes proliferation and confers chemoresistance to breast cancer cells through activation of the NF-κB pathway. J Cancer 2018; 9(8): 1349-56.
[http://dx.doi.org/10.7150/jca.22390] [PMID: 29721043]

[160] Liu Y, Du F, Chen W, Yao M, Lv K, Fu P. EIF5A2 is a novel chemoresistance gene in breast cancer. Breast Cancer 2015; 22(6): 602-7.
[http://dx.doi.org/10.1007/s12282-014-0526-2] [PMID: 24638963]

[161] Calin GA, Croce CM. MicroRNA signatures in human cancers. Nat Rev Cancer 2006; 6(11): 857-66.
[http://dx.doi.org/10.1038/nrc1997] [PMID: 17060945]

[162] Wang YW, Zhang W, Ma R. Bioinformatic identification of chemoresistance-associated microRNAs in breast cancer based on microarray data. Oncol Rep 2018; 39(3): 1003-10.
[http://dx.doi.org/10.3892/or.2018.6205] [PMID: 29328395]

[163] Hu W, Tan C, He Y, Zhang G, Xu Y, Tang J. Functional miRNAs in breast cancer drug resistance. OncoTargets Ther 2018; 11: 1529-41.
[http://dx.doi.org/10.2147/OTT.S152462] [PMID: 29593419]

[164] Wang J, Yang M, Li Y, Han B. The role of MicroRNAs in the chemoresistance of breast cancer. Drug Dev Res 2015; 76(7): 368-74.
[http://dx.doi.org/10.1002/ddr.21275] [PMID: 26310899]

[165] Hanahan D, Weinberg RA. Hallmarks of cancer: the next generation. Cell 2011; 144(5): 646-74.
[http://dx.doi.org/10.1016/j.cell.2011.02.013] [PMID: 21376230]

[166] Coleman RE, Gregory W, Marshall H, Wilson C, Holen I. The metastatic microenvironment of breast cancer: clinical implications. Breast 2013; 22(22) (Suppl. 2): S50-6.
[http://dx.doi.org/10.1016/j.breast.2013.07.010] [PMID: 24074793]

[167] Tan W, Zhang W, Strasner A, *et al.* Tumour-infiltrating regulatory T cells stimulate mammary cancer metastasis through RANKL-RANK signalling. Nature 2011; 470(7335): 548-53.
[http://dx.doi.org/10.1038/nature09707] [PMID: 21326202]

[168] Fertig EJ, Lee E, Pandey NB, Popel AS. Analysis of gene expression of secreted factors associated with breast cancer metastases in breast cancer subtypes. Sci Rep 2015; 5: 12133.
[http://dx.doi.org/10.1038/srep12133] [PMID: 26173622]

[169] Tsuyada A, Chow A, Wu J, *et al.* CCL2 mediates cross-talk between cancer cells and stromal fibroblasts that regulates breast cancer stem cells. Cancer Res 2012; 72(11): 2768-79.
[http://dx.doi.org/10.1158/0008-5472.CAN-11-3567] [PMID: 22472119]

[170] Velaei K, Samadi N, Barazvan B, Soleimani Rad J. Tumor microenvironment-mediated chemoresistance in breast cancer. Breast 2016; 30: 92-100.
[http://dx.doi.org/10.1016/j.breast.2016.09.002] [PMID: 27668856]

[171] Zhang Z, Ni C, Chen W, *et al.* Expression of CXCR4 and breast cancer prognosis: a systematic review and meta-analysis. BMC Cancer 2014; 14: 49.
[http://dx.doi.org/10.1186/1471-2407-14-49] [PMID: 24475985]

[172] Lin L, Chen YS, Yao YD, *et al.* CCL18 from tumor-associated macrophages promotes angiogenesis in breast cancer. Oncotarget 2015; 6(33): 34758-73.
[http://dx.doi.org/10.18632/oncotarget.5325] [PMID: 26416449]

[173] Liu S, Ginestier C, Ou SJ, *et al.* Breast cancer stem cells are regulated by mesenchymal stem cells through cytokine networks. Cancer Res 2011; 71(2): 614-24.
[http://dx.doi.org/10.1158/0008-5472.CAN-10-0538] [PMID: 21224357]

[174] Daverey A, Drain AP, Kidambi S. Physical intimacy of breast cancer cells with mesenchymal stem cells elicits trastuzumab resistance through Src activation. Sci Rep 2015; 5: 13744.
[http://dx.doi.org/10.1038/srep13744] [PMID: 26345302]

[175] Folgueira MA, Maistro S, Katayama ML, *et al.* Markers of breast cancer stromal fibroblasts in the primary tumour site associated with lymph node metastasis: a systematic review including our case series. Biosci Rep 2013; 33(6): 33.
[http://dx.doi.org/10.1042/BSR20130060] [PMID: 24229053]

[176] Soysal SD, Tzankov A, Muenst SE. Role of the tumor microenvironment in breast cancer. Pathobiology 2015; 82(3-4): 142-52.
[http://dx.doi.org/10.1159/000430499] [PMID: 26330355]

[177] Busch S, Acar A, Magnusson Y, Gregersson P, Rydén L, Landberg G. TGF-beta receptor type-2 expression in cancer-associated fibroblasts regulates breast cancer cell growth and survival and is a prognostic marker in pre-menopausal breast cancer. Oncogene 2015; 34(1): 27-38.
[http://dx.doi.org/10.1038/onc.2013.527] [PMID: 24336330]

[178] Yasuda K, Torigoe T, Mariya T, *et al.* Fibroblasts induce expression of FGF4 in ovarian cancer stem-like cells/cancer-initiating cells and upregulate their tumor initiation capacity. Lab Invest 2014; 94(12): 1355-69.
[http://dx.doi.org/10.1038/labinvest.2014.122] [PMID: 25329002]

[179] Solinas G, Germano G, Mantovani A, Allavena P. Tumor-associated macrophages (TAM) as major players of the cancer-related inflammation. J Leukoc Biol 2009; 86(5): 1065-73.
[http://dx.doi.org/10.1189/jlb.0609385] [PMID: 19741157]

[180] Wolfe AR, Trenton NJ, Debeb BG, *et al.* Mesenchymal stem cells and macrophages interact through IL-6 to promote inflammatory breast cancer in pre-clinical models. Oncotarget 2016; 7(50): 82482-92.
[http://dx.doi.org/10.18632/oncotarget.12694] [PMID: 27756885]

[181] da Cunha A, Michelin MA, Murta EF. Pattern response of dendritic cells in the tumor microenvironment and breast cancer. World J Clin Oncol 2014; 5(3): 495-502.
[http://dx.doi.org/10.5306/wjco.v5.i3.495] [PMID: 25114862]

[182] Aspord C, Pedroza-Gonzalez A, Gallegos M, *et al.* Breast cancer instructs dendritic cells to prime interleukin 13-secreting CD4+ T cells that facilitate tumor development. J Exp Med 2007; 204(5): 1037-47.
[http://dx.doi.org/10.1084/jem.20061120] [PMID: 17438063]

[183] Mahmoud SM, Paish EC, Powe DG, *et al.* Tumor-infiltrating CD8+ lymphocytes predict clinical outcome in breast cancer. J Clin Oncol 2011; 29(15): 1949-55.
[http://dx.doi.org/10.1200/JCO.2010.30.5037] [PMID: 21483002]

[184] Ma XJ, Dahiya S, Richardson E, Erlander M, Sgroi DC. Gene expression profiling of the tumor microenvironment during breast cancer progression. Breast Cancer Res 2009; 11(1): R7.
[http://dx.doi.org/10.1186/bcr2222] [PMID: 19187537]

[185] Bainer R, Frankenberger C, Rabe D, An G, Gilad Y, Rosner MR. Gene expression in local stroma reflects breast tumor states and predicts patient outcome. Sci Rep 2016; 6: 39240.
[http://dx.doi.org/10.1038/srep39240] [PMID: 27982086]

[186] Natrajan R, Sailem H, Mardakheh FK, *et al.* Microenvironmental heterogeneity parallels breast cancer progression: a histology-genomic integration analysis. PLoS Med 2016; 13(2): e1001961.
[http://dx.doi.org/10.1371/journal.pmed.1001961] [PMID: 26881778]

[187] Wahl MC, Will CL, Lührmann R. The spliceosome: design principles of a dynamic RNP machine. Cell 2009; 136(4): 701-18.
[http://dx.doi.org/10.1016/j.cell.2009.02.009] [PMID: 19239890]

[188] Hegele A, Kamburov A, Grossmann A, *et al.* Dynamic protein-protein interaction wiring of the human spliceosome. Mol Cell 2012; 45(4): 567-80.
[http://dx.doi.org/10.1016/j.molcel.2011.12.034] [PMID: 22365833]

[189] Xiping Z, Qingshan W, Shuai Z, Hongjian Y, Xiaowen D. A summary of relationships between alternative splicing and breast cancer. Oncotarget 2017; 8(31): 51986-93.
[http://dx.doi.org/10.18632/oncotarget.17727] [PMID: 28881705]

[190] Anczuków O, Krainer AR. Splicing-factor alterations in cancers. RNA 2016; 22(9): 1285-301.
[http://dx.doi.org/10.1261/rna.057919.116] [PMID: 27530828]

[191] Gökmen-Polar Y, Neelamraju Y, Goswami CP, *et al.* Splicing factor *ESRP1* controls ER-positive breast cancer by altering metabolic pathways. EMBO Rep 2019; 20(2): 20.
[http://dx.doi.org/10.15252/embr.201846078] [PMID: 30665944]

[192] Hu Y, Sun Z, Deng J, *et al.* Splicing factor hnRNPA2B1 contributes to tumorigenic potential of breast cancer cells through STAT3 and ERK1/2 signaling pathway. Tumour Biol 2017; 39(3): 1010428317694318.
[http://dx.doi.org/10.1177/1010428317694318] [PMID: 28351333]

[193] Yang J, Bennett BD, Luo S, *et al.* LIN28A modulates splicing and gene expression programs in breast cancer cells. Mol Cell Biol 2015; 35(18): 3225-43.
[http://dx.doi.org/10.1128/MCB.00426-15] [PMID: 26149387]

[194] Ke H, Zhao L, Zhang H, *et al.* Loss of TDP43 inhibits progression of triple-negative breast cancer in

coordination with SRSF3. Proc Natl Acad Sci USA 2018; 115(15): E3426-35.
[http://dx.doi.org/10.1073/pnas.1714573115] [PMID: 29581274]

[195] Gökmen-Polar Y, Neelamraju Y, Goswami CP, *et al.* Expression levels of SF3B3 correlate with prognosis and endocrine resistance in estrogen receptor-positive breast cancer. Mod Pathol 2015; 28(5): 677-85.
[http://dx.doi.org/10.1038/modpathol.2014.146] [PMID: 25431237]

[196] Hatami R, Sieuwerts AM, Izadmehr S, *et al.* KLF6-SV1 drives breast cancer metastasis and is associated with poor survival. Sci Transl Med 2013; 5(169): 169ra12.
[http://dx.doi.org/10.1126/scitranslmed.3004688] [PMID: 23345610]

[197] Singh A, Karnoub AE, Palmby TR, Lengyel E, Sondek J, Der CJ. Rac1b, a tumor associated, constitutively active Rac1 splice variant, promotes cellular transformation. Oncogene 2004; 23(58): 9369-80.
[http://dx.doi.org/10.1038/sj.onc.1208182] [PMID: 15516977]

[198] Mavaddat N, Antoniou AC, Easton DF, Garcia-Closas M. Genetic susceptibility to breast cancer. Mol Oncol 2010; 4(3): 174-91.
[http://dx.doi.org/10.1016/j.molonc.2010.04.011] [PMID: 20542480]

[199] Siewit CL, Gengler B, Vegas E, Puckett R, Louie MC. Cadmium promotes breast cancer cell proliferation by potentiating the interaction between ERalpha and c-Jun. Mol Endocrinol 2010; 24(5): 981-92.
[http://dx.doi.org/10.1210/me.2009-0410] [PMID: 20219890]

[200] Snedeker SM. Pesticides and breast cancer risk: a review of DDT, DDE, and dieldrin. Environ Health Perspect 2001; 109(109) (Suppl. 1): 35-47.
[PMID: 11250804]

[201] Negri E, Bosetti C, Fattore E, La Vecchia C. Environmental exposure to polychlorinated biphenyls (PCBs) and breast cancer: a systematic review of the epidemiological evidence. Eur J Cancer Prev 2003; 12(6): 509-16.
[http://dx.doi.org/10.1097/00008469-200312000-00010] [PMID: 14639129]

[202] Mandal PK. Dioxin: a review of its environmental effects and its aryl hydrocarbon receptor biology. J Comp Physiol B 2005; 175(4): 221-30.
[http://dx.doi.org/10.1007/s00360-005-0483-3] [PMID: 15900503]

[203] Mukherjee S, Koner BC, Ray S, Ray A. Environmental contaminants in pathogenesis of breast cancer. Indian J Exp Biol 2006; 44(8): 597-617.
[PMID: 16924830]

[204] Jenkins S, Wang J, Eltoum I, Desmond R, Lamartiniere CA. Chronic oral exposure to bisphenol A results in a nonmonotonic dose response in mammary carcinogenesis and metastasis in MMTV-erbB2 mice. Environ Health Perspect 2011; 119(11): 1604-9.
[http://dx.doi.org/10.1289/ehp.1103850] [PMID: 21988766]

[205] Dairkee SH, Luciani-Torres MG, Moore DH, Goodson WH III. Bisphenol-A-induced inactivation of the p53 axis underlying deregulation of proliferation kinetics, and cell death in non-malignant human breast epithelial cells. Carcinogenesis 2013; 34(3): 703-12.
[http://dx.doi.org/10.1093/carcin/bgs379] [PMID: 23222814]

[206] Dhimolea E, Wadia PR, Murray TJ, *et al.* Prenatal exposure to BPA alters the epigenome of the rat mammary gland and increases the propensity to neoplastic development. PLoS One 2014; 9(7): e99800.
[http://dx.doi.org/10.1371/journal.pone.0099800] [PMID: 24988533]

[207] Doherty LF, Bromer JG, Zhou Y, Aldad TS, Taylor HS. *In utero* exposure to diethylstilbestrol (DES) or bisphenol-A (BPA) increases EZH2 expression in the mammary gland: an epigenetic mechanism linking endocrine disruptors to breast cancer. Horm Cancer 2010; 1(3): 146-55.
[http://dx.doi.org/10.1007/s12672-010-0015-9] [PMID: 21761357]

[208] Bhan A, Hussain I, Ansari KI, Bobzean SA, Perrotti LI, Mandal SS. Bisphenol-A and diethylstilbestrol exposure induces the expression of breast cancer associated long noncoding RNA HOTAIR *in vitro* and *in vivo.* J Steroid Biochem Mol Biol 2014; 141: 160-70.
[http://dx.doi.org/10.1016/j.jsbmb.2014.02.002] [PMID: 24533973]

[209] Charles AK, Darbre PD. Combinations of parabens at concentrations measured in human breast tissue can increase proliferation of MCF-7 human breast cancer cells. J Appl Toxicol 2013; 33(5): 390-8.
[http://dx.doi.org/10.1002/jat.2850] [PMID: 23364952]

[210] Darbre PD, Harvey PW. Parabens can enable hallmarks and characteristics of cancer in human breast epithelial cells: a review of the literature with reference to new exposure data and regulatory status. J Appl Toxicol 2014; 34(9): 925-38.
[http://dx.doi.org/10.1002/jat.3027] [PMID: 25047802]

[211] Rodgers KM, Udesky JO, Rudel RA, Brody JG. Environmental chemicals and breast cancer: An updated review of epidemiological literature informed by biological mechanisms. Environ Res 2018; 160: 152-82.
[http://dx.doi.org/10.1016/j.envres.2017.08.045] [PMID: 28987728]

[212] Yilmaz B, Ssempebwa J, Mackerer CR, Arcaro KF, Carpenter DO. Effects of polycyclic aromatic hydrocarbon-containing oil mixtures on generation of reactive oxygen species and cell viability in MCF-7 breast cancer cells. J Toxicol Environ Health A 2007; 70(13): 1108-15.
[http://dx.doi.org/10.1080/15287390701208545] [PMID: 17558805]

[213] Mordukhovich I, Rossner P Jr, Terry MB, *et al.* Associations between polycyclic aromatic hydrocarbon-related exposures and p53 mutations in breast tumors. Environ Health Perspect 2010; 118(4): 511-8.
[http://dx.doi.org/10.1289/ehp.0901233] [PMID: 20064791]

[214] Castillo-Sanchez R, Villegas-Comonfort S, Galindo-Hernandez O, Gomez R, Salazar EP. Benzo-[a]-pyrene induces FAK activation and cell migration in MDA-MB-231 breast cancer cells. Cell Biol Toxicol 2013; 29(4): 303-19.
[http://dx.doi.org/10.1007/s10565-013-9254-1] [PMID: 23955088]

[215] Chen Y, Huang C, Bai C, *et al.* Benzo[α]pyrene repressed DNA mismatch repair in human breast cancer cells. Toxicology 2013; 304: 167-72.
[http://dx.doi.org/10.1016/j.tox.2013.01.003] [PMID: 23313663]

[216] Byrne C, Divekar SD, Storchan GB, Parodi DA, Martin MB. Cadmium--a metallohormone? Toxicol Appl Pharmacol 2009; 238(3): 266-71.
[http://dx.doi.org/10.1016/j.taap.2009.03.025] [PMID: 19362102]

[217] Byrne C, Divekar SD, Storchan GB, Parodi DA, Martin MB. Metals and breast cancer. J Mammary Gland Biol Neoplasia 2013; 18(1): 63-73.
[http://dx.doi.org/10.1007/s10911-013-9273-9] [PMID: 23338949]

[218] Ebrahim AM, Eltayeb MA, Shaat MK, Mohmed NM, Eltayeb EA, Ahmed AY. Study of selected trace elements in cancerous and non-cancerous human breast tissues from Sudanese subjects using instrumental neutron activation analysis. Sci Total Environ 2007; 383(1-3): 52-8.
[http://dx.doi.org/10.1016/j.scitotenv.2007.04.047] [PMID: 17570463]

[219] Alatise OI, Schrauzer GN. Lead exposure: a contributing cause of the current breast cancer epidemic in Nigerian women. Biol Trace Elem Res 2010; 136(2): 127-39.
[http://dx.doi.org/10.1007/s12011-010-8608-2] [PMID: 20195925]

[220] Mulware SJ. The mammary gland carcinogens: the role of metal compounds and organic solvents. Int J Breast Cancer 2013; 2013: 640851.
[http://dx.doi.org/10.1155/2013/640851] [PMID: 23762568]

[221] Toriola AT, Colditz GA. Trends in breast cancer incidence and mortality in the United States: implications for prevention. Breast Cancer Res Treat 2013; 138(3): 665-73.

[http://dx.doi.org/10.1007/s10549-013-2500-7] [PMID: 23546552]

[222] Ferlay J, Soerjomataram I, Dikshit R, *et al.* Cancer incidence and mortality worldwide: sources, methods and major patterns in GLOBOCAN 2012. Int J Cancer 2015; 136(5): E359-86.
[http://dx.doi.org/10.1002/ijc.29210] [PMID: 25220842]

[223] Mukherjee S. The Emperor of All Maladies: A Biography of Cancer 2010.
Scribner publication New York. [ISBN: 978-1-4391-0795-9]

[224] Jiang YZ, Ma D, Suo C, *et al.* Genomic and transcriptomic landscape of triple-negative breast cancers: subtypes and treatment strategies. Cancer Cell 2019; 35(428-440): e425.

[225] Lo PK, Sukumar S. Epigenomics and breast cancer. Pharmacogenomics 2008; 9(12): 1879-902.
[http://dx.doi.org/10.2217/14622416.9.12.1879] [PMID: 19072646]

[226] Lawrence RT, Perez EM, Hernández D, *et al.* The proteomic landscape of triple-negative breast cancer. Cell Rep 2015; 11(6): 990.
[http://dx.doi.org/10.1016/j.celrep.2015.04.059] [PMID: 28843283]

[227] Dai C, Arceo J, Arnold J, *et al.* Metabolomics of oncogene-specific metabolic reprogramming during breast cancer. Cancer Metab 2018; 6: 5.
[http://dx.doi.org/10.1186/s40170-018-0175-6] [PMID: 29619217]

CHAPTER 7

Perspectives of Deregulated Metabolism in Breast Cancer

Shankar Suman[*]

Cancer Comprehensive Centre, The Ohio State University, West 12th Avenue, Columbus 43210, Ohio, USA

Abstract: Cancer cells devise different mechanisms to undergo aberrant cell division. Dysregulated signaling pathways and metabolic reprogramming are the two key mechanisms leading to cancer development. The role of metabolic dysregulation has been well known in cell proliferation, metastasis, and resistance to therapy, eventually leading to tumor progression. The dysregulation of enzyme activity and biochemical pathways have emerged as major factors in the metabolic reprogramming of breast cancer. The abnormal changes in the level of metabolites are mechanistically associated with the metabolism of cancer. Quantitative research studies have provided a list of metabolic biomarkers, which have a promising role in the early detection of breast cancer as well as in its therapy. Many of the current research studies are directed towards understanding the intricacies of metabolism in cancer cell proliferation. This chapter gives an overview of breast cancer metabolism with updated information and describes how deregulated metabolism plays a key role in the oncogenic cascade leading to the neoplastic transformation of cells.

Keywords: Amino acid, Cancer, Carbohydrate, Glycolytic pathways, Immunometabolism, Lipid, Metabolism, TCA cycle.

INTRODUCTION

Breast cancer (BC) is a major health concern all around the world [1]. Cancer is well known to be caused by abnormal cells that possess unregulated proliferative potential. Such abnormalities are associated with deregulated metabolism in cancer cells. The alterations of metabolic pathways in cancer support their atypical growth [2, 3]. Many cancers, including BC, are considered lifestyle-related diseases, and great emphasis has been laid on understanding the role of lifestyle and environmental factors in cancer development. Cell metabolism and signaling pathways in BC are complicated, but their knowledge helps understand

---

[*] **Correspondence Shankar Suman:** Cancer Comprehensive Centre, West 12th Avenue, The Ohio State University, Columbus, OH-43210, Department of Biochemistry and Immunology, Meharry Medical College, Dr. D.B. Todd Jr Blvd. Nashville, TN-37209, Ohio, USA; E-mail: shankarsuman.suman@gmail.com

the interactions of genes with the environment. Studies show that nutrient uptake and change in nutrient absorption play an important role in BC metabolism. The role of trace metals and enzymatic functions are also gaining more importance, and their roles are emerging in current scientific research. Recent studies have revealed the impact of altered metabolism in cancer progression. It has been also shown that diet restriction could influence cancer progression, and there is a positive effect of glucose restriction on controlling cancer [4]. A plethora of evidence from the metabolomics research has shown that several metabolites can potentially act as diagnostic, prognostic, and therapeutic biomarkers in BC. The discovery of metabolic biomarkers is rising with the advancement in sophisticated technologies in metabolomics research due to increased sensitivity of detecting novel metabolites using newer techniques. The role of deregulated metabolites is also deciphered in the metabolism of cancer, which assist in the new therapeutic developments of BC.

Studies show that the alteration of several metabolic pathways in cancer has a pivotal role in the carcinogenesis; specifically, the changes of glycolytic flux in the cancer are one of the major alterations. In particular, aerobic glycolysis is more prevalent in cancer cells rather than normal cells. The altered glycolytic process in cancer is known to induce acidity (lowering pH) in the tumor mass and trigger oncogenic signaling pathways [5]. Otto Warburg's hypothesis is the most simplified in the glycolytic pathway of cancer. The hypothesis demonstrates that cancer cells undergo glycolysis at a higher rate, even in the presence of oxygen with a lowered mitochondria-mediated oxidation process [6]. The hypothesis can also elucidate the differences in cellular metabolism in cancer and normal cells. The clinical tumor imaging of primary and metastatic cancers can also corroborate the altered metabolic pathways and accept the Warburg hypothesis universally [7]. Cancer cells sustain a high rate of proliferation through metabolic alterations, for example, glucose and glutamine uptake in cancer cells is altered as compared to normal cells, which is considered to be one of the hallmarks of cancer [8]. Researchers also believe that the persistent glucose to lactate metabolism even in the presence of sufficient oxygen confers an adaptation to hypoxic conditions in early malignant lesions. The upregulated glycolysis may lead to form acidic microenvironment; thereby, it induces resistant cell phenotypes in cancer against acidosis [5]. Furthermore, these mechanisms enable cancer progression. In cancer cells, few reasons are understood, which increase the aerobic glycolysis. Mitochondrial dysfunction is one of them. The high glycolytic process in cancer leads to the accumulation of phospho-metabolites, which can further lead to the activation of nucleic acid and lipid biosynthesis *via* the pentose phosphate pathway [9]. The high glycolytic activity also produces lactate, which is exported in the extracellular microenvironment to promote tumor aggressiveness. Tumor cells also overexpress monocarboxylate transport (MCTs) and Na^+/H^+ exchanger to remove large H^+ ions [10]. In general, cancer cell aggressiveness is either directly or indirectly associated with glycolytic pathways. Studies have shown the impact of changes in the expressions of genes by the transcriptional regulation during the initiation and progression of carcinogenesis in BC. Hormonal defects also control BC progression by involving several steroid-responsive molecules. The changes in hormonal responsiveness show altered transcriptional activation by various protein kinases. There are several hormonal receptors deregulated in BC.Among them, the estrogen receptor (ER), progesterone receptor (PR) and human epidermal receptor 2 (HER2) are commonly talked about in the clinical setting. To develop a better diagnostic, prognostic, and therapeutic approach, BCs can be classified into different subtypes based on the expression patterns of these receptors. These BC subtypes also possess a unique set of protein signatures in the patient's samples [11]. For the treatment of a certain type of BC, antagonists to the receptors mentioned above are being currently used in the clinic as hormonal therapy. However, there is also one of the BC subtypes, which does not respond to any nuclear receptor (NR) antagonist due to lack of ER, PR, and HERexpressions and thus known as triple-negative BC. Triple-negative BC is highly aggressive among all other BC subtypes. One of the causes of aggressiveness of this subtype is because of adaptive metabolic pathways. Moreover, the metabolic pathways in all the hormonal BC subtypes are not common, and many more discoveries have to be made to classify BC based on metabolic differences. The metabolism in various BC subtypes mediates different oncogenic pathways associated with transcriptional regulators,most commonly through the kinase-dependent signalling pathway. Studies reveal that several unique metabolites act as mediators of oncogenic pathways. The activation of many oncogenic signalling is mediated through nuclear receptors and transcriptional co-regulators. Researchers have given more emphasis on linking the intricacy of cellular signaling pathways and epigenetics in cancer cell metabolism. Nowadays, there is a growing interest in studying the BC stem cells (present as a rare population in BC tumor mass) [12]. These cells have the ability to self-renew and differentiate into the different phenotypes;and pose a challenge in the current therapeutic approach [13]. This hypothesis is supported by the results of multiple studies and reveal the fact that BC stem cells are transformed into a new state and sustain prolonged stress in tumor microenvironment even during therapy. These cells have shown unique metabolic features and are burning topics in the ongoing research [14]. It has been anticipated that anew line of therapy can be developed that can target BC stem cells by disrupting metabolic pathways. Furthermore, BC stage progression can also be predicted through changes in the metabolic pathways, and our study in the past has revealed the changes in metabolic signature with BC stage progression [15]. In general, the dysregulated metabolic activities in BC assist in acquiring drug resistance and multiple cellular phenotypes through different energy-related pathways. This chapter will confer all details of altered metabolism associated with molecular signaling, including immunological prospects. The altered energy associated metabolism in BC has been discussed in detailin this chapter,particularly the role of carbohydrate, fatty acid, amino acid,and nucleotide metabolism and how metabolic restriction can be useful in BC therapy and ongoing research.In addition,it has been our effort to bring together different pieces of data covering the metabolic reprogramming of BC, in this chapter.

GENOMIC ALTERATIONS IN METABOLIC REPROGRAMMING OF BC

Metabolic reprogramming is one of the common features of BC. The changes in metabolic pathways in BC are directly controlled by certain genes, which regulate carbohydrate, fatty, amino acid, and nucleotide metabolism. These genes are muted and/or overexpressed among BC patients. In clinical settings, several mutant genes are reported in even germline cells. It has also been well known that the immortal and rapidly proliferating cancer cells have high-energy requirements. Cancer cells grow in the hypoxic conditions and have to rely more on the non-oxidative source such as glycolysis for energy. Furthermore, the dividing cells acquire a high rate of lipogenesis, particularly for membrane biosynthesis. Therefore, the expression of several genes is upregulated in cancer, especially those playing a role in lipogenesis. Cancer cells continuously acquire mutations in cancer microenvironment to sustain high oxidative stress and hypoxic conditions. There quite a lot of data showing that the cancer cells protect themselves from the cytotoxicity of the drug through acquired mutations and metabolic changes and further develop drug-resistant clones against a variety of chemotherapeutic drugs. The gain in function mutation in genes (oncogene) and loss of function mutation in tumor suppressor genes are major factors in the dysregulation of the cell cycle in cancer cells. Changes in gene regulation in cancer cells also allow reprogramming in cancer cell homeostasis.

Epigenetic Modifications

Epigenetic modifications may alter many enzymatic functions and metabolic pathways in cancer. The epigenetic modification affects gene expression level, which modulates the process of BC progression and metastasis. Epigenetic modification corresponds to the changes in the level of acetylation, methylation, and other modifications associated with DNA and histone proteins, which can alter the expression of genes. There are several studies available, showing that epigenetic modifications regulate gluconeogenesis, amino acid, fatty acid, and nucleic acid associated metabolic pathways in proliferating tumor cells [16]. The methylation of DNA and histones is one of the important epigenetic modifications, which is carried out by DNA-methyl transferases (DNMT) and histone methyltransferases (HMT). These enzymes transfer the methyl group mostly from S-adenosyl methionine (SAM) or folate to DNA or Histone. Studies show that low folate levels in the diet can cause hypomethylation, which is a major risk factor for BC, particularly in postmenopausal women [17, 18]. Histone deacetylase is a very important enzyme for epigenetic modification. Sirtuin family of genes (SIRT) is one of the histone deacetylases that have shown to destabilize HIF-1α and affect many genes of the glycolytic pathway. Several oncogenes are hypomethylated, and several tumor suppressor genes are hyper-methylated in BC. These genes regulate DNA repair mechanism, chronic inflammation, and other deregulations *via* the complicated molecular signaling and metabolic pathways. In glycolysis, the epigenetic modification of promoters of hexokinase, fructose 1,6-bisphosphatase (FBP), Pyruvate kinase M2 isoform can affect glucose metabolism [19]. Studies have shown that hypermethylation of the FBP1 promoter activates the gene expression and increases glycolytic pathways in BC [20]. Moreover, promoter hypo-methylation can also silence FBP expression. The pyruvate kinase activity of M2 isoform (PKM2) is reduced in cancer due to hyper-acetylation, which leads to increase biosynthesis of macromolecules (Nucleic acids, lipids, and amino acids) required for cancer cells [21]. The hypo-methylation PKM2 promoters can also regulate the function and thereby affect glycolysis. PKM2 is also involved in the regulation of anabolic processes by changing the glycolytic flux into the pentose phosphate pathways and serine biosynthetic pathways [22]. Several modifications in chromatin (DNA and histones) are directly correlated with changes in metabolic pathways [23]. These interactions are highly dynamic changes with physiological concentrations of metabolites [24]. In the network of biochemical pathways, NAD^+, $NADH^+$, acetyl coenzyme A, alpha-ketoglutarate, *S*-adenosylhomocysteine (SAH), fumarate, lactate, glutamate and many more are among those metabolites, which bear epigenetic modification in cancer. Acetyl Coenzyme A synthase is overexpressed in BC and also known to take part in the histone acetylation and take part in epigenetic modification [25].

Oncogenic Regulators

Breast cancer is a heterogeneous and complex disease. BC cells orchestrate transformed gene expression patterns, controlled by various regulators and co-regulators. There are several regulators and co-regulators of transcriptional activities in BC studied so far, which cross-talks in cell signaling pathways and the metabolism of cancer cells. Among the hormone-dependent BC, mutations in transcriptional regulators transform normal cells by inducing oncogenic pathways. The major regulators are nuclear receptors. Among them, estrogen receptor and progesterone receptors are key receptors in BC. However, there are several other nuclear receptors also known to be involved in the BC progression, for example, receptors of steroid hormone, particularly corticosteroids and androgens, fatty acids, vitamins (A & D), *etc.*, [26]. Nuclear receptors are often associated with epidermal growth factor signaling and activate downstream signaling kinases. These kinases may also communicate in metabolic deregulation in BC. Interestingly, the different specific BC subtypes have different sets of kinases activation, more specifically, because of different mutations carried in kinases. Studies have shown that in HER2+ BC, p53 and myc mutations are very common, and in luminal BC cases, ~ 50% of genes of PI3K/AKT/mTOR pathways are mutated [27 - 29]. It has also been investigated that the metabolic enzymes associated with various biochemical pathways are modulated in the different BC subtypes or hormone-dependent BC. For instance, the mutation of enzymes of glycolysis and pentose phosphate pathways are mutated in ER- BC subtypes [30]. Altered levels of some of the metabolites may lay the foundation for epigenetic changes in the regulation of the metabolic gene in cancer. For example, mutations in isocitrate dehydrogenase alter its function, and then it cannot decarboxylase α-ketoglutarate to isocitrate, but it increases 2-hydroxyglutarate, which acts as an antagonist of α-ketoglutarate dependent dioxygenases [31]. Furthermore, the antagonist behavior of 2-hydroxyglutarate against dioxygenases can change the DNA/Histone methylation patterns in cancer. Apart from 2-hydroxyglutarate, succinate, and fumarate also act as antagonists against α ketoglutarate dependent dioxygenases [32].

Steroid receptor coactivator-3(SRC3) is an oncogenic coregulatory agent of BC, which is regulated by phosphofructokinase and FBP, and SRC activation is critical in aggressive BC [33]. The overexpression of SRC 3 has also been reported to be associated with resistance of tamoxifen/aromatase inhibitor [34]. Phosphofructokinase is a key enzyme to increase fructose bisphosphate level, which is elevated in BC, and it plays a key role in BC associated metabolism [35]. Furthermore, SRC mediates the binding of the ATF4 transcription factor to increase purine synthesis in BC [33]. In the *in vitro* study on the BC model, it has been revealed that phosphoglycerate mutase 1 (PGAM1) is modulated, which can be altered interactions with cytoskeleton [50].

PGAM1 interacts with α-smooth muscle actin and actin filament to maintain integrity. PGAM1 converts 3- phosphoglycerate to 2-phosphoglycerate in the glycolytic pathway. Study shows that knockdown of PGAM1 decreases BC metastasis *in vivo* study [50]. There are several reports available, describing the role of responsive genes in deregulated metabolism in BC, given above in Table **1**.

Table 1. Role of differential expression of genes in BC.

Genes/Enzymes	Role in breast cancer	References
Glucose-6-phosphate dehydrogenase (G6PD)	HER2 + inflammatory early BC	[36]
Glucose phosphate isomerase (PGI)	Epithelial-mesenchymal transition regulation	[37]
Acetyl-CoA carboxylase (ACC1)	Controls BC metastasis and Recurrence	[38]
Fatty acid synthase(FASN)	Estrogen receptor-α signalling in BC	[39]
Thymidylate synthase (TYMS)	Maintains the de-differentiated state of triple-negative BC	[40]
Cysteine dioxygenase type 1 (CDO1) and homeobox only protein homeobox (HOPX)	Clinical potential as prognostic biomarkers in BC	[41]
Sterol regulatory element-binding protein 1 (SREBP1)	Regulate fatty acid synthesis	[42]
Cbp/p300-interacting transactivator, with Glu/Asp-rich carboxy-terminal domain, 2 (CITED 2)	Augment BC	[43]
Phosphofructokinase 1 (PFK1)	PFK1 isoenzyme patterns and glycolytic efficiency	[44]
Phosphoglycerate mutase (PGM)	Increased activity in BC	[45]
Pyruvate kinase (PKM1 and PKM2)	Increased in cancer-associated fibroblasts and tumor growth	[46]
Pyruvate kinase muscle isozyme M2 (PKM2)	Glucose metabolism through let-7--5p/Stat3/hnRNP-A1 feedback loop in BC	[47]
Fatty acid synthase (FASN)	Regulates estrogen receptor-α signalling	[39]
Stearoyl-coa desaturase (SCD)-1, 5	Progression, migration and a novel pro-cell survival in BC	[48]
glucose-6-phosphate dehydrogenase (G6PDH) and 6-phosphogluconolactonase (6PGL)	Differentially expressed in BC subtypes and highly expressed in HER-2 subtype.	[30]
Fatty acid-binding protein 4 (FABP4)	Decreased survival in triple-negative BC	[49]
Phosphoglycerate mutase 1 (PGAM1)	Increase metastasis	[50]

CARBOHYDRATE METABOLISM

Carbohydrate breaks down into glucose in the digestion process, which turns into a key molecule involved in the overall metabolic process in the cell. There is a central process involved in the glucose metabolism named as glycolysis. Besides, glucose concentration can be increased in blood from non-carbohydrate sources also through gluconeogenesis. During the physiological digestion of dietary nutrients, studies suggest that delayed absorption of carbohydrates can cause several types of metabolic disorders including cancer [51]. Undigested carbohydrates in the intestine are further fermented by microbiota in the colon and lead to short-chain fatty acids, SCFA (acetic, butyric, and propionic acid) production [52]. Some specific SCFA has very high nutritional values in lowering disease risks [52]. Recent investigations have also drawn much more attention towards the strategy of lowing down the digestion of carbohydrates to increase fermentation, which has the potency to decrease the risk for chronic diseases like cancer [51]. Prebiotics, like inulin and oligofructose, can promote specific bacteria such as bifidobacteria, lactobacillus, *etc.*, which can play an important role in impeding disease risks [53]. Current research studies emphasize that food with low glycaemic index (GI) (a quantitative value for the classification of carbohydrate foods based on its absorption in the intestine) can prevent the occurrence of diabetes, cardiovascular disease, and many types of cancers [54, 55]. Deregulation of carbohydrate metabolism has been shown to have an important link to cancer progression [3]. Several research articles have also revealed the link of sugar or sucrose, milk products, and lactose in cancer and delineated the impact of changing the glycaemic index with many cancers [56 - 58]. There are specific cases of carbohydrate related metabolic syndrome like hyperinsulinemia that show that the stimulation of insulin growth factor 1 is associated with both deregulated cell proliferation and cell death mechanisms [59]. Numerous studies have been carried out which give evidence of an altered carbohydrate related metabolic pathways in cancer [2, 3]. The mechanism of the deregulated process has been studied in the clinical and biological models, indicating a complex network of carbohydrate associated metabolic pathways in the carcinogenesis steps carrying a variety of molecular-level changes. It has been understood since the early days that weight loss in cancer patients is associated with abnormalities in carbohydrate metabolism. Subsequent studies deciphered that cancer therapeutic agents could modulate glucose metabolism in cancer is reviewed by Jang *et al.,* [60]. In 1921, Braunstein observed that those diabetic patients who develop cancer in their lifetime were found to have reduced glucose levels in urine. Furthermore, they also reported that cancer cells have a higher consumption of glucose as compared to liver and muscles[4]. H. G. Crabtree explained the consumption of carbohydrates by tumor cells in 1929 [61]. His observation is highly relevant in explaining glucose metabolism in cancer. According to Crabtree's observation, normal cells can increase the rate of respiration in the presence of glucose. However, in cancer, the presence of glucose inhibits oxygen uptake in tumor cells. This effect was later known as Crabtree effect. Moreover, the investigations also showed that, this effect is not only specific to cancer, but this effect has also been observed in fast dividing cells such as thymocytes, spermatozoa, and embryonic stem cells. In the later years of studies, the accumulation of lactate was observed in the tumor mass, an essential component for the cancer progression [62]. Otto Warburg demonstrated a high rate of glycolysis and high amounts of glucose to lactate conversion even under aerobic conditions in tumor tissues, which is different from normal cells [63]. However, in contrast to it, the Pasteur effect explains the decrease in the rate of glucose uptake and lactate formation in the absence of oxygen in normal cells [64]. Both of these explanations illustrate the important differences between normal and cancer cells. The glycolysis process uses glucose to yield two molecules of pyruvate, ATP and NADPH. In normoxic conditions, healthy cells generate pyruvate, which is oxidized to acetyl coenzyme A, and used in the tricarboxylic acid cycle or Kreb's cycle. Complete oxidation of glucose *via* glycolysis and Kreb's cycle generates ~32 ATP. However, in the case of insufficient oxygen, lactate is produced by lactate dehydrogenase A (LDHA) which is upregulated in cancer cells.. Pentose phosphate pathway, required for nucleotide precursor and NADPH production is another catabolic process which is upregulated in the BC. The enzyme associated with this pathway is modulated in BC (Fig. **1**). For example, Glucose-6-phosphate dehydrogenase-6-phosphoglu-conolactonase (G6PDH) and 6-phosphogluconolactonase (6PGL) are modulated in BC subtypes [30].

LIPID METABOLISM IN BC

Lipid metabolism is a crucial part of cancer progression as cancer cells need a high content of lipid to increase cell proliferation. Lipogenesis in BC is increased to maintain the anabolic process in BC. In cancer, several metabolic pathways associated with lipogenesis are upregulated since lipid building blocks are in increased demand in cancer. In the *de novo* lipid synthesis, acetyl coenzyme A (CoA), ribose 5- phosphate, and NADH requirement are increased. In the process, citrate is catabolized to acetyl CoA through an enzyme called ATP citrate lyase (ACLY) [65]. In BC, ACLY is upregulated to meet the demand of *de novo* lipogenesis [66]. Cancer cells utilize more amount of glucose and glutamine in the metabolic process and, as discussed in the previous sections.

The metabolic process in BC increases the level of acetyl CoA by utilizing a high amount of glucose. The increased acetyl CoA can regulate histone acetylation and alter the expressions of oncogenes and prepare for metabolic reprogramming [67]. It has been investigated that in mammary epithelial cells, phosphoACLY can be increased by Akt, which recruits BRCA1 in DNA double-strand break repair [68]. Serum lipids and lipoproteins are associated with BC risk. The reduction of Non-HDL-C or elevation in HDL-C is also important in BC risk assessment apart from cardiac risk investigation [69]. In BC, mitochondrial isocitrate dehydrogenase (IDH) is mutated [70]. The mutations in isocitrate dehydrogenase 1 (IDH1) and IDH2 fail to catalyze alpha KG to isocitrate but help in increasing the levels of 2 hydroxyglutarate, which is in carcinogenesis [71]. The levels of sphingolipids particularly glycosphingolipids, are increased and correlated with tumor progression. Glycosphingolipids like SSEA3/SSEA4/Globo-H make a complex with FAK/CAV1/AKT/RIP to participate in tumor progression [72]. The free fatty acid is correlated with the aggressiveness of ER +BC cells as it activates ER and mTOR pathways. It is interesting to look at the impact of blocking these pathways, particularly in ER+BC in postmenopausal women [73]. In the hypoxic microenvironment, the production of acetyl CoA is increased, which can relate to the increased biogenesis process in BC [74]. BC cells utilize acetate to convert into acetyl CoA by acetyl CoA synthase. Acetyl CoA takes part in fatty acid synthesis, which is increased in BC. Studies reveal that there is an increased expression of multiple genes regulating lipogenesis in BC. The increased production of acetyl CoA plays multiple roles in BC including cell transformation, migration, *etc.*

In recent years, fatty acid synthase (FASN), a part of the lipogenesis process, has emerged as a major player in the BC progression. It is currently being investigated as a therapeutic target for BC [75]. A recent study also shows that FASN crosstalk with Osteoprotegerin (OPG), COX2 in the carcinogenesis event [76]. The increased expression of (acyl-CoA oxidase) ACOX1 and FASN have shown in the brain metastasis [77]. In cancer cells, fatty acid synthesis and oxidation play a pivotal role in cellular proliferation. An altered lipid-metabolism takes part in metastatic cancer, as well. An investigative study on lipid biosynthesis showed that the degradation of the unused part of acetyl CoA by mitochondria leads to the transfer of reducing potential from the cytoplasm to mitochondria [78]. Several genes are responsible for lipid metabolism; among them, N-myc downstream-regulated gene (NDRG1) is critically involved in BC lipid metabolism. It has also been reported that NDRG1 is associated with poor prognosis in BC patients [79]. It has been shown that fatty acid synthesis is increased in the cytoplasm, and long-chain fatty acid plays a pivotal role in BC. Elongation of very-long-chain fatty acids protein (ELOVL) is different in triple-negative as compared to ER-positive, PR-positive, HER2-negative BC patients [80].

AMINO ACID METABOLISM

Several studies have revealed that glucose is not the only source of cancer cell proliferation, but amino acid is a principal source of cancer metabolism also. Cancer cells are broadly dependent upon amino acid metabolism in the phase of initiation, progression, and metastasis. The metabolic reprogramming in BC is highly established on amino acid metabolism. The most common set of amino acids in breast carcinogenesis reported so far are glutamine, serine, glycine, *etc.* We have investigated that there are several amino acids altered in the stage progression in BC [15]. Glutamine is one of the key metabolic sources of energy for the growth of cancer cells. It is utilized as a source for carbon or nitrogen consumptions. Glutaminolysis is a key process regulating function in cancer cells metabolism. The presence of glutamine is increased in blood circulation during cancer progression. Glutamine can convert to α-Ketoglutarate through glutamate dehydrogenase and take part in the citric acid cycle. Glutaminase, an enzyme that converts glutamine to glutamate, is increased in BC. Thus, glutamine enters into cells and converts into glutamate and increase glutamate level in the cytoplasm. A study explains that blocking the glutaminase can inhibit the proliferation of BC cells [81]. Serine is also another important amino acid for cancer. Cancer cells depend on the extracellular source for serine, and it can also increase serine biosynthesis pathways to fulfill the serine demands. Serine supports in cancer cells for the transport system, nucleotide, and folate metabolism, and redox homeostasis [82]. Phosphoglycerate dehydrogenase (PHGDH), an enzyme, plays a key role in 3-phosphoglycerate into 3-phosphohydroxypyruvate transition in L-serine biosynthetic pathways. PHGDH is overexpressed in BC, particularly triple-negative BC [83]. There are several enzymes (PGDH, PSP, and SHMT) responsible for serine biosynthesis that are overexpressed in ER+ BC as compared to ER- BC [84]. Another amino acid, methionine derivatives S-adenosyl methionine is one of the methyl donors in methylation, can execute epigenetic modification, and alter transcriptome to govern cancer-related pathways [85]. In BC, amino acid metabolisms are diversified in different BC subtypes. MYC genes are amplified in BC that can increase the uptake of glutamine in BC cells more specifically [86]. Studies revealed that MYC increases the one-carbon metabolism in serine, glycine, tryptophan and it also upregulates uptake of amino acids in BC cells [87] which can lead to affect TCA cycle.

Further, ASCT2/SLC1A5 mediated transport is also increased in BC, which helps to increase glutamine transport [88, 89]. Unfortunately, the inhibitor against the transporter reduces in triple-negative BC only as compared to other luminal subtypes [89]. An interesting study has revealed that an altered amino acid and lipid metabolism shifts the tumor cells opposite to Warburg effect [90]. In cancer cells, the conversion of serine to glycine and *vice versa* is very common due to one-carbon metabolism in cancer. The one-carbon unit limits the biosynthesis of nucleotides. In the *de-novo* nucleotide synthesis process, one carbon unit *via* folate exchanges conversion of serine to glycine. In the purine biosynthesis conversion of precursor glycinamide ribonucleotide (GAR) to AMP or GMP acquire additional carbon from folate [91]. Hence, the changes in the serine to glycine metabolism can enhance the proliferation of cancer cells.

NUCLEOTIDE METABOLISM IN BC

Nucleotides are essentially an important part of the cells. The imbalance of nucleotides leads to a diverse category of diseases, including BC. A nucleotide is a monomeric unit of nucleic acid, made of a nitrogenous base, sugar, and phosphate. Nitrogenous bases are purine (adenine and guanine) and pyrimidine (cytosine, thiamine, and uracil). Nucleic acid, deoxyribose, or nucleic ribose acid are life forms in the universe. The roles of genes and epigenetics regulation of cells through metabolic pathways have already been discussed in the previous paragraphs. Nucleoside triphosphate (ATP, CTP, GTP, UTP) are understood to be a currency of energy in the life forms and take part in all source of metabolism in cells. Apart from these, nucleotides essentially play a role in cell signaling. Cyclic AMP, cyclic GMP and many of the cofactors are derived from nucleotides, for example, coenzyme A, FAD, FMN, and NAD, *etc.*, are among key molecules involved in the molecular signaling and metabolic pathways of the cell. It has a very crucial role in cancer, as well. The nucleotides are biosynthesized through *de novo* and salvage pathways in cells. Folate or vitamin B9 is an important source of nucleotide synthesis. Cancer cells highly express folate receptors, which may be associated with high nucleotide demands in cancer cells. Methylenetetrahydrofolate dehydrogenase/cyclohydrolase (MTHFD) is a crucial enzyme, taking part in folate metabolism. Study shows that MTHFD2 is overexpressed in cancer, linked with aggressiveness and poor survival of BC [92, 93]. Literature shows that an imbalance of dNTP levels exists in the BC, which is probably due to mutagenic BC cells regulated by oncogenic signaling like mTOR, cMyc, p53, *etc.* It encompasses the imbalance of dNTP metabolism in BC. Several chemotherapeutic drugs targeted to control the dNTP biosynthesis process in cancer [94]. In the cancer cell proliferation, *de novo* purine biosynthesis and purine metabolism are impaired. During *de novo* purine biosynthesis in various steps, six enzymes are required to convert phosphoribosyl pyrophosphate to inosine 5'-monophosphate. The cluster of all these enzymes around mitochondria/microtubules forms a purinosome assisted in nucleotide synthesis in cancer. The formation of the purinosome is regulated by mTOR [95]. On the other hand, *de novo* pyrimidine biosynthesis is also increased in BC [96]. In the investigation, the *de novo* pyrimidine biosynthesis in MCF7 BC cells is increased by a 4.4-fold change compared to control MCF10A breast cells. Three enzymes, carbamoyl-phosphate synthetase 2, aspartate transcarbamylase, and dihydroorotase (CAD), are involved in the pyrimidine biosynthesis in 6-steps. In MCF- 7 cells, intracellular CAD is increased to 3.5-4 folds to enhance the pyrimidine biosynthesis pathway. The enhanced CAD level in BC cells is a result of increased MAP kinase activity [96]. Folate has a protective effect on ER+ PR+ and HER2- BC subtypes; however, thiamine has a protective effect in HER2+ BC subtypes [97].

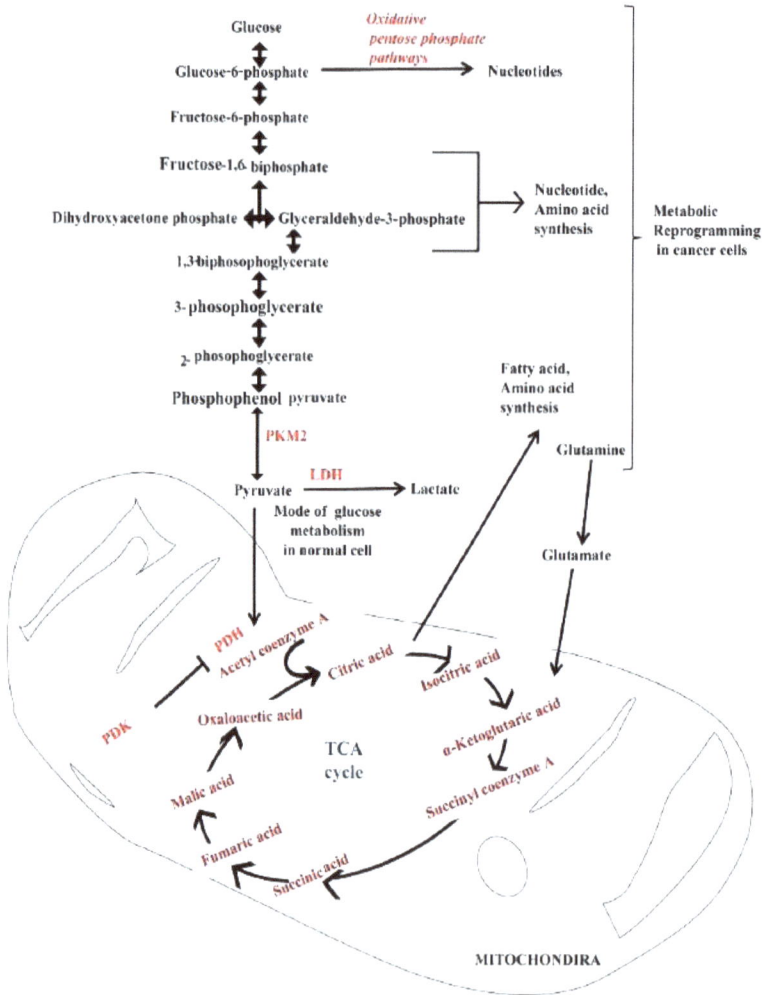

Fig. (1). Summary of metabolic pathways for glucose metabolism in normal and cancer cells; Cancer cells proliferate in the presence of an upregulated glucose catabolic process. Studies in the recent past have also emphasized the role of glutamine in aggressive cancer. Glutaminolysis is upregulated in cancer cells.It leads to the deamination of glutamine to glutamate and then α-ketoglutaric acid, which is subsequently incorporated into the TCA cycle. These mechanisms may also facilitate macromolecular synthesis in cancer cells. As discussed, cancer cells are more dependent on aerobic glycolysis and drive cancer cell proliferation through glycolytic modulated enzymes such as pyruvate kinase PKM2 isoenzyme and lactate dehydrogenase (LDH). The accumulated lactate is secreted out in extracellular space through monocarboxylate transporter (MCT). Besides, there are many metabolic pathways deregulated in cancer through oncogenic activation, which may further prevent the TCA cycle and promote glycolysis. For example, unregulated pyruvate dehydrogenase kinase (PDK) expression impedes pyruvate dehydrogenase (PDH) activity, declines the TCA cycle, and enhances glycolytic flux in cancer cells. In tumor cells, the pentose phosphate pathway (PPP) is activated, which generates NADPH with five-carbon sugar. The secretion of citrate from mitochondria to cytosol is also reported, which can help to turn on lipid and amino acid synthesis pathways.

METABOLIC ALTERATIONS MEDIATED MOLECULAR CARCINO-GENESIS

Hypoxia

Oxidative stress is an important factor in the neoplastic transformation. In the sustained hypoxic microenvironment, the metabolic process is significantly affected, which is known to be involved in cancer development. Oxidative stress is caused by the generation of reactive oxygen species (ROS), free radicals majorly in the form of H_2O_2, OH^-, O_2^-, *etc.,* [98]. Mitochondria produce the quantity of ROS generation, damaged membranes, and some oxidase (NADPH oxidase, NOX), which are mutagenic [99]. In the normal cells, the ROS generation is controlled by a variety of enzymes including superoxide dismutase, catalase, *etc.* However, in tumor cells, the imbalances of ROS levels can alter metabolic pathways, which can ultimately lead to support cancer progression. For instance, high ROS can modify the sulfhydryl group of pyruvate kinase M2 (PKM2), which resulted in changes in glucose pathways towards the pentose phosphate pathway (PPP) [100]. Tumor cells are known to produce abundant lactic acid with an accelerated glycolysis process. The accumulated lactic acid is likely to involve in the pH reduction in aggravated tumors. A study has shown that the production of >40 end products (amines, alcohols, acids, aldehydes, or ketones) are produced by malignant neuroblastoma under accelerated glycolysis condition [101]. Mazzio *et al.* suggested that the existence of active pyruvate–alanine transaminase or phosphotransacetylase/acetyl-CoA synthetase pathway participates in the anaerobic energy metabolism of cancer cells [101]. Hypoxia in cancer cells actively involved in the proliferation of cancer cells. Hypoxia directly controls the changes in the metabolism, especially like shifting from the oxidative phosphorylation to glycolysis, prevent fatty acid desaturation, changes of enzyme expression, and activation of HIF, *etc.,* to support maintaining tumor microenvironment. Studies also show that activation of HIF promotes aerobic glycolysis lead to increase glucose uptake and L lactate synthesis in cancer. More precisely, HIF1α acts as inducers of aerobic glycolysis in stromal cells but suppressor in cancer cells, but HIF2α acts as a promoter in cancer cells. HIF1α drives aerobic glycolysis in stromal cells to support cancer cell growth *via* producing L-lactate to feed cancer cells.

Interestingly, HIF1α linked aerobic glycolysis inhibits tumorigenesis. HIF1α can be repressed in its transcriptional activity by binding with FBP1 [102]. The level of FBP1 in reduced in breast tumor tissue, particularly in basal subtypes of BC as compared to the luminal BC [103].

Glucose Transporters

Glucose transporters are known to play an important role in cancer. It is because increased glucose metabolism is key to maintaining a high proliferation rate in cancer. Since cancer cells require a high amount of glucose to sustain the high metabolic rate, and therefore, cancer cells transport a high amount of glucose by using facilitated glucose transporters (GLUTs). GLUTs are energy independent transporters of glucose through the plasma membrane. There are 13 GLUTs investigated. These are coded by the genes of solute carrier 2A family(SLC2A) are grouped under three classes [104]. Among them, GLUT 1 – 4 belong to Class I, GLUT 5, 7, 9 and 11 to class II, and GLUT 6, 8, 10, 12, and H^+/myo-inositol transporter (HMIT) belong to Class III groups. The transmembrane domains of GLUTs have a high degree of homology among them. Ongoing studies on cancer have suggested the cancer cells have upregulated levels of glucose transporters such as GLUT1 and GLUT3, as well as glycolytic enzymes to increase the glycolytic flux in for low glucose concentration [105]. It is clear that the increased glucose consumption and increased GLUT1 and GLUT3 levels in cancer cells highly contribute to their proliferation rate. GLUT1 is highly increased in invasive BC and found overexpressed in BC cells [106]. Hypoxia in BC can induce GLUT1 level and glucose uptake in BC. Oncogenes like src and ras activate GLUT1 expressions [107]. A study also shows that the glycosylation of GLUT1 can increase its efficiency for glucose transport [108]. Recent investigation delineated that GLUT12 is overexpressed in the BC cell line and involved in glucose sensing and migration [109]. The transporter is present in both intracellularly and extracellularly. *In vitro* study shows that adding estradiol and epidermal growth factor in culture media increase GLUT12 expression [110].

Other Transporters in BC

Together with GLUTs, ion transporters also play an important part in BC progression. Cancer cells utilize various cellular transporters in the development of aggressive phenotype. Studies have revealed that ion channels and various other transporters, including aquaporin, helps cancer to get motility through volume homeostasis. Ion channels and transporters are not only involved in cellular metabolism in BC, but they can also assist in the oncogenic signaling. Change in pH intracellularly and extracellularly in BC compared to normal cells also show a major metabolic shift. Ion transporters are key agents to deregulate pH shifts in cancer. The role of various ion transporters in pH homeostasis and maintaining favorable tumor microenvironment in cancer is still not well elucidated, and the investigation is still ongoing to delineate their roles in BC. It has been observed that in the tumor microenvironment, acid extruding from cancer cells makes intracellular pH more alkaline compared to normal cells and favors cancer cell migration and characteristics like drug resistance.

Association of Deregulated Signaling Pathways in BC Metabolism

There are several deregulated signaling pathways involved in metabolic reprogramming. The mitochondria are key organelle, which regulates the energy associated pathways in cells. Mitochondrial damage or dysfunction and alterations has been oxidative phosphorylation (OXPHOS) genes are known to enhance oxidative stress and alter the energy-related pathway in tumor cells [111]. In cancer cells, TCA cycle intermediate like succinate or fumarate accumulated in mitochondria, which stabilizes hypoxia-inducible factor (HIF)-1α, which in turn activates oncogenic (PI3K/Akt/mTOR) signaling pathways and distorts tumor suppressor (P53 and PTEN) signaling pathways [112, 113]. These signaling cascades take part in cancer cell proliferation through metabolic reprogramming; for example, Akt targets β-oxidation of fatty acids [114]. Akt is involved in cell survival signaling pathways, including activation of mTOR pathway, insulin growth factor pathways, *etc.,* and also in aerobic glycolysis [115, 116]. Further, this activation may lead to the upregulation of myc and HIF 1 and modulation of pyruvate kinase M2 expression, which has a very crucial function in cancer cells [117]. As above mentioned, hypoxia in cancer induces changes in molecular phenotypes in the tumor loci, which make tumor microenvironment. HIF-1α and some of the glycolytic enzymes, such as hexokinase II, are overexpressed in cancer, which generates angiogenic stimuli to initiate angiogenesis [118]. The phenomena, including high glycolysis and alterations in OXPHOS, could be the major factor for mitochondrial dysfunction, which may suffice for Warburg effects. The gene, c-myc, is shown to be a key regulator for glutaminolysis in cancer. Glutamine catabolizes to α ketoglutaric acid, known as a carbon source for the Kerbs cycle, which is involved in amino acid, nucleotide, and lipid biosynthesis [119]. Thereby, these processes support cancer cells to proliferate at a fast rate. Investigations also evidenced that high insulin-like growth factor receptor, insulin receptor, PI3K, Akt and mTOR signaling pathways are activated in cancer, which is associated with tumor metabolism [114, 120]. Wnt signaling cascade was first studied in the murine cancer model in the 1980s [121] and is also further well recognized in carbohydrate metabolic pathways [122]. Infrequent aberrant mutations of phosphoinositide-3-kinase (PI3K) pathways can cause constituent activation in BC. PI3K inhibitors act as immunomodulatory and show a pleiotropic effect in the tumor microenvironment [123]. Cells are highly correlated with methionine dependency in oncogenic mutation in PI3K of cancer cells [124]. An oncogenic mutation in lipid kinase PI3Kα transcriptionally repressed the expression of SLC7A1 (a cysteine transporter) and elicits metabolic reprogramming of cancer cells [124]. For the sensing of cellular fuel, the hexosamine biosynthesis pathway is well recognized [125], and it relates to glycolytic pathways. Glutamine/fructose-6-phosphate aminotransferase converts fructose six phosphates to glucosamine-6-phosphate, and UDP-GlcNAC is formed at the end of hexosamine biosynthesis pathway, which leads to the glycosylation of protein, preferentially O-linked glycosylation to intracellular, and N-linked glycosylation to the extracellular proteins or receptors [125]. The hexosamine biosynthesis pathway is associated with Wnt/β-catenin signaling [126]. There is a plethora of evidence showing that the Wnt/β-catenin signaling involved in many cancer including BC. Notch signaling is also now understood to be a critical player of cancer cell metabolic reprogramming, as it is fundamental signaling in cell-to-cell communication. A study reveals that Notch signaling participates in vascular remodeling through VEGF [127].

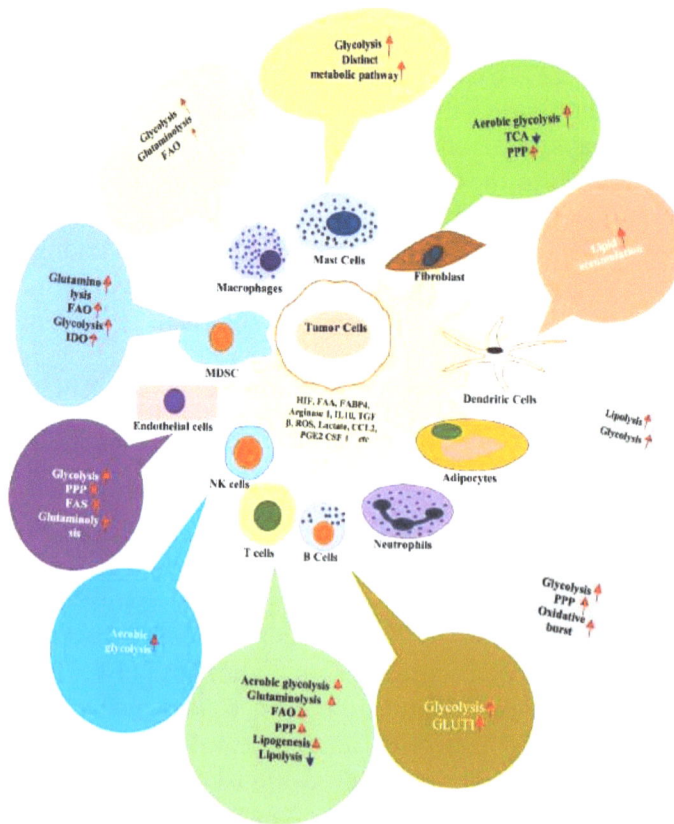

Fig. (2). An overview of immunometabolism in cancer. Cancer cells secrete several cytokines, chemokines to attract immune cells to generate an immunosuppressive microenvironment to grow tumor cells. These cells respond with metabolic alterations mediated through glycolysis, glutaminolysis, and oxidative pentose phosphate pathways (PPP), Fatty acid oxidation (FAO), and lipogenesis and lipolysis in the distinct cancer-associated cells. In general, the fate of cancer is determined by the immunosuppressive tumor microenvironment.

IMMUNOMETABOLISM IN CANCER

The changes in the metabolism of immune cells are highly important because the alteration of immunometabolism leads to create favorable immunosuppressive tumor microenvironment to support tumor growth in BC. The role of immune cells in the oncogenic modulation has been well decoded. The cancer cells can get detected during active immune surveillance mechanisms, and are destroyed by immune cells in the early tumorigenesis [128]. However, cancer cells get support from the extracellular matrices, adipocytes, fibroblasts, endothelial cells, and other immune-inflammatory cells to generate an evading mechanism through intercellular communications of various signaling metabolites and growth factors. Cytotoxic T cells can trigger cancer cell destruction, but these cells are evaded during tumor growth. This immunomodulation is regulated by several metabolites such as kynurenine, lactate, two hydroxyl butyrates, *etc.* regulated by stromal and immune cells [129]. Cancer cell metabolism widely utilize secretive metabolites to manifest the immunosuppressive effect of immune cells, for example, lactate and kynurenine are immunosuppressive [129] and their high levels in tumor microenvironment increase resistance towards therapy. The dependency of immune cells on metabolites is well recognized. However, in cancer, the behavior of immune cells changes due to the development of tumor microenvironment for cancer progression. The changes in the level of cytokines and growth factor rewire immunometabolism in cancer towards tumor growth. Immunometabolism is a key dimension to unravel the mechanism of tumor progression. Immune cells, like B cells and T cells, macrophages, natural killer cells, *etc.*, have different roles in cancer initiation and progression. Immune cell surface receptors assist in this process. For example, normal T cell receptors trigger glycolytic or glutaminolysis pathways in the MYC dependent manner, not on HIF dependent manner as it observed in cancer [130]. M1 macrophages and M2 macrophages have different roles understood in which M1 form can be pro-inflammatory, and M2 macrophages relatively act as an anti-inflammatory. The level of M2 macrophages compared to M1 macrophages are known to be higher in the advanced cancerous form. The M1 and M2 macrophages differ in their metabolism. M1 macrophages prefer anabolic metabolism, but M2 macrophages do the catabolic process. Thus the dependency of M1 macrophages on anaerobic glycolysis, fatty acid synthesis is higher, but M2 macrophages possess oxidative phosphorylation [131]. Thus, in cancer, macrophage behavior is a highly contributing factor in producing the tumor microenvironment. Myeloid cells play a protective role during the early events of cancer, but it transforms into myeloid-derived suppressor cells in the tumor microenvironment. Myeloid-derived suppressor cells have a different metabolic role as they increase fatty acid uptake and fatty acid oxidation by enhancing associated enzyme activity in cancer [132]. This metabolism also leads to developing the anti-tumor activity of myeloid-derived suppressor cells.

Regulatory T cells (Treg) are studied as supporting cells for immunosuppression and building tumor microenvironment. Treg and myeloid suppressor cells have anti-inflammatory and pro-tumorigenic roles in tumor growth. These cells rely more on fatty acid oxidation rather than glycolytic pathways. The oxidative states create a more favorable tumorigenic environment, for example, metformin, an inhibitor of a mitochondrial oxidative metabolic pathway, acts as anti-tumorigenic also. As discussed in the previous paragraphs, cancer cells have high glucose uptake and glycolysis. A study shows that an increase in glycolysis related gene expression in cancer cells could deplete the anti-tumor activity of T cells [133]. In recent years, it has also been observed that the increase in glucose metabolism in cancer induces T cell-mediated tumor rejection in patients [133]. Hypoxia and hypoglycemia can also increase the inactivity of tumor-infiltrating lymphocytes due to low intracellular glucose levels in cancer [134]. Overall, the changes of immunometabolism in cancer make a favorable tumor microenvironment to progress cancer cells in the presence of immunosuppressive behavior of immune cells and other associated cells (Fig. **2**).

TARGETING METABOLISM IN CANCER

Numerous investigations have delineated the differences between normal and cancer cell metabolism. Ongoing studies on cancer cell metabolism reveal the contribution of glucose, fatty acid, and amino acid, like glutamine, in cancer cell proliferation. Further, the altered level of metabolites is becoming an obvious interest for cancer researchers. The concept of myc oncogene stimulated tumorigenesis suggests that deregulated myc expression in cancer cells can make cancer cells activated for the uptake of nutrients (glucose and glutamine), and the deprivation of these nutrients can lead to cancer cell death [135]. However, in normal cells, over-expression of myc can attenuate normal cells. Some studies have revealed that myc associated transformed cancer cells addicted to nutrients, in which the growth can be impeded by using LDHA and glutaminase inhibitors [135, 136]. Moreover, the modulations in the expression of glycolytic enzymes could be another notable point in cancer metabolism. As discussed in the above paragraphs, PKM1 is switched to PKM2 isoenzyme for pyruvate in the tumor tissues, which makes it an attractive target in cancer metabolism [137]. Furthermore, LDHA, PHDH, GLDC expressions are also increased in most cancers [138]. The specific inhibitors against this isoenzyme can provide a therapeutic opportunity. Scientists have always been targeting HIF, to control fast-dividing cancer cells [139], HIF has an influence on enzymes such as carbonic anhydrase IX, MCT 4, hence targeting these can be useful for cancer control [140]. Since the 1950s, metformin gained importance as a drug for hyperglycaemic patients, and it is also recommended as the first line of oral therapy of type 2 diabetes [141]. However, recent studies have revealed the importance of this drug in cancer treatments as well. It is being tested for clinical trials, not only for therapy but also to prevent increased risk. Epidemiological evidence of cancer incidence in diabetes patients showed that metformin inhibits mitochondrial complex (I) showed a higher reduction in cancer compared to those patients who took insulin [142]. Hence, targeting deregulated carbohydrate metabolism could be a new strategy for the development of anti-cancer drugs. Many metabolic pathways have been studied in BC, which are now boosting the discovery of novel pathways. Not all metabolic pathways are good targets used for therapy, but there has been a good success in targeting a few of them. For example, IDO1 blockade can affect immune cell interaction and change tumor microenvironment. Furthermore, studies were also conducted to reveal the role of dendritic cells in cancer progression. Studies also revealed that IDO1 inhibitors with dendritic cells vaccine have advanced chemo-sensitization effects in cancer [143, 144]. Many studies were conducted to reveal the effect of blocking IDO1 with immune checkpoint inhibitors and data show an impressive result.

SUMMARY, CONCLUSIONS AND FUTURE DIRECTIONS

In the present scenario, the rising incidence of BC has become a global concern for clinicians and researchers. Studies have advocated that improper dietary habits and lifestyles are one of the important reasons for the development of chronic diseases like cancer. The metabolic reprogramming is one of the facts in cancer, which is governed by dysregulation in cell energetics and cell signaling pathways. Several pieces of evidence for an altered metabolic portrait in BC cells have defined that BC is a metabolic disease. Numerous studies have propounded the intricacy of metabolic pathways in cancer cells. Here in this chapter, an overview of various metabolic pathways has been outlined, and the details of metabolism involved in cancer, which can be associated with oncogenic cell signaling cascades, have been discussed. The metabolic signatures and genomic markers in cancer perspectives have also been discussed. It has also been detailed how immune cells contribute to the maintenance of tumor microenvironment for cancer. Some investigations have described molecular as well as metabolic switches, which can assist in targeting oncogenic pathways, and thereby, it can help to control cancer cell proliferation. The metabolic advances from the ongoing studies also open a new therapeutic window for cancer prevention. However, there are still many challenges that persist for intensive research on altered metabolic and molecular interactions in cancer. Metabolic studies can assist in decoding the complexity in the tumor microenvironment, mainly governed by oncogenic signaling and immunomodulation. In the future, this endeavor can be a giant step towards deciphering the mechanism of breast carcinogenesis and developing novel metabolic targets for cancer control.

CONSENT FOR PUBLICATION

Not applicable.

CONFLICT OF INTEREST

The authors confirm that the contents of this chapter have no conflict of interest.

ACKNOWLEDGEMENTS

I am thankful to doctoral and postdoctoral advisors for all supports. Meharry Medical College and Ohio State University are also greatly acknowledged for providing research opportunities and financial supports.

REFERENCES

[1]   Ferlay J, Soerjomataram I, Dikshit R, *et al.* Cancer incidence and mortality worldwide: sources, methods and major patterns in GLOBOCAN 2012. Int J Cancer 2015; 136(5): E359-86.
[http://dx.doi.org/10.1002/ijc.29210] [PMID: 25220842]

[2]   Key TJ, Spencer EA. Carbohydrates and cancer: an overview of the epidemiological evidence. Eur J Clin Nutr 2007; 61 (Suppl. 1): S112-21.
[http://dx.doi.org/10.1038/sj.ejcn.1602941] [PMID: 17992182]

[3]   Dang CV. Links between metabolism and cancer. Genes Dev 2012; 26(9): 877-90.
[http://dx.doi.org/10.1101/gad.189365.112] [PMID: 22549953]

[4]   Klement RJ, Kämmerer U. Is there a role for carbohydrate restriction in the treatment and prevention of cancer? Nutr Metab (Lond) 2011; 8: 75.
[http://dx.doi.org/10.1186/1743-7075-8-75] [PMID: 22029671]

[5]   Choi SY, Collins CC, Gout PW, Wang Y. Cancer-generated lactic acid: a regulatory, immunosuppressive metabolite? J Pathol 2013; 230(4): 350-5.
[http://dx.doi.org/10.1002/path.4218] [PMID: 23729358]

[6]   Vander Heiden MG, Cantley LC, Thompson CB. Understanding the Warburg effect: the metabolic requirements of cell proliferation. Science 2009; 324(5930): 1029-33.
[http://dx.doi.org/10.1126/science.1160809] [PMID: 19460998]

[7]   Gatenby RA, Gillies RJ. Why do cancers have high aerobic glycolysis? Nat Rev Cancer 2004; 4(11): 891-9.
[http://dx.doi.org/10.1038/nrc1478] [PMID: 15516961]

[8]   Pavlova NN, Thompson CB. The emerging hallmarks of cancer metabolism. Cell Metab 2016; 23(1): 27-47.
[http://dx.doi.org/10.1016/j.cmet.2015.12.006] [PMID: 26771115]

[9]   Patra KC, Hay N. The pentose phosphate pathway and cancer. Trends Biochem Sci 2014; 39(8): 347-54.
[http://dx.doi.org/10.1016/j.tibs.2014.06.005] [PMID: 25037503]

[10]   Damaghi M, Wojtkowiak JW, Gillies RJ. pH sensing and regulation in cancer. Front Physiol 2013; 4: 370.
[http://dx.doi.org/10.3389/fphys.2013.00370] [PMID: 24381558]

[11]   Suman S, Basak T, Gupta P, *et al.* Quantitative proteomics revealed novel proteins associated with molecular subtypes of breast cancer. J Proteom 2016; 148: 183-93.
[http://dx.doi.org/10.1016/j.jprot.2016.07.033] [PMID: 27498393]

[12]   Kakarala M, Wicha MS. Implications of the cancer stem-cell hypothesis for breast cancer prevention and therapy. J Clin Oncol 2008; 26(17): 2813-20.
[http://dx.doi.org/10.1200/JCO.2008.16.3931] [PMID: 18539959]

[13]   Saeg F, Anbalagan M. Breast cancer stem cells and the challenges of eradication: a review of novel therapies. Stem Cell Investig 2018; 5: 39.
[http://dx.doi.org/10.21037/sci.2018.10.05] [PMID: 30498750]

[14]   Snyder V, Reed-Newman TC, Arnold L, Thomas SM, Anant S. Cancer stem cell metabolism and potential therapeutic targets. Front Oncol 2018; 8: 203.
[http://dx.doi.org/10.3389/fonc.2018.00203] [PMID: 29922594]

[15]   Suman S, Sharma RK, Kumar V, Sinha N, Shukla Y. Metabolic fingerprinting in breast cancer stages through ^{1}H NMR spectroscopy-based metabolomic analysis of plasma. J Pharm Biomed Anal 2018; 160: 38-45.
[http://dx.doi.org/10.1016/j.jpba.2018.07.024] [PMID: 30059813]

[16]   Wong CC, Qian Y, Yu J. Interplay between epigenetics and metabolism in oncogenesis: mechanisms and therapeutic approaches. Oncogene 2017; 36(24): 3359-74.
[http://dx.doi.org/10.1038/onc.2016.485] [PMID: 28092669]

[17]   Teegarden D, Romieu I, Lelièvre SA. Redefining the impact of nutrition on breast cancer incidence: is epigenetics involved? Nutr Res Rev 2012; 25(1): 68-95.
[http://dx.doi.org/10.1017/S0954422411000199] [PMID: 22853843]

[18]   Stolzenberg-Solomon RZ, Chang SC, Leitzmann MF, *et al.* Folate intake, alcohol use, and postmenopausal breast cancer risk in the Prostate, Lung, Colorectal, and Ovarian Cancer Screening Trial. Am J Clin Nutr 2006; 83(4): 895-904.
[http://dx.doi.org/10.1093/ajcn/83.4.895] [PMID: 16600944]

[19]   Kaelin WG Jr, McKnight SL. Influence of metabolism on epigenetics and disease. Cell 2013; 153(1): 56-69.
[http://dx.doi.org/10.1016/j.cell.2013.03.004] [PMID: 23540690]

[20]   Dong C, Yuan T, Wu Y, *et al.* Loss of FBP1 by Snail-mediated repression provides metabolic advantages in basal-like breast cancer. Cancer Cell 2013; 23(3): 316-31.
[http://dx.doi.org/10.1016/j.ccr.2013.01.022] [PMID: 23453623]

[21]   Lv L, Li D, Zhao D, *et al.* Acetylation targets the M2 isoform of pyruvate kinase for degradation through chaperone-mediated autophagy and promotes tumor growth. Mol Cell 2011; 42(6): 719-30.
[http://dx.doi.org/10.1016/j.molcel.2011.04.025] [PMID: 21700219]

[22]   Jiang P, Du W, Wu M. Regulation of the pentose phosphate pathway in cancer. Protein Cell 2014; 5(8): 592-602.
[http://dx.doi.org/10.1007/s13238-014-0082-8] [PMID: 25015087]

[23]   Schvartzman JM, Thompson CB, Finley LWS. Metabolic regulation of chromatin modifications and gene expression. J Cell Biol 2018; 217(7): 2247-59.
[http://dx.doi.org/10.1083/jcb.201803061] [PMID: 29760106]

[24]   Etchegaray JP, Mostoslavsky R. Interplay between metabolism and epigenetics: A nuclear adaptation to environmental changes. Mol Cell 2016; 62(5): 695-711.
[http://dx.doi.org/10.1016/j.molcel.2016.05.029] [PMID: 27259202]

[25]   Carrer A, Wellen KE. Metabolism and epigenetics: a link cancer cells exploit. Curr Opin Biotechnol 2015; 34: 23-9.
[http://dx.doi.org/10.1016/j.copbio.2014.11.012] [PMID: 25461508]

[26]   Conzen SD. Minireview: nuclear receptors and breast cancer. Mol Endocrinol 2008; 22(10): 2215-28.
[http://dx.doi.org/10.1210/me.2007-0421] [PMID: 18417735]

[27]   Fallah Y, Brundage J, Allegakoen P, Shajahan-Haq AN. MYC-driven pathways in breast cancer

subtypes. Biomolecules 2017; 7(3): E53.
[http://dx.doi.org/10.3390/biom7030053] [PMID: 28696357]

[28] Feng Y, Spezia M, Huang S, *et al.* Breast cancer development and progression: Risk factors, cancer stem cells, signaling pathways, genomics, and molecular pathogenesis. Genes Dis 2018; 5(2): 77-106.
[http://dx.doi.org/10.1016/j.gendis.2018.05.001] [PMID: 30258937]

[29] Schettini F, Buono G, Trivedi MV, De Placido S, Arpino G, Giuliano M. PI3K/mTOR inhibitors in the treatment of luminal breast cancer. Why, when and to whom? Breast Care (Basel) 2017; 12(5): 290-4.
[http://dx.doi.org/10.1159/000481657] [PMID: 29234247]

[30] Choi J, Kim ES, Koo JS. Expression of pentose phosphate pathway-related proteins in breast cancer. Dis Markers 2018; 2018: 9369358.
[http://dx.doi.org/10.1155/2018/9369358] [PMID: 29682102]

[31] Xu W, Yang H, Liu Y, *et al.* Oncometabolite 2-hydroxyglutarate is a competitive inhibitor of α-ketoglutarate-dependent dioxygenases. Cancer Cell 2011; 19(1): 17-30.
[http://dx.doi.org/10.1016/j.ccr.2010.12.014] [PMID: 21251613]

[32] Xiao M, Yang H, Xu W, *et al.* Inhibition of α-KG-dependent histone and DNA demethylases by fumarate and succinate that are accumulated in mutations of FH and SDH tumor suppressors. Genes Dev 2012; 26(12): 1326-38.
[http://dx.doi.org/10.1101/gad.191056.112] [PMID: 22677546]

[33] Dasgupta S, Rajapakshe K, Zhu B, *et al.* Metabolic enzyme PFKFB4 activates transcriptional coactivator SRC-3 to drive breast cancer. Nature 2018; 556(7700): 249-54.
[http://dx.doi.org/10.1038/s41586-018-0018-1] [PMID: 29615789]

[34] Chang M. Tamoxifen resistance in breast cancer. Biomol Ther (Seoul) 2012; 20(3): 256-67.
[http://dx.doi.org/10.4062/biomolther.2012.20.3.256] [PMID: 24130921]

[35] Ros S, Schulze A. Balancing glycolytic flux: the role of 6-phosphofructo-2-kinase/fructose 2,6-bisphosphatases in cancer metabolism. Cancer Metab 2013; 1(1): 8.
[http://dx.doi.org/10.1186/2049-3002-1-8] [PMID: 24280138]

[36] Cunquero-Tomas AJ, Avila-Andrade CD, Milara J, Javier K, Iranzo V, Camps C. Safe neoadjuvant trastuzumab-based treatment in HER2 + inflammatory early breast cancer in a glucose 6-phosphate dehydrogenase-deficient postmenopausal woman: A case report and review of the literature. J Oncol Pharm Pract 2020; 26(2): 492-5.
[PMID: 31260379]

[37] Ahmad A, Aboukameel A, Kong D, *et al.* Phosphoglucose isomerase/autocrine motility factor mediates epithelial-mesenchymal transition regulated by miR-200 in breast cancer cells. Cancer Res 2011; 71(9): 3400-9.
[http://dx.doi.org/10.1158/0008-5472.CAN-10-0965] [PMID: 21389093]

[38] Rios Garcia M, Steinbauer B, Srivastava K, *et al.* Acetyl-CoA carboxylase 1-dependent protein acetylation controls breast cancer metastasis and recurrence. Cell Metab 2017; 26(6): 842-55.: e5.

[39] Menendez JA, Lupu R. Fatty acid synthase regulates estrogen receptor-α signaling in breast cancer cells. Oncogenesis 2017; 6(2): e299.
[http://dx.doi.org/10.1038/oncsis.2017.4] [PMID: 28240737]

[40] Siddiqui A, Gollavilli PN, Schwab A, *et al.* Thymidylate synthase maintains the de-differentiated state of triple negative breast cancers. Cell Death Differ 2019; 26(11): 2223-36.
[http://dx.doi.org/10.1038/s41418-019-0289-6] [PMID: 30737477]

[41] Tanaka Y, Kosaka Y, Waraya M, *et al.* Differential prognostic relevance of promoter DNA methylation of *CDO1* and *HOPX* in primary breast cancer. Anticancer Res 2019; 39(5): 2289-98.
[http://dx.doi.org/10.21873/anticanres.13345] [PMID: 31092420]

[42] Yang Yu, Morin PJ, Han WF, *et al.* Regulation of fatty acid synthase expression in breast cancer by sterol regulatory element binding protein-1c. Exp Cell Res 2003; 282(2): 132-7.

[http://dx.doi.org/10.1016/S0014-4827(02)00023-X] [PMID: 12531699]

[43] Minemura H, Takagi K, Sato A, *et al.* CITED2 in breast carcinoma as a potent prognostic predictor associated with proliferation, migration and chemoresistance. Cancer Sci 2016; 107(12): 1898-908.
[http://dx.doi.org/10.1111/cas.13081] [PMID: 27627783]

[44] Wang G, Xu Z, Wang C, *et al.* Differential phosphofructokinase-1 isoenzyme patterns associated with glycolytic efficiency in human breast cancer and paracancer tissues. Oncol Lett 2013; 6(6): 1701-6.
[http://dx.doi.org/10.3892/ol.2013.1599] [PMID: 24260065]

[45] Durany N, Joseph J, Jimenez OM, *et al.* Phosphoglycerate mutase, 2,3-bisphosphoglycerate phosphatase, creatine kinase and enolase activity and isoenzymes in breast carcinoma. Br J Cancer 2000; 82(1): 20-7.
[http://dx.doi.org/10.1054/bjoc.1999.0871] [PMID: 10638961]

[46] Chiavarina B, Whitaker-Menezes D, Martinez-Outschoorn UE, *et al.* Pyruvate kinase expression (PKM1 and PKM2) in cancer-associated fibroblasts drives stromal nutrient production and tumor growth. Cancer Biol Ther 2011; 12(12): 1101-13.
[http://dx.doi.org/10.4161/cbt.12.12.18703] [PMID: 22236875]

[47] Yao A, Xiang Y, Si YR, *et al.* PKM2 promotes glucose metabolism through a let-7a-5p/Stat3/hnRP-A1 regulatory feedback loop in breast cancer cells. J Cell Biochem 2019; 120(4): 6542-54.
[http://dx.doi.org/10.1002/jcb.27947] [PMID: 30368881]

[48] Angelucci C, D'Alessio A, Iacopino F, *et al.* Pivotal role of human stearoyl-CoA desaturases (SCD1 and 5) in breast cancer progression: oleic acid-based effect of SCD1 on cell migration and a novel pro-cell survival role for SCD5. Oncotarget 2018; 9(36): 24364-80.
[http://dx.doi.org/10.18632/oncotarget.25273] [PMID: 29849946]

[49] Kim S, Lee Y, Koo JS. Differential expression of lipid metabolism-related proteins in different breast cancer subtypes. PLoS One 2015; 10(3): e0119473.
[http://dx.doi.org/10.1371/journal.pone.0119473] [PMID: 25751270]

[50] Zhang D, Jin N, Sun W, *et al.* Phosphoglycerate mutase 1 promotes cancer cell migration independent of its metabolic activity. Oncogene 2017; 36(20): 2900-9.
[http://dx.doi.org/10.1038/onc.2016.446] [PMID: 27991922]

[51] Wong JM, Jenkins DJ. Carbohydrate digestibility and metabolic effects. J Nutr 2007; 137(11) (Suppl.): 2539S-46S.
[http://dx.doi.org/10.1093/jn/137.11.2539S] [PMID: 17951499]

[52] Ríos-Covián D, Ruas-Madiedo P, Margolles A, Gueimonde M, de Los Reyes-Gavilán CG, Salazar N. Intestinal short chain fatty acids and their link with diet and human health. Front Microbiol 2016; 7: 185.
[http://dx.doi.org/10.3389/fmicb.2016.00185] [PMID: 26925050]

[53] Slavin J. Fiber and prebiotics: mechanisms and health benefits. Nutrients 2013; 5(4): 1417-35.
[http://dx.doi.org/10.3390/nu5041417] [PMID: 23609775]

[54] Pi-Sunyer FX. Glycemic index and disease. Am J Clin Nutr 2002; 76(1): 290S-8S.
[http://dx.doi.org/10.1093/ajcn/76.1.290S] [PMID: 12081854]

[55] Venn BJ, Green TJ. Glycemic index and glycemic load: measurement issues and their effect on diet-disease relationships. Eur J Clin Nutr 2007; 61 (Suppl. 1): S122-31.
[http://dx.doi.org/10.1038/sj.ejcn.1602942] [PMID: 17992183]

[56] Wang Z, Uchida K, Ohnaka K, *et al.* Sugars, sucrose and colorectal cancer risk: the Fukuoka colorectal cancer study. Scand J Gastroenterol 2014; 49(5): 581-8.
[http://dx.doi.org/10.3109/00365521.2013.822091] [PMID: 24716480]

[57] Larsson SC, Orsini N, Wolk A. Milk, milk products and lactose intake and ovarian cancer risk: a meta-analysis of epidemiological studies. Int J Cancer 2006; 118(2): 431-41.
[http://dx.doi.org/10.1002/ijc.21305] [PMID: 16052536]

[58]   Gnagnarella P, Gandini S, La Vecchia C, Maisonneuve P. Glycemic index, glycemic load, and cancer risk: a meta-analysis. Am J Clin Nutr 2008; 87(6): 1793-801.
[http://dx.doi.org/10.1093/ajcn/87.6.1793] [PMID: 18541570]

[59]   Roberts CK, Hevener AL, Barnard RJ. Metabolic syndrome and insulin resistance: underlying causes and modification by exercise training. Compr Physiol 2013; 3(1): 1-58.
[http://dx.doi.org/10.1002/cphy.c110062] [PMID: 23720280]

[60]   Jang M, Kim SS, Lee J. Cancer cell metabolism: implications for therapeutic targets. Exp Mol Med 2013; 45: e45.
[http://dx.doi.org/10.1038/emm.2013.85] [PMID: 24091747]

[61]   Crabtree HG. Observations on the carbohydrate metabolism of tumours. Biochem J 1929; 23(3): 536-45.
[http://dx.doi.org/10.1042/bj0230536] [PMID: 16744238]

[62]   Dhup S, Dadhich RK, Porporato PE, Sonveaux P. Multiple biological activities of lactic acid in cancer: influences on tumor growth, angiogenesis and metastasis. Curr Pharm Des 2012; 18(10): 1319-30.
[http://dx.doi.org/10.2174/138161212799504902] [PMID: 22360558]

[63]   Warburg O, Wind F, Negelein E. The metabolism of tumors in the body. J Gen Physiol 1927; 8(6): 519-30.
[http://dx.doi.org/10.1085/jgp.8.6.519] [PMID: 19872213]

[64]   Barker J, Khan MA, Solomos T. Mechanism of the pasteur effect. Nature 1964; 201: 1126-7.
[http://dx.doi.org/10.1038/2011126a0] [PMID: 14152792]

[65]   Icard P, Lincet H. A global view of the biochemical pathways involved in the regulation of the metabolism of cancer cells. Biochim Biophys Acta 2012; 1826(2): 423-33.
[PMID: 22841746]

[66]   Milgraum LZ, Witters LA, Pasternack GR, Kuhajda FP. Enzymes of the fatty acid synthesis pathway are highly expressed in in situ breast carcinoma. Clin Cancer Res 1997; 3(11): 2115-20.
[PMID: 9815604]

[67]   Miranda-Gonçalves V, Lameirinhas A, Henrique R, Jerónimo C. Metabolism and epigenetic interplay in cancer: regulation and putative therapeutic targets. Front Genet 2018; 9: 427.
[http://dx.doi.org/10.3389/fgene.2018.00427] [PMID: 30356832]

[68]   Sivanand S, Rhoades S, Jiang Q, *et al.* Nuclear acetyl-coa production by acly promotes homologous recombination. Mol Cell 2017; 67(2): 252-65.: e6.
[http://dx.doi.org/10.1016/j.molcel.2017.06.008]

[69]   Martin LJ, Melnichouk O, Huszti E, *et al.* Serum lipids, lipoproteins, and risk of breast cancer: a nested case-control study using multiple time points. J Natl Cancer Inst 2015; 107(5): djv032.
[http://dx.doi.org/10.1093/jnci/djv032] [PMID: 25817193]

[70]   Clark O, Yen K, Mellinghoff IK. Molecular pathways: Isocitrate dehydrogenase mutations in cancer. Clin Cancer Res 2016; 22(8): 1837-42.
[http://dx.doi.org/10.1158/1078-0432.CCR-13-1333] [PMID: 26819452]

[71]   Lin AP, Abbas S, Kim SW, *et al.* D2HGDH regulates alpha-ketoglutarate levels and dioxygenase function by modulating IDH2. Nat Commun 2015; 6: 7768.
[http://dx.doi.org/10.1038/ncomms8768] [PMID: 26178471]

[72]   Chuang PK, Hsiao M, Hsu TL, *et al.* Signaling pathway of globo-series glycosphingolipids and β1,3-galactosyltransferase V (β3GalT5) in breast cancer. Proc Natl Acad Sci USA 2019; 116(9): 3518-23.
[http://dx.doi.org/10.1073/pnas.1816946116] [PMID: 30808745]

[73]   Madak-Erdogan Z, Band S, Zhao YC, *et al.* Free fatty acids rewire cancer metabolism in obesity-associated breast cancer *via* estrogen receptor and mTOR signaling. Cancer Res 2019; 79(10): 2494-

510.
[http://dx.doi.org/10.1158/0008-5472.CAN-18-2849] [PMID: 30862719]

[74]   Corbet C, Feron O. Emerging roles of lipid metabolism in cancer progression. Curr Opin Clin Nutr
       Metab Care 2017; 20(4): 254-60.
       [http://dx.doi.org/10.1097/MCO.0000000000000381] [PMID: 28403011]

[75]   Menendez JA, Lupu R. Fatty acid synthase (FASN) as a therapeutic target in breast cancer. Expert
       Opin Ther Targets 2017; 21(11): 1001-16.
       [http://dx.doi.org/10.1080/14728222.2017.1381087] [PMID: 28922023]

[76]   Goswami S, Sharma-Walia N. Crosstalk between osteoprotegerin (OPG), fatty acid synthase (FASN)
       and, cycloxygenase-2 (COX-2) in breast cancer: implications in carcinogenesis. Oncotarget 2016;
       7(37): 58953-74.
       [http://dx.doi.org/10.18632/oncotarget.9835] [PMID: 27270654]

[77]   Jung YY, Kim HM, Koo JS. Expression of lipid metabolism-related proteins in metastatic breast
       cancer. PLoS One 2015; 10(9): e0137204.
       [http://dx.doi.org/10.1371/journal.pone.0137204] [PMID: 26334757]

[78]   Mikalayeva V, Ceslevičienė I, Sarapinienė I, *et al.* Fatty acid synthesis and degradation interplay to
       regulate the oxidative stress in cancer cells. Int J Mol Sci 2019; 20(6): E1348.
       [http://dx.doi.org/10.3390/ijms20061348] [PMID: 30889783]

[79]   Sevinsky CJ, Khan F, Kokabee L, Darehshouri A, Maddipati KR, Conklin DS. NDRG1 regulates
       neutral lipid metabolism in breast cancer cells. Breast Cancer Res 2018; 20(1): 55.
       [http://dx.doi.org/10.1186/s13058-018-0980-4] [PMID: 29898756]

[80]   Yamashita Y, Nishiumi S, Kono S, Takao S, Azuma T, Yoshida M. Differences in elongation of very
       long chain fatty acids and fatty acid metabolism between triple-negative and hormone receptor-
       positive breast cancer. BMC Cancer 2017; 17(1): 589.
       [http://dx.doi.org/10.1186/s12885-017-3554-4] [PMID: 28851309]

[81]   Sheikh TN, Patwardhan PP, Cremers S, Schwartz GK. Targeted inhibition of glutaminase as a
       potential new approach for the treatment of *NF1* associated soft tissue malignancies. Oncotarget 2017;
       8(55): 94054-68.
       [http://dx.doi.org/10.18632/oncotarget.21573] [PMID: 29212209]

[82]   Mattaini KR, Sullivan MR, Vander Heiden MG. The importance of serine metabolism in cancer. J Cell
       Biol 2016; 214(3): 249-57.
       [http://dx.doi.org/10.1083/jcb.201604085] [PMID: 27458133]

[83]   Gromova I, Gromov P, Honma N, *et al.* High level PHGDH expression in breast is predominantly
       associated with keratin 5-positive cell lineage independently of malignancy. Mol Oncol 2015; 9(8):
       1636-54.
       [http://dx.doi.org/10.1016/j.molonc.2015.05.003] [PMID: 26026368]

[84]   Possemato R, Marks KM, Shaul YD, *et al.* Functional genomics reveal that the serine synthesis
       pathway is essential in breast cancer. Nature 2011; 476(7360): 346-50.
       [http://dx.doi.org/10.1038/nature10350] [PMID: 21760589]

[85]   Wang Y, Sun Z, Szyf M. S-adenosyl-methionine (SAM) alters the transcriptome and methylome and
       specifically blocks growth and invasiveness of liver cancer cells. Oncotarget 2017; 8(67): 111866-81.
       [http://dx.doi.org/10.18632/oncotarget.22942] [PMID: 29340097]

[86]   Camarda R, Williams J, Goga A. *In vivo* reprogramming of cancer metabolism by MYC. Front Cell
       Dev Biol 2017; 5: 35.
       [http://dx.doi.org/10.3389/fcell.2017.00035] [PMID: 28443280]

[87]   Locasale JW. Serine, glycine and one-carbon units: cancer metabolism in full circle. Nat Rev Cancer
       2013; 13(8): 572-83.
       [http://dx.doi.org/10.1038/nrc3557] [PMID: 23822983]

[88]   Scalise M, Pochini L, Console L, Losso MA, Indiveri C. The human SLC1A5 (ASCT2) amino acid transporter: From function to structure and role in cell biology. Front Cell Dev Biol 2018; 6: 96.
[http://dx.doi.org/10.3389/fcell.2018.00096] [PMID: 30234109]

[89]   van Geldermalsen M, Wang Q, Nagarajah R, *et al.* ASCT2/SLC1A5 controls glutamine uptake and tumour growth in triple-negative basal-like breast cancer. Oncogene 2016; 35(24): 3201-8.
[http://dx.doi.org/10.1038/onc.2015.381] [PMID: 26455325]

[90]   Luis C, Duarte F, Faria I, *et al.* Warburg Effect Inversion: Adiposity shifts central primary metabolism in MCF-7 breast cancer cells. Life Sci 2019; 223: 38-46.
[http://dx.doi.org/10.1016/j.lfs.2019.03.016] [PMID: 30862570]

[91]   Zhao H, French JB, Fang Y, Benkovic SJ. The purinosome, a multi-protein complex involved in the *de novo* biosynthesis of purines in humans. Chem Commun (Camb) 2013; 49(40): 4444-52.
[http://dx.doi.org/10.1039/c3cc41437j] [PMID: 23575936]

[92]   Nilsson R, Jain M, Madhusudhan N, *et al.* Metabolic enzyme expression highlights a key role for MTHFD2 and the mitochondrial folate pathway in cancer. Nat Commun 2014; 5: 3128.
[http://dx.doi.org/10.1038/ncomms4128] [PMID: 24451681]

[93]   Liu F, Liu Y, He C, *et al.* Increased MTHFD2 expression is associated with poor prognosis in breast cancer. Tumour Biol 2014; 35(9): 8685-90.
[http://dx.doi.org/10.1007/s13277-014-2111-x] [PMID: 24870594]

[94]   Buj R, Aird KM. Deoxyribonucleotide triphosphate metabolism in cancer and metabolic disease. Front Endocrinol (Lausanne) 2018; 9: 177.
[http://dx.doi.org/10.3389/fendo.2018.00177] [PMID: 29720963]

[95]   Yin J, Ren W, Huang X, Deng J, Li T, Yin Y. Potential mechanisms connecting purine metabolism and cancer therapy. Front Immunol 2018; 9: 1697.
[http://dx.doi.org/10.3389/fimmu.2018.01697] [PMID: 30105018]

[96]   Sigoillot FD, Sigoillot SM, Guy HI. Breakdown of the regulatory control of pyrimidine biosynthesis in human breast cancer cells. Int J Cancer 2004; 109(4): 491-8.
[http://dx.doi.org/10.1002/ijc.11717] [PMID: 14991569]

[97]   Cancarini I, Krogh V, Agnoli C, *et al.* Micronutrients involved in one-carbon metabolism and risk of breast cancer subtypes. PLoS One 2015; 10(9): e0138318.
[http://dx.doi.org/10.1371/journal.pone.0138318] [PMID: 26376452]

[98]   Liou GY, Storz P. Reactive oxygen species in cancer. Free Radic Res 2010; 44(5): 479-96.
[http://dx.doi.org/10.3109/10715761003667554] [PMID: 20370557]

[99]   Block K, Gorin Y. Aiding and abetting roles of NOX oxidases in cellular transformation. Nat Rev Cancer 2012; 12(9): 627-37.
[http://dx.doi.org/10.1038/nrc3339] [PMID: 22918415]

[100]   Anastasiou D, Poulogiannis G, Asara JM, *et al.* Inhibition of pyruvate kinase M2 by reactive oxygen species contributes to cellular antioxidant responses. Science 2011; 334(6060): 1278-83.
[http://dx.doi.org/10.1126/science.1211485] [PMID: 22052977]

[101]   Mazzio EA, Smith B, Soliman KF. Evaluation of endogenous acidic metabolic products associated with carbohydrate metabolism in tumor cells. Cell Biol Toxicol 2010; 26(3): 177-88.
[http://dx.doi.org/10.1007/s10565-009-9138-6] [PMID: 19784859]

[102]   Kang Y, Zhu X, Xu Y, *et al.* Energy stress-induced lncRNA HAND2-AS1 represses HIF1α-mediated energy metabolism and inhibits osteosarcoma progression. Am J Cancer Res 2018; 8(3): 526-37.
[PMID: 29637006]

[103]   Shi L, Zhao C, Pu H, Zhang Q. FBP1 expression is associated with basal-like breast carcinoma. Oncol Lett 2017; 13(5): 3046-56.
[http://dx.doi.org/10.3892/ol.2017.5860] [PMID: 28529559]

[104] Joost HG, Bell GI, Best JD, *et al.* Nomenclature of the GLUT/SLC2A family of sugar/polyol transport facilitators. Am J Physiol Endocrinol Metab 2002; 282(4): E974-6.
[http://dx.doi.org/10.1152/ajpendo.00407.2001] [PMID: 11882521]

[105] Krzeslak A, Wojcik-Krowiranda K, Forma E, *et al.* Expression of GLUT1 and GLUT3 glucose transporters in endometrial and breast cancers. Pathol Oncol Res 2012; 18(3): 721-8.
[http://dx.doi.org/10.1007/s12253-012-9500-5] [PMID: 22270867]

[106] Grover-McKay M, Walsh SA, Seftor EA, Thomas PA, Hendrix MJ. Role for glucose transporter 1 protein in human breast cancer. Pathol Oncol Res 1998; 4(2): 115-20.
[http://dx.doi.org/10.1007/BF02904704] [PMID: 9654596]

[107] Flier JS, Mueckler MM, Usher P, Lodish HF. Elevated levels of glucose transport and transporter messenger RNA are induced by ras or src oncogenes. Science 1987; 235(4795): 1492-5.
[http://dx.doi.org/10.1126/science.3103217] [PMID: 3103217]

[108] Asano T, Katagiri H, Takata K, *et al.* The role of N-glycosylation of GLUT1 for glucose transport activity. J Biol Chem 1991; 266(36): 24632-6.
[PMID: 1761560]

[109] Matsui C, Takatani-Nakase T, Maeda S, Nakase I, Takahashi K. Potential roles of GLUT12 for glucose sensing and cellular migration in MCF-7 human breast cancer cells under high glucose conditions. Anticancer Res 2017; 37(12): 6715-22.
[PMID: 29187448]

[110] Macheda ML, Rogers S, Best JD. Molecular and cellular regulation of glucose transporter (GLUT) proteins in cancer. J Cell Physiol 2005; 202(3): 654-62.
[http://dx.doi.org/10.1002/jcp.20166] [PMID: 15389572]

[111] Yu L, Lu M, Jia D, *et al.* Modeling the genetic regulation of cancer metabolism: interplay between glycolysis and oxidative phosphorylation. Cancer Res 2017; 77(7): 1564-74.
[http://dx.doi.org/10.1158/0008-5472.CAN-16-2074] [PMID: 28202516]

[112] Wittig R, Coy JF. The role of glucose metabolism and glucose-associated signalling in cancer. Perspect Medicin Chem 2007; 1: 64-82.
[http://dx.doi.org/10.1177/1177391X0700100006]

[113] Papa A, Pandolfi PP. The PTEN−PI3K axis in cancer. Biomolecules 2019; 9(4): E153.
[http://dx.doi.org/10.3390/biom9040153] [PMID: 30999672]

[114] Buzzai M, Bauer DE, Jones RG, *et al.* The glucose dependence of Akt-transformed cells can be reversed by pharmacologic activation of fatty acid beta-oxidation. Oncogene 2005; 24(26): 4165-73.
[http://dx.doi.org/10.1038/sj.onc.1208622] [PMID: 15806154]

[115] Makinoshima H, Takita M, Saruwatari K, *et al.* Signaling through the Phosphatidylinositol 3-Kinase (PI3K)/Mammalian Target of Rapamycin (mTOR) Axis Is Responsible for Aerobic Glycolysis mediated by Glucose Transporter in Epidermal Growth Factor Receptor (EGFR)-mutated Lung Adenocarcinoma. J Biol Chem 2015; 290(28): 17495-504.
[http://dx.doi.org/10.1074/jbc.M115.660498] [PMID: 26023239]

[116] Lyons A, Coleman M, Riis S, *et al.* Insulin-like growth factor 1 signaling is essential for mitochondrial biogenesis and mitophagy in cancer cells. J Biol Chem 2017; 292(41): 16983-98.
[http://dx.doi.org/10.1074/jbc.M117.792838] [PMID: 28821609]

[117] Yang W, Lu Z. Pyruvate kinase M2 at a glance. J Cell Sci 2015; 128(9): 1655-60.
[http://dx.doi.org/10.1242/jcs.166629] [PMID: 25770102]

[118] Masoud GN, Li W. HIF-1α pathway: role, regulation and intervention for cancer therapy. Acta Pharm Sin B 2015; 5(5): 378-89.
[http://dx.doi.org/10.1016/j.apsb.2015.05.007] [PMID: 26579469]

[119] Yin C, Qie S, Sang N. Carbon source metabolism and its regulation in cancer cells. Crit Rev Eukaryot

Gene Expr 2012; 22(1): 17-35.
[http://dx.doi.org/10.1615/CritRevEukarGeneExpr.v22.i1.20] [PMID: 22339657]

[120] Matsuda S, Kobayashi M, Kitagishi Y. Roles for PI3K/AKT/PTEN pathway in cell signaling of nonalcoholic fatty liver disease. ISRN Endocrinol 2013; 2013: 472432.
[http://dx.doi.org/10.1155/2013/472432] [PMID: 23431468]

[121] Nusse R, Varmus HE. Many tumors induced by the mouse mammary tumor virus contain a provirus integrated in the same region of the host genome. Cell 1982; 31(1): 99-109.
[http://dx.doi.org/10.1016/0092-8674(82)90409-3] [PMID: 6297757]

[122] Chafey P, Finzi L, Boisgard R, *et al.* Proteomic analysis of beta-catenin activation in mouse liver by DIGE analysis identifies glucose metabolism as a new target of the Wnt pathway. Proteom 2009; 9(15): 3889-900.
[http://dx.doi.org/10.1002/pmic.200800609] [PMID: 19639598]

[123] Qin H, Liu L, Sun S, *et al.* The impact of PI3K inhibitors on breast cancer cell and its tumor microenvironment. PeerJ 2018; 6: e5092.
[http://dx.doi.org/10.7717/peerj.5092] [PMID: 29942710]

[124] Lien EC, Ghisolfi L, Geck RC, Asara JM, Toker A. Oncogenic PI3K promotes methionine dependency in breast cancer cells through the cystine-glutamate antiporter xCT. Sci Signal 2017; 10(510): eaao6604.
[http://dx.doi.org/10.1126/scisignal.aao6604] [PMID: 29259101]

[125] de Queiroz RM, Oliveira IA, Piva B, *et al.* Hexosamine biosynthetic pathway and glycosylation regulate cell migration in melanoma cells. Front Oncol 2019; 9(116): 116.
[http://dx.doi.org/10.3389/fonc.2019.00116] [PMID: 30891426]

[126] Anagnostou SH, Shepherd PR. Glucose induces an autocrine activation of the Wnt/beta-catenin pathway in macrophage cell lines. Biochem J 2008; 416(2): 211-8.
[http://dx.doi.org/10.1042/BJ20081426] [PMID: 18823284]

[127] Roca C, Adams RH. Regulation of vascular morphogenesis by Notch signaling. Genes Dev 2007; 21(20): 2511-24.
[http://dx.doi.org/10.1101/gad.1589207] [PMID: 17938237]

[128] Suman S, Sharma PK, Rai G, *et al.* Current perspectives of molecular pathways involved in chronic inflammation-mediated breast cancer. Biochem Biophys Res Commun 2016; 472(3): 401-9.
[http://dx.doi.org/10.1016/j.bbrc.2015.10.133] [PMID: 26522220]

[129] Dang CV, Kim JW. Convergence of Cancer Metabolism and Immunity: an Overview. Biomol Ther (Seoul) 2018; 26(1): 4-9.
[http://dx.doi.org/10.4062/biomolther.2017.194] [PMID: 29212301]

[130] Wang R, Dillon CP, Shi LZ, *et al.* The transcription factor Myc controls metabolic reprogramming upon T lymphocyte activation. Immunity 2011; 35(6): 871-82.
[http://dx.doi.org/10.1016/j.immuni.2011.09.021] [PMID: 22195744]

[131] Ho PC, Liu PS. Metabolic communication in tumors: a new layer of immunoregulation for immune evasion. J Immunother Cancer 2016; 4: 4.
[http://dx.doi.org/10.1186/s40425-016-0109-1] [PMID: 26885366]

[132] Al-Khami AA, Zheng L, Del Valle L, *et al.* Exogenous lipid uptake induces metabolic and functional reprogramming of tumor-associated myeloid-derived suppressor cells. OncoImmunology 2017; 6(10): e1344804.
[http://dx.doi.org/10.1080/2162402X.2017.1344804] [PMID: 29123954]

[133] Cascone T, McKenzie JA, Mbofung RM, *et al.* Increased tumor glycolysis characterizes immune resistance to adoptive T cell therapy Cell Metab 2018; 27(5): 977-87.: e4.

[134] Zhang Y, Ertl HC. Starved and asphyxiated: How can CD8(+) T cells within a tumor microenvironment prevent tumor progression. Front Immunol 2016; 7: 32.

[http://dx.doi.org/10.3389/fimmu.2016.00032] [PMID: 26904023]

[135] Dang CV. MYC, metabolism, cell growth, and tumorigenesis. Cold Spring Harb Perspect Med 2013; 3(8): a014217.
[http://dx.doi.org/10.1101/cshperspect.a014217] [PMID: 23906881]

[136] Wise DR, Thompson CB. Glutamine addiction: a new therapeutic target in cancer. Trends Biochem Sci 2010; 35(8): 427-33.
[http://dx.doi.org/10.1016/j.tibs.2010.05.003] [PMID: 20570523]

[137] Wong N, De Melo J, Tang D. PKM2, a central point of regulation in cancer metabolism. Int J Cell Biol 2013; 2013: 242513.
[http://dx.doi.org/10.1155/2013/242513] [PMID: 23476652]

[138] Cantor JR, Sabatini DM. Cancer cell metabolism: one hallmark, many faces. Cancer Discov 2012; 2(10): 881-98.
[http://dx.doi.org/10.1158/2159-8290.CD-12-0345] [PMID: 23009760]

[139] Ajduković J. HIF-1--a big chapter in the cancer tale. Exp Oncol 2016; 38(1): 9-12.
[http://dx.doi.org/10.31768/2312-8852.2016.38(1):9-12] [PMID: 27031712]

[140] McDonald PC, Winum JY, Supuran CT, Dedhar S. Recent developments in targeting carbonic anhydrase IX for cancer therapeutics. Oncotarget 2012; 3(1): 84-97.
[http://dx.doi.org/10.18632/oncotarget.422] [PMID: 22289741]

[141] Viollet B, Guigas B, Sanz Garcia N, Leclerc J, Foretz M, Andreelli F. Cellular and molecular mechanisms of metformin: an overview. Clin Sci (Lond) 2012; 122(6): 253-70.
[http://dx.doi.org/10.1042/CS20110386] [PMID: 22117616]

[142] Wheaton WW, Weinberg SE, Hamanaka RB, *et al.* Metformin inhibits mitochondrial complex I of cancer cells to reduce tumorigenesis. eLife 2014; 3: e02242.
[http://dx.doi.org/10.7554/eLife.02242] [PMID: 24843020]

[143] Soliman H, Rawal B, Fulp J, *et al.* Analysis of indoleamine 2-3 dioxygenase (IDO1) expression in breast cancer tissue by immunohistochemistry. Cancer Immunol Immunother 2013; 62(5): 829-37.
[http://dx.doi.org/10.1007/s00262-013-1393-y] [PMID: 23344392]

[144] Jung KH, LoRusso P, Burris H, *et al.* Phase I study of the indoleamine 2,3-dioxygenase 1 (IDO1) inhibitor navoximod (GDC-0919) administered with PD-L1 inhibitor (atezolizumab) in advanced solid tumors. Clin Cancer Res 2019; 25(11): 3220-8.
[http://dx.doi.org/10.1158/1078-0432.CCR-18-2740] [PMID: 30770348]

CHAPTER 8

Oxidative Stress and Lifestyle-based Changes in Breast Cancer Progression

Vipendra K. Singh[1, 2] and Pradeep K. Sharma[1, 2,*]

[1] *Environmental Carcinogenesis Laboratory, Food Drug and Chemical Toxicology Group, CSIR-Indian Institute of Toxicology Research (CSIR-IITR), India*

[2] *Academy of Scientific and Innovative Research, Ghaziabad-201002, India*

Abstract: Lifestyle-based changes such as diet, physical inactivity, smoking, and alcohol consumption are some key risk factors of breast cancer among women. Changes in the lifestyle disrupt redox homeostasis, particularly decreasing the ability of the body to detoxify harmful free radicals. Therefore, an imbalance between these finely tuned mechanisms results in the formation of excessive reactive oxygen species (ROS). These elevated levels of ROS may promote breast cancer development and progression. Over the centuries, the way of living has changed drastically worldwide, and several lifestyle factors have evolved as a threat and risk factor for cancer in humans. Most of these lifestyle factors, *e.g.*, smoking, alcohol consumption, physical inactivity, poor nutrition, *etc.*, have been associated with the rise in breast cancer incidences globally. A large number of accumulating evidence from clinical and epidemiological studies strongly suggest the link between lifestyle factors and the incidence of breast cancer in women. Some changes in lifestyles increase the risk of breast cancer in both premenopausal and postmenopausal women. However, the period between menarche to the birth of the first child is the most vulnerable phase in women's lives. Lifestyle factors drive carcinogenesis through various mechanisms. Among them, ROS-mediated oxidative damage plays a significant role in breast cancer development. Here, in this chapter, we have discussed the most relevant lifestyle factors associated with breast carcinogenesis in women. Also, we have discussed how these lifestyle factors modulate redox homeostasis to elicit oxidative damage-induced carcinogenesis. A better understanding of the association between lifestyle factors and breast cancer may enable us to identify critical factors that can play a significant role in breast carcinogenesis.

Keywords: Breast cancer, Diet, Lifestyle factors, Oxidative stress, Reactive oxygen species.

* Corresponding author: Pradeep K. Sharma: Environmental Carcinogenesis Laboratory, Food, Drug, and Chemical Toxicology Group, CSIR-Indian Institute of Toxicology Research, Vishvigyan Bhawan, 31, Mahatma Gandhi Marg, Lucknow-226001, Uttar Pradesh, India; Tel: +91 5222217645; Fax +91-5222628227; E-mails: drpksiitr@gmail.com, pradeep.sharma@iitr.res.in

Shankar Suman, Garima Suman and Sanjay Mishra (Eds.)

INTRODUCTION

Lifestyle is the way of living of an individual or a population in a defined ecosystem, which is usually characterized by several parameters like geographical distribution, socioeconomic status, political, cultural and religious context, behavioral orientation, interests, and opinions, *etc.* Lifestyle is defined by a combination of intangible and physical factors and may, therefore, vary from rural to urban, low to the high socioeconomic group, and country to country. In recent decades, lifestyle has emerged as a measure of an individual's health and quality of life. Epidemiological data strongly suggest that the lifestyle is tightly associated with the health and happiness of individuals. However, an unhealthy lifestyle is a significant risk factor for a large number of diseases such as diabetes, obesity, cardiovascular disorders, hypertension, muscular-skeletal problems, and cancer.

Breast cancer is the second leading cause of cancer-related mortality and morbidity in women worldwide [1]. Approximately 2.08 million new breast cancer cases are diagnosed every year, and 0.6 million mortalities were reported worldwide in 2018 [2]. Breast cancer has emerged as the most significant cancer burden in women over the last few decades, and a large number of clinical trials are conducted on breast cancer as compared to other gynecological malignancies [3]. Genetic predisposition, mutations, oncogene activation, DNA damage, and high estrogen levels are some established risk factors for breast cancer. Most of these factors get influenced by environmental or lifestyle factors and, therefore, lifestyle patterns may play a crucial role in breast carcinogenesis. Epidemiological studies suggest that lifestyle factors play a role in the progression of breast cancer. For example, Asian females who have migrated to the US have more chances of developing breast cancer due to the changes in lifestyle and diet [4]. Approximately 5-10% of breast cancer incidences are associated with genetic defects, while 90-95% of breast cancers are due to environmental and lifestyle factors.

Interestingly, two major lifestyle factors, namely diet, and obesity contribute to approximately 30–35% and 10–20% of breast cancer incidences, respectively [5]. Lifestyle is not a single entity but characterized by a combination of several factors that define the way by which a particular individual or a population lives. Critical factors such as diet and nutrition, physical activity, other activities such as alcohol consumption, smoking, oral contraceptives, steroids, drug abuse, *etc.*, play a significant role in defining one's lifestyle. As such, there are no established criteria of a healthy lifestyle, but certain factors such as a healthy diet, physical activity, *etc.*, have been shown to protect humans from various ailments and diseases, including cancer. Changes in lifestyle factors may influence the health of an individual and link to a range of pathophysiological conditions. In this chapter, a summary of lifestyle factors and lifestyle-induced oxidative stress is presented that may underlie the mechanisms of carcinogenesis in breast tissue. Also, we have described an association between various lifestyle factors and breast cancer based on the evidence from clinical trials and epidemiological studies.

FREE RADICALS (REACTIVE OXYGEN AND NITROGEN SPECIES) AND OXIDATIVE STRESS

The existence of free radicals is well-known in chemistry since the starting of the 20th century [6], but the involvement of free radicals in the biological system was discovered in 1954 [7]. The isolation of enzyme superoxide dismutase (SOD) in 1969 tremendously increased our knowledge of free radicals biology [8]. Oxidizing free radicals such as reactive nitrogen species (RNS) and reactive oxygen species (ROS) arise from either exogenous or endogenous sources. Free radicals encompass reactive species that are derived from free oxygen and nitrogen, consisting of a large variety of reactive radicals such as superoxide anions ($O_2^{\cdot-}$), singlet oxygen ($^1O_2$), hydrogen peroxide (H_2O_2), hydroxyl radicals ($^{\cdot}OH$), organic radicals ($R^{\cdot}$), alkoxyl radicals ($RO^{\cdot}$), peroxyl radicals ($ROO^{\cdot}$), nitric oxide ($NO^{\cdot}$), ozone/trioxygen (O_3), organic hydroperoxides ($ROOH$), hypochlorite ($HOCl$), peroxynitrite (ONO^-), nitronium (NO_2^+), dinitrogen dioxide (N_2O_2), *etc.*, [9]. Both the ROS and RNS are generated as a part of naturally occurring metabolism in the body and cause oxidative damage to tissues [10].

During oxidative phosphorylation (*i.e.*, the process of ATP production) in mitochondria, ROS are generated through the leakage of electrons from the electron transport chain (ETC) directly to an oxygen molecule. The ETC chain comprises several electron donors and acceptors that carry out the transportation of free electrons to the electronegative oxygen to create a proton gradient, which is used for the production of ATP. However, during oxidative phosphorylation, not all the electrons pass through all the complexes of ETC, and some percentage of electrons leak out from the ETC and react with oxygen to form highly reactive oxygen radicals such as superoxide anions [11]. Approximately 80% of superoxide anions are generated from ETC complex I and III, and 20% from the mitochondrial matrix [9, 12, 13]. The other endogenous sources of ROS are endoplasmic reticulum and peroxisome.

ROS play a critical role in various physiological and pathological conditions, including cancer. ROS are tightly coupled to carcinogenesis, and ROS-mediated signaling is well understood in cellular transformations (as shown in Fig. **1**). Excessive ROS generation with antioxidant defense results in a physiological condition called oxidative stress. ROS have dual roles, depending on their concentration. They may exert both beneficial or harmful effects. For example, ROS can activate various signaling pathways at a low concentration that promote proliferation or survival. However, a higher level of ROS can damage or kill cells by irreversibly damaging macromolecules such as proteins, lipids, and nucleic acids [14 - 16]. Cells possess a well-defined antioxidant defense mechanism to protect themselves from oxidative insult. Cellular antioxidant protection is provided by both enzymatic and non-enzymatic antioxidants. Multiple enzymatic antioxidants (such as superoxide dismutase, catalase, glutathione peroxide, thioredoxin peroxidase, *etc.*) and non-enzymatic defense (glutathione, thioredoxin, glutaredoxin, NADPH, pyruvate, *etc.*) quench oxidative stress and render free radicals harmless [17 - 19].

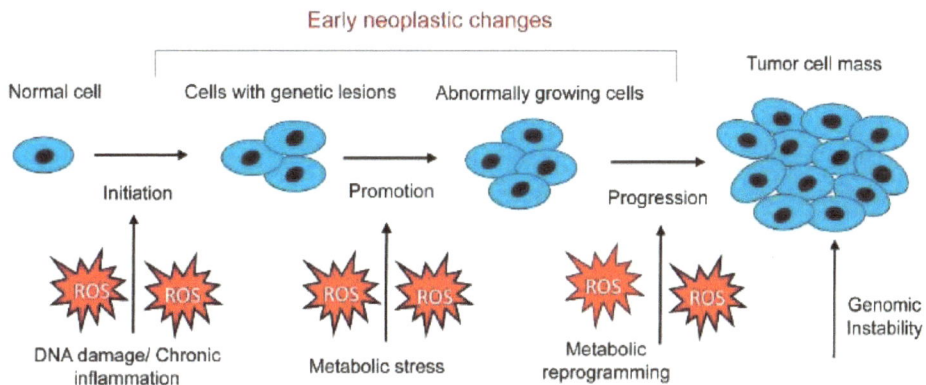

Fig. (1). Reactive oxygen species (ROS)-induced oxidative damage plays a central role in carcinogenesis. Excessive ROS due to chemical exposure, unhealthy lifestyle, or other pathologic conditions can cause oxidative damage to DNA as well as chronic inflammation in normal cells. ROS play a critical role in all the stages of carcinogenesis, from initiation to metastasis. ROS-induced genomic instability leads to altered cell cycle regulations, which subsequently give rise to an expansion of abnormally proliferating cancer cells.

ASSOCIATION AMID LIFESTYLE FACTORS, ROS, AND CANCER

Environmental and lifestyle factors such as physical activity and dietary intake are coupled to the generation of oxidative stress and affect the health of individuals throughout their life [20]. Inadequate or excessive dietary intake of nutrients enhances oxidative stress that may play a significant role in chronic diseases like cancer and metabolic disorders [21 - 23]. Nutrition is a mediator of oxidative stress and plays a substantial role in both cancer progression and cancer therapy, probably by activating several signaling cascades due to oxidative damage [24]. Oxidative DNA damage and associated signaling are central to the progression of various cancers, including breast, lung, liver, and colon, *etc.* [25 - 27]. Nutrition mediated oxidative stress is another player in carcinogenesis, which is an addition to the known carcinogens that directly interact and bind with DNA to initiate carcinogenesis. Ethanol is a known carcinogen and strongly associated with breast cancer [28, 29]. Dietary intake of alcohol leads to the production of ROS, resulting in the accumulation of acetaldehyde, a carcinogen that causes severe damage to DNA and dysfunction to other signaling molecules [30]. Folate deficiency due to alcohol abuse is also an identified risk factor for breast cancer in women [31]. Dietary intake of carbohydrates and fatty acids can also generate an oxidizing micro-environment, a potential risk factor for breast cancer, as evident in several clinical and epidemiological studies [32, 33]. Based on the observations from European Prospective Investigation into Cancer and Nutrition (EPIC) and Women's Health Initiative (WHI) studies, excessive dietary carbohydrate and glycemic burden were strongly linked with breast cancer incidences in women with ER-/PR- and ER- status [34, 35]. However, an inverse relationship between dietary uptake of fibers and breast cancer was noted in a meta-analysis [36].

Both ROS and RNS play a significant role in carcinogenesis. The sustained level of nitric oxide causes chronic inflammation, which may be mutagenic. Nitric oxide causes structural alterations in DNA, such as chromosomal alterations, mutations in DNA *via* rearrangements, deletion, insertion in base pairs, *etc.* [37, 38]. Nitric oxide is predominantly expressed in all types of tumors and regulates various types of physiological processes through multiple pathways such as soluble guanylyl-cyclase–cGMP pathway, S-nitrosylation, enhanced level of cyclooxygenase-2, hypoxia-inducible factor-1, *etc*. Moreover, activation of signaling pathways such as phosphoinositide 3-kinase/protein kinase B (PI3K/Akt), mitogen-activated protein kinase (MAPK), epidermal growth factor receptor (EGFR), and Ras-mediated transformation also underlies nitric oxide-induced cytotoxicity and genotoxicity [39, 40]. ROS/RNS-mediated oxidative stress can suppress antioxidant defense mechanisms and may further promote angiogenesis and progression of cancer [41]. Cancer cells exhibit relatively a higher level of ROS, such as superoxide anions and H_2O_2 as compared to their normal counterparts [42]. ROS serve as signaling molecules to control proliferation-related responses, including angiogenesis. Angiogenesis is primarily regulated by vascular endothelial growth factor (VEGF) that confers survival advantages to the progression of tumors. NADPH oxidase generates ROS that are involved in VEGFR2 autophosphorylation, which regulates various genes and transcription factors involved in angiogenesis [43, 44]. NADPH oxidase-mediated ROS stimulate proliferation and metastasis in endothelial cells *via* the expression of VEGF receptor type2 (VEGFR2, Flk1/KDR). Chronic oxidative stress damages DNA and induces mutations to drive carcinogenesis [45]. Recent studies related to oxidative stress suggest that lifestyle factors such as poor nutritional profile like high fat intake and low antioxidant enhance ROS level [46]. Unhealthy or sedentary lifestyles such as poor nutrition, smoking, obesity, and physical inactivity, *etc*. can alter redox homeostasis [47]. Studies have shown that obese people with a high intake of fatty diets may experience more acute oxidative stress as compared to non-obese individuals [48]. The interplay between lifestyle factors, generation of oxidative stress, and the progression of breast cancer is summarized in Fig. (**2**).

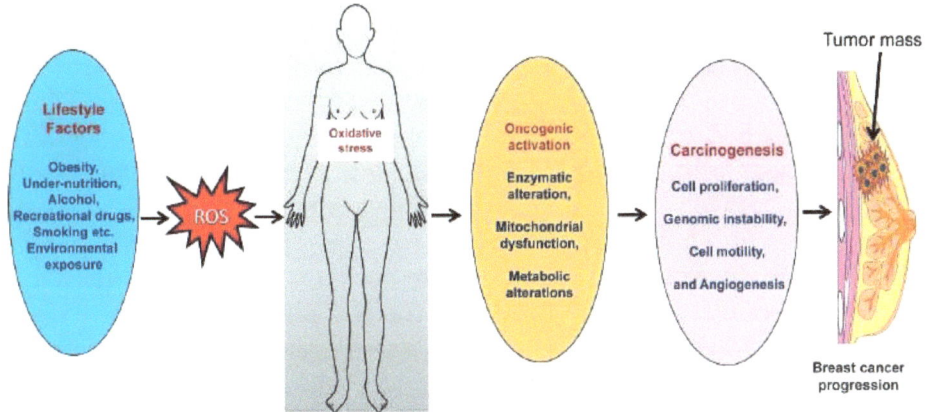

Fig. (2). Lifestyle is tightly coupled to the generation or accumulation of ROS, resulting in various pathophysiological conditions, including cancer. Some lifestyle factors such as obesity, alcohol consumption, recreational drugs, smoking, physical inactivity, poor nutrition, and diet, *etc.*, can cause generation or accumulation of reactive oxygen species irreversibly in the human body. Oxidative stress-induced by enhanced ROS leads to various cellular alterations such as oncogenic activation, genomic instability, angiogenesis, *etc.* that play a significant role in ROS-mediated carcinogenesis in different organs and tissues, including breast cancer.

LIFESTYLE FACTORS AND RISK FOR BREAST CANCER: EVIDENCE FROM EPIDEMIOLOGICAL AND CLINICAL STUDIES

Cancer-related deaths are the leading cause of mortality worldwide in women of all income groups. The burden of cancer is rising across the globe due to the increased life expectancy and aging of the population. Interestingly, cancer burden in low-middle income countries is also growing nowadays as the general public health has improved in these countries due to effective control of infectious diseases and reduction in maternal and childhood mortality in the recent past. Cancer risk factors other than genetic predispositions and mutations such as smoking, obesity, low or no physical activity, and changes in reproductive life patterns, such as late age pregnancies and childbirths have become quite prevalent in low-income countries also and therefore rate of cancer incidence and its related deaths are increasing in these countries as well. Various established modifiable (lifestyle) and non-modifiable (genetic) factors that increase the risk of breast cancer include a family history, BRCA1 or 2 mutations, reproductive factors (early age at menarche, late menopause, and late age at first full-term pregnancy), smoking, alcohol drinking, physical inactivity, obesity, use of oral contraceptives and menopausal hormone replacement therapy, and exposure to high-dose radiation. Here, in this chapter, we describe the link between several common modifiable lifestyle factors and breast cancer.

Physical Inactivity and Breast Cancer

Any bodily movement that uses skeletal muscles and consumes energy can be defined as physical activity. Physical activity maintains a balance between the number of calories consumed and the number of calories burnt. Inadequate physical activity has been convincingly linked to increased risk of various disorders such as obesity, diabetes, and cancers, including breast cancer. Earlier observations on reduced risk of breast cancer in athletes led scientists to explore the plausible connection between physical activity and breast cancer etiology [49, 50]. Various clinical studies have shown a decreasing trend of breast cancer incidence in a population of females with higher physical activity [51 - 58]. However, some studies have also suggested that there is no association between physical activity and the risk of breast cancer [59 - 62]. Complications in measuring physical activity and inconsistent observations and other anthropogenic factors may partly be related to this non-correlation.

Moreover, only a limited number of clinical studies have been performed so far to assess the association between physical activity and the risk of breast cancer in women. Some case-control studies have been reported to suggest physical inactivity as a plausible risk factor in breast cancer. Regular physical activity reduces the risk of breast cancer in women [55]. Both vigorous and moderate physical activities have been shown to interrupt the menstrual cycle and may, therefore, reduce the level as well exposure to endogenous hormones such as estrogens and progesterone, thereby inhibiting carcinogenesis in breast tissues. However, evidence showing the direct effect of breast carcinogenesis is obscure and needs to be evaluated thoroughly. Determining the impact of physical activity is a challenging task and whether or not a certain type(s) or duration of exercise have an impact on curbing breast cancer incidence is not well known so far. However, the data suggest a considerable risk of breast cancer in women with poor physical activity or a sedentary lifestyle. Moreover, physical activity performed in the premenopausal age is more beneficial in preventing cancer [63 - 66].

Obesity and Breast Cancer

Estrogens play an essential role in the etiology of breast cancer [67]. The molecular evidence of estrogenic carcinogenesis is poorly known. Past evidence showed that excess estrogen exposure is directly proportional to the generation of ROS through the estrogen receptor or the alteration of metabolic pathways and

DNA damage in breast cancer [68]. Scientific evidence linked excess body weight with breast cancer, but there is no common consensus on this correlation [69]. According to Chan *et al.*, obesity is a serious concern that affects hundreds of millions of people across the globe [70]. Lifestyle-based changes such as western lifestyle are associated with both obesity and overweight, which are associated with poorer overall breast cancer survival in pre- and postmenopausal breast cancer [70]. Increased oxidative stress is associated with obesity, and a high level of ROS has been shown to denature macromolecules such as lipids, proteins, and nucleic acids that lead to genetic instability driven neoplastic changes in breast cells and tissues *via* triggering the oncogenic PI3K/AKT pathway [71]. Gene polymorphism has also been associated with obesity as well as breast cancer.

Moreover, mutations in BRCA1 and BRCA2 [72], phosphatase and tensin homologs (PTEN) [73], as well as serine-threonine kinase-11 (STK11/LKB1) [74], and cadherin 1-type 1 (CDH1) genes [75] are also tightly associated with breast cancer. However, the role of these mutations is relatively unknown in the context of obesity. Genetic predisposition due to hereditary factors may account for the inter-individual differences that enhance the vulnerability of breast cancer in developed countries; however, the impact of mutations appears to be implicated in less than 10% of all breast cancer patients [76]. The role of obesity-related genes in breast cancer initiation is poorly known, and only a few studies have reported that obesity-related genes stimulated the benign breast disease to an aggressiveness form of cancer. Simone *et al.*, described several polymorphisms in obesity-associated genes coupled to the unpredictable risk of breast cancer occurrence [77].

Alcohol Consumption and Breast Cancer

Alcohol consumption is one of the integral parts of daily lifestyle in western countries, and this trend is also increasing in Asian countries like India. The significant acute ill effects of alcohol drinking on humans are liver diseases, impaired cognitive behavior, blurred vision, poor judgment or decision making, and, most importantly, humans with regular intake get addicted to alcoholic drinks [78 - 86]. On the other hand, chronic exposure to alcohol may increase the risk of various types of cancers [87]. International Agency for Research on Cancer (IARC) has categorized ethanol as a probable carcinogen and is causally related to the risk of several types of cancers, including breast cancer [88]. Epidemiological evidence and experimental data suggest a clear link between alcohol intake and the chance of breast cancer incidence in adult women consuming at least 10 g of alcohol daily [89 - 93]. The risk of alcohol-induced breast cancer has been noted equally in both pre- and postmenopausal women [94, 95]. The risk of breast cancer usually increases upto 15% in women with low alcohol intake, while no such increase in the risk of cancer to other organs is noted [90, 96, 97]. The aforementioned data indicates the higher susceptibility of breast tissue for developing cancer upon alcohol exposure in adult women.

Alcohol consumption during adolescence and premenopause is significantly associated with the risk of breast cancer. However, the highest risk has been observed in women below the age of 30, up to 34% of increased risk for the intake of every 13g/day alcohol (≈1 drink/day) [98 - 101]. Women who abstain from alcohol have less chances of breast cancer than those with alcohol intake of ≥ 15g/ day before their first pregnancy [93, 100]. The threat of breast cancer further increases in women having a considerably more extended period between menarche and first pregnancy. For every 10 g/day of alcohol consumption, the risk of breast cancer increases by up to 14% in women with an interval of fewer than 14 years between the menarche and their first pregnancy. Interestingly, the risk further increases by 25% among the women having a gap of more than 15 years between the menarche and their first pregnancy.

Moreover, the drinking pattern, such as binge drinking ie. drinking four or more drinks in one sitting, may also increase the risk of breast cancer in women significantly [100]. As per the study, the intake of alcohol before the diagnosis of breast cancer is considered a significant risk factor, and some cohort and case-control studies have also suggested that alcohol intake is associated with cancer recurrence [102]. All in all, studies conducted so far have shown positive, negative, and no correlation between alcohol intake and breast cancer incidence in women [100]. Similarly, mixed results are also reported with alcohol intake and breast cancer recurrence.

Alcohol can influence the threat of breast cancer, probably by altering estrogen metabolism and increasing endogenous estrogen levels in both pre- and postmenopausal women. Moreover, alcohol (ethanol) gets oxidized and metabolized into a potent carcinogen, namely acetaldehyde *via* the action of alcohol dehydrogenase (ALDH) and cytochrome P450 2E1 (CYP2E1) [103]. Acetaldehyde strongly binds to DNA and forms DNA adducts resulting in DNA cross-linking and mutations [91, 100, 104]. Also, acetaldehyde interferes with the repair mechanism involved in the repairing of oxidative DNA damage [105]. Several *in vitro* and *in vivo* studies have demonstrated that ethanol promotes mammary carcinogenesis, stimulates cell proliferation, migration, invasion, and epithelial-mesenchymal transition in breast cancer cells [90, 92, 106 - 110].

Human breast cancer cells or mammary epithelial cells that exhibit high expression of receptor tyrosine-protein kinase ErbB2 respond quickly to ethanol and stimulate cell invasion and ROS generation [108, 111, 112]. Epidemiological studies show that alcohol intake is associated with highly invasive breast carcinoma, suggesting that alcohol may also regulate the invasiveness of breast cancer. Matrix metalloproteinases (MMPs) are known to be involved in carcinogenesis and malignant transformation, and several studies have demonstrated that MMPs are the target of ethanol [107, 108, 113]. Therefore, ethanol-induced modulation in MMPs expression might play a significant role in disease metastasis and recurrence.

Smoking and Breast Cancer

Tobacco smoke is highly carcinogenic and primarily an etiological factor for lung cancer in both males and females worldwide [114]. Tobacco smoking-induced risk of breast cancer is mostly inconsistent across the globe [114 - 117]. However, recent epidemiological studies support the decisive role of smoking in breast carcinogenesis with the highest risk in female smokers who begin smoking at early adolescence or who have been a chronic smoker before the first pregnancy [118 - 120]. In a very recent multi-ethnic cohort study, this risk of breast cancer related to smoking was found to be similar across the racial/ethnic groups and estrogen receptor-positive (ER+) and progesterone-receptor positive (PR+) subtypes. These observations indicate that smoking may be a significant risk factor for breast cancer [121]. In another collaborative cohort study in African-American women, the relationship between the risk of breast cancer and cigarette smoking depending on menopausal status was studied. The risk of breast cancer was higher in postmenopausal women with a smoking duration of more than 20 years and also was more apparent in the ER^+ phenotype.

Interestingly, no such correlation was reported in the premenopausal women between the duration and intensity of smoking and the risk of breast cancer. Moreover, these results were similar in different subtypes such as ER+, ER- and triple-negative breast cancers [122]. Several other cohorts and population-based case-control studies have also established a significant linkage between tobacco smoking and the threat of breast cancer [123 - 127]. However, the results obtained from studies on the association of breast cancer risk with tobacco smoking in pre- or postmenopausal women are mixed [117, 128].

Radiation Exposure and Breast Cancer

The mammary gland is quite sensitive to ionizing radiation-associated carcinogenesis, particularly at an early age [129, 130]. Data from several epidemiological studies obtained from cohort or population-based studies on radiation exposure from medical exposures and Japanese atomic bomb survivors demonstrated an increased risk of breast cancer. Medical radiations (diagnostic or therapeutic) account for up to 14% of all radiation exposure, including low dose diagnostic X-rays (10 mGy) to high dose radiation (20-60 Gy; for therapy in cancer) [130, 131]. Epidemiological data from long-term follow-up studies of the medically exposed population revealed that the increased risk was noted among the patients who were exposed to high-dose radiations during radiotherapy for Hodgkin lymphoma [132, 133], or breast cancer [134 - 136] or childhood cancer survivors exposed to high dose chest radiations [137, 138]. The risk of developing cancer also increases in the population undergoing radiotherapy for the enlarged thymus gland during infancy or childhood, skin hemangioma, and other medical conditions like scoliosis, tuberculosis, *etc.*, [139 - 143]. Follow-up of the Japanese population who survived after the atomic bomb explosion also revealed similar trends in breast cancer risk following high exposure to radiation. The risk was the highest in women below the age of 20 years exposed to radiation, and this risk further increases due to an increase in the dose of exposure at this age [129, 144].

Moreover, women with large breasts might be at a higher risk of radiation-induced breast cancer [145]. After reanalyzing the dosimetry in a cohort (Swedish hemangioma)-based study, Eidemüller *et al.*, reported that the chance of developing breast cancer is high in women after exposure to radiations. The Swedish hemangioma cohort is a unique radio-epidemiological cohort where subjects from the very first exposure to radiation after birth to the age of 18 months were available and this cohort was ideal for the study of radiation-induced risk assessment after exposure in infancy or early ages during their lifetime [146]. However, no data suggest whether radiation exposure enhanced the frequency in the genetically predisposed population and also whether the low dose exposure during diagnostic chest X-ray contributes to breast carcinogenesis [130, 147, 148].

Furthermore, limited data are available that can correlate breast cancer risk in women who are exposed to low dose radiations during the diagnosis of other clinical conditions such as pneumonia, interstitial lung disease, *etc.* For a better understanding of the risk of breast cancer due to low-dose radiation exposure, more studies on large populations are warranted. Overall, based on the epidemiological data, ionizing radiation is an established risk factor for breast cancer. The risk of breast cancer has been shown to increase linearly with the increase in radiation dose. The window of highest susceptibility to radiation-induced breast cancer is seen for females of young age (*i.e.*, exposed before 20 years of the age) while women exposed after menopause were found to be at reduced risk of developing breast cancer. However, determining the role of radiation-induced genomic instability in breast carcinogenesis is quite challenging and needs to be studied further at the molecular level to consider it as a risk factor for breast cancer.

Vitamin D and Breast Cancer

Vitamin D plays an essential role in maintaining calcium homeostasis, bone metabolism, and other physiological systems such as reproductive system, cardiovascular system, and immune system. Deficiency of vitamin D is quite common worldwide nowadays and contributes to serious health concerns like diabetes, arthritis, osteoporosis, bone fractures, *etc.* [149]. The high serum concentration of vitamin D is linked inversely with many cancers, including breast cancer. Vitamin D plays a vital role in milk production and calcium transport during lactation in mammary glands by interacting with vitamin D receptor (VDR) [150]. Serum concentrations of vitamin D have been shown to protect against breast cancer [151]. Various case-controlled epidemiological studies have demonstrated an inverse relationship between high vitamin D concentration and breast cancer risk in women [152 - 158]. Chen *et al.* have also revealed that a higher serum concentration of 25-hydroxyvitamin D (25(OH) D) is linked with the reduced risk of breast cancer in women [159]. A case-control study also suggested a positive correlation in postmenopausal women than premenopausal women [160]. However, serum deficiency of vitamin D is reported to increase the risk of breast cancer in both premenopausal and postmenopausal women [156, 161]. A large number of case-control studies, meta-analysis and pooled studies have established a significant linkage between the deficiency of vitamin D and breast cancer incidences. However, a limited number of randomized controlled trials (RCTs) have also supported an inverse relationship between vitamin D deficiency and breast cancer [162, 163]. Therefore, due to the limited availability of studies, it is quite challenging to conclude the role of vitamin D and risk of breast cancer and needs more RCTs to be conducted worldwide with proper study design. In a recent study, a revised model has been developed that can be used in planning and evaluating vitamin D related RCTs for breast cancer incidence [164].

In a study, the level of vitamin D was measured at the time of the diagnosis of breast cancer and the study reported that a high serum level of vitamin D at the time of early breast cancer diagnosis was associated with smaller tumor size, better overall survival rate and improved cancer-specific outcomes particularly in postmenopausal women [165]. Whereas, a concentration of 25 (OH) D <20 ng/mL was linked with poor prognosis and these patients developed metastasis frequently, and approximately 73% died due to advanced disease [166]. Interestingly, in early-stage breast cancer, the level of 25 (OH) D was found to be significantly higher than the advanced stage cancer patients [167]. In most of the studies, a low level of 25 (OH) D was highly associated with the smaller tumor size, lower grade as well as lesser metastatic disease in both pre- as well as postmenopausal patients [168 - 170]. However, some exceptional studies have also shown that there is no correlation between the level of serum 25 (OH) D and breast cancer risk [171]. This inconsistency may be due to the limited sample size that has been considered in studies correlating the risk of breast cancer and lifestyle and ethnicity. Moreover, menopausal status is also closely related to the level of vitamin D; therefore, polymorphism of VDR must be considered in meta-analysis studies.

Various *in vitro* and animal studies have suggested a linkage between vitamin D and the risk of breast cancer. Interestingly, these studies have demonstrated the anticancer role of vitamin D, where it exerts both anti-proliferative and pro-apoptotic actions [172 - 174]. Upon binding to VDR, vitamin D enhances the level of pro-apoptotic proteins (*e.g.*, Bax and Bak) and also diminishes the expression of anti-apoptotic proteins (*e.g.* Bcl-2/Bcl-XL) [174]. The enzymatic reaction carried out by 1-α-hydroxylase in breast tissue generates active vitamin D metabolite from its circulating precursor (25 hydroxyvitamin D). Moreover, the presence of VDR in breast tissues suggests an autocrine action of vitamin D [175]. Vitamin D can regulate the transcription of multiple genes that can restrict growth inhibitory and antineoplastic effects on cells [150, 176]. Low vitamin D level results in the growth and development of cancer and neo-angiogenesis. Studies with VDR knockout animals have also shown an increase in the rate of preneoplastic lesions in mammary tissues [177]. A recent study has explained that vitamin D receptor regulates autophagy in the healthy mammary epithelial cells and luminal breast cancer cells and could serve as a potential mechanism for cancer prevention. This further strengthens the and between vitamin D linkbreast cancer [178]. So far, most of the studies on vitamin D and breast cancer risk showed that deficiency of vitamin D is correlated with increased risk of breast cancer in both pre- and postmenopausal women. Moreover, the reduced vitamin D level also correlated well with disease aggressiveness and poor prognosis in breast cancer patients. However, some inconsistent reports are also available, which show that increased serum concentration of 25 (OH) D is linked to a higher risk of breast cancer [179]. Therefore, there is a need to design better RCTs that may address the linkage between vitamin D and the risk of breast cancer.

Oral Contraceptives and Breast Cancer

Oral contraceptives are hormone-containing pills that are taken orally to prevent unwanted pregnancies. These hormone-containing pills inhibit ovulation as well as block the sperm from penetrating the cervix. Epidemiological data from the nurses' health study, which had approximately 116,000 female nurses between the ages group of 24 to 43 years enrolled in the study in 1989, suggested that the participants who used oral contraceptives had a slightly higher risk of breast cancer [180, 181]. However, the correlation between breast cancer and oral contraceptives is poorly known. The epidemiological studies suggest that postmenopausal women who take oral contraceptives before menopause have a higher breast cancer incidence [182, 183]. Premenopausal women who have used hormonal contraceptives for longer times than the women who have used oral contraceptives for short periods are at higher risk of developing breast cancer [180, 184, 185].

SUMMARY

Lifestyle factors are associated with various pathophysiological disorders. Interestingly, most of the metabolic diseases such as diabetes, obesity, thyroid dysfunction, vascular disorders, *etc.*, are influenced by the change in lifestyle. Most importantly, cancer also occurs due to the change in lifestyle factors. In the past few decades, lifestyle factors have gained much importance as a threat for several malignancies, including breast cancer. Some lifestyle factors, *e.g.*, diet, obesity, alcohol consumption, tobacco use, vitamin D, oral contraceptives, *etc.* have been found to be associated with the increased incidence of different types of cancers. These lifestyle factors are coupled with oxidative stress, which is central to carcinogenesis induced by them. A large number of accumulating evidence have revealed that the reactive oxygen species alter cellular metabolisms that play a central role in the progression of breast cancer. Lifestyle-based carcinogenesis is significantly associated with acute or chronic levels of oxidative stress. An unhealthy lifestyle, and the onset of menstruation at an early age lead to obesity in adult life and thus pose a significant threat to develop breast cancer in women. In the past few decades, several epidemiological and clinical studies have been conducted that signify the carcinogenic role of various lifestyle factors in both pre- and postmenopausal women. Moreover, the period between menarche to the birth of the first child in women represents the most sensitive period for the risk of breast cancer. Various lifestyle factors such as obesity, diet, vitamin D deficiency, alcohol consumption, *etc.*, affect women in this phase, thereby increasing the rate of breast cancer incidence. Some lifestyle factors such as obesity also play a role in the prognosis of this disease as premenopausal obesity is highly associated with aggressive cancer with poor prognosis. Several randomized controlled trials have shown that a healthier lifestyle, higher level of physical activity, less alcohol consumption, abstinence from smoking and, a healthy and nutritious diet can prevent women from the risk of breast cancer. Also, these modifiable risk factors also play a role in the patients' post-treatment by preventing recurrence and metastasis. By adopting a healthy lifestyle, indeed, we can curtail the rate of breast cancer incidence as a number of clinical evidence indicate that individuals with a balanced lifestyle are at a lower risk of developing cancer. Though individual risk factor-based studies have been conducted in the past, studies focusing on multiple co-existing components of the lifestyle are quite limited.

Also, it is quite challenging to determine the role of lifestyle factors in carcinogenesis as large numbers of studies with extended duration are required to comprehend the risk. For this, some comprehensive and comparative randomized trials are needed to be performed on different population groups for a considerably longer duration. A better understanding of the interplay between lifestyle factors and the risk of breast cancer might play a significant role in reducing the incidence of cancer in women worldwide.

ABBREVIATIONS

ROS	Reactive oxygen species
Bcl-2	B-cell lymphoma-2
ER+	Estrogen receptor-positive
PR+	Progesterone receptor-positive
RNS	Reactive nitrogen species
PTEN	Phosphatase and tensin homologs
SOD	Superoxide dismutase
EPIC	European Prospective Investigation into Cancer and Nutrition
WHI	Women's Health Initiative
BRCA1	Breast cancer 1
MMPs	Matrix metalloproteinases
mGy	milligray
RCTs	Randomized controlled trials
VDR	Vitamin D receptor
ETC	Electron transport chain
IARC	International Agency for Research on Cancer
PI3K/Akt	Phosphoinositide 3-kinase/protein kinase B
MAPK	Mitogen-activated protein kinase
EGFR	Epidermal growth factor receptor
ALDH	Alcohol dehydrogenase

CONSENT FOR PUBLICATION

Not applicable.

CONFLICT OF INTEREST

The authors confirm that the contents of this chapter have no conflict of interest.

ACKNOWLEDGEMENT

Vipendra Kumar Singh is a recipient of the DST-INSPIRE senior research fellowship.

REFERENCES

[1]   Siegel RL, Miller KD, Jemal A. Cancer statistics, 2018. CA Cancer J Clin 2018; 68(1): 7-30.
       [http://dx.doi.org/10.3322/caac.21442] [PMID: 29313949]

[2]   Bray F, Ferlay J, Soerjomataram I, Siegel RL, Torre LA, Jemal A. Global cancer statistics 2018: GLOBOCAN estimates of incidence and mortality worldwide for 36 cancers in 185 countries. CA Cancer J Clin 2018; 68(6): 394-424.
       [http://dx.doi.org/10.3322/caac.21492] [PMID: 30207593]

[3]   Dieterich M, Stubert J, Reimer T, Erickson N, Berling A. Influence of lifestyle factors on breast cancer risk. Breast Care (Basel) 2014; 9(6): 407-14.
       [http://dx.doi.org/10.1159/000369571] [PMID: 25759623]

[4]   Ziegler RG, Hoover RN, Pike MC, *et al.* Migration patterns and breast cancer risk in Asian-American women. J Natl Cancer Inst 1993; 85(22): 1819-27.
       [http://dx.doi.org/10.1093/jnci/85.22.1819] [PMID: 8230262]

[5]   Anand P, Kunnumakkara AB, Sundaram C, *et al.* Cancer is a preventable disease that requires major lifestyle changes. Pharm Res 2008; 25(9): 2097-116.
       [http://dx.doi.org/10.1007/s11095-008-9661-9] [PMID: 18626751]

[6]   Gomberg M. An instance of trivalent carbon: Triphenylmethyl. J Am Chem Soc 1900; 22(11): 757-71.
       [http://dx.doi.org/10.1021/ja02049a006]

[7]   Commoner B, Townsend J, Pake GE. Free radicals in biological materials. Nature 1954; 174(4432): 689-91.
       [http://dx.doi.org/10.1038/174689a0] [PMID: 13213980]

[8]   McCord JM, Fridovich I. Superoxide dismutase. An enzymic function for erythrocuprein (hemocuprein). J Biol Chem 1969; 244(22): 6049-55.
       [PMID: 5389100]

[9]   Liou GY, Storz P. Reactive oxygen species in cancer. Free Radic Res 2010; 44(5): 479-96.
       [http://dx.doi.org/10.3109/10715761003667554] [PMID: 20370557]

[10]   Pan MH, Ho CT. Chemopreventive effects of natural dietary compounds on cancer development. Chem Soc Rev 2008; 37(11): 2558-74.
       [http://dx.doi.org/10.1039/b801558a] [PMID: 18949126]

[11]   Sarniak A, Lipińska J, Tytman K, Lipińska S. Endogenous mechanisms of reactive oxygen species (ROS) generation. Postepy Hig Med Dosw 2016; 70(0): 1150-65.
       [http://dx.doi.org/10.5604/17322693.1224259] [PMID: 27892899]

[12]   Han D, Williams E, Cadenas E. Mitochondrial respiratory chain-dependent generation of superoxide anion and its release into the intermembrane space. Biochem J 2001; 353(Pt 2): 411-6.
       [http://dx.doi.org/10.1042/bj3530411] [PMID: 11139407]

[13]   Kumari S, Badana AK, G MM, G S, Malla R. Reactive oxygen species: A key constituent in cancer survival. Biomark Insights 2018; 13: 1177271918755391.
       [http://dx.doi.org/10.1177/1177271918755391] [PMID: 29449774]

[14]   Gill JG, Piskounova E, Morrison SJ. Cancer, Oxidative Stress, and Metastasis. Cold Spring Harb Symp Quant Biol 2016; 81: 163-75.
       [http://dx.doi.org/10.1101/sqb.2016.81.030791] [PMID: 28082378]

[15]   Hippert MM, O'Toole PS, Thorburn A. Autophagy in cancer: good, bad, or both? Cancer Res 2006; 66(19): 9349-51.
[http://dx.doi.org/10.1158/0008-5472.CAN-06-1597] [PMID: 17018585]

[16]   Di Meo S, Reed TT, Venditti P, Victor VM. Role of ROS and RNS Sources in Physiological and Pathological Conditions. Oxid Med Cell Longev 2016; 2016: 1245049.
[http://dx.doi.org/10.1155/2016/1245049] [PMID: 27478531]

[17]   Devasagayam TP, Tilak JC, Boloor KK, Sane KS, Ghaskadbi SS, Lele RD. Free radicals and antioxidants in human health: current status and future prospects. J Assoc Physicians India 2004; 52: 794-804.
[PMID: 15909857]

[18]   Valko M, Leibfritz D, Moncol J, Cronin MT, Mazur M, Telser J. Free radicals and antioxidants in normal physiological functions and human disease. Int J Biochem Cell Biol 2007; 39(1): 44-84.
[http://dx.doi.org/10.1016/j.biocel.2006.07.001] [PMID: 16978905]

[19]   Patlevič P, Vašková J, Švorc P Jr, Vaško L, Švorc P. Reactive oxygen species and antioxidant defense in human gastrointestinal diseases. Integr Med Res 2016; 5(4): 250-8.
[http://dx.doi.org/10.1016/j.imr.2016.07.004] [PMID: 28462126]

[20]   Lambrinoudaki I, Ceasu I, Depypere H, *et al.* EMAS position statement: Diet and health in midlife and beyond. Maturitas 2013; 74(1): 99-104.
[http://dx.doi.org/10.1016/j.maturitas.2012.10.019] [PMID: 23200515]

[21]   Saha SK, Lee SB, Won J, *et al.* Correlation between Oxidative Stress, Nutrition, and Cancer Initiation. Int J Mol Sci 2017; 18(7): E1544.
[http://dx.doi.org/10.3390/ijms18071544] [PMID: 28714931]

[22]   World Cancer Research Fund / American Institute for Cancer Research. Food, Nutrition, Physical Activity, and the Prevention of Cancer: a Global Perspective. Washington, DC: AICR 2007.

[23]   Wellen KE, Thompson CB. Cellular metabolic stress: considering how cells respond to nutrient excess. Mol Cell 2010; 40(2): 323-32.
[http://dx.doi.org/10.1016/j.molcel.2010.10.004] [PMID: 20965425]

[24]   Diamanti-Kandarakis E, Papalou O, Kandaraki EA, Kassi G. MECHANISMS IN ENDOCRINOLOGY: Nutrition as a mediator of oxidative stress in metabolic and reproductive disorders in women. Eur J Endocrinol 2017; 176(2): R79-99.
[http://dx.doi.org/10.1530/EJE-16-0616] [PMID: 27678478]

[25]   Lee JD, Cai Q, Shu XO, Nechuta SJ. The role of biomarkers of oxidative stress in breast cancer risk and prognosis: a systematic review of the epidemiologic literature. J Womens Health (Larchmt) 2017; 26(5): 467-82.
[http://dx.doi.org/10.1089/jwh.2016.5973] [PMID: 28151039]

[26]   Saijo H, Hirohashi Y, Torigoe T, *et al.* Plasticity of lung cancer stem-like cells is regulated by the transcription factor HOXA5 that is induced by oxidative stress. Oncotarget 2016; 7(31): 50043-56.
[http://dx.doi.org/10.18632/oncotarget.10571] [PMID: 27418136]

[27]   Wang Z, Li Z, Ye Y, Xie L, Li W. Oxidative stress and liver cancer: etiology and therapeutic targets. Oxid Med Cell Longev 2016; 2016: 7891574.
[http://dx.doi.org/10.1155/2016/7891574] [PMID: 27957239]

[28]   Brooks PJ, Zakhari S. Moderate alcohol consumption and breast cancer in women: from epidemiology to mechanisms and interventions. Alcohol Clin Exp Res 2013; 37(1): 23-30.
[http://dx.doi.org/10.1111/j.1530-0277.2012.01888.x] [PMID: 23072454]

[29]   Arranz S, Chiva-Blanch G, Valderas-Martínez P, Medina-Remón A, Lamuela-Raventós RM, Estruch R. Wine, beer, alcohol and polyphenols on cardiovascular disease and cancer. Nutrients 2012; 4(7): 759-81.
[http://dx.doi.org/10.3390/nu4070759] [PMID: 22852062]

[30]   Kandi S, Deshpande N, Pinnelli VBK, Devaki R, Rao P, Ramana K. Alcoholism and its role in the development of oxidative stress and DNA damage: An Insight. Am J Med Sci Med 2014; 2: 64-6.
[http://dx.doi.org/10.12691/ajmsm-2-3-3]

[31]   Varela-Rey M, Woodhoo A, Martinez-Chantar ML, Mato JM, Lu SC. Alcohol, DNA methylation, and cancer. Alcohol Res 2013; 35(1): 25-35.
[PMID: 24313162]

[32]   Gregersen S, Samocha-Bonet D, Heilbronn LK, Campbell LV. Inflammatory and oxidative stress responses to high-carbohydrate and high-fat meals in healthy humans. J Nutr Metab 2012; 2012: 238056.
[http://dx.doi.org/10.1155/2012/238056] [PMID: 22474579]

[33]   Michels KB, Mohllajee AP, Roset-Bahmanyar E, Beehler GP, Moysich KB. Diet and breast cancer: a review of the prospective observational studies. Cancer 2007; 109(12) (Suppl.): 2712-49.
[http://dx.doi.org/10.1002/cncr.22654] [PMID: 17503428]

[34]   Romieu I, Ferrari P, Rinaldi S, *et al.* Dietary glycemic index and glycemic load and breast cancer risk in the European Prospective Investigation into Cancer and Nutrition (EPIC). Am J Clin Nutr 2012; 96(2): 345-55.
[http://dx.doi.org/10.3945/ajcn.111.026724] [PMID: 22760570]

[35]   Shikany JM, Redden DT, Neuhouser ML, *et al.* Dietary glycemic load, glycemic index, and carbohydrate and risk of breast cancer in the Women's Health Initiative. Nutr Cancer 2011; 63(6): 899-907.
[http://dx.doi.org/10.1080/01635581.2011.587227] [PMID: 21714685]

[36]   Aune D, Chan DS, Greenwood DC, *et al.* Dietary fiber and breast cancer risk: a systematic review and meta-analysis of prospective studies. Ann Oncol 2012; 23(6): 1394-402.
[http://dx.doi.org/10.1093/annonc/mdr589] [PMID: 22234738]

[37]   Cerutti PA. Oxy-radicals and cancer. Lancet 1994; 344(8926): 862-3.
[http://dx.doi.org/10.1016/S0140-6736(94)92832-0] [PMID: 7916406]

[38]   Lala PK, Chakraborty C. Role of nitric oxide in carcinogenesis and tumour progression. Lancet Oncol 2001; 2(3): 149-56.
[http://dx.doi.org/10.1016/S1470-2045(00)00256-4] [PMID: 11902565]

[39]   Fukumura D, Kashiwagi S, Jain RK. The role of nitric oxide in tumour progression. Nat Rev Cancer 2006; 6(7): 521-34.
[http://dx.doi.org/10.1038/nrc1910] [PMID: 16794635]

[40]   Basudhar D, Somasundaram V, de Oliveira GA, *et al.* Nitric oxide synthase-2-derived nitric oxide drives multiple pathways of breast cancer progression. Antioxid Redox Signal 2017; 26(18): 1044-58.
[http://dx.doi.org/10.1089/ars.2016.6813] [PMID: 27464521]

[41]   Nourazarian AR, Kangari P, Salmaninejad A. Roles of oxidative stress in the development and progression of breast cancer. Asian Pac J Cancer Prev 2014; 15(12): 4745-51.
[http://dx.doi.org/10.7314/APJCP.2014.15.12.4745] [PMID: 24998536]

[42]   Aykin-Burns N, Ahmad IM, Zhu Y, Oberley LW, Spitz DR. Increased levels of superoxide and H2O2 mediate the differential susceptibility of cancer cells *versus* normal cells to glucose deprivation. Biochem J 2009; 418(1): 29-37.
[http://dx.doi.org/10.1042/BJ20081258] [PMID: 18937644]

[43]   Ushio-Fukai M, Nakamura Y. Reactive oxygen species and angiogenesis: NADPH oxidase as target for cancer therapy. Cancer Lett 2008; 266(1): 37-52.
[http://dx.doi.org/10.1016/j.canlet.2008.02.044] [PMID: 18406051]

[44]   Brown NS, Bicknell R. Hypoxia and oxidative stress in breast cancer. Oxidative stress: its effects on the growth, metastatic potential and response to therapy of breast cancer. Breast Cancer Res 2001; 3(5): 323-7.

[http://dx.doi.org/10.1186/bcr315] [PMID: 11597322]

[45] Sander CS, Chang H, Hamm F, Elsner P, Thiele JJ. Role of oxidative stress and the antioxidant network in cutaneous carcinogenesis. Int J Dermatol 2004; 43(5): 326-35.
[http://dx.doi.org/10.1111/j.1365-4632.2004.02222.x] [PMID: 15117361]

[46] Kang DH. Oxidative stress, DNA damage, and breast cancer. AACN Clin Issues 2002; 13(4): 540-9.
[http://dx.doi.org/10.1097/00044067-200211000-00007] [PMID: 12473916]

[47] Navab M, Gharavi N, Watson AD. Inflammation and metabolic disorders. Curr Opin Clin Nutr Metab Care 2008; 11(4): 459-64.
[http://dx.doi.org/10.1097/MCO.0b013e32830460c2] [PMID: 18542007]

[48] Bloomer RJ, Fisher-Wellman KH. Systemic oxidative stress is increased to a greater degree in young, obese women following consumption of a high fat meal. Oxid Med Cell Longev 2009; 2(1): 19-25.
[http://dx.doi.org/10.4161/oxim.2.1.7860] [PMID: 20046641]

[49] Frisch RE, Wyshak G, Albright NL, *et al.* Lower prevalence of breast cancer and cancers of the reproductive system among former college athletes compared to non-athletes. Br J Cancer 1985; 52(6): 885-91.
[http://dx.doi.org/10.1038/bjc.1985.273] [PMID: 4074640]

[50] Gammon MD, John EM, Britton JA. Recreational and occupational physical activities and risk of breast cancer. J Natl Cancer Inst 1998; 90(2): 100-17.
[http://dx.doi.org/10.1093/jnci/90.2.100] [PMID: 9450570]

[51] Pukkala E, Poskiparta M, Apter D, Vihko V. Life-long physical activity and cancer risk among Finnish female teachers. Eur J Cancer Prev 1993; 2(5): 369-76.
[http://dx.doi.org/10.1097/00008469-199309000-00002] [PMID: 8401170]

[52] Bernstein L, Henderson BE, Hanisch R, Sullivan-Halley J, Ross RK. Physical exercise and reduced risk of breast cancer in young women. J Natl Cancer Inst 1994; 86(18): 1403-8.
[http://dx.doi.org/10.1093/jnci/86.18.1403] [PMID: 8072034]

[53] Friedenreich CM, Rohan TE. Physical activity and risk of breast cancer. Eur J Cancer Prev 1995; 4(2): 145-51.
[http://dx.doi.org/10.1097/00008469-199504000-00004] [PMID: 7767240]

[54] McTiernan A, Stanford JL, Weiss NS, Daling JR, Voigt LF. Occurrence of breast cancer in relation to recreational exercise in women age 50-64 years. Epidemiology 1996; 7(6): 598-604.
[http://dx.doi.org/10.1097/00001648-199611000-00006] [PMID: 8899385]

[55] Thune I, Brenn T, Lund E, Gaard M. Physical activity and the risk of breast cancer. N Engl J Med 1997; 336(18): 1269-75.
[http://dx.doi.org/10.1056/NEJM199705013361801] [PMID: 9113929]

[56] Hu YH, Nagata C, Shimizu H, Kaneda N, Kashiki Y. Association of body mass index, physical activity, and reproductive histories with breast cancer: a case-control study in Gifu, Japan. Breast Cancer Res Treat 1997; 43(1): 65-72.
[http://dx.doi.org/10.1023/A:1005745824388] [PMID: 9065600]

[57] Coogan PF, Newcomb PA, Clapp RW, Trentham-Dietz A, Baron JA, Longnecker MP. Physical activity in usual occupation and risk of breast cancer (United States). Cancer Causes Control 1997; 8(4): 626-31.
[http://dx.doi.org/10.1023/A:1018402615206] [PMID: 9242479]

[58] Mezzetti M, La Vecchia C, Decarli A, Boyle P, Talamini R, Franceschi S. Population attributable risk for breast cancer: diet, nutrition, and physical exercise. J Natl Cancer Inst 1998; 90(5): 389-94.
[http://dx.doi.org/10.1093/jnci/90.5.389] [PMID: 9498489]

[59] Sesso HD, Paffenbarger RS Jr, Lee IM. Physical activity and breast cancer risk in the College Alumni Health Study (United States). Cancer Causes Control 1998; 9(4): 433-9.
[http://dx.doi.org/10.1023/A:1008827903302] [PMID: 9794176]

[60]   Paffenbarger RS Jr, Hyde RT, Wing AL. Physical activity and incidence of cancer in diverse populations: a preliminary report. Am J Clin Nutr 1987; 45(1) (Suppl.): 312-7.
[http://dx.doi.org/10.1093/ajcn/45.1.312] [PMID: 3799521]

[61]   Gammon MD, Schoenberg JB, Britton JA, *et al.* Recreational physical activity and breast cancer risk among women under age 45 years. Am J Epidemiol 1998; 147(3): 273-80.
[http://dx.doi.org/10.1093/oxfordjournals.aje.a009447] [PMID: 9482502]

[62]   Rockhill B, Willett WC, Hunter DJ, *et al.* Physical activity and breast cancer risk in a cohort of young women. J Natl Cancer Inst 1998; 90(15): 1155-60.
[http://dx.doi.org/10.1093/jnci/90.15.1155] [PMID: 9701365]

[63]   Wu Y, Zhang D, Kang S. Physical activity and risk of breast cancer: a meta-analysis of prospective studies. Breast Cancer Res Treat 2013; 137(3): 869-82.
[http://dx.doi.org/10.1007/s10549-012-2396-7] [PMID: 23274845]

[64]   Fournier A, Dos Santos G, Guillas G, *et al.* Recent recreational physical activity and breast cancer risk in postmenopausal women in the E3N cohort. Cancer Epidemiol Biomarkers Prev 2014; 23(9): 1893-902.
[http://dx.doi.org/10.1158/1055-9965.EPI-14-0150] [PMID: 25114017]

[65]   Hildebrand JS, Gapstur SM, Campbell PT, Gaudet MM, Patel AV. Recreational physical activity and leisure-time sitting in relation to postmenopausal breast cancer risk. Cancer Epidemiol Biomarkers Prev 2013; 22(10): 1906-12.
[http://dx.doi.org/10.1158/1055-9965.EPI-13-0407] [PMID: 24097200]

[66]   Eliassen AH, Hankinson SE, Rosner B, Holmes MD, Willett WC. Physical activity and risk of breast cancer among postmenopausal women. Arch Intern Med 2010; 170(19): 1758-64.
[http://dx.doi.org/10.1001/archinternmed.2010.363] [PMID: 20975025]

[67]   Hankinson SE, Willett WC, Manson JE, *et al.* Plasma sex steroid hormone levels and risk of breast cancer in postmenopausal women. J Natl Cancer Inst 1998; 90(17): 1292-9.
[http://dx.doi.org/10.1093/jnci/90.17.1292] [PMID: 9731736]

[68]   Mobley JA, Brueggemeier RW. Estrogen receptor-mediated regulation of oxidative stress and DNA damage in breast cancer. Carcinogenesis 2004; 25(1): 3-9.
[http://dx.doi.org/10.1093/carcin/bgg175] [PMID: 14514655]

[69]   Kruk J. Overweight, obesity, oxidative stress and the risk of breast cancer. Asian Pac J Cancer Prev 2014; 15(22): 9579-86.
[http://dx.doi.org/10.7314/APJCP.2014.15.22.9579] [PMID: 25520070]

[70]   Chan DS, Vieira AR, Aune D, *et al.* Body mass index and survival in women with breast cancer-systematic literature review and meta-analysis of 82 follow-up studies. Ann Oncol 2014; 25(10): 1901-14.
[http://dx.doi.org/10.1093/annonc/mdu042] [PMID: 24769692]

[71]   Seibold P, Hein R, Schmezer P, *et al.* Polymorphisms in oxidative stress-related genes and postmenopausal breast cancer risk. Int J Cancer 2011; 129(6): 1467-76.
[http://dx.doi.org/10.1002/ijc.25761] [PMID: 21792883]

[72]   Newman B, Austin MA, Lee M, King MC. Inheritance of human breast cancer: evidence for autosomal dominant transmission in high-risk families. Proc Natl Acad Sci USA 1988; 85(9): 3044-8.
[http://dx.doi.org/10.1073/pnas.85.9.3044] [PMID: 3362861]

[73]   García JM, Silva J, Peña C, *et al.* Promoter methylation of the PTEN gene is a common molecular change in breast cancer. Genes Chromosomes Cancer 2004; 41(2): 117-24.
[http://dx.doi.org/10.1002/gcc.20062] [PMID: 15287024]

[74]   Chen J, Lindblom A. Germline mutation screening of the STK11/LKB1 gene in familial breast cancer with LOH on 19p. Clin Genet 2000; 57(5): 394-7.
[http://dx.doi.org/10.1034/j.1399-0004.2000.570511.x] [PMID: 10852375]

[75]   Kuusisto KM, Bebel A, Vihinen M, Schleutker J, Sallinen SL. Screening for BRCA1, BRCA2, CHEK2, PALB2, BRIP1, RAD50, and CDH1 mutations in high-risk Finnish BRCA1/2-founder mutation-negative breast and/or ovarian cancer individuals. Breast Cancer Res 2011; 13(1): R20.
[http://dx.doi.org/10.1186/bcr2832] [PMID: 21356067]

[76]   Lichtenstein P, Holm NV, Verkasalo PK, *et al.* Environmental and heritable factors in the causation of cancer--analyses of cohorts of twins from Sweden, Denmark, and Finland. N Engl J Med 2000; 343(2): 78-85.
[http://dx.doi.org/10.1056/NEJM200007133430201] [PMID: 10891514]

[77]   Simone V, D'Avenia M, Argentiero A, *et al.* Obesity and Breast Cancer: Molecular Interconnections and Potential Clinical Applications. Oncologist 2016; 21(4): 404-17.
[http://dx.doi.org/10.1634/theoncologist.2015-0351] [PMID: 26865587]

[78]   Bosron WF, Li TK. Genetic polymorphism of human liver alcohol and aldehyde dehydrogenases, and their relationship to alcohol metabolism and alcoholism. Hepatology 1986; 6(3): 502-10.
[http://dx.doi.org/10.1002/hep.1840060330] [PMID: 3519419]

[79]   Gao B, Bataller R. Alcoholic liver disease: pathogenesis and new therapeutic targets. Gastroenterology 2011; 141(5): 1572-85.
[http://dx.doi.org/10.1053/j.gastro.2011.09.002] [PMID: 21920463]

[80]   Osna NA, Donohue TM Jr, Kharbanda KK. Alcoholic Liver Disease: Pathogenesis and Current Management. Alcohol Res 2017; 38(2): 147-61.
[PMID: 28988570]

[81]   Goodwin DW, Othmer E, Halikas JA, Freemon F. Loss of short term memory as a predictor of the alcoholic "blackout". Nature 1970; 227(5254): 201-2.
[http://dx.doi.org/10.1038/227201a0] [PMID: 4913709]

[82]   Kunchulia M, Pilz KS, Herzog MH. How alcohol intake affects visual temporal processing. Vision Res 2012; 66: 11-6.
[http://dx.doi.org/10.1016/j.visres.2012.06.010] [PMID: 22733012]

[83]   Camchong J, Endres M, Fein G. Decision making, risky behavior, and alcoholism. Handb Clin Neurol 2014; 125: 227-36.
[http://dx.doi.org/10.1016/B978-0-444-62619-6.00014-8] [PMID: 25307578]

[84]   Ferraguti G, Pascale E, Lucarelli M. Alcohol addiction: a molecular biology perspective. Curr Med Chem 2015; 22(6): 670-84.
[http://dx.doi.org/10.2174/0929867321666141229103158] [PMID: 25544474]

[85]   Azevedo CA, Mammis A. Neuromodulation therapies for alcohol addiction: a literature review. Neuromodulation 2018; 21(2): 144-8.
[http://dx.doi.org/10.1111/ner.12548] [PMID: 28055126]

[86]   Rehm J. The risks associated with alcohol use and alcoholism. Alcohol Res Health 2011; 34(2): 135-43.
[PMID: 22330211]

[87]   LoConte NK, Brewster AM, Kaur JS, Merrill JK, Alberg AJ. Alcohol and cancer: a statement of the american society of clinical oncology. J Clin Oncol 2018; 36(1): 83-93.
[http://dx.doi.org/10.1200/JCO.2017.76.1155] [PMID: 29112463]

[88]   IARC Working Group on the Evaluation of Carcinogenic Risk to Humans. Alcohol consumption and ethyl carbamate. Lyon (FR): international agency for research on cancer. IARC Monogr Eval Carcinog Risks Hum 2010; 96: 3-1383.

[89]   Chen WY, Rosner B, Hankinson SE, Colditz GA, Willett WC. Moderate alcohol consumption during adult life, drinking patterns, and breast cancer risk. JAMA 2011; 306(17): 1884-90.
[http://dx.doi.org/10.1001/jama.2011.1590] [PMID: 22045766]

[90]   Seitz HK, Pelucchi C, Bagnardi V, La Vecchia C. Epidemiology and pathophysiology of alcohol and breast cancer: Update 2012. Alcohol Alcohol 2012; 47(3): 204-12.
[http://dx.doi.org/10.1093/alcalc/ags011] [PMID: 22459019]

[91]   Dumitrescu RG, Shields PG. The etiology of alcohol-induced breast cancer. Alcohol 2005; 35(3): 213-25.
[http://dx.doi.org/10.1016/j.alcohol.2005.04.005] [PMID: 16054983]

[92]   Singletary KW, Gapstur SM. Alcohol and breast cancer: review of epidemiologic and experimental evidence and potential mechanisms. JAMA 2001; 286(17): 2143-51.
[http://dx.doi.org/10.1001/jama.286.17.2143] [PMID: 11694156]

[93]   Smith-Warner SA, Spiegelman D, Yaun SS, *et al.* Alcohol and breast cancer in women: a pooled analysis of cohort studies. JAMA 1998; 279(7): 535-40.
[http://dx.doi.org/10.1001/jama.279.7.535] [PMID: 9480365]

[94]   Liu Y, Tamimi RM, Colditz GA, Bertrand KA. Alcohol consumption across the life course and mammographic density in premenopausal women. Breast Cancer Res Treat 2018; 167(2): 529-35.
[http://dx.doi.org/10.1007/s10549-017-4517-9] [PMID: 28952004]

[95]   Flom JD, Ferris JS, Tehranifar P, Terry MB. Alcohol intake over the life course and mammographic density. Breast Cancer Res Treat 2009; 117(3): 643-51.
[http://dx.doi.org/10.1007/s10549-008-0302-0] [PMID: 19184416]

[96]   Bagnardi V, Rota M, Botteri E, *et al.* Light alcohol drinking and cancer: a meta-analysis. Ann Oncol 2013; 24(2): 301-8.
[http://dx.doi.org/10.1093/annonc/mds337] [PMID: 22910838]

[97]   Hamajima N, Hirose K, Tajima K, *et al.* Collaborative Group on Hormonal Factors in Breast Cancer. Alcohol, tobacco and breast cancer--collaborative reanalysis of individual data from 53 epidemiological studies, including 58,515 women with breast cancer and 95,067 women without the disease. Br J Cancer 2002; 87(11): 1234-45.
[http://dx.doi.org/10.1038/sj.bjc.6600596] [PMID: 12439712]

[98]   Liu Y, Colditz GA, Rosner B, *et al.* Alcohol intake between menarche and first pregnancy: a prospective study of breast cancer risk. J Natl Cancer Inst 2013; 105(20): 1571-8.
[http://dx.doi.org/10.1093/jnci/djt213] [PMID: 23985142]

[99]   Jayasekara H, MacInnis RJ, Hodge AM, *et al.* Is breast cancer risk associated with alcohol intake before first full-term pregnancy? Cancer Causes Control 2016; 27(9): 1167-74.
[http://dx.doi.org/10.1007/s10552-016-0789-3] [PMID: 27437703]

[100] Liu Y, Nguyen N, Colditz GA. Links between alcohol consumption and breast cancer: a look at the evidence. Womens Health (Lond) 2015; 11(1): 65-77.
[http://dx.doi.org/10.2217/WHE.14.62] [PMID: 25581056]

[101] Rosner B, Colditz GA, Willett WC. Reproductive risk factors in a prospective study of breast cancer: the Nurses' Health Study. Am J Epidemiol 1994; 139(8): 819-35.
[http://dx.doi.org/10.1093/oxfordjournals.aje.a117079] [PMID: 8178795]

[102] Kwan ML, Chen WY, Flatt SW, *et al.* Postdiagnosis alcohol consumption and breast cancer prognosis in the after breast cancer pooling project. Cancer Epidemiol Biomarkers Prev 2013; 22(1): 32-41.
[http://dx.doi.org/10.1158/1055-9965.EPI-12-1022] [PMID: 23150063]

[103] Heit C, Dong H, Chen Y, Thompson DC, Deitrich RA, Vasiliou VK. The role of CYP2E1 in alcohol metabolism and sensitivity in the central nervous system. Subcell Biochem 2013; 67: 235-47.
[http://dx.doi.org/10.1007/978-94-007-5881-0_8] [PMID: 23400924]

[104] Nakamura K, Iwahashi K, Furukawa A, *et al.* Acetaldehyde adducts in the brain of alcoholics. Arch Toxicol 2003; 77(10): 591-3.
[http://dx.doi.org/10.1007/s00204-003-0465-8] [PMID: 14574447]

[105]   Lorenti Garcia C, Mechilli M, Proietti De Santis L, Schinoppi A, Kobos K, Palitti F. Relationship between DNA lesions, DNA repair and chromosomal damage induced by acetaldehyde. Mutat Res 2009; 662(1-2): 3-9.
[http://dx.doi.org/10.1016/j.mrfmmm.2008.11.008] [PMID: 19084543]

[106]   Hong J, Holcomb VB, Tekle SA, Fan B, Núñez NP. Alcohol consumption promotes mammary tumor growth and insulin sensitivity. Cancer Lett 2010; 294(2): 229-35.
[http://dx.doi.org/10.1016/j.canlet.2010.02.004] [PMID: 20202743]

[107]   Aye MM, Ma C, Lin H, Bower KA, Wiggins RC, Luo J. Ethanol-induced *in vitro* invasion of breast cancer cells: the contribution of MMP-2 by fibroblasts. Int J Cancer 2004; 112(5): 738-46.
[http://dx.doi.org/10.1002/ijc.20497] [PMID: 15386367]

[108]   Luo J. Role of matrix metalloproteinase-2 in ethanol-induced invasion by breast cancer cells. J Gastroenterol Hepatol 2006; 21 (Suppl. 3): S65-8.
[http://dx.doi.org/10.1111/j.1440-1746.2006.04578.x] [PMID: 16958676]

[109]   Izevbigie EB, Ekunwe SI, Jordan J, Howard CB. Ethanol modulates the growth of human breast cancer cells *in vitro.* Exp Biol Med (Maywood) 2002; 227(4): 260-5.
[http://dx.doi.org/10.1177/153537020222700406] [PMID: 11910048]

[110]   Meng Q, Gao B, Goldberg ID, Rosen EM, Fan S. Stimulation of cell invasion and migration by alcohol in breast cancer cells. Biochem Biophys Res Commun 2000; 273(2): 448-53.
[http://dx.doi.org/10.1006/bbrc.2000.2942] [PMID: 10873626]

[111]   Xu M, Bower KA, Chen G, *et al.* Ethanol enhances the interaction of breast cancer cells over-expressing ErbB2 with fibronectin. Alcohol Clin Exp Res 2010; 34(5): 751-60.
[http://dx.doi.org/10.1111/j.1530-0277.2010.01147.x] [PMID: 20201928]

[112]   Ma C, Lin H, Leonard SS, Shi X, Ye J, Luo J. Overexpression of ErbB2 enhances ethanol-stimulated intracellular signaling and invasion of human mammary epithelial and breast cancer cells *in vitro.* Oncogene 2003; 22(34): 5281-90.
[http://dx.doi.org/10.1038/sj.onc.1206675] [PMID: 12917629]

[113]   Ke Z, Lin H, Fan Z, *et al.* MMP-2 mediates ethanol-induced invasion of mammary epithelial cells over-expressing ErbB2. Int J Cancer 2006; 119(1): 8-16.
[http://dx.doi.org/10.1002/ijc.21769] [PMID: 16450376]

[114]   IARC Working Group on the Evaluation of Carcinogenic Risks to Humans. Tobacco smoke and involuntary smoking. IARC Monogr Eval Carcinog Risks Hum 2004; 83: 1-1438.
[PMID: 15285078]

[115]   Terry PD, Rohan TE. Cigarette smoking and the risk of breast cancer in women: a review of the literature. Cancer Epidemiol Biomarkers Prev 2002; 11(10 Pt 1): 953-71.
[PMID: 12376493]

[116]   Secretan B, Straif K, Baan R, *et al.* WHO International Agency for Research on Cancer Monograph Working Group. A review of human carcinogens--Part E: tobacco, areca nut, alcohol, coal smoke, and salted fish. Lancet Oncol 2009; 10(11): 1033-4.
[http://dx.doi.org/10.1016/S1470-2045(09)70326-2] [PMID: 19891056]

[117]   Jones ME, Schoemaker MJ, Wright LB, Ashworth A, Swerdlow AJ. Smoking and risk of breast cancer in the Generations Study cohort. Breast Cancer Res 2017; 19(1): 118.
[http://dx.doi.org/10.1186/s13058-017-0908-4] [PMID: 29162146]

[118]   Johnson KC, Miller AB, Collishaw NE, *et al.* Active smoking and secondhand smoke increase breast cancer risk: the report of the canadian expert panel on tobacco smoke and breast cancer risk (2009). Tob Control 2011; 20(1): e2.
[http://dx.doi.org/10.1136/tc.2010.035931] [PMID: 21148114]

[119]   Reynolds P. Smoking and breast cancer. J Mammary Gland Biol Neoplasia 2013; 18(1): 15-23.
[http://dx.doi.org/10.1007/s10911-012-9269-x] [PMID: 23179580]

[120] Gaudet MM, Gapstur SM, Sun J, Diver WR, Hannan LM, Thun MJ. Active smoking and breast cancer risk: original cohort data and meta-analysis. J Natl Cancer Inst 2013; 105(8): 515-25.
[http://dx.doi.org/10.1093/jnci/djt023] [PMID: 23449445]

[121] Gram IT, Park SY, Maskarinec G, Wilkens LR, Haiman CA, Le Marchand L. Smoking and breast cancer risk by race/ethnicity and oestrogen and progesterone receptor status: the Multiethnic Cohort (MEC) study. Int J Epidemiol 2019; 48(2): 501-11.
[http://dx.doi.org/10.1093/ije/dyy290] [PMID: 30668861]

[122] Park SY, Palmer JR, Rosenberg L, *et al.* A case-control analysis of smoking and breast cancer in African American women: findings from the AMBER Consortium. Carcinogenesis 2016; 37(6): 607-15.
[http://dx.doi.org/10.1093/carcin/bgw040] [PMID: 27207658]

[123] Palmer JR, Rosenberg L. Cigarette smoking and the risk of breast cancer. Epidemiol Rev 1993; 15(1): 145-56.
[http://dx.doi.org/10.1093/oxfordjournals.epirev.a036098] [PMID: 8405197]

[124] Bjerkaas E, Parajuli R, Weiderpass E, *et al.* Smoking duration before first childbirth: an emerging risk factor for breast cancer? Results from 302,865 Norwegian women. Cancer Causes Control 2013; 24(7): 1347-56.
[http://dx.doi.org/10.1007/s10552-013-0213-1] [PMID: 23633026]

[125] Dossus L, Boutron-Ruault MC, Kaaks R, *et al.* Active and passive cigarette smoking and breast cancer risk: results from the EPIC cohort. Int J Cancer 2014; 134(8): 1871-88.
[http://dx.doi.org/10.1002/ijc.28508] [PMID: 24590452]

[126] Nyante SJ, Gierach GL, Dallal CM, *et al.* Cigarette smoking and postmenopausal breast cancer risk in a prospective cohort. Br J Cancer 2014; 110(9): 2339-47.
[http://dx.doi.org/10.1038/bjc.2014.132] [PMID: 24642621]

[127] Kawai M, Malone KE, Tang MT, Li CI. Active smoking and the risk of estrogen receptor-positive and triple-negative breast cancer among women ages 20 to 44 years. Cancer 2014; 120(7): 1026-34.
[http://dx.doi.org/10.1002/cncr.28402] [PMID: 24515648]

[128] Personal habits and indoor combustions. Volume 100 E. A review of human carcinogens IARC Monogr Eval Carcinog Risks Hum 2012; 100(Pt E): 1-538.

[129] Preston DL, Mattsson A, Holmberg E, Shore R, Hildreth NG, Boice JD Jr. Radiation effects on breast cancer risk: a pooled analysis of eight cohorts. Radiat Res 2002; 158(2): 220-35.
[http://dx.doi.org/10.1667/0033-7587(2002)158[0220:REOBCR]2.0.CO;2] [PMID: 12105993]

[130] John EM, Phipps AI, Knight JA, *et al.* Medical radiation exposure and breast cancer risk: findings from the Breast Cancer Family Registry. Int J Cancer 2007; 121(2): 386-94.
[http://dx.doi.org/10.1002/ijc.22668] [PMID: 17372900]

[131] UNSCEAR. Sources and Effects of Ionizing Radiation, United Nations Scientific Committee on the Effects of Atomic Radiation (UNSCEAR). UN, New York: Report to the General Assembly, with Scientific Annexes-Sources 2000; Volume I.

[132] Hancock SL, Tucker MA, Hoppe RT. Breast cancer after treatment of Hodgkin's disease. J Natl Cancer Inst 1993; 85(1): 25-31.
[http://dx.doi.org/10.1093/jnci/85.1.25] [PMID: 8416252]

[133] Aisenberg AC, Finkelstein DM, Doppke KP, Koerner FC, Boivin JF, Willett CG. High risk of breast carcinoma after irradiation of young women with Hodgkin's disease. Cancer 1997; 79(6): 1203-10.
[http://dx.doi.org/10.1002/(SICI)1097-0142(19970315)79:6<1203::AID-CNCR20>3.0.CO;2-2] [PMID: 9070499]

[134] Boice JD Jr, Harvey EB, Blettner M, Stovall M, Flannery JT. Cancer in the contralateral breast after radiotherapy for breast cancer. N Engl J Med 1992; 326(12): 781-5.
[http://dx.doi.org/10.1056/NEJM199203193261201] [PMID: 1538720]

[135] Mattsson A, Rudén BI, Hall P, Wilking N, Rutqvist LE. Radiation-induced breast cancer: long-term follow-up of radiation therapy for benign breast disease. J Natl Cancer Inst 1993; 85(20): 1679-85. [http://dx.doi.org/10.1093/jnci/85.20.1679] [PMID: 8411245]

[136] Shore RE, Hildreth N, Woodard E, Dvoretsky P, Hempelmann L, Pasternack B. Breast cancer among women given X-ray therapy for acute postpartum mastitis. J Natl Cancer Inst 1986; 77(3): 689-96. [http://dx.doi.org/10.1093/jnci/77.3.689] [PMID: 3462410]

[137] Swerdlow AJ, Barber JA, Hudson GV, *et al.* Risk of second malignancy after Hodgkin's disease in a collaborative British cohort: the relation to age at treatment. J Clin Oncol 2000; 18(3): 498-509. [http://dx.doi.org/10.1200/JCO.2000.18.3.498] [PMID: 10653865]

[138] Kenney LB, Yasui Y, Inskip PD, *et al.* Breast cancer after childhood cancer: a report from the Childhood Cancer Survivor Study. Ann Intern Med 2004; 141(8): 590-7. [http://dx.doi.org/10.7326/0003-4819-141-8-200410190-00006] [PMID: 15492338]

[139] Hildreth NG, Shore RE, Dvoretsky PM. The risk of breast cancer after irradiation of the thymus in infancy. N Engl J Med 1989; 321(19): 1281-4. [http://dx.doi.org/10.1056/NEJM198911093211901] [PMID: 2797100]

[140] Boice JD Jr, Preston D, Davis FG, Monson RR. Frequent chest X-ray fluoroscopy and breast cancer incidence among tuberculosis patients in Massachusetts. Radiat Res 1991; 125(2): 214-22. [http://dx.doi.org/10.2307/3577890] [PMID: 1996380]

[141] Holmberg E, Holm LE, Lundell M, Mattsson A, Wallgren A, Karlsson P. Excess breast cancer risk and the role of parity, age at first childbirth and exposure to radiation in infancy. Br J Cancer 2001; 85(3): 362-6. [http://dx.doi.org/10.1054/bjoc.2001.1868] [PMID: 11487266]

[142] Hoffman DA, Lonstein JE, Morin MM, Visscher W, Harris BS III, Boice JD Jr. Breast cancer in women with scoliosis exposed to multiple diagnostic x rays. J Natl Cancer Inst 1989; 81(17): 1307-12. [http://dx.doi.org/10.1093/jnci/81.17.1307] [PMID: 2769783]

[143] Modan B, Chetrit A, Alfandary E, Katz L. Increased risk of breast cancer after low-dose irradiation. Lancet 1989; 1(8639): 629-31. [http://dx.doi.org/10.1016/S0140-6736(89)92140-5] [PMID: 2564456]

[144] Land CE, Tokunaga M, Koyama K, *et al.* Incidence of female breast cancer among atomic bomb survivors, Hiroshima and Nagasaki, 1950-1990. Radiat Res 2003; 160(6): 707-17. [http://dx.doi.org/10.1667/RR3082] [PMID: 14640793]

[145] Miglioretti DL, Lange J, van den Broek JJ, *et al.* Radiation-induced breast cancer incidence and mortality from digital mammography screening: a modeling study. Ann Intern Med 2016; 164(4): 205-14. [http://dx.doi.org/10.7326/M15-1241] [PMID: 26756460]

[146] Eidemüller M, Holmberg E, Jacob P, Lundell M, Karlsson P. Breast cancer risk and possible mechanisms of radiation-induced genomic instability in the Swedish hemangioma cohort after reanalyzed dosimetry. Mutat Res 2015; 775: 1-9. [http://dx.doi.org/10.1016/j.mrfmmm.2015.03.002] [PMID: 25839758]

[147] Hill DA, Preston-Martin S, Ross RK, Bernstein L. Medical radiation, family history of cancer, and benign breast disease in relation to breast cancer risk in young women, USA. Cancer Causes Control 2002; 13(8): 711-8. [http://dx.doi.org/10.1023/A:1020201106117] [PMID: 12420949]

[148] Ron E. Cancer risks from medical radiation. Health Phys 2003; 85(1): 47-59. [http://dx.doi.org/10.1097/00004032-200307000-00011] [PMID: 12852471]

[149] Atoum M, Alzoughool F. Vitamin D and breast cancer: latest evidence and future steps. Breast Cancer (Auckl) 2017; 11: 1178223417749816. [http://dx.doi.org/10.1177/1178223417749816] [PMID: 29434472]

[150] Khan MI, Bielecka ZF, Najm MZ, *et al.* Vitamin D receptor gene polymorphisms in breast and renal cancer: current state and future approaches (review). Int J Oncol 2014; 44(2): 349-63. [review].
[http://dx.doi.org/10.3892/ijo.2013.2204] [PMID: 24297042]

[151] Eliassen AH, Warner ET, Rosner B, *et al.* Plasma 25-hydroxyvitamin D and risk of breast cancer in women followed over 20 years. Cancer Res 2016; 76(18): 5423-30.
[http://dx.doi.org/10.1158/0008-5472.CAN-16-0353] [PMID: 27530324]

[152] Bilinski K, Boyages J. Association between 25-hydroxyvitamin D concentration and breast cancer risk in an Australian population: an observational case-control study. Breast Cancer Res Treat 2013; 137(2): 599-607.
[http://dx.doi.org/10.1007/s10549-012-2381-1] [PMID: 23239153]

[153] Park S, Lee DH, Jeon JY, *et al.* Serum 25-hydroxyvitamin D deficiency and increased risk of breast cancer among Korean women: a case-control study. Breast Cancer Res Treat 2015; 152(1): 147-54.
[http://dx.doi.org/10.1007/s10549-015-3433-0] [PMID: 26037255]

[154] Colagar AH, Firouzjah HM, Halalkhor S. Vitamin D receptor Poly(A) microsatellite polymorphism and 25-hydroxyvitamin d serum levels: association with susceptibility to breast cancer. J Breast Cancer 2015; 18(2): 119-25.
[http://dx.doi.org/10.4048/jbc.2015.18.2.119] [PMID: 26155287]

[155] Bertrand KA, Rosner B, Eliassen AH, *et al.* Premenopausal plasma 25-hydroxyvitamin D, mammographic density, and risk of breast cancer. Breast Cancer Res Treat 2015; 149(2): 479-87.
[http://dx.doi.org/10.1007/s10549-014-3247-5] [PMID: 25543181]

[156] Kim Y, Franke AA, Shvetsov YB, *et al.* Plasma 25-hydroxyvitamin D3 is associated with decreased risk of postmenopausal breast cancer in whites: a nested case-control study in the multiethnic cohort study. BMC Cancer 2014; 14: 29.
[http://dx.doi.org/10.1186/1471-2407-14-29] [PMID: 24438060]

[157] Jamshidinaeini Y, Akbari ME, Abdollahi M, Ajami M, Davoodi SH. Vitamin D status and risk of breast cancer in iranian women: a case-control study. J Am Coll Nutr 2016; 35(7): 639-46.
[http://dx.doi.org/10.1080/07315724.2015.1127786] [PMID: 27331363]

[158] Estébanez N, Gómez-Acebo I, Palazuelos C, Llorca J, Dierssen-Sotos T. Vitamin D exposure and Risk of Breast Cancer: a meta-analysis. Sci Rep 2018; 8(1): 9039.
[http://dx.doi.org/10.1038/s41598-018-27297-1] [PMID: 29899554]

[159] Chen P, Hu P, Xie D, Qin Y, Wang F, Wang H. Meta-analysis of vitamin D, calcium and the prevention of breast cancer. Breast Cancer Res Treat 2010; 121(2): 469-77.
[http://dx.doi.org/10.1007/s10549-009-0593-9] [PMID: 19851861]

[160] Bauer SR, Hankinson SE, Bertone-Johnson ER, Ding EL. Plasma vitamin D levels, menopause, and risk of breast cancer: dose-response meta-analysis of prospective studies. Medicine (Baltimore) 2013; 92(3): 123-31.
[http://dx.doi.org/10.1097/MD.0b013e3182943bc2] [PMID: 23625163]

[161] Bidgoli SA, Azarshab H. Role of vitamin D deficiency and lack of sun exposure in the incidence of premenopausal breast cancer: a case control study in Sabzevar, Iran. Asian Pac J Cancer Prev 2014; 15(8): 3391-6.
[http://dx.doi.org/10.7314/APJCP.2014.15.8.3391] [PMID: 24870727]

[162] Bolland MJ, Grey A, Gamble GD, Reid IR. Calcium and vitamin D supplements and health outcomes: a reanalysis of the Women's Health Initiative (WHI) limited-access data set. Am J Clin Nutr 2011; 94(4): 1144-9.
[http://dx.doi.org/10.3945/ajcn.111.015032] [PMID: 21880848]

[163] McDonnell SL, Baggerly C, French CB, *et al.* Serum 25-hydroxyvitamin D concentrations ≥40 ng/ml are associated with >65% lower cancer risk: pooled analysis of randomized trial and prospective cohort study. PLoS One 2016; 11(4): e0152441.

[http://dx.doi.org/10.1371/journal.pone.0152441] [PMID: 27049526]

[164]   Grant WB, Boucher BJ. Randomized controlled trials of vitamin D and cancer incidence: A modeling study. PLoS One 2017; 12(5): e0176448.
[http://dx.doi.org/10.1371/journal.pone.0176448] [PMID: 28459861]

[165]   Hatse S, Lambrechts D, Verstuyf A, *et al*. Vitamin D status at breast cancer diagnosis: correlation with tumor characteristics, disease outcome, and genetic determinants of vitamin D insufficiency. Carcinogenesis 2012; 33(7): 1319-26.
[http://dx.doi.org/10.1093/carcin/bgs187] [PMID: 22623648]

[166]   Imtiaz S, Siddiqui N, Raza SA, Loya A, Muhammad A. Vitamin D deficiency in newly diagnosed breast cancer patients. Indian J Endocrinol Metab 2012; 16(3): 409-13.
[http://dx.doi.org/10.4103/2230-8210.95684] [PMID: 22629509]

[167]   Palmieri C, MacGregor T, Girgis S, Vigushin D. Serum 25-hydroxyvitamin D levels in early and advanced breast cancer. J Clin Pathol 2006; 59(12): 1334-6.
[http://dx.doi.org/10.1136/jcp.2006.042747] [PMID: 17046848]

[168]   Janbabai G, Shekarriz R, Hassanzadeh H, Aarabi M, Borhani SS. A survey on the relationship between serum 25-hydroxy vitamin D level and tumor characteristics in patients with breast cancer. Int J Hematol Oncol Stem Cell Res 2016; 10(1): 30-6.
[PMID: 27047648]

[169]   Yao S, Kwan ML, Ergas IJ, *et al*. Association of serum level of vitamin d at diagnosis with breast cancer survival: a case-cohort analysis in the pathways study. JAMA Oncol 2017; 3(3): 351-7.
[http://dx.doi.org/10.1001/jamaoncol.2016.4188] [PMID: 27832250]

[170]   de Sousa Almeida-Filho B, De Luca Vespoli H, Pessoa EC, Machado M, Nahas-Neto J, Nahas EAP. Vitamin D deficiency is associated with poor breast cancer prognostic features in postmenopausal women. J Steroid Biochem Mol Biol 2017; 174: 284-9.
[http://dx.doi.org/10.1016/j.jsbmb.2017.10.009] [PMID: 29031688]

[171]   Imtiaz S, Siddiqui N. Vitamin-D status at breast cancer diagnosis: correlation with social and environmental factors and dietary intake. J Ayub Med Coll Abbottabad 2014; 26(2): 186-90.
[PMID: 25603674]

[172]   Simboli-Campbell M, Narvaez CJ, Tenniswood M, Welsh J. 1,25-Dihydroxyvitamin D3 induces morphological and biochemical markers of apoptosis in MCF-7 breast cancer cells. J Steroid Biochem Mol Biol 1996; 58(4): 367-76.
[http://dx.doi.org/10.1016/0960-0760(96)00055-6] [PMID: 8903420]

[173]   Welsh J. Induction of apoptosis in breast cancer cells in response to vitamin D and antiestrogens. Biochem Cell Biol 1994; 72(11-12): 537-45.
[http://dx.doi.org/10.1139/o94-072] [PMID: 7654327]

[174]   James SY, Mackay AG, Colston KW. Effects of 1,25 dihydroxyvitamin D3 and its analogues on induction of apoptosis in breast cancer cells. J Steroid Biochem Mol Biol 1996; 58(4): 395-401.
[http://dx.doi.org/10.1016/0960-0760(96)00048-9] [PMID: 8903423]

[175]   Khan QJ, Kimler BF, Fabian CJ. The relationship between vitamin D and breast cancer incidence and natural history. Curr Oncol Rep 2010; 12(2): 136-42.
[http://dx.doi.org/10.1007/s11912-010-0081-8] [PMID: 20425599]

[176]   Mohr SB, Gorham ED, Alcaraz JE, *et al*. Serum 25-hydroxyvitamin D and prevention of breast cancer: pooled analysis. Anticancer Res 2011; 31(9): 2939-48.
[PMID: 21868542]

[177]   Matthews D, LaPorta E, Zinser GM, Narvaez CJ, Welsh J. Genomic vitamin D signaling in breast cancer: Insights from animal models and human cells. J Steroid Biochem Mol Biol 2010; 121(1-2): 362-7.
[http://dx.doi.org/10.1016/j.jsbmb.2010.03.061] [PMID: 20412854]

[178] Tavera-Mendoza LE, Westerling T, Libby E, *et al.* Vitamin D receptor regulates autophagy in the normal mammary gland and in luminal breast cancer cells. Proc Natl Acad Sci USA 2017; 114(11): E2186-94.
[http://dx.doi.org/10.1073/pnas.1615015114] [PMID: 28242709]

[179] Ordóñez-Mena JM, Schöttker B, Fedirko V, *et al.* Pre-diagnostic vitamin D concentrations and cancer risks in older individuals: an analysis of cohorts participating in the CHANCES consortium. Eur J Epidemiol 2016; 31(3): 311-23.
[http://dx.doi.org/10.1007/s10654-015-0040-7] [PMID: 25977096]

[180] Hunter DJ, Colditz GA, Hankinson SE, *et al.* Oral contraceptive use and breast cancer: a prospective study of young women. Cancer Epidemiol Biomarkers Prev 2010; 19(10): 2496-502.
[http://dx.doi.org/10.1158/1055-9965.EPI-10-0747] [PMID: 20802021]

[181] Bhupathiraju SN, Grodstein F, Stampfer MJ, Willett WC, Hu FB, Manson JE. Exogenous hormone use: oral contraceptives, postmenopausal hormone therapy, and health outcomes in the nurses' health study. Am J Public Health 2016; 106(9): 1631-7.
[http://dx.doi.org/10.2105/AJPH.2016.303349] [PMID: 27459451]

[182] Collaborative Group on Hormonal Factors in Breast Cancer. Breast cancer and hormonal contraceptives: collaborative reanalysis of individual data on 53 297 women with breast cancer and 100 239 women without breast cancer from 54 epidemiological studies. Lancet 1996; 347(9017): 1713-27.
[http://dx.doi.org/10.1016/S0140-6736(96)90806-5] [PMID: 8656904]

[183] Hannaford PC, Selvaraj S, Elliott AM, Angus V, Iversen L, Lee AJ. Cancer risk among users of oral contraceptives: cohort data from the Royal College of General Practitioner's oral contraception study. BMJ 2007; 335(7621): 651.
[http://dx.doi.org/10.1136/bmj.39289.649410.55] [PMID: 17855280]

[184] Shantakumar S, Terry MB, Paykin A, *et al.* Age and menopausal effects of hormonal birth control and hormone replacement therapy in relation to breast cancer risk. Am J Epidemiol 2007; 165(10): 1187-98.
[http://dx.doi.org/10.1093/aje/kwm006] [PMID: 17337757]

[185] Rosenberg L, Zhang Y, Coogan PF, Strom BL, Palmer JR. A case-control study of oral contraceptive use and incident breast cancer. Am J Epidemiol 2009; 169(4): 473-9.
[http://dx.doi.org/10.1093/aje/kwn360] [PMID: 19074777]

CHAPTER 9

Epithelial-Mesenchymal Transition (EMT) in Breast Cancer: An Overview

Manish Charan[1,*], **Bhavana Kushwaha**[2], **Sanjay Mishra**[1] and **Ramesh K Ganju**[1]

[1] Department of Pathology, The Ohio State University, Columbus, OH, USA

[2] Endocrinology Division, CSIR-Central Drug Research Institute, Jankipuram Extension, Sitapur Road, Lucknow 226031, India

Abstract: The epithelial to mesenchymal transition (EMT) is a key cellular event that plays a pivotal role in promoting metastatic disease and tumor recurrence among solid malignances. EMT is involved not only in essential cellular processes, including embryonic development and tissue remodeling, but also in inducing tumorigenesis. Breast cancer (BC) is the most prevalent cancer in women globally, and the main causes of breast cancer mortality are metastasis and recurrence. EMT plays an imperative role in enhancing invasion, following metastasis. Integrated changes in several cell signaling events lead to an epithelial to mesenchymal phenotypic shift and provide cells with more migratory and invasive properties that eventually results in metastatic colonization at a secondary site. However, the present knowledge about the cross-talk of multi-faceted signaling pathways and associated crucial transcription factors is yet to be understood. Understanding the cellular complexities of EMT will provide valuable insights for the therapeutic targeting of aggressive breast cancers, and in the development of novel biomarkers to delimit malignancies with greater chances of metastasis and recurrence.

Keywords: Breast cancer, Biomarker, Cell signaling, Cancer stem cells, Circulating tumor cells, EMT, Invasion, Metastasis, Migration, Tumor growth.

INTRODUCTION

Breast cancer (BC) is the most common cancer in women across the globe. Secondary spread of BC cells to distant sites in the body is the main cause of BC related death in patients [1]. Although, exact causes of BC are not well defined, but several risk factors promoting the growth of BC have been identified. Sex, racial disparity, age and family history comprise an important portion of risk fac-

---

* **Corresponding author Manish Charan:** Department of Pathology, The Ohio State University, Columbus 43210, OH, USA; E-mail: Manish.charan@osumc.edu

tors that influence BC growth and treatment outcomes [2]. However, a majority of primary breast tumors are treatable with current therapeutic options but the management of metastatic and recurrence of BC is still unmet. Various factors have been recognized that are crucial for metastasis, and recurrence of the disease includes the existence of cancer stem cells (CSCs) in the circulation and the constant genomic evolution of cancer cells leading to the development of intratumor heterogeneity, which makes it worse for treatment.

Early, in all solid tumors, the only leading cause of mortality is distant metastasis [3, 4]. Metastasis is the process of migration of tumor cells from the primary site of growth to distant secondary sites in the body and subsequent colonization [3, 5, 6]. The process of metastasis is a multistep and complex event, which is influenced by the amount of cell mutational burden and micro-environmental niches. Cancer metastasis remains the most imperfectly reviewed hallmark of cancer [7]. Metastatic cascade involves following sequential events: a) Disruption of adjacent tissue (local invasion), entering lymph and blood circulation (intravasation), survival in the circulation, and transmigration to secondary sites (extravasation), and eventually leading to proliferation (colonization) [5 - 7]. BC cells can metastasize to distant sites such as lungs, liver, bone, brain, and skin [8 - 12], but not all sites support the growth of disseminated cells. Interaction between CTCs and microenvironment of secondary metastatic organs decide the successful colonization of circulating tumor cells. However, very little is known about the regulation of these processes.

Till now, EMT has been attributed to metastasis of epithelial cancers, including BC. The characteristic features of EMT include the destruction of cellular tight junctions and loss of cell-cell contact. These events will enable the cells to attain mesenchymal properties. Thus, cells show an enhanced self-renewal and an increased heterogeneous subpopulation. These features provide the cells with increased motility and promote shedding from the primary epithelial site [11, 12]. Understanding the underlying mechanism of BC metastasis will lead to the identification of novel biomarkers for early diagnosis and in the development of targeted therapy against aggressive BC. In depth knowledge and insights about the underlying molecular events and signaling pathways indispensable for the initiation and progression of BC metastases would lead to the identification and development of more effective and targeted treatment.

EPITHELIAL-TO-MESENCHYMAL TRANSITION (EMT) AND BC METASTASIS

Breast cancers are epithelial-derived carcinomas and possess intact tight and adherents junctions with the apical and basal polarity of cells that are separated from the primary tissues underneath by lining of extracellular matrix; basement membrane [12]. Mesenchymal cells are loosely connected and a disorganized layer of cells without cellular tight and adherents junctions [13]. These cells can differentiate into a variety of cell types. Mesenchymal properties allow the cells to migrate and invade better.

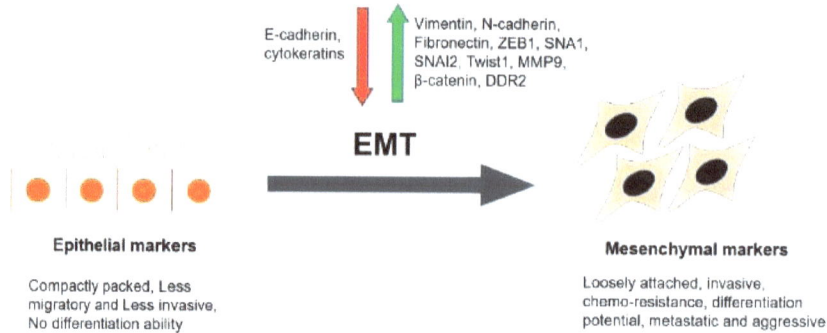

E-cadherin, cytokeratins

Vimentin, N-cadherin, Fibronectin, ZEB1, SNA1, SNAI2, Twist1, MMP9, β-catenin, DDR2

EMT

Epithelial markers

Compactly packed, Less migratory and Less invasive, No differentiation ability

Mesenchymal markers

Loosely attached, invasive, chemo-resistance, differentiation potential, metastatic and aggressive

Fig. (1). Schematic diagram showing characteristic EMT of breast cancer.

The epithelial-to-mesenchymal transition (EMT) is a highly dynamic process by which epithelial cells can convert into a mesenchymal phenotype [13]. However, it is also involved in tumor progression with metastatic expansion and the generation of tumor cells with stem cell properties that play a major role in resistance to cancer treatment [14 - 16]. EMT has been tremendously believed to contribute to breast tumor metastasis (Fig. **1**). However, the exact function or association of EMT and distant tumor metastases has been mostly centered on analysis from cancer cell lines. Importantly, the significance of EMT in clinical settings needs to be confirmed to declare its indispensability in promoting BC metastasis.

One of the first and foremost hurdles is to track cells in real-time that are shedding off the primary tumor or are about cast off the primary site. As the majority of the cells have either not gone through the EMT or already surpassed the transition during a histopathological assessment. Thus, the transition stage is very hard to be construed and scrutinized at a particular point of the tumor growth phase. EMT is the principal mechanism by which epithelial cancer cells acquire mesenchymal properties that foster metastasis. Typical EMT process includes the loss of epithelial cell-adhesion proteins such as E-cadherin and cytokeratin along with the attainment of mesenchymal markers such as vimentin, N-cadherin, and fibronectin [17].

EMT is believed to be the very first crucial step of primary cancer towards a metastatic cascade. The level of EMT biomarkers in clinical breast cancer tissues undertaking EMT has not been entirely established. Although its role in breast cancer metastases has been debated [18]. EMT cascade leading to malignancy, invasion, and metastasis is also known as EMT type 3 (Fig. **2**), whereas type 1 and type 2EMT are related to embryogenesis and tissue regeneration respectively [13, 19]. IHC (Immunohistochemistry has detected the expression of EMT associated proteins; N-cadherin, Vimentin, Snail, Slug, and Twist in a variety of cancers including breast cancer [13, 15]. BC patient data on EMT markers suggested higher expression of EMT related proteins were more inclined towards basal-like subtype of breast cancers [20].

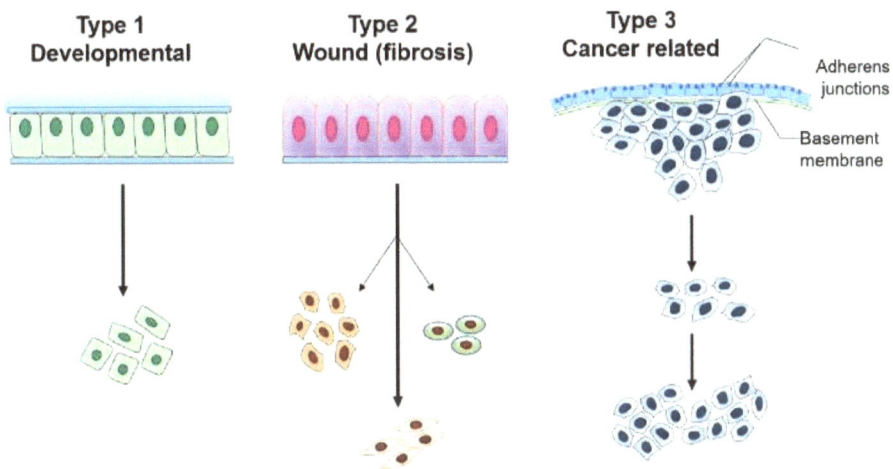

Fig. (2). Schematic representation of different EMT types.

EMT transition happens to occur selectively to a few clonally selected cells from the primary tumor mass and does not apply to all cancer cells. Tumor cells remain in mixed transitional states and differentially express genes. This amalgam of cells with partly EMT signature phenotype can travel together as clusters, and render more aggressive compared to cells showing complete EMT characteristics [21, 22]. In the early stage of the tumor, metastatic cancer cells shed off the primary tumor and gain malignant invasive properties and get access to the blood and lymphatic systems to spread to other metastatic sites in the body for colonization. Such tumor cells are denoted as circulating tumor cells (CTCs) [21, 23, 24].

This event is abetted by neoangiogenic processes and remodeling of the basement membrane [23]. In circulation within the bloodstream and lymphatic system, only a few numbers of CTCs survive and eventually enter distant secondary metastatic sites, such as bone, lungs, liver, skin, and brain [8, 12]. This whole course is achieved largely by the mesenchymal-epithelial transition (MET), a process contrasting to EMT at the primary tumor growth site. This interplay of tumor cells undergoing different phenotypical changes substantially impacts the secondary metastatic colonization [25 - 27]. Such dynamic transitional states, EMT/MET, plays a key role in distant tumor metastasis.

In many types of cancers, hypoxia, tumor microenvironment, stromal cell cross-talk, cytokines, growth factors, innate and adaptive immune responses, and treatment with anti-tumor chemotherapeutic drugs induce the cells to undergo EMT. Differential gene expression switch during the EMT is achieved by an intricate regulatory network of transcriptional regulators such as SNAI1 and SNAI2, ZEB1 and ZEB2, Twist, and E12/E47. It has also been shown that non-coding RNAs (miRNAs and long non-coding RNAs), chromatin modifications, alternative splicing, post-translational regulation, protein stability, and subcellular localization also impacts MT transition [28 - 31].

EMT conversion has been believed as a hallmark for the plasticity of a stem cell population, pertinent to tumors. Considering the profound role of EMT in tumor metastasis, it is becoming an attractive target against all types of tumors, including BC [31]. Most recent molecular classification, mammary tumors can be divided into six sub-groups. These entail normal (expression profile similar to the noncancerous breast tissue); luminal A and B (generally estrogen receptor (ER)-positive tumors, with expression of epithelial markers; luminal B shows a higher Ki67 index and poor prognosis compared to luminal A); HER2 positive (overexpressing ERBB2 oncogene); basal-like (expressing basal cytokeratin and other markers characteristic of the myoepithelium of the normal mammary gland); and claudin-low (enriched in EMT characteristics).

Basal-like and claudin-low subtypes fall into the cluster of triple-negative breast cancer (TNBC), characterized by the lack of progesterone receptor (PR), ER and HER2 expression, and have a high incidence rate of distant metastatic recurrence [32, 33]. About 10–20% of BC reports fall into the category of basal-like subtype. These tumors demonstrate a high rate of the proliferative index, elevated histological grading, and worse prognosis. Basal-like tumors could develop triple-negative subtype with a higher incidence of TP53 mutations along with the loss of Rb1 [34, 35]. Nevertheless, all basal-like cancers lead to triple-negative breast cancers; it has been reported that up to 45% of a basal-like subtype is positive for ER, while approximately 14% of them show expression of Her2/Neu [36].

TNBC per se is a broad group with diverse malignancies that can be further classified into several additional subtypes. Studies have reported that TNBC patient datasets show differential expression of thousands of genes and show mixed subtypes such as basal-like (BL1 and BL2), mesenchymal stem cell-like, immunomodulatory, luminal androgen receptor-like [37]. In modern times, basal-like subtypes are on top priority for further investigation among all subtypes considering their aggressive nature. RNA in situ hybridization assay has been utilized to characterize EMT in circulating tumor cells (CTCs) from a pool of breast cancer patients [38]. Only a rare number of primary tumors show both EMT and MET related biomarkers, whereas CTCs were replete in mesenchymal related markers.

Importantly, it was observed that only clusters of CTCs were highly enriched in mesenchymal markers rather than the single migratory cells. These findings established that in human breast cancers the route of dissemination of CTCs undergoing EMT is *via* blood circulatory system. Furthermore, several studies established that the EMT event can be traced out by analyzing the detached CTCs in the circulation [39].

Several clinical studies on metastatic breast and prostate cancer have confirmed the presence of both the epithelial and mesenchymal markers that indicates that CTCs are transitioning and detected expression of various epithelial markers such as EpCAM, cytokeratins (CKs), and E-cadherin and mesenchymal markers vimentin, N-cadherin, O-cadherin, and the stem cell marker CD133 [39, 40]. Recent reports do support the idea of EMT contributes to the metastatic cascade in human breast cancers. Although tumor heterogeneity of CTCs and procedural difficulties make it hard to isolate and detect CTCs.

This book chapter aims to underscore the emerging fact that EMT plays a crucial role in the inception of metastatic events and cascades of breast cancer. A number of EMT-associated proteins, microRNAs and epigenetic modifications promote EMT to enhance breast cancer invasion and distant metastasis. However, none of the available literature has ever reconciled the vitality of EMT markers in the progression of breast cancer invasion and metastasis. In this book chapter, the relationship between EMT biomarkers and breast cancer metastasis will be thoroughly reviewed.

RELEVANCE OF EMT AND ITS ASSOCIATED MOLECULAR SIGNALING PATHWAYS IN BREAST CARCINOMAS

A myriad of biomarkers is known that are indicative of EMT in breast cancer (Fig. **1**). In this section, we will review the most common proteins associated with the EMT process, where some of the proteins get augmented, and a few get diminished during the event of a transition. Cadherin calcium-dependent proteins and represent a type of cell adhesion molecule (CAM) plays an important function in building adherens junctions to firmly hold cells with each other. Cadherins fall into a group of type-1 transmembrane proteins. E-cadherin is one such protein that helps in binding the epithelial cells with each other [41].

E-cadherin

E-cadherin is a well-known epithelial marker, and any significant change in the amount of E-cadherin is indicative of cells going through the EMT phenotype. Loss of E-cadherin level or the function enables the cell to go into mesenchymal morphology and led to the loosening of cell connections that promotes migration, invasion, and metastasis [42]. Human breast cancers involving the fractional or complete loss of E-cadherin expression is associated with loss of cell-differentiation, increased invasiveness, high tumor grade, aggressive metastatic behavior and worse prognosis [42, 43]. Human breast cancers involving the fractional or complete loss of E-cadherin expression is associated with loss of cell-differentiation, increased invasiveness, high tumor grade, aggressive metastatic behavior and worse prognosis [44]. Moreover, its diminished expression has been linked with aggressive metastatic breast tumors [45]. Several studies have established the fact that E-cadherin expression is being used to estimate EMT.

N-cadherin

N-cadherin is also a transmembrane protein that mediates cell-cell adhesion. The expression level of E-cadherin and N-cadherin are used to evaluate EMT during tumor progression. The switch of these markers enhances cell migration, invasion, and metastasis of breast cancers [31]. Besides, N-cadherin levels rise to correlate positively with EMT and increase metastatic properties of tumor cells. E-cadherin levels are indicative of cells going through MET. In BC liver or lung metastasis cells originally were low in E-cadherin, show stable expression of E-cadherin after colonizing the metastatic site [45].

CD44

A cluster of differentiation (CD) 44 is a cell-surface receptor that regulates an array of cellular signaling *via* different receptor tyrosine kinases (RTKs). It plays a key role in BC metastasis [46]. And various studies have confirmed its higher expression is found in highly aggressive metastatic cell lines [47]. High CD44 and N-cadherin expression are detected in high-grade human breast cancers [46].

Discoidin Domain Receptors

Discoidin domain receptors (DDRs) are commonly found as collagen receptors like other receptor tyrosine kinases and get activated after collagen-binding through autophosphorylation of the receptor. Discoidin domain receptor 2 (DDR2) is an odd receptor tyrosine kinase and a biomarker for the altered ECM microenvironment regarding EMT [48]. Commonly DDR2 expression is limited to smooth muscles and fibroblasts but it gets upregulated in certain metastatic cancer events, including breast, lung and prostate cancers [49]. DDR2 acts *via* collagen type1, and since collagen can promote EMT, the role of DDR2 in promoting EMT and metastasis during tumor growth and progression cannot be overlooked.

DDR2 expression associates in parallel with aggravated invasiveness and migration potential of human breast cancer cells and turns out to be inevitable for metastasis and a marker for monitoring the status of EMT [50]. Tumor related studies have reported that DDR2 is involved in the activity and stability of Snail1 protein stability *via* activating extracellular signal-regulated kinase 2 (ERK2). Thus, activated ERK2 directly phosphorylates Snail1 and stabilizes it by inhibiting its ubiquitination as a result. DDR2 led stabilized Snail1 contributes to enhancing the invasive and metastatic properties of BC cells [51]. Recent research suggests an important role of DDR2 in mediating TGF-β stimulated EMT in kidney epithelial cells and lung carcinomas, considering the important functions of DDR2; it could become an attractive drug target against various types of cancer. However, the exact mechanism of DDR2 regulation during the process of EMT still needs to be addressed.

β-catenin

β-catenin, another important element of cells undergoing EMT transition, a cell adhesion protein, and a transcription factor important in the expression of EMT and metastatic genes [52]. β-catenin is part of the adherens junctions component and remains associated with E-cadherin in both normal epithelial cells and cancer cells [53]. In case of activation, such as cells going through EMT or metastasis, β-catenin gets stabilized in the cytoplasm and translocate to the nucleus of cells where it can induce the expression of EMT or metastasis-related genes [53, 54].

Matrix Metalloproteinase

Matrix metalloproteinase (MMPs) are indispensable for tissue remodelings such as wound healing, cellular growth, and embryogenesis [55]. Also, their capability to disrupt nearly all components of the extracellular matrix and basement membrane of different organs highlights their essentiality in various malignancies including breast cancer. The acquisition of high expression of MMPs endows the cells with more invasive and metastatic potential.

TGF-β has been reported to induce the expression of MMP2 and 9 [55, 56] in breast cancers, which make the disease more invasive and aggressive in nature. Consistently, MMP3 has been known to promote EMT in various cancers and alone increases breast and lung fibrosis [57, 58]. Moreover, deeper insights of TGF dependent EMT stimulation and MMP upregulation related changes in E-cadherin, vimentin, and snail would allow us to better understand the biology for efficient targeting of the metastatic tumors.

Notch

Notch signaling is involved homeostasis of cell proliferation, cell differentiation, and programmed cell death [59]. It is known to stimulate NF-κB signaling, and also regulate TGF-β induced EMT. In normal mammary glands, notch signaling regulates cell survival and has been associated with tumor growth progression [60]. Recent reports on human breast cancers have demonstrated the crucial role of Notch signaling in the sustenance of cancer stem cell-like population [61].

Notch signaling modulates the expression of snail protein *via* direct transcriptional upregulation or by lysyl oxidase mediated activation to promote EMT cascade [62]. Notch expression correlates with poor prognosis in several malignancies, including breast cancer [63, 64]. Notch inhibition is a promising strategy for aggressive metastatic cancers including breast cancers.

Receptor Tyrosine Kinase (RTK) Signaling Pathway

RTKs are cell surface receptors for different growth factors, peptides, cytokines, and hormones [65, 66]. These receptors carry out essential functions and physiological processes in cells such as cell survival, proliferation, migration, cell cycle progression, and metabolism [66, 67]. Intrinsic enzymatic activity of RTKs makes them unique among all other cell surface receptors.

Cellular signaling events are mostly studied and analyzed for promoting the EMT program. Besides signaling molecules, several RTKs are also involved in contributing EMT and metastasis [68]. Many growth factors such as hepatocyte growth factor (HGF) and epidermal growth factor (EGF) can modulate [67]. EMT; such effects are also mediated partly through RTKs [69 - 71]. Although RTKs are known to influence oncogenic signaling events and affect tumor progression but apart from this, RTKs are significantly involved in inducing EMT phenotype [70].

Transforming Growth Factor (TGF-β)

TGF-β is a cytokine that plays important role in various cellular and physiological processes. Its diverse role during cell growth, differentiation, apoptosis, cellular homeostasis, and embryogenesis marks the essentiality of this multifunctional cytokine in cellular signaling. It has been reported to affect the process of EMT [72]. Mammalian cells encode three distinct isoforms of TGF-β; TGF-β1, TGF-β2, and TGF-β3 [73], with three different types of receptors: types I, II and III.

Binding of TGF-β to its receptor activates classical Smad 2/3-dependent signaling [73, 74]. TGF-β is known to induce EMT *via* both canonical and non-canonical pathways involving activation of Smad 2 and Smad 3, which further gets complexed with Smad 4. Such a complex will lead to the transcriptional activation of EMT related genes [75, 76].

Higher expression levels of Smad 2 and Smad 3 correlates with EMT phenotype, while lower levels of their expression correlate with reduced metastatic ability of cells. Non-canonical TGF-β signaling mediates by several pathways such as NF-κB, GTPases, PI3K/AKT/TOR, and MAPKs [77].

Non-classical TGF-β signaling activates the ZEB-1 transcription factor that is known to regulate EMT genes in various carcinomas [78]. These pathways highly affect cellular signaling, such as ECM organization, survival, migration, and invasion [75, 76, 78]. TGF-β also stimulates EMT by activating gene expression of Snail (SNAI1 and SNAI2), Twist and six families of proteins [79].

Tumor Necrosis Factor-Alpha (TNF-α)

TNF-α is a vital secreted cytokine for various cellular processes like inflammation, tumor progression, and homeostasis [80, 81]. It is known to enhance the aggressiveness of a tumor by increasing invasion and angiogenesis. It is known to promote EMT program by downregulating E-cadherin and increasing MMP9 expression [82]. However, the mechanism of EMT induction by TNF-α indicates a correlation of Twist-1 that might be involved in supporting EMT [83]. Higher levels of TNF-α have been shown to positively correlate with increased metastatic potential and invasiveness of human breast cancers [84]. In renal cell carcinomas (RCC), TNF-α stimulated EMT acts by repressing the expression of E-cadherin and activating MMP9 which results in increased invasive and metastatic abilities of cancer cells [82]. TNF-α mediated Twist-1 overexpression has been linked with an increase in stemness and EMT program of tumor cells, including breast cancers, which highlights the presence of a signaling axis to promote cancer invasion and metastasis [85].

EMT AND PROMISING TARGETED THERAPEUTIC APPROACHES

Even though with the advent of computational and experimental analysis of cellular signaling over the last few decades, critical steps in the cell signaling pathway have been identified. Considering the diverse role of EMT in inducing invasion and metastatic potential in several carcinomas including breast cancers, has drawn attention towards the EMT program and its chemotherapeutic intervention to curb tumor metastasis. Tumor heterogeneity has made gene targeting a formidable task as several transcription factors contribute to the transcriptional regulation of key signaling molecules. Thus, many inhibitors are being explored, particularly EMT related transcription factors that are indispensable for the EMT transition.

In melanoma patients, such chemical inhibitors are used in combination with checkpoint inhibitor drugs such as anti-PD-1 and anti-CTLA-4 to improve the overall and progression-free survival [86]. A phytochemical; Baicalein, targets Wnt/β-catenin, downregulated Wnt1 and β-catenin protein levels, had also shown a suppressive effect on growth, migration, and invasion of MDA-MB-231 cells both *in vitro* and *in vivo* [87]. Moreover, in breast cancers, EMT inhibition has been achieved by using various small molecule chemical inhibitors; they decrease the expression level of crucial EMT inducing factors like NF-κB and Snail [88]. Dasatinib; Src kinase inhibitor, inhibits the growth and progression of breast cancer cells exhibiting the EMT signature [89].

Moscatilin; targets Akt-Twist-dependent pathway, recently showed an inhibitory effect on migration and metastasis of MDA MB 231 breast cancer cells. Also, an inhibitor LY2157299 (galunisertib), targets TGFβ, which is in phase II clinical studies against glioblastoma and hepatocellular carcinoma [90, 91]. In addition to the chemotherapeutic strategies to target EMT and related transcriptional factors, monoclonal antibodies are also being used to target essential EMT transcription factors [92] selectively.

These antibodies bind to cell surface receptors and secreted growth factors or signaling proteins and disrupt their downstream functions. Especially, small molecule chemical inhibitors are of high interest, as they easily permeate across the cell membrane and target the specific protein and inhibit its function in the cell. Largely, optimized combinations of chemotherapeutic drugs and small molecule inhibitors would be emphatic in targeting the tumors linked with EMT and improving the prognosis of the disease.

CONCLUDING REMARKS

The knowledge and understanding of EMT transition in human breast cancer have grown over the last few years, right from the role of E-cadherin repression to integrated, multifaceted molecular signaling events. The process of EMT enables the tumor cells with novel gain of functions such as augmented invasive traits *via* modulating the function and expression levels of oncogenes and by repressing tumor suppressors leading to atypical signaling pathways.

In this book chapter, we have reviewed the complex events of EMT and documented a clear understanding of the composite underlying molecular mechanisms that drive the transition from an epithelial cell phenotype to a mesenchymal phenotype. Our reviewed chapter will broaden the understanding of the process of EMT in human breast cancer and provides detailed information on prognostic biomarkers of EMT and shed more light on its novel therapeutic intervention strategies.

CONSENT FOR PUBLICATION

Not applicable.

CONFLICT OF INTEREST

The authors confirm that the contents of this chapter have no conflict of interest.

ACKNOWLEDGEMENTS

Declare none.

REFERENCES

[1]   Siegel RL, Miller KD, Jemal A. Cancer Statistics, 2017. CA Cancer J Clin 2017; 67(1): 7-30.
        [http://dx.doi.org/10.3322/caac.21387] [PMID: 28055103]

[2]   Williams F, Thompson E. Disparities in breast cancer stage at diagnosis: Importance of race, Poverty and Age. J Health Dispar Res Pract 2017; 10(3): 34-45.
        [PMID: 30637180]

[3]   Chitty JL, Filipe EC, Lucas MC, Herrmann D, Cox TR, Timpson P. Recent advances in understanding the complexities of metastasis. F1000 Res 2018; 7: 7.
        [http://dx.doi.org/10.12688/f1000research.15064.2] [PMID: 30135716]

[4]   Steeg PS. Tumor metastasis: mechanistic insights and clinical challenges. Nat Med 2006; 12(8): 895-904.
        [http://dx.doi.org/10.1038/nm1469] [PMID: 16892035]

[5]   Kai F, Drain AP, Weaver VM. The extracellular matrix modulates the metastatic journey. Dev Cell 2019; 49(3): 332-46.
        [http://dx.doi.org/10.1016/j.devcel.2019.03.026] [PMID: 31063753]

[6]   Mierke CT. The matrix environmental and cell mechanical properties regulate cell migration and contribute to the invasive phenotype of cancer cells. Rep Prog Phys 2019; 82(6): 064602.
        [http://dx.doi.org/10.1088/1361-6633/ab1628] [PMID: 30947151]

[7]   Chaffer CL, Weinberg RA. A perspective on cancer cell metastasis. Science 2011; 331(6024): 1559-64.
        [http://dx.doi.org/10.1126/science.1203543] [PMID: 21436443]

[8]   Chen W, Hoffmann AD, Liu H, Liu X. Organotropism: new insights into molecular mechanisms of breast cancer metastasis. NPJ Precis Oncol 2018; 2(1): 4.
        [http://dx.doi.org/10.1038/s41698-018-0047-0] [PMID: 29872722]

[9]   Bittencourt MdeJ, Carvalho AH, Nascimento BA, Freitas LK, Parijós AM. Cutaneous metastasis of a breast cancer diagnosed 13 years before. An Bras Dermatol 2015; 90(3) (Suppl. 1): 134-7.
[http://dx.doi.org/10.1590/abd1806-4841.20153842] [PMID: 26312696]

[10]   Bos PD, Zhang XH, Nadal C, *et al.* Genes that mediate breast cancer metastasis to the brain. Nature 2009; 459(7249): 1005-9.
[http://dx.doi.org/10.1038/nature08021] [PMID: 19421193]

[11]   Cominetti MR, Altei WF, Selistre-de-Araujo HS. Metastasis inhibition in breast cancer by targeting cancer cell extravasation. Breast Cancer (Dove Med Press) 2019; 11: 165-78.
[http://dx.doi.org/10.2147/BCTT.S166725] [PMID: 31114313]

[12]   Drekolias D, Mamounas EP. Metaplastic breast carcinoma: Current therapeutic approaches and novel targeted therapies. Breast J 2019; 25(6): 1192-7.
[http://dx.doi.org/10.1111/tbj.13416] [PMID: 31250492]

[13]   Fedele M, Cerchia L, Chiappetta G. The epithelial-to-mesenchymal transition in breast cancer: focus on basal-like carcinomas. Cancers (Basel) 2017; 9(10): E134.
[http://dx.doi.org/10.3390/cancers9100134] [PMID: 28974015]

[14]   Liao TT, Yang MH. Revisiting epithelial-mesenchymal transition in cancer metastasis: the connection between epithelial plasticity and stemness. Mol Oncol 2017; 11(7): 792-804.
[http://dx.doi.org/10.1002/1878-0261.12096] [PMID: 28649800]

[15]   Pastushenko I, Blanpain C. EMT transition states during tumor progression and metastasis. Trends Cell Biol 2019; 29(3): 212-26.
[http://dx.doi.org/10.1016/j.tcb.2018.12.001] [PMID: 30594349]

[16]   Jia D, Li X, Bocci F, *et al.* Quantifying cancer epithelial-mesenchymal plasticity and its association with stemness and immune response. J Clin Med 2019; 8(5): E725.
[http://dx.doi.org/10.3390/jcm8050725] [PMID: 31121840]

[17]   Santamaria PG, Moreno-Bueno G, Portillo F, Cano A. EMT: Present and future in clinical oncology. Mol Oncol 2017; 11(7): 718-38.
[http://dx.doi.org/10.1002/1878-0261.12091] [PMID: 28590039]

[18]   Zheng X, Carstens JL, Kim J, *et al.* Epithelial-to-mesenchymal transition is dispensable for metastasis but induces chemoresistance in pancreatic cancer. Nature 2015; 527(7579): 525-30.
[http://dx.doi.org/10.1038/nature16064] [PMID: 26560028]

[19]   Felipe Lima J, Nofech-Mozes S, Bayani J, Bartlett JM. EMT in breast carcinoma-a review. J Clin Med 2016; 5(7): E65.
[http://dx.doi.org/10.3390/jcm5070065] [PMID: 27429011]

[20]   Choi Y, Lee HJ, Jang MH, *et al.* Epithelial-mesenchymal transition increases during the progression of in situ to invasive basal-like breast cancer. Hum Pathol 2013; 44(11): 2581-9.
[http://dx.doi.org/10.1016/j.humpath.2013.07.003] [PMID: 24055090]

[21]   Au SH, Storey BD, Moore JC, *et al.* Clusters of circulating tumor cells traverse capillary-sized vessels. Proc Natl Acad Sci USA 2016; 113(18): 4947-52.
[http://dx.doi.org/10.1073/pnas.1524448113] [PMID: 27091969]

[22]   Jolly MK, Boareto M, Huang B, *et al.* Implications of the hybrid epithelial/mesenchymal phenotype in metastasis. Front Oncol 2015; 5: 155.
[http://dx.doi.org/10.3389/fonc.2015.00155] [PMID: 26258068]

[23]   Chambers AF, Groom AC, MacDonald IC. Dissemination and growth of cancer cells in metastatic sites. Nat Rev Cancer 2002; 2(8): 563-72.
[http://dx.doi.org/10.1038/nrc865] [PMID: 12154349]

[24]   Woodhouse EC, Chuaqui RF, Liotta LA. General mechanisms of metastasis. Cancer 1997; 80(8) (Suppl.): 1529-37.

[http://dx.doi.org/10.1002/(SICI)1097-0142(19971015)80:8+<1529::AID-CNCR2>3.0.CO;2-F]
[PMID: 9362419]

[25]   Chao YL, Shepard CR, Wells A. Breast carcinoma cells re-express E-cadherin during mesenchymal to epithelial reverting transition. Mol Cancer 2010; 9: 179.
[http://dx.doi.org/10.1186/1476-4598-9-179] [PMID: 20609236]

[26]   Nan X, Wang J, Liu HN, Wong STC, Zhao H. Epithelial-mesenchymal plasticity in organotropism metastasis and tumor immune escape. J Clin Med 2019; 8(5): E747.
[http://dx.doi.org/10.3390/jcm8050747] [PMID: 31130637]

[27]   Gao Y, Bado I, Wang H, Zhang W, Rosen JM, Zhang XH. Metastasis organotropism: Redefining the congenial soil. Dev Cell 2019; 49(3): 375-91.
[http://dx.doi.org/10.1016/j.devcel.2019.04.012] [PMID: 31063756]

[28]   De Craene B, Berx G. Regulatory networks defining EMT during cancer initiation and progression. Nat Rev Cancer 2013; 13(2): 97-110.
[http://dx.doi.org/10.1038/nrc3447] [PMID: 23344542]

[29]   Hu Y, Tang H. MicroRNAs regulate the epithelial to mesenchymal transition (EMT) in cancer progression. MicroRNA 2014; 3(2): 108-17.
[http://dx.doi.org/10.2174/2211536603666141010115102] [PMID: 25323025]

[30]   Brozovic A. The relationship between platinum drug resistance and epithelial-mesenchymal transition. Arch Toxicol 2017; 91(2): 605-19.
[http://dx.doi.org/10.1007/s00204-016-1912-7] [PMID: 28032148]

[31]   Sciacovelli M, Frezza C. Metabolic reprogramming and epithelial-to-mesenchymal transition in cancer. FEBS J 2017; 284(19): 3132-44.
[http://dx.doi.org/10.1111/febs.14090] [PMID: 28444969]

[32]   Kast K, Link T, Friedrich K, *et al.* Impact of breast cancer subtypes and patterns of metastasis on outcome. Breast Cancer Res Treat 2015; 150(3): 621-9.
[http://dx.doi.org/10.1007/s10549-015-3341-3] [PMID: 25783184]

[33]   Zeichner SB, Herna S, Mani A, *et al.* Survival of patients with *de-novo* metastatic breast cancer: analysis of data from a large breast cancer-specific private practice, a university-based cancer center and review of the literature. Breast Cancer Res Treat 2015; 153(3): 617-24.
[http://dx.doi.org/10.1007/s10549-015-3564-3] [PMID: 26358708]

[34]   Manié E, Vincent-Salomon A, Lehmann-Che J, *et al.* High frequency of TP53 mutation in BRCA1 and sporadic basal-like carcinomas but not in BRCA1 luminal breast tumors. Cancer Res 2009; 69(2): 663-71.
[http://dx.doi.org/10.1158/0008-5472.CAN-08-1560] [PMID: 19147582]

[35]   Holstege H, Joosse SA, van Oostrom CT, Nederlof PM, de Vries A, Jonkers J. High incidence of protein-truncating TP53 mutations in BRCA1-related breast cancer. Cancer Res 2009; 69(8): 3625-33.
[http://dx.doi.org/10.1158/0008-5472.CAN-08-3426] [PMID: 19336573]

[36]   Seal MD, Chia SK. What is the difference between triple-negative and basal breast cancers? Cancer J 2010; 16(1): 12-6.
[http://dx.doi.org/10.1097/PPO.0b013e3181cf04be] [PMID: 20164685]

[37]   Masuda H, Baggerly KA, Wang Y, *et al.* Differential response to neoadjuvant chemotherapy among 7 triple-negative breast cancer molecular subtypes. Clin Cancer Res 2013; 19(19): 5533-40.
[http://dx.doi.org/10.1158/1078-0432.CCR-13-0799] [PMID: 23948975]

[38]   Yu M, Bardia A, Wittner BS, *et al.* Circulating breast tumor cells exhibit dynamic changes in epithelial and mesenchymal composition. Science 2013; 339(6119): 580-4.
[http://dx.doi.org/10.1126/science.1228522] [PMID: 23372014]

[39]   Gorges TM, Tinhofer I, Drosch M, *et al.* Circulating tumour cells escape from EpCAM-based detection due to epithelial-to-mesenchymal transition. BMC Cancer 2012; 12: 178.

[http://dx.doi.org/10.1186/1471-2407-12-178] [PMID: 22591372]

[40] Mego M, Cierna Z, Janega P, *et al.* Relationship between circulating tumor cells and epithelial to mesenchymal transition in early breast cancer. BMC Cancer 2015; 15: 533.
[http://dx.doi.org/10.1186/s12885-015-1548-7] [PMID: 26194471]

[41] Dewitz C, Duan X, Zampieri N. Organization of motor pools depends on the combined function of N-cadherin and type II cadherins. Development 2019; 146(13): dev180422.
[http://dx.doi.org/10.1242/dev.180422] [PMID: 31235635]

[42] Aiello NM, Maddipati R, Norgard RJ, *et al.* EMT subtype influences epithelial plasticity and mode of cell migration. Dev Cell 2018; 45(6): 681-95.: e4.
[http://dx.doi.org/10.1016/j.devcel.2018.05.027]

[43] Heimann R, Lan F, McBride R, Hellman S. Separating favorable from unfavorable prognostic markers in breast cancer: the role of E-cadherin. Cancer Res 2000; 60(2): 298-304.
[PMID: 10667580]

[44] Takenoshita Y, Ishibashi H, Oka M. Comparison of functional recovery after nonsurgical and surgical treatment of condylar fractures. J Oral Maxillofac Surg 1990; 48(11): 1191-5.
[http://dx.doi.org/10.1016/0278-2391(90)90535-A] [PMID: 2213313]

[45] Chao Y, Wu Q, Acquafondata M, Dhir R, Wells A. Partial mesenchymal to epithelial reverting transition in breast and prostate cancer metastases. Cancer Microenviron 2012; 5(1): 19-28.
[http://dx.doi.org/10.1007/s12307-011-0085-4] [PMID: 21892699]

[46] Preca BT, Bajdak K, Mock K, *et al.* A self-enforcing CD44s/ZEB1 feedback loop maintains EMT and stemness properties in cancer cells. Int J Cancer 2015; 137(11): 2566-77.
[http://dx.doi.org/10.1002/ijc.29642] [PMID: 26077342]

[47] Leth-Larsen R, Lund R, Hansen HV, *et al.* Metastasis-related plasma membrane proteins of human breast cancer cells identified by comparative quantitative mass spectrometry. Mol Cell Proteom 2009; 8(6): 1436-49.
[http://dx.doi.org/10.1074/mcp.M800061-MCP200] [PMID: 19321434]

[48] Carafoli F, Hohenester E. Collagen recognition and transmembrane signalling by discoidin domain receptors. Biochim Biophys Acta 2013; 1834(10): 2187-94.
[http://dx.doi.org/10.1016/j.bbapap.2012.10.014] [PMID: 23128141]

[49] Anurag M, Punturi N, Hoog J, Bainbridge MN, Ellis MJ, Haricharan S. Comprehensive profiling of DNA repair defects in breast cancer identifies a novel class of endocrine therapy resistance drivers. Clin Cancer Res 2018; 24(19): 4887-99.
[http://dx.doi.org/10.1158/1078-0432.CCR-17-3702] [PMID: 29793947]

[50] Toy KA, Valiathan RR, Núñez F, *et al.* Tyrosine kinase discoidin domain receptors DDR1 and DDR2 are coordinately deregulated in triple-negative breast cancer. Breast Cancer Res Treat 2015; 150(1): 9-18.
[http://dx.doi.org/10.1007/s10549-015-3285-7] [PMID: 25667101]

[51] Ren T, Zhang W, Liu X, *et al.* Discoidin domain receptor 2 (DDR2) promotes breast cancer cell metastasis and the mechanism implicates epithelial-mesenchymal transition programme under hypoxia. J Pathol 2014; 234(4): 526-37.
[http://dx.doi.org/10.1002/path.4415] [PMID: 25130389]

[52] Basu S, Cheriyamundath S, Ben-Ze'ev A. Cell-cell adhesion: linking Wnt/β-catenin signaling with partial EMT and stemness traits in tumorigenesis. F1000 Res 2018; 7: 7.
[http://dx.doi.org/10.12688/f1000research.15782.1] [PMID: 30271576]

[53] Tian X, Liu Z, Niu B, *et al.* E-cadherin/β-catenin complex and the epithelial barrier. J Biomed Biotechnol 2011; 2011: 567305.
[http://dx.doi.org/10.1155/2011/567305] [PMID: 22007144]

[54] Onder TT, Gupta PB, Mani SA, Yang J, Lander ES, Weinberg RA. Loss of E-cadherin promotes

metastasis *via* multiple downstream transcriptional pathways. Cancer Res 2008; 68(10): 3645-54.
[http://dx.doi.org/10.1158/0008-5472.CAN-07-2938] [PMID: 18483246]

[55]   Gong Y, Chippada-Venkata UD, Oh WK. Roles of matrix metalloproteinases and their natural inhibitors in prostate cancer progression. Cancers (Basel) 2014; 6(3): 1298-327.
[http://dx.doi.org/10.3390/cancers6031298] [PMID: 24978435]

[56]   Gialeli C, Theocharis AD, Karamanos NK. Roles of matrix metalloproteinases in cancer progression and their pharmacological targeting. FEBS J 2011; 278(1): 16-27.
[http://dx.doi.org/10.1111/j.1742-4658.2010.07919.x] [PMID: 21087457]

[57]   Radisky ES, Radisky DC. Matrix metalloproteinase-induced epithelial-mesenchymal transition in breast cancer. J Mammary Gland Biol Neoplasia 2010; 15(2): 201-12.
[http://dx.doi.org/10.1007/s10911-010-9177-x] [PMID: 20440544]

[58]   Lin CY, Tsai PH, Kandaswami CC, *et al.* Matrix metalloproteinase-9 cooperates with transcription factor Snail to induce epithelial-mesenchymal transition. Cancer Sci 2011; 102(4): 815-27.
[http://dx.doi.org/10.1111/j.1349-7006.2011.01861.x] [PMID: 21219539]

[59]   Bray SJ. Notch signalling in context. Nat Rev Mol Cell Biol 2016; 17(11): 722-35.
[http://dx.doi.org/10.1038/nrm.2016.94] [PMID: 27507209]

[60]   Kontomanolis EN, Kalagasidou S, Pouliliou S, *et al.* The notch pathway in breast cancer progression. Sci World J 2018; 2018: 2415489.
[http://dx.doi.org/10.1155/2018/2415489] [PMID: 30111989]

[61]   Wang J, Sullenger BA, Rich JN. Notch signaling in cancer stem cells. Adv Exp Med Biol 2012; 727: 174-85.
[http://dx.doi.org/10.1007/978-1-4614-0899-4_13] [PMID: 22399347]

[62]   Xiao Q, Ge G. Lysyl oxidase, extracellular matrix remodeling and cancer metastasis. Cancer Microenviron 2012; 5(3): 261-73.
[http://dx.doi.org/10.1007/s12307-012-0105-z] [PMID: 22528876]

[63]   Ye J, Wen J, Ning Y, Li Y. Higher notch expression implies poor survival in pancreatic ductal adenocarcinoma: A systematic review and meta-analysis. Pancreatology 2018; 18(8): 954-61.
[http://dx.doi.org/10.1016/j.pan.2018.09.014] [PMID: 30297095]

[64]   Zhong Y, Shen S, Zhou Y, *et al.* NOTCH1 is a poor prognostic factor for breast cancer and is associated with breast cancer stem cells. OncoTargets Ther 2016; 9: 6865-71.
[http://dx.doi.org/10.2147/OTT.S109606] [PMID: 27853380]

[65]   Lemmon MA, Schlessinger J. Cell signaling by receptor tyrosine kinases. Cell 2010; 141(7): 1117-34.
[http://dx.doi.org/10.1016/j.cell.2010.06.011] [PMID: 20602996]

[66]   Du Z, Lovly CM. Mechanisms of receptor tyrosine kinase activation in cancer. Mol Cancer 2018; 17(1): 58.
[http://dx.doi.org/10.1186/s12943-018-0782-4] [PMID: 29455648]

[67]   Yamaoka T, Kusumoto S, Ando K, Ohba M, Ohmori T. Receptor tyrosine kinase-targeted cancer therapy. Int J Mol Sci 2018; 19(11): E3491.
[http://dx.doi.org/10.3390/ijms19113491] [PMID: 30404198]

[68]   Butti R, Das S, Gunasekaran VP, Yadav AS, Kumar D, Kundu GC. Receptor tyrosine kinases (RTKs) in breast cancer: signaling, therapeutic implications and challenges. Mol Cancer 2018; 17(1): 34.
[http://dx.doi.org/10.1186/s12943-018-0797-x] [PMID: 29455658]

[69]   Organ SL, Tsao MS. An overview of the c-MET signaling pathway. Ther Adv Med Oncol 2011; 3(1) (Suppl.): S7-S19.
[http://dx.doi.org/10.1177/1758834011422556] [PMID: 22128289]

[70]   Cruickshanks N, Zhang Y, Yuan F, Pahuski M, Gibert M, Abounader R. Role and therapeutic targeting of the HGF/MET pathway in glioblastoma. Cancers (Basel) 2017; 9(7): E87.

[http://dx.doi.org/10.3390/cancers9070087] [PMID: 28696366]

[71] Wee P, Wang Z. Epidermal growth factor receptor cell proliferation signaling pathways. Cancers (Basel) 2017; 9(5): E52.
[PMID: 28513565]

[72] Syed V. TGF-β signaling in cancer. J Cell Biochem 2016; 117(6): 1279-87.
[http://dx.doi.org/10.1002/jcb.25496] [PMID: 26774024]

[73] Okubo M, Chiba R, Karakida T, *et al.* Potential function of TGF-β isoforms in maturation-stage ameloblasts. J Oral Biosci 2019; 61(1): 43-54.
[http://dx.doi.org/10.1016/j.job.2018.12.002] [PMID: 30929801]

[74] Cabezas F, Farfán P, Marzolo MP. Participation of the SMAD2/3 signalling pathway in the down regulation of megalin/LRP2 by transforming growth factor beta (TGF-ß1). PLoS One 2019; 14(5): e0213127.
[http://dx.doi.org/10.1371/journal.pone.0213127] [PMID: 31120873]

[75] Ioannou M, Kouvaras E, Papamichali R, Samara M, Chiotoglou I, Koukoulis G. Smad4 and epithelial-mesenchymal transition proteins in colorectal carcinoma: an immunohistochemical study. J Mol Histol 2018; 49(3): 235-44.
[http://dx.doi.org/10.1007/s10735-018-9763-6] [PMID: 29468299]

[76] Zhao M, Mishra L, Deng CX. The role of TGF-β/SMAD4 signaling in cancer. Int J Biol Sci 2018; 14(2): 111-23.
[http://dx.doi.org/10.7150/ijbs.23230] [PMID: 29483830]

[77] Zhang YE. Non-smad signaling pathways of the TGF-β family. Cold Spring Harb Perspect Biol 2017; 9(2): a022129.
[http://dx.doi.org/10.1101/cshperspect.a022129] [PMID: 27864313]

[78] Joseph JV, Conroy S, Tomar T, *et al.* TGF-β is an inducer of ZEB1-dependent mesenchymal transdifferentiation in glioblastoma that is associated with tumor invasion. Cell Death Dis 2014; 5: e1443.
[http://dx.doi.org/10.1038/cddis.2014.395] [PMID: 25275602]

[79] Aomatsu K, Arao T, Sugioka K, *et al.* TGF-β induces sustained upregulation of SNAI1 and SNAI2 through Smad and non-Smad pathways in a human corneal epithelial cell line. Invest Ophthalmol Vis Sci 2011; 52(5): 2437-43.
[http://dx.doi.org/10.1167/iovs.10-5635] [PMID: 21169525]

[80] Leong KG, Karsan A. Signaling pathways mediated by tumor necrosis factor alpha. Histol Histopathol 2000; 15(4): 1303-25.
[PMID: 11005254]

[81] Aggarwal BB. Signalling pathways of the TNF superfamily: a double-edged sword. Nat Rev Immunol 2003; 3(9): 745-56.
[http://dx.doi.org/10.1038/nri1184] [PMID: 12949498]

[82] Ho MY, Tang SJ, Chuang MJ, *et al.* TNF-α induces epithelial-mesenchymal transition of renal cell carcinoma cells *via* a GSK3β-dependent mechanism. Mol Cancer Res 2012; 10(8): 1109-19.
[http://dx.doi.org/10.1158/1541-7786.MCR-12-0160] [PMID: 22707636]

[83] Wang H, Wang HS, Zhou BH, *et al.* Epithelial-mesenchymal transition (EMT) induced by TNF-α requires AKT/GSK-3β-mediated stabilization of snail in colorectal cancer. PLoS One 2013; 8(2): e56664.
[http://dx.doi.org/10.1371/journal.pone.0056664] [PMID: 23431386]

[84] Mikami S, Mizuno R, Kosaka T, Saya H, Oya M, Okada Y. Expression of TNF-α and CD44 is implicated in poor prognosis, cancer cell invasion, metastasis and resistance to the sunitinib treatment in clear cell renal cell carcinomas. Int J Cancer 2015; 136(7): 1504-14.
[http://dx.doi.org/10.1002/ijc.29137] [PMID: 25123505]

[85]   Li CW, Xia W, Huo L, *et al.* Epithelial-mesenchymal transition induced by TNF-α requires NF-κ--mediated transcriptional upregulation of Twist1. Cancer Res 2012; 72(5): 1290-300.
[http://dx.doi.org/10.1158/0008-5472.CAN-11-3123] [PMID: 22253230]

[86]   Seidel JA, Otsuka A, Kabashima K. Anti-PD-1 and anti-CTLA-4 therapies in cancer: mechanisms of action, efficacy, and limitations. Front Oncol 2018; 8: 86.
[http://dx.doi.org/10.3389/fonc.2018.00086] [PMID: 29644214]

[87]   Ma X, Yan W, Dai Z, *et al.* Baicalein suppresses metastasis of breast cancer cells by inhibiting EMT *via* downregulation of SATB1 and Wnt/β-catenin pathway. Drug Des Devel Ther 2016; 10: 1419-41.
[http://dx.doi.org/10.2147/DDDT.S102541] [PMID: 27143851]

[88]   Malek R, Wang H, Taparra K, Tran PT. Therapeutic targeting of epithelial plasticity programs: focus on the epithelial-mesenchymal transition. Cells Tissues Organs (Print) 2017; 203(2): 114-27.
[http://dx.doi.org/10.1159/000447238] [PMID: 28214899]

[89]   Kennedy LC, Gadi V. Dasatinib in breast cancer: Src-ing for response in all the wrong kinases. Ann Transl Med 2018; 6 (Suppl. 1): S60.
[http://dx.doi.org/10.21037/atm.2018.10.26] [PMID: 30613635]

[90]   Pai HC, Chang LH, Peng CY, *et al.* Moscatilin inhibits migration and metastasis of human breast cancer MDA-MB-231 cells through inhibition of Akt and Twist signaling pathway. J Mol Med (Berl) 2013; 91(3): 347-56.
[http://dx.doi.org/10.1007/s00109-012-0945-5] [PMID: 22961111]

[91]   Herbertz S, Sawyer JS, Stauber AJ, *et al.* Clinical development of galunisertib (LY2157299 monohydrate), a small molecule inhibitor of transforming growth factor-beta signaling pathway. Drug Des Devel Ther 2015; 9: 4479-99.
[PMID: 26309397]

[92]   Rezaei M, Ghaderi A. Monoclonal antibody production against vimentin by whole cell immunization in a mouse model. Iranian J Biotechnol 2018; 16(2): e1802.
[http://dx.doi.org/10.21859/ijb.1802] [PMID: 30805388]

miRNA Biology in Breast Cancer Progression

Sanjay Mishra[*], **Manish Charan**, **Swati Misri**, **Dinesh Ahirwar** and **Ramesh K. Ganju**

Department of Pathology, The Ohio State University, Columbus, Ohio, 43210, USA

Abstract: Among the plethora of human malignancies, breast cancer is one of the most prevalent cancers diagnosed in women worldwide. The early detection of breast cancer with current techniques has significantly reduced the mortality rate in the last decade. Nonetheless, various drawbacks presented by these techniques remain as one of the foremost hurdles in the proper clinical management of the condition. The discovery and utilization of highly specific, minimally invasive unique biomarkers would greatly aid an efficient diagnosis and prognosis of breast cancer. The differential expressions of miRNAs also play well-studied roles in the progression and metastasis of the condition. The chapter outlines the clinical importance of miRNAs-based biomarkers in the early detection and prognosis of breast cancer and reviews the different subtypes involved. The role of miRNAs in modulating various cellular processes during the progression and metastasis of breast cancer has been discussed. Finally, the importance of an integrated omics approach in identifying novel targets of miRNAs is also elaborated upon.

Keywords: Autophagy, Apoptosis, Biomarker, Breast cancer, Cancer stem cells, Metabolomics, miRNA, Proteomics, Senescence.

INTRODUCTION

MicroRNAs or miRNAs are a class of short (~15-22 nucleotides) non-coding RNAs that mediate the post-translational gene silencing (PTGS) of target genes [1]. The discovery of the first miRNA in *Caenorhabditis elegans* in 1993 did little in elucidating their functional roles in different cancers [2]. Moreover, the importance of miRNAs in breast cancer progression and metastasis has not been fully explored.

Many experimental studies have reported dysregulated expression of miRNAs in different human malignancies, especially in comparison studies conducted between sporadic breast tumors and normal breast tissue [3 - 10]. One study

---

[*] **Corresponding Author: Sanjay Mishra**: Department of Pathology, The Ohio State University, Columbus, Ohio, 43210, USA; E-mail: sanjay.mishra@osumc.edu

Shankar Suman, Garima Suman and Sanjay Mishra (Eds.)

revealed the altered expression of numerous miRNA signatures in 86 breast tumor tissues to adjacent normal tissues, thus suggesting these miRNA markers defined a specific discriminating signature panel between malignant breast cancer and normal individuals [4]. Recently, an increasing number of experimental studies based on the different molecular technologies also reported the deregulated expressions of miRNA in breast cancer cases [11 - 15]. In this book chapter, we will describe the altered expression, biological functions, and therapeutic application of different miRNAs in breast cancer progression and metastasis. This book chapter will also discuss the application of an integrated omics approach in identifying the novel targets of miRNAs deregulated in breast cancer.

miRNA BIOGENESIS AND FUNCTIONS

Despite the discovery of thousands of human miRNAs to date, none of their functions are well understood [16]. miRNAs regulate target gene expression either by mRNA degradation or translational repression, depending on the degree of complementarities between seed sequence of miRNA and 3' or 5'-UTR of mRNA transcripts [17, 18]. The bulk of miRNA encoding genes are transcribed in the nucleus by RNA polymerase type II enzyme (Pol II), after which the resulting primary miRNAs (pri-miRNAs) are capped, spliced and polyadenylated similar to messenger RNA (Fig. **1**) [19]. It was reported that around 30% of miRNAs encoding genes are transcribed from introns of protein-encoding genes, while the majority of miRNAs are processed from specific miRNA gene loci [1]. An individual primary-miRNA can either generate a single miRNA molecule or may comprise a cluster of two or more miRNAs [1]. These long primary-miRNAs are then processed by a microprocessor, which includes a double-stranded RNase III enzyme (DROSHA) and its important cofactor, the double-stranded RNA (dsRNA)-binding protein DiGeorge syndrome critical region 8 (DGCR8) [20 - 23]. DROSHA has two RNase III domains, each of which cleaves one strand of the dsRNA towards the base of stem-loop secondary structures contained within pri-miRNAs to process ~60-70 nucleotide hairpin-shaped precursor miRNAs (pre-miRNAs) [20 - 23]. The single-stranded RNA stem junction and the distance from the terminal loop region of single-stranded RNA-stem junction are recognized by this microprocessor complex, which specifically cleaves the dsRNA at approximately 11 bp from the junction with the flanking ssRNA [20 - 23]. This cleavage produces the hairpin-shaped structure of pre-miRNAs with an overhang at the 3′ end of either two nucleotides (group I) or one nucleotide (group II) [24 - 27]. The pre-miRNAs are then exported to cytoplasm from the nucleus by exportin 5 (XPO5) complex, and then further processed by RNase III DICER1 enzyme, which measures the pre-miRNA from its 5′ to 3′ ends [28 - 30]. The catalytic RNase III domains of DICER1 enzyme located to the end of the pre-miRNA, so that asymmetrical cleavage of the dsRNA stem, located close to the terminal loop sequence, generates a mature (~22-nucleotides) miRNA duplex with two-nucleotide 3′ overhangs [31]. DICER1 enzyme has also been found to associate with transactivation-responsive RNA-binding protein (TARBP2), which binds with dsRNA [32]. The primary function of the TRBP enzyme is to enhance the fidelity of DICER1-regulated cleavage of a subset of pre-miRNAs in a structure-dependent fashion, thus modulating the miRNA guide-strand selection by causing the formation of iso-miRNAs [33, 34]. Iso-miRNAs are 1 nucleotide longer than regular miRNAs [33, 34]. TRBP plays additional important roles in physically bridging DICER1 with different Argonaute proteins (AGO-1, 2, 3 or 4) and contributing to the formation of the miRNA-induced silencing complex (miRISC) [32]. Consequently, a single strand of the mature miRNA will be bound to a Argonaute protein, known as a "guide strand", and this strand remains in the RISC complex. This miRNA guide strand with RISC assembly will then bind to the complementary sequence of target mRNA transcripts with other members of the GW182 family of proteins [1]. The resultant complex causes post transcriptional gene silencing in processing bodies (P-bodies), which are cytoplasmic foci formed post- mRNA silencing and decay. Nonetheless, they are not essential for miRNA-mediated post-transcriptional gene silencing [35, 36].

miRNA MISREGULATION IN BREAST CANCER PATHOGENESIS

Although some discrepancies exist in the expression of a few specific miRNAs in breast cancer, many miRNAs (*e.g.*, let-7a, miR-100, miR-21, miR-34a, miR-125a, miR-145, miR-125b, miR-143, miR-10b, miR-101, miR-205, miR-210, miR-29b, miR-99a, miR-497, miR-99b) show the same reproducible differential expression pattern in sporadic breast cancer cases [10, 37]. Indeed, a few of them, such as let-7 family, miR-21, miR-34a, miR-145, and miR-155 are also altered in different types of human malignancies, including lung, colon, and liver cancers [38]. Besides these, the differential expression of miRNAs was also found to correlate with histopathological features of breast tumors such as progesterone and estrogen receptor status (miR-30) and tumor stages (miR-203 and miR-213) [39, 40]. The altered expression pattern of different isoforms of let-7 was also found to be associated with lymph node metastasis (let-7a-2, let-7a-3, and let-7f-1), histopathological features including progesterone receptor status (let-7c), or high proliferation index (let-7c and let-7d) in breast cancer samples [4]. Mattie *et al.* have also identified a distinctive set of miRNA signatures associated with breast cancer cases of ER/PR or HER2 profile [41].

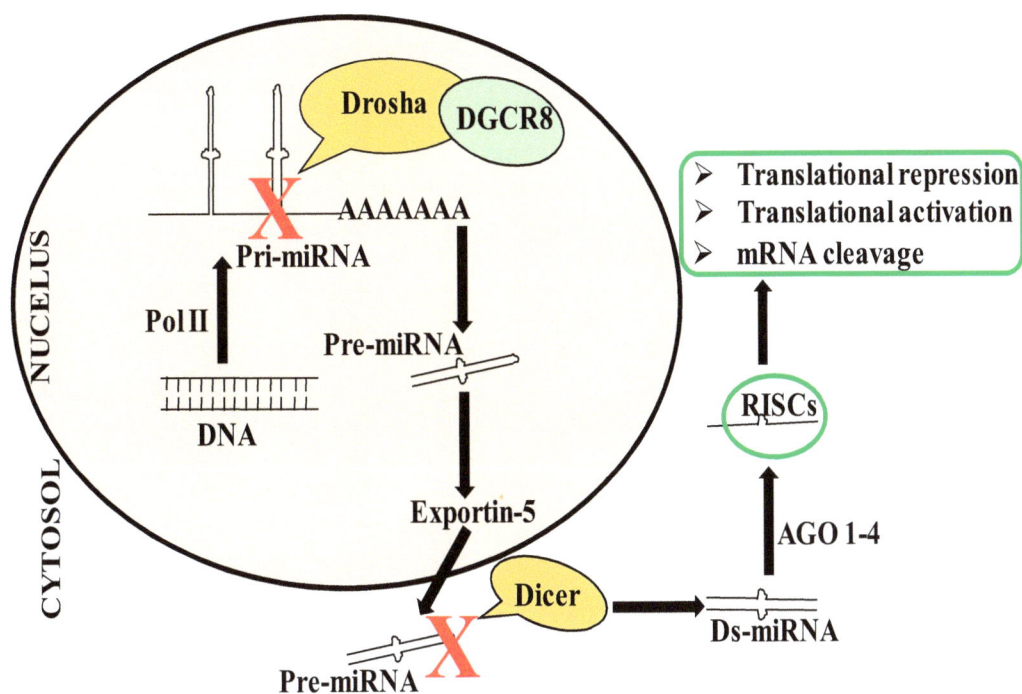

Fig. (1). Schematic diagram showing the biogenesis and molecular function of miRNA. miRNA encoding genes are transcribed by RNA polymerase II (Pol II) into primary miRNA (Pri-miRNA) in the nucleus. Pri-miRNA is then processed into Pre-miRNA by the RNase III enzyme called Drosha and RNA binding protein DGCR8. Pre-miRNAs are then exported to the cytosol from the nucleus by Exportin-5 and cleaved into double-stranded miRNAs by another RNase III enzyme called Dicer. Finally, mature miRNAs require ribonucleoprotein complexes, termed as RNA-induced silencing complexes (RISCs), and mature single-stranded miRNAs exert their functions by interacting with Argonaute proteins (AGO 1-4) in RISCs complex.

Several experimental studies also explored the functional role of miRNAs in regulating different biological processes altered during breast cancer pathogenesis. A specific panel of miRNAs (miR-221, miR-222and miR-206) was reported as a set of potent modulators of ER expression, and their expressions were found to be upregulated in ER-negative tumors [42, 43]. The downregulated expressions of miR-335 and miR-126 were also found to be associated with increased metastatic potential and relapse of breast cancer cases [44]. Moreover, differential expression of miRNAs has also been found to be very specific and defined, comparable to gene expression profiling of coding genes, differential hormonal subtypes (luminal A, luminal B, basal-like, and HER2+) and differential histological grades (lobular/ductal, ER+/ER-).

Currently, reports on the functional importance of miRNAs in familial breast cancer cases remain paucal. The altered expression of miRNA signatures in hereditary breast cancer could be used to classify different types of breast cancer and delineate the role of miRNAs in hereditary breast cancer [45] BRCAX breast tumors have shown specific altered miRNAs expression pattern that could be used to identify histological and molecular heterogeneity of these tumors [10, 46]. In summary, the misregulation of several miRNAs is potentially associated with breast cancer pathogenesis, and these altered miRNA signatures could be successfully used to develop the potential diagnostic and therapeutic markers for breast cancer diagnosis and treatment.

ROLE OF miRNAS IN DIFFERENT CELLULAR PROCESSES ASSOCIATED WITH BREAST CANCER PATHOGENESIS

As elaborated, miRNAs are potential regulators of diverse cellular and molecular processes associated with different human cancers, including breast cancer. The altered expression of miRNAs is associated with aberrant breast cancer cell proliferation and survival. It has been reported that overexpression of miR-199a-3p increased the proliferation rate and survival of breast cancer and endothelial cells by regulating the caveolin-2 gene [47]. On the other hand, miR-193a was found to suppress the proliferation and metastasis of breast cancer cells by inhibiting the WT1 gene [48]. The amplification of chromosomal locus encoding miR-191/425 was reported to increase the proliferation and metastasis of breast cancer by targeting the DICER1 protein [49]. Apart from its role in the proliferation and survival of breast cancer cells, miRNAs have also been reported to regulate apoptosis in normal and cancer cells. miR-101 was found to attenuate the growth and proliferation of breast cancer cells by inducing apoptosis *via* regulation of the Sex-Determining Region Y-box 2 gene [50]. Breunig *et al.* also showed that overexpression of miR-519a-3p is linked to reduced survival probability of breast cancer subjects [51]. They also found that the high level of miR-519a-3p in breast cancer cells causes resistivity to apoptosis mediated by granzyme-B, FasL and TRAIL by attenuating the apoptosis machinery in breast cancer cells [51].

Moreover, miR-519a-3p also suppressed breast cancer cell killing by modulating the natural killer (NK) cells through the inhibition of NKG2D ligands (MICA and ULBP2) expressed on the surface of breast cancer cells [51]. These ligands are essential for the recognition of cancer cells by NK cells [51]. miR-372 and 449 inhibit proliferation and cause apoptosis by directly targeting the E2F1 in different human breast cancer cell types [52, 53]. The increased expression of miR-32 has been shown to induce breast cancer cell proliferation and migration *via* inhibition of FBXW7 [54]. Furthermore, a high level of miR-224 has also been shown to induce the TNBC progression *via* inhibition of Caspase-9 [55]. Few studies also highlighted the essential role of miRNAs in regulating autophagy in breast cancer cells. It has been shown that the downregulation of miR-26b can promote irradiation-induced autophagy in these cells [56]. One similar study also analyzed the role of miR-30a in breast cancer cells by inhibiting the expression of beclin 1 activated by rapamycin [57]. Moreover, miR-25 has also been shown to regulate the chemoresistance-associated autophagy in breast cancer cells [58]. The differential expressions of miRNAs have also been found to be associated with the induction of cellular senescence in different *in-vitro* and *in-vivo* models. One study identified the sets of miRNAs (miR-376a*, miR-486-5p, miR-210, miR-542-5p, and miR-494) found to induce cellular senescence in normal fibroblasts by causing double-strand DNA breakage and ROS generation [59]. The overexpression of miR-22 and miR-203 were also found to induce senescence in different cancer cell lines [60, 61]. The exogenous expression of miR-34a and let-7 were reported to cause cellular senescence in various normal, as well as cancer cells [60, 61]. However, to date, little is understood about the functional role of miRNAs in mediating sustained SASPs in *in-vitro* and *in-vivo* systems despite a few studies suggesting the potential role of miR-34a and miR-146a/b in causing SASPs in different normal cells [62, 63]. Yet no previous study has been performed to investigate the functional significance of miRNAs, especially of miR-34a in mediating the sustained SASPs in drug-induced pseudo-senescent TNBC cells.

CIRCULATING miRNAS AS POTENTIAL BIOMARKER IN BREAST CANCER

As misregulation of miRNAs expression is potentially coupled with breast cancer pathogenesis, therefore, miRNAs (especially circulating miRNAs) hold great potential for use as clinical molecular biomarkers. There are several reasons, which highlighted the high clinical impact of miRNA global profiling as compared to conventional mRNA expression analysis [64]. It was found that miRNAs are well preserved in formalin-fixed paraffin-embedded (FFPE) tissue tissues up to several years and exceptional high stability of miRNAs in different bodily fluids (blood, urine, sputum, and saliva) also permitting the retroactive examination of cancer patient samples [65]. The small size of miRNAs also makes them potent circulating biomarkers for the detection of different human malignancies, including breast cancer [66]. Due to their small length, they are also found to extremely resistant to degradation and thus can be extracted from any sample sources. Moreover, the detection of miRNAs requires a very low concentration of total RNA for analysis by quantitative real-time PCR and thus has the possibility to be developed as an unvarying clinical biomarker for breast cancer detection. It was also reported that circulating miRNAs could be effortlessly quantified in whole blood or serum sample and several experimental studies revealed the cancer-specific alteration of circulating miRNAs in different cancer patients and thus, provide a huge possibility of using them as a minimally invasive biomarker of different human cancers [67, 68]. Furthermore, the identification of miRNAs as potent modulators of different target genes associated with breast cancer pathogenesis also identifies them as novel potential diagnostic, prognostic or therapeutic markers. The altered expression of miRNA in serum was initially described in cancer patients with diffuse large B-cell lymphoma in 2008 [69]. The circulating miRNAs have the broad potential to serve as candidate molecular signatures for the diagnosis of any human malignancies, because circulating miRNAs can be easily quantified in the circulation and that levels might directly or indirectly reflect miRNA expression in tumors [68, 70, 71]. The area of circulating miRNA research in breast cancer pathogenesis is just currently rising and is generating lots of enthusiasm in clinical as well as scientific communities. Following this, few experimental evidence has revealed the differential miRNAs expression's profile in both tissue and body fluids samples of different molecular subtypes of breast cancer [4, 39]. The blood samples of different biological cohorts of breast cancer cases have also revealed a direct positive correlation between increased levels of circulating miRNAs (miR-195 and let-7a) and the probability of having breast cancer [72]. Moreover, miR-376c, miR-148b, miR-801, and miR-409-3p have been suggested as potential candidate biomarkers in blood plasma for early diagnosis of breast cancer [3]. Likewise, circulating miRNAs such as miR-34a, miR-155 and miR-10b have also been reported as a potential molecular signature of primary and metastatic breast-cancer cases [73]. It has been reported that miR-195-5p and miR-495 miRNAs can be used as potential molecular markers for the early stages of breast cancer [74]. McGuire *et al.*, have also reviewed the clinical importance of several miRNAs in metastatic breast cancer [75]. In this review, they have highlighted the role of different miRNAs (miRNAs-10b, 155, 34a, 200a/b/c, 141, 429, 209, 31, 373, 214, 199a) in breast cancer cells proliferation, extravasation, dissemination and invasion [75]. Furthermore, it has also been reported that let-7 miRNA showed increased expression in luminal breast cancer patients, regardless of different breast cancer subtypes. The high expression of miR-195 was also observed in the blood plasma of TNBC patients [76]. Adhami *et al.*, also reported a novel panel of miRNAs that can be used for the early diagnosis and prognosis of breast cancer. In this study, they have identified altered expressions of miR-21, miR-145, miR-139-5p, miR-195, miR-205, miR-99a, miR-210 and miR-497 in breast tissues samples of breast cancer patients [77]. The Cancer Genome Atlas (TCGA) analysis of retrieved miRNA-sequence datasets of 1,052 breast cancer samples showed upregulated expressions of miR-18a and miR-205 and have found that the increased expression of miR-744 was associated with improved survival of breast cancer patients [78]. Further analysis showed that increased expressions of miR-205, miR-18a, and miR-744 with ER, PR positive and lymph node-negative had a significant better survivability [78]. Shimomura *et al.*, have also analysed the expression profiles of miRNAs in 1280 serum samples of several large cohorts to identify unique miRNA panel which can be used for the early detection of breast cancer [79]. In this study, authors have compared the altered expressions of miRNA between patients with breast cancer and non-breast cancer. After analysis, a panel of five miRNAs (miR-4634, miR-1307-3p, miR-6875-5p, miR-1246 and miR-6861-5p) were found to be differentially expressed and could be used for diagnosis of breast cancer subjects. This panel of 5 miRNAs showed specificity of 82.9%, sensitivity of 97.3%, with an accuracy of 89.7% for breast cancer patients in the test cohort. Moreover, this combination could also be used to detect the early stage breast cancer with sensitivity of 98.0%. Several studies also highlighted the differential expressions of miRNAs for different molecular intrinsic subtypes of breast cancers [80]. It has been shown that altered expression of miRNAs correlated with endocrine therapy resistivity with differ the ent hormonal subtypes of breast cancer [80]. In this study, authors have also elaborated the functional importance of deregulated miRNAs expressions with triple-negative breast cancer (TNBC) progression, BRCA mutations, EMT, cancer stem cells (CSCs) generation and also functioning of the immune system. The names of differentially expressed miRNAs associated with breast tumor development and different molecular subtypes are given in Table **1**. In summarily, these few experimental studies have highlighted the potential novel role of circulating miRNAs as key markers for diagnosis and prognosis of breast-cancer cases.

REGULATORY ROLE OF miRNA IN SELF-RENEWAL, TUMORIGENICITY OF BCSCS

MicroRNAs play a key role in CSCs maintenance, including BCSCs [81 - 83]. Among all CSCs reported so far from different tumors, BCSCs are the most studied CSCs because breast cancer is the most common cancer and the second leading cause of cancer-related deaths in Europe and the USA [84]. In 2007, for the first time, Yu *et al.* performed the microarray analysis of BCSCs, isolated from the primary tumors or breast cancer cell lines [85]. They found that let-7 miRNA family (let-7a, let-7b, let-7c, let-7d, let-7f, let-7i) resided at chromosome 9, a region frequently deleted in many human cancers [85].

Table 1. Name of miRNAs linked with different molecular subtypes of breast cancer.

miRNAs	Molecular Subtypes	References
let-7c, let-7f, miR-206, miR-10a miR-15b, miR-191, miR-107, miR-26, miR-103, miR-190b, miR-99a, miR-130, miR-126, miR-136, miR-146b, miR-100	Luminal A-like (HR-positive and HER2-negative and low proliferation)	[4, 41, 80, 86, 87]

(Table 1) cont.....

miRNAs	Molecular Subtypes	References
miR-342, miR-100, miR-15b, miR-99a, miR-107, miR-130, miR-103, miR-126, miR-136, miR-146b,	Luminal B-like (HR-positive and HER2-negative and high proliferation)	[39, 41, 80]
miR-142-3p, miR-125a/b, miR-150	HR-negative and HER2-positive	[41, 80, 86]
miR18a/b, miR-29, miR-135b, miR-190b, miR-93, miR-155, miR-17-92	TNBC	[80, 86, 87]

They also observed that the ectopic expression of let-7 miRNA decreased mammospheres formation by suppressing the expression of HRAS, which is responsible for the self-renewal potentiality and HMGA2, which regulates the differentiation capability of the BCSCs [85]. In breast cancer, let-7 was also shown to inhibit brain metastasis by suppressing the KLF4 [88]. Another miRNA reported to regulate the stem cell phenotype in basal breast cancer cell lines (SUM159, HCC1954) is miR-93, and this miRNA was found to inhibit the self-renewal capability of by inducing the differentiation of these BCSCs and thus making them more sensitive to cytotoxic drugs [89]. It was suggested that miR-93 regulates the BCSCs subpopulations by simultaneously targeting a set of BCSCs regulatory genes such as SOX4, JAK1, STAT3, AKT, HMGA2, and E2H1 [89]. It was also found that the exogenous expression of this miRNA in these cells inhibited the relapse of breast tumors in NOD/SCID mice [89]. Although miR-93 was reported as an anti-oncomir in breast cancer cells, surprisingly, opposite effects were noticed in luminal breast cancer cells like MCF7 cell line, where it promotes the stem cell phenotype of BCSCs [89]. Thereby, this study suggested the complexity of miRNAs regulation, where the same miRNAs can have completely opposite roles in different cellular contexts of similar cancer. Few studies also reported the downregulation of miR-200 family members (miR-200a, miR-200b, miR-200c, miR-141, and miR-429) together with miR-145 and miR-146 in BCSCs [90, 91]. These miRNAs were found to inhibit the EMT in BCSCs in response to TGF-β, an essential component required for the maintenance of BCSCs [90, 91]. The ectopic expression of miR-200b in combination with chemotherapy was found to inhibit the mammospheres formation and also prevent tumor growth and relapse in the xenograft mouse model [90, 91]. The expression of miR-200 family members was also found to be decreased in metaplastic breast cancer cases lacking E-cadherin (an important marker of MET) [90, 92 - 94]. The global miRNAs profiling study also revealed the altered expression of 37 miRNAs in CD44[+]/CD24[-/low] BCSCs and three downregulated miRNAs clusters (miR-200c-miR-141, miR-200a,b-miR-429, and miR-96-miR-182-miR-183) with same seed sequences were identified [82, 95]. Out of 37 miRNAs, two miRNAs (miR-146a and miR-146b) were found to be downregulated in highly metastatic human breast cancer cell line, MDA-MB-231 [82, 95]. The ectopic expression of these two miRNAs was found to inhibit the invasion, and migration capabilities of MDA MB-231 derived BCSCs by downregulating IL-1 receptor-associated kinase and TNF receptor-associated factor-6 [82, 95]. Besides this, increased expression of miR-181 family members were also observed in mammospheres grown in undifferentiating conditions [96, 97]. These miRNA families target the mutated ataxia-telangiectasia (ATM) gene, showing the reduced expression in mammospheres formation upon TGF-β treatment [96, 97]. The exogenous expression of miR-181a/b is sufficient to induce the mammospheres formation in breast cancer cells, thus providing them with BCSCs properties [96, 97]. One study also reported the downregulation of miR-34a in MCF 7 derived BCSCs, and it was found that miR-34a negatively regulated cell proliferation, migration, invasion, and propagation of BCSCs by downregulating the Notch1 signaling [83, 98, 99]. The differential expression of miR-34a was also found to negatively correlate with tumor stages, metastasis, and Notch1 expression in tissue sections of breast cancer cases [83, 98, 99]. Moreover, the ectopic of miR-34a in MCF7 derived tumorspheres increased the chemosensitivity to paclitaxel (PTX) drug by suppressing the Notch1 pathway [83, 98, 99]. The formation of tumorspheres and expression of the ALDH1 were also decreased in the BCSCs treated with miR-34a mimics and PTX compared to those treated with PTX alone [83, 98, 99]. It has also been found that MCF-7 derived spheroids showed differential expressions of 134 miRNAs as compared to parental cells analyzed by using miRNA-NGS [100]. This study showed 109 under-expressed and 25 overexpressed miRNAs such as miR-4492, miR-4532, miR-381, miR-4508, miR-4448, miR-1296, and miR-365a [100]. These miRNAs have been reported to associate with self-renewal capability and chemoresistance in breast cancer [101]. Similarly, one study also highlighted the deregulated expression of 33 miRNAs in MCF-7 multicellular tumor spheroids [101]. In this study, miRNA-221-3p and miR-187 were found to be linked with the increased migration/invasion abilities, stemness, self-renewal and cell cycle phase regulation of BCSCs [101]. Thus, the differential expression of miRNA is closely linked with self-renewal and tumorigenicity of BCSCs (Table **2**) and can be used as potential targets for the successful prevention and therapy of breast cancer.

Table 2. Name of miRNAs regulate self-renewal, stemness, and resistance of BCSCs.

miRNAs	Target Genes	Functions	References
miR-146	ZNRF3/NUMB/Frizzled	Wnt/Notch Signaling	[102, 103]
miR-142	APC	Wnt Signaling	[102, 104]
miR-141	β-catenin	Wnt Signaling	[102, 105]
miR-34	Notch, HDAC	Wnt Signaling	[102, 106, 107]

(Table 2) cont.....

miRNAs	Target Genes	Functions	References
miR-200	STAT5a, Zeb	EMT and BCSCs	[102, 108]
miR-205	Notch2	EMT and BCSCs	[102, 109]
miR-106	SMAD7	TGF-β signaling	[102, 110]
miR-21	PTEN	Akt signaling	[102, 111, 112]
miR-140	ALDH1	BCSCs maintenance	[102, 113]
miR-221	ATXN1	Invasion and metastasis	[102, 114]
miR-7	KLF4	Invasion and metastasis	[88, 102]
miR-33b	Twist1, HMGA2	Invasion and metastasis	[102, 115]
miR-495	E-cadherin	EMT	[102, 116]
miR-22	TET family	Methylation	[102, 117]
miR-888	E-cadherin	EMT	[102, 118]
miR-16	Wip1	Drug resistivity	[102, 119]
Let-7	RAS, HMGA2	BCSCs proliferation	[85, 102, 120]
miR-31	PKCε	BCSCs proliferation	[102, 121]
miR-335	SOX4, TNC	BCSCs proliferation	[102, 122, 123]
miR-760	Nanog	BCSCs proliferation	[102, 124]

APPLICATION OF INTEGRATED OMICS APPROACH FOR IDENTIFICATION OF miRNA TARGETS ASSOCIATED WITH BREAST CANCER PATHOGENESIS

At present days, different *in-silico* tools are used to predict the potential miRNA targets that primarily based on the sequence complementarity between the 5' end of the mature miRNA and the 3' or 5'UTR of target genes [125]. But, all of these computational tools show the increased rate of false-negative and false-positive results, as most of the miRNAs contain an imperfect match to their mRNA targets in different cultured cells [126]. Although several high-throughput approaches based on mRNA profiling study have been broadly used for miRNA target identification, this technique also has some limits, like other computational algorithms [126]. As the microarray-based studies relied on the relative abundance of target mRNAs at transcripts level, but it was reported that in most of the cases, miRNA regulate gene expression by translational repression rather than mRNA degradation [126, 127]. Thus, this type of approach will neglect the miRNA targets repressed only at the translational level. Consequently, some novel proteomics approaches such as 2D-DIGE, pulse-SILAC, and iTRAQ based analysis are needed to perform to explore the potent mRNA targets at translational level with increased specificity and sensitivity [126, 128 - 130]. Integrated metabolomics and quantitative proteomics approach can be very useful in identifying the potential targets of miRNAs in BCSCs because target proteins regulating deregulated metabolism might be novel targeted for the successful eradication of BCSCs. Already, numerous proteomics studies are used to identify the potential targets of different differentially expressed miRNAs by using several breast cancer cells [126, 131], but none of them have identified the miRNAs in BCSCs. Besides this, no integrated proteomics and metabolomics analysis has been done to identify the potent miRNA targets that regulate the altered metabolism of BCSCs subpopulations as compared to non-BCSCs. Although, one this type of integrated study is used to identify the potent altered proteins and metabolites for the diagnosis of colorectal cancer [132], but none study has been done to predict the miRNAs targets in BCSCs using this type of integrated approach. Micro-RNAs have been reported to modulate the tumor cell's metabolism, which is mainly associated with an increased uptake of cellular glucose *via* glycolysis followed by the conversion of glycolytic pyruvate into lactate (a process called as Warburg Effect). It has been shown that miR-27b regulates the levels of different metabolites (such as pyruvate, lactate, and citrate) by downregulating the PDHX in breast cancer cells [133]. In this study, the authors also reported that miR-27b attenuates mitochondrial oxidation and promoting extracellular acidification by suppressing the PDHX and, thus, increases the proliferation of breast cancer cells [133]. They have also observed the decreased expression of PDHX with the worst survival probability in breast cancer patients [133]. Similarly, the metabolic analysis of miR-155 deleted breast cancer cells showed decreased uptake of glucose and thus, attenuates the glycolytic pathway through the inhibition of different glucose transporters and metabolic enzymes such as LDHA, PKM2, and HK2 [134]. In this study, the authors revealed the functional role of miR-155 in regulating glucose metabolism *via* (PIK3R1)-PDK1/AKT-FOXO3a pathway. The stable overexpression of miR-155 in TNBC patient-derived cells revealed increased glucose metabolism, while downregulation of miR-155 in these cells showed suppressed glucose metabolism and thus, reduced tumor burden *in a vivo* mouse model. Interestingly, specific uptake value (SUV) of PET analysis of 50 TNBC subjects showed a positive correlation between the glucose uptake and miR-155 expression. In summary, this study revealed the novel functional importance of miR-155 in regulating the glucose metabolism in TNBC by regulating different metabolic enzymes.

Similarly, many studies also applied the high-throughput proteomics approaches to identify the novel targets of miRNAs in breast cancer. One study used an integrated omics approach to identify the differentially expressed miRNAs and their targets by using formalin-fixed, paraffin-embedded tumors obtained from 71 estrogen receptor-positive (ER+) and 25 triple-negative breast cancer (TNBC) samples [135]. In this study, the combined approach of miRNAs profiling and protein expressions showed a complex molecular process that could be associated with the initiation and progression of different subtypes of breast cancer. The authors also revealed the complex and unique metabolic profile, which can be used as therapeutic targets for the treatment of breast cancer. Similarly, one study also identified the novel targets of miR-21 in breast cancer cells by using proteomics, and they have reported that the downregulation of miR-21 in MCF-7 cells showed increased expression of 58 proteins [126]. Further validation by other molecular methods revealed the direct translational inhibition of 6 targets in MCF-7 cells. In another study, Ouchida *et al.*, identified the novel target of miR-20a, miR-19a, and miR-92-1 in MCF-7 breast cancer cells by a quantitative proteomic strategy [131]. The stable downregulation of miR-20a, miR-19a, and miR-92-1 showed significantly overexpression of IMPDH1, ARHGAP1, PPP2R2A and NPEPL1 in breast cancer cells as identified by two-dimensional electrophoresis and a mass spectrometric approach [131]. After validation by luciferase assays and other experimental approaches, authors have identified the IMPDH1 and NPEPL1 as direct targets of miR-19a in breast cancer cells. Moreover, this kind of proteomic approaches were found to be novel technologies for identifying the direct miRNA targets in breast cancer cells. Interestingly, one study revealed the novel targets of an oncogenic miR-373 in breast cancer by using SILAC-based quantitative proteomics approach [136]. In this study, the authors have identified the 335 differentially regulated proteins targeted by miR-373 out of 3666 proteins in breast cancer cells [136]. After in-depth validation by using different molecular approaches, authors have found that miR-373 target RABEP1, TXNIP, GRHL2, HIP1, and TRPS1 by translational repression rather than mRNA degradation in breast cancer cells [136]. Another important study discovered the novel targets of miR-200c in breast cancer cells as its loss associated with aggressive breast cancer subtypes and the worst response to chemotherapeutic treatments [137]. To identify the novel targets of miR-200c in MCF-7 cells, authors have generated a TALENs knock out (KO) of miR-200c by using MCF-7 breast cancer cells. They have identified the novel 26 target proteins associated with different metabolic and cytoskeleton processes. Out of these 26 targets, six targets (SCIN, AGR2, GSTM3, ALDH7A1, and FLNA/B) have been found to regulate at mRNA level in breast cancer cells. In summary, this proteomics study revealed novel targets of miR-200c in regulating the migration of deregulated metabolism and chemotherapeutic resistivity in breast cancer cells. These findings provide novel insights into miR-200c and pave the way for further studies. Furthermore, one study also identified the novel targets of miR-21 in breast cancer cells and tumor tissues by using a quasi-direct liquid chromatography-tandem mass spectrometry (LC-MS/MS)-based targeted proteomics study [138].

SUMMARY AND CONCLUDING REMARKS

The early diagnosis of breast cancer by different existing techniques have significantly decreased the mortality rate over the last few decades. However, these techniques have some limitations like poor sensitivity and specificity, and thus represent one of the major hurdles in the efficient management of this disease. Therefore, the identification of highly specific, minimally invasive distinctive molecular markers is instantaneously needed for the struggle against breast cancer. Besides the proficient diagnosis, effective therapy of breast cancer is also necessary to avoid further relapse of breast cancer. Doxorubicin, a well-known anti-cancer drug, can induce cellular senescence, autophagy, and apoptosis in different types of human cancer cells including breast cancer. Now a day, miRNAs are reported as a big player in regulating the different cellular and molecular processes during breast cancer pathogenesis. Thus, it is very important to uncover the impact of miRNAs as a circulating biomarker and also its regulation in different biological processes, including autophagy, apoptosis, and cellular senescence during breast cancer development and progression. Above all, it is also necessary to identify the novel targets of miRNAs having a role in breast cancer pathogenesis. Now, most of the computational tools predict miRNA targets based mostly on sequence complementarities between the 5' end of the mature miRNA and only the 3' and 5'-UTRs of target genes. But this approach has several limitations like high rates of false negatives and false positives results. High-throughput techniques based on DNA microarrays, which rely on the changes in the abundance of target mRNA, also have some drawbacks because most miRNAs are supposed to modulate the gene expression by translationally repression rather than mRNA degradation. In this book chapter, we have addressed and discusses all the discoveries related to novel functional and translation impact of miRNAs in breast cancer. In summary, this book chapter delineated the diagnostic, prognostic, and therapeutic significance of miRNAs in the successful management of breast cancer. Shortly, the basic concepts generated by these outcomes can be used to diagnose and treat breast cancer patients and also to prevent the relapse of breast tumors in females worldwide. Although, it's a big challenge to effectively and efficiently translate miRNAs based novel biomarkers to enter into daily clinical practice, and thus, it requires a multidisciplinary efforts of scientists and also clinicians from a different branch of medical science.

CONSENT FOR PUBLICATION

Not applicable.

CONFLICT OF INTEREST

The authors confirm that the contents of this chapter have no conflict of interest.

ACKNOWLEDGEMENTS

Declared none.

REFERENCES

[1]   Lin S, Gregory RI. MicroRNA biogenesis pathways in cancer. Nat Rev Cancer 2015; 15(6): 321-33.
        [http://dx.doi.org/10.1038/nrc3932] [PMID: 25998712]

[2]   Lee RC, Feinbaum RL, Ambros V. The C. elegans heterochronic gene lin-4 encodes small RNAs with
        antisense complementarity to lin-14. Cell 1993; 75(5): 843-54.
        [http://dx.doi.org/10.1016/0092-8674(93)90529-Y] [PMID: 8252621]

[3]   Cuk K, Zucknick M, Heil J, *et al.* Circulating microRNAs in plasma as early detection markers for
        breast cancer. Int J Cancer 2013; 132(7): 1602-12.
        [http://dx.doi.org/10.1002/ijc.27799] [PMID: 22927033]

[4]   Iorio MV, Ferracin M, Liu CG, *et al.* MicroRNA gene expression deregulation in human breast cancer.
        Cancer Res 2005; 65(16): 7065-70.
        [http://dx.doi.org/10.1158/0008-5472.CAN-05-1783] [PMID: 16103053]

[5]   Volinia S, Calin GA, Liu CG, *et al.* A microRNA expression signature of human solid tumors defines
        cancer gene targets. Proc Natl Acad Sci USA 2006; 103(7): 2257-61.
        [http://dx.doi.org/10.1073/pnas.0510565103] [PMID: 16461460]

[6]   Xing L, Todd NW, Yu L, Fang H, Jiang F. Early detection of squamous cell lung cancer in sputum by
        a panel of microRNA markers. Mod Pathol 2010; 23(8): 1157-64.
        [http://dx.doi.org/10.1038/modpathol.2010.111] [PMID: 20526284]

[7]   Cummins JM, He Y, Leary RJ, *et al.* The colorectal microRNAome. Proc Natl Acad Sci USA 2006;
        103(10): 3687-92.
        [http://dx.doi.org/10.1073/pnas.0511155103] [PMID: 16505370]

[8]   Eder M, Scherr M. MicroRNA and lung cancer. N Engl J Med 2005; 352(23): 2446-8.
        [http://dx.doi.org/10.1056/NEJMcibr051201] [PMID: 15944431]

[9]   Murakami Y, Yasuda T, Saigo K, *et al.* Comprehensive analysis of microRNA expression patterns in
        hepatocellular carcinoma and non-tumorous tissues. Oncogene 2006; 25(17): 2537-45.
        [http://dx.doi.org/10.1038/sj.onc.1209283] [PMID: 16331254]

[10]   Yan M, Shield-Artin K, Byrne D, *et al.* kConFab Investigators, kConFab. Comparative microRNA
        profiling of sporadic and BRCA1 associated basal-like breast cancers. BMC Cancer 2015; 15: 506.
        [http://dx.doi.org/10.1186/s12885-015-1522-4] [PMID: 26152113]

[11]   Farazi TA, Horlings HM, Ten Hoeve JJ, *et al.* MicroRNA sequence and expression analysis in breast
        tumors by deep sequencing. Cancer Res 2011; 71(13): 4443-53.
        [http://dx.doi.org/10.1158/0008-5472.CAN-11-0608] [PMID: 21586611]

[12]   Fassan M, Baffa R, Palazzo JP, *et al.* MicroRNA expression profiling of male breast cancer. Breast
        Cancer Res 2009; 11(4): R58.
        [http://dx.doi.org/10.1186/bcr2348] [PMID: 19664288]

[13]   Persson H, Kvist A, Rego N, *et al.* Identification of new microRNAs in paired normal and tumor
        breast tissue suggests a dual role for the ERBB2/Her2 gene. Cancer Res 2011; 71(1): 78-86.
        [http://dx.doi.org/10.1158/0008-5472.CAN-10-1869] [PMID: 21199797]

[14]   Sempere LF, Christensen M, Silahtaroglu A, *et al.* Altered MicroRNA expression confined to specific epithelial cell subpopulations in breast cancer. Cancer Res 2007; 67(24): 11612-20.
[http://dx.doi.org/10.1158/0008-5472.CAN-07-5019] [PMID: 18089790]

[15]   Volinia S, Galasso M, Sana ME, *et al.* Breast cancer signatures for invasiveness and prognosis defined by deep sequencing of microRNA. Proc Natl Acad Sci USA 2012; 109(8): 3024-9.
[http://dx.doi.org/10.1073/pnas.1200010109] [PMID: 22315424]

[16]   Kozomara A, Griffiths-Jones S. miRBase: integrating microRNA annotation and deep-sequencing data. Nucleic Acids Res 2011; 39(Database issue): D152-7.
[http://dx.doi.org/10.1093/nar/gkq1027] [PMID: 21037258]

[17]   Bartel DP. MicroRNAs: target recognition and regulatory functions. Cell 2009; 136(2): 215-33.
[http://dx.doi.org/10.1016/j.cell.2009.01.002] [PMID: 19167326]

[18]   Lytle JR, Yario TA, Steitz JA. Target mRNAs are repressed as efficiently by microRNA-binding sites in the 5′ UTR as in the 3′ UTR. Proc Natl Acad Sci USA 2007; 104(23): 9667-72.
[http://dx.doi.org/10.1073/pnas.0703820104] [PMID: 17535905]

[19]   Lee Y, Kim M, Han J, *et al.* MicroRNA genes are transcribed by RNA polymerase II. EMBO J 2004; 23(20): 4051-60.
[http://dx.doi.org/10.1038/sj.emboj.7600385] [PMID: 15372072]

[20]   Gregory RI, Yan KP, Amuthan G, *et al.* The Microprocessor complex mediates the genesis of microRNAs. Nature 2004; 432(7014): 235-40.
[http://dx.doi.org/10.1038/nature03120] [PMID: 15531877]

[21]   Denli AM, Tops BB, Plasterk RH, Ketting RF, Hannon GJ. Processing of primary microRNAs by the Microprocessor complex. Nature 2004; 432(7014): 231-5.
[http://dx.doi.org/10.1038/nature03049] [PMID: 15531879]

[22]   Lee Y, Ahn C, Han J, *et al.* The nuclear RNase III Drosha initiates microRNA processing. Nature 2003; 425(6956): 415-9.
[http://dx.doi.org/10.1038/nature01957] [PMID: 14508493]

[23]   Han J, Lee Y, Yeom KH, Kim YK, Jin H, Kim VN. The Drosha-DGCR8 complex in primary microRNA processing. Genes Dev 2004; 18(24): 3016-27.
[http://dx.doi.org/10.1101/gad.1262504] [PMID: 15574589]

[24]   Han J, Lee Y, Yeom KH, *et al.* Molecular basis for the recognition of primary microRNAs by the Drosha-DGCR8 complex. Cell 2006; 125(5): 887-901.
[http://dx.doi.org/10.1016/j.cell.2006.03.043] [PMID: 16751099]

[25]   Zeng Y, Yi R, Cullen BR. Recognition and cleavage of primary microRNA precursors by the nuclear processing enzyme Drosha. EMBO J 2005; 24(1): 138-48.
[http://dx.doi.org/10.1038/sj.emboj.7600491] [PMID: 15565168]

[26]   Burke JM, Kelenis DP, Kincaid RP, Sullivan CS. A central role for the primary microRNA stem in guiding the position and efficiency of Drosha processing of a viral pri-miRNA. RNA 2014; 20(7): 1068-77.
[http://dx.doi.org/10.1261/rna.044537.114] [PMID: 24854622]

[27]   Heo I, Ha M, Lim J, *et al.* Mono-uridylation of pre-microRNA as a key step in the biogenesis of group II let-7 microRNAs. Cell 2012; 151(3): 521-32.
[http://dx.doi.org/10.1016/j.cell.2012.09.022] [PMID: 23063654]

[28]   Yi R, Qin Y, Macara IG, Cullen BR. Exportin-5 mediates the nuclear export of pre-microRNAs and short hairpin RNAs. Genes Dev 2003; 17(24): 3011-6.
[http://dx.doi.org/10.1101/gad.1158803] [PMID: 14681208]

[29]   Lund E, Güttinger S, Calado A, Dahlberg JE, Kutay U. Nuclear export of microRNA precursors. Science 2004; 303(5654): 95-8.

[http://dx.doi.org/10.1126/science.1090599] [PMID: 14631048]

[30] Park JG, Yoo JY, Jeong SJ, *et al.* Peroxiredoxin 2 deficiency exacerbates atherosclerosis in apolipoprotein E-deficient mice. Circ Res 2011; 109(7): 739-49.
[http://dx.doi.org/10.1161/CIRCRESAHA.111.245530] [PMID: 21835911]

[31] Bernstein E, Caudy AA, Hammond SM, Hannon GJ. Role for a bidentate ribonuclease in the initiation step of RNA interference. Nature 2001; 409(6818): 363-6.
[http://dx.doi.org/10.1038/35053110] [PMID: 11201747]

[32] Chendrimada TP, Gregory RI, Kumaraswamy E, *et al.* TRBP recruits the Dicer complex to Ago2 for microRNA processing and gene silencing. Nature 2005; 436(7051): 740-4.
[http://dx.doi.org/10.1038/nature03868] [PMID: 15973356]

[33] Lee HY, Doudna JA. TRBP alters human precursor microRNA processing *in vitro*. RNA 2012; 18(11): 2012-9.
[http://dx.doi.org/10.1261/rna.035501.112] [PMID: 23006623]

[34] Kim Y, Yeo J, Lee JH, *et al.* Deletion of human tarbp2 reveals cellular microRNA targets and cell-cycle function of TRBP. Cell Rep 2014; 9(3): 1061-74.
[http://dx.doi.org/10.1016/j.celrep.2014.09.039] [PMID: 25437560]

[35] Liu J, Valencia-Sanchez MA, Hannon GJ, Parker R. MicroRNA-dependent localization of targeted mRNAs to mammalian P-bodies. Nat Cell Biol 2005; 7(7): 719-23.
[http://dx.doi.org/10.1038/ncb1274] [PMID: 15937477]

[36] Eulalio A, Behm-Ansmant I, Schweizer D, Izaurralde E. P-body formation is a consequence, not the cause, of RNA-mediated gene silencing. Mol Cell Biol 2007; 27(11): 3970-81.
[http://dx.doi.org/10.1128/MCB.00128-07] [PMID: 17403906]

[37] Bertoli G, Cava C, Castiglioni I. MicroRNAs: New biomarkers for diagnosis, prognosis, therapy prediction and therapeutic tools for breast cancer. Theranostics 2015; 5(10): 1122-43.
[http://dx.doi.org/10.7150/thno.11543] [PMID: 26199650]

[38] Lujambio A, Lowe SW. The microcosmos of cancer. Nature 2012; 482(7385): 347-55.
[http://dx.doi.org/10.1038/nature10888] [PMID: 22337054]

[39] Lowery AJ, Miller N, Devaney A, *et al.* MicroRNA signatures predict oestrogen receptor, progesterone receptor and HER2/neu receptor status in breast cancer. Breast Cancer Res 2009; 11(3): R27.
[http://dx.doi.org/10.1186/bcr2257] [PMID: 19432961]

[40] Donadelli M, Dando I, Zaniboni T, *et al.* Gemcitabine/cannabinoid combination triggers autophagy in pancreatic cancer cells through a ROS-mediated mechanism. Cell Death Dis 2011; 2: e152.
[http://dx.doi.org/10.1038/cddis.2011.36] [PMID: 21525939]

[41] Mattie MD, Benz CC, Bowers J, *et al.* Optimized high-throughput microRNA expression profiling provides novel biomarker assessment of clinical prostate and breast cancer biopsies. Mol Cancer 2006; 5: 24.
[http://dx.doi.org/10.1186/1476-4598-5-24] [PMID: 16784538]

[42] Foekens JA, Sieuwerts AM, Smid M, *et al.* Four miRNAs associated with aggressiveness of lymph node-negative, estrogen receptor-positive human breast cancer. Proc Natl Acad Sci USA 2008; 105(35): 13021-6.
[http://dx.doi.org/10.1073/pnas.0803304105] [PMID: 18755890]

[43] Zhao JJ, Lin J, Yang H, *et al.* MicroRNA-221/222 negatively regulates estrogen receptor alpha and is associated with tamoxifen resistance in breast cancer. J Biol Chem 2008; 283(45): 31079-86.
[http://dx.doi.org/10.1074/jbc.M806041200] [PMID: 18790736]

[44] Tavazoie SF, Alarcón C, Oskarsson T, *et al.* Endogenous human microRNAs that suppress breast cancer metastasis. Nature 2008; 451(7175): 147-52.
[http://dx.doi.org/10.1038/nature06487] [PMID: 18185580]

[45]   Tanic M, Yanowsky K, Rodriguez-Antona C, *et al.* Deregulated miRNAs in hereditary breast cancer revealed a role for miR-30c in regulating KRAS oncogene. PLoS One 2012; 7(6): e38847.
[http://dx.doi.org/10.1371/journal.pone.0038847] [PMID: 22701724]

[46]   Danza K, De Summa S, Pilato B, *et al.* Combined microRNA and ER expression: a new classifier for familial and sporadic breast cancer patients. J Transl Med 2014; 12: 319.
[http://dx.doi.org/10.1186/s12967-014-0319-6] [PMID: 25406994]

[47]   Shatseva T, Lee DY, Deng Z, Yang BB. MicroRNA miR-199a-3p regulates cell proliferation and survival by targeting caveolin-2. J Cell Sci 2011; 124(Pt 16): 2826-36.
[http://dx.doi.org/10.1242/jcs.077529] [PMID: 21807947]

[48]   Xie F, Hosany S, Zhong S, *et al.* MicroRNA-193a inhibits breast cancer proliferation and metastasis by downregulating WT1. PLoS One 2017; 12(10): e0185565.
[http://dx.doi.org/10.1371/journal.pone.0185565] [PMID: 29016617]

[49]   Zhang X, Wu M, Chong QY, *et al.* Amplification of hsa-miR-191/425 locus promotes breast cancer proliferation and metastasis by targeting DICER1. Carcinogenesis 2018; 39(12): 1506-16.
[http://dx.doi.org/10.1093/carcin/bgy102] [PMID: 30084985]

[50]   Wang J, Zeng H, Li H, *et al.* MicroRNA-101 inhibits growth, proliferation and migration and induces apoptosis of breast cancer cells by targeting sex-determining region Y-box 2. Cell Physiol Biochem 2017; 43(2): 717-32.
[http://dx.doi.org/10.1159/000481445] [PMID: 28946143]

[51]   Breunig C, Pahl J, Küblbeck M, *et al.* MicroRNA-519a-3p mediates apoptosis resistance in breast cancer cells and their escape from recognition by natural killer cells. Cell Death Dis 2017; 8(8): e2973.
[http://dx.doi.org/10.1038/cddis.2017.364] [PMID: 28771222]

[52]   Tormo E, Ballester S, Adam-Artigues A, *et al.* The miRNA-449 family mediates doxorubicin resistance in triple-negative breast cancer by regulating cell cycle factors. Sci Rep 2019; 9(1): 5316.
[http://dx.doi.org/10.1038/s41598-019-41472-y] [PMID: 30926829]

[53]   Zhao YX, Liu HC, Ying WY, *et al.* microRNA-372 inhibits proliferation and induces apoptosis in human breast cancer cells by directly targeting E2F1. Mol Med Rep 2017; 16(6): 8069-75.
[http://dx.doi.org/10.3892/mmr.2017.7591] [PMID: 28944922]

[54]   Xia W, Zhou J, Luo H, *et al.* MicroRNA-32 promotes cell proliferation, migration and suppresses apoptosis in breast cancer cells by targeting FBXW7. Cancer Cell Int 2017; 17: 14.
[http://dx.doi.org/10.1186/s12935-017-0383-0] [PMID: 28149200]

[55]   Zhang L, Zhang X, Wang X, He M, Qiao S. MicroRNA-224 promotes tumorigenesis through downregulation of caspase-9 in triple-negative breast cancer. Dis Markers 2019; 2019: 7378967.
[http://dx.doi.org/10.1155/2019/7378967] [PMID: 30886656]

[56]   Meng C, Liu Y, Shen Y, *et al.* MicroRNA-26b suppresses autophagy in breast cancer cells by targeting DRAM1 mRNA, and is downregulated by irradiation. Oncol Lett 2018; 15(2): 1435-40.
[PMID: 29399189]

[57]   Zhu H, Wu H, Liu X, *et al.* Regulation of autophagy by a beclin 1-targeted microRNA, miR-30a, in cancer cells. Autophagy 2009; 5(6): 816-23.
[http://dx.doi.org/10.4161/auto.9064] [PMID: 19535919]

[58]   Wang Z, Wang N, Liu P, *et al.* MicroRNA-25 regulates chemoresistance-associated autophagy in breast cancer cells, a process modulated by the natural autophagy inducer isoliquiritigenin. Oncotarget 2014; 5(16): 7013-26.
[http://dx.doi.org/10.18632/oncotarget.2192] [PMID: 25026296]

[59]   Faraonio R, Salerno P, Passaro F, *et al.* A set of miRNAs participates in the cellular senescence program in human diploid fibroblasts. Cell Death Differ 2012; 19(4): 713-21.
[http://dx.doi.org/10.1038/cdd.2011.143] [PMID: 22052189]

[60]   Xu D, Takeshita F, Hino Y, *et al.* miR-22 represses cancer progression by inducing cellular senescence. J Cell Biol 2011; 193(2): 409-24.
[http://dx.doi.org/10.1083/jcb.201010100] [PMID: 21502362]

[61]   Noguchi S, Mori T, Otsuka Y, *et al.* Anti-oncogenic microRNA-203 induces senescence by targeting E2F3 protein in human melanoma cells. J Biol Chem 2012; 287(15): 11769-77.
[http://dx.doi.org/10.1074/jbc.M111.325027] [PMID: 22354972]

[62]   Bhaumik D, Scott GK, Schokrpur S, *et al.* MicroRNAs miR-146a/b negatively modulate the senescence-associated inflammatory mediators IL-6 and IL-8. Aging (Albany NY) 2009; 1(4): 402-11.
[http://dx.doi.org/10.18632/aging.100042] [PMID: 20148189]

[63]   Badi I, Burba I, Ruggeri C, *et al.* MicroRNA-34a induces vascular smooth muscle cells senescence by SIRT1 downregulation and promotes the expression of age-associated pro-inflammatory secretory factors. J Gerontol A Biol Sci Med Sci 2015; 70(11): 1304-11.
[http://dx.doi.org/10.1093/gerona/glu180] [PMID: 25352462]

[64]   Esquela-Kerscher A, Slack FJ. Oncomirs - microRNAs with a role in cancer. Nat Rev Cancer 2006; 6(4): 259-69.
[http://dx.doi.org/10.1038/nrc1840] [PMID: 16557279]

[65]   Del Vescovo V, Grasso M, Barbareschi M, Denti MA. MicroRNAs as lung cancer biomarkers. World J Clin Oncol 2014; 5(4): 604-20.
[http://dx.doi.org/10.5306/wjco.v5.i4.604] [PMID: 25302165]

[66]   Shalaby T, Fiaschetti G, Baumgartner M, Grotzer MA. MicroRNA signatures as biomarkers and therapeutic target for CNS embryonal tumors: the pros and the cons. Int J Mol Sci 2014; 15(11): 21554-86.
[http://dx.doi.org/10.3390/ijms151121554] [PMID: 25421247]

[67]   Mar-Aguilar F, Mendoza-Ramírez JA, Malagón-Santiago I, *et al.* Serum circulating microRNA profiling for identification of potential breast cancer biomarkers. Dis Markers 2013; 34(3): 163-9.
[http://dx.doi.org/10.1155/2013/259454] [PMID: 23334650]

[68]   Mo MH, Chen L, Fu Y, Wang W, Fu SW. Cell-free Circulating miRNA Biomarkers in Cancer. J Cancer 2012; 3: 432-48.
[http://dx.doi.org/10.7150/jca.4919] [PMID: 23074383]

[69]   Lawrie CH, Gal S, Dunlop HM, *et al.* Detection of elevated levels of tumour-associated microRNAs in serum of patients with diffuse large B-cell lymphoma. Br J Haematol 2008; 141(5): 672-5.
[http://dx.doi.org/10.1111/j.1365-2141.2008.07077.x] [PMID: 18318758]

[70]   Brase JC, Wuttig D, Kuner R, Sültmann H. Serum microRNAs as non-invasive biomarkers for cancer. Mol Cancer 2010; 9: 306.
[http://dx.doi.org/10.1186/1476-4598-9-306] [PMID: 21110877]

[71]   Matamala N, Vargas MT, González-Cámpora R, *et al.* Tumor microRNA expression profiling identifies circulating microRNAs for early breast cancer detection. Clin Chem 2015; 61(8): 1098-106.
[http://dx.doi.org/10.1373/clinchem.2015.238691] [PMID: 26056355]

[72]   Heneghan HM, Miller N, Kerin MJ. Circulating miRNA signatures: promising prognostic tools for cancer. J Clin Oncol 2010; 28(29): e573-4.
[http://dx.doi.org/10.1200/JCO.2010.29.8901] [PMID: 20697097]

[73]   Roth C, Rack B, Müller V, Janni W, Pantel K, Schwarzenbach H. Circulating microRNAs as blood-based markers for patients with primary and metastatic breast cancer. Breast Cancer Res 2010; 12(6): R90.
[http://dx.doi.org/10.1186/bcr2766] [PMID: 21047409]

[74]   Mishra S, Srivastava AK, Suman S, Kumar V, Shukla Y. Circulating miRNAs revealed as surrogate molecular signatures for the early detection of breast cancer. Cancer Lett 2015; 369(1): 67-75.
[http://dx.doi.org/10.1016/j.canlet.2015.07.045] [PMID: 26276721]

[75] McGuire A, Brown JA, Kerin MJ. Metastatic breast cancer: the potential of miRNA for diagnosis and treatment monitoring. Cancer Metastasis Rev 2015; 34(1): 145-55.
[http://dx.doi.org/10.1007/s10555-015-9551-7] [PMID: 25721950]

[76] Qattan A, Intabli H, Alkhayal W, Eltabache C, Tweigieri T, Amer SB. Robust expression of tumor suppressor miRNA's let-7 and miR-195 detected in plasma of Saudi female breast cancer patients. BMC Cancer 2017; 17(1): 799.
[http://dx.doi.org/10.1186/s12885-017-3776-5] [PMID: 29183284]

[77] Adhami M, Haghdoost AA, Sadeghi B, Malekpour Afshar R. Candidate miRNAs in human breast cancer biomarkers: a systematic review. Breast Cancer 2018; 25(2): 198-205.
[http://dx.doi.org/10.1007/s12282-017-0814-8] [PMID: 29101635]

[78] Kim SY, Kawaguchi T, Yan L, Young J, Qi Q, Takabe K. Clinical relevance of microRNA expressions in breast cancer validated using the cancer genome atlas (TCGA). Ann Surg Oncol 2017; 24(10): 2943-9.
[http://dx.doi.org/10.1245/s10434-017-5984-2] [PMID: 28766230]

[79] Shimomura A, Shiino S, Kawauchi J, *et al.* Novel combination of serum microRNA for detecting breast cancer in the early stage. Cancer Sci 2016; 107(3): 326-34.
[http://dx.doi.org/10.1111/cas.12880] [PMID: 26749252]

[80] Kurozumi S, Yamaguchi Y, Kurosumi M, Ohira M, Matsumoto H, Horiguchi J. Recent trends in microRNA research into breast cancer with particular focus on the associations between microRNAs and intrinsic subtypes. J Hum Genet 2017; 62(1): 15-24.
[http://dx.doi.org/10.1038/jhg.2016.89] [PMID: 27439682]

[81] Takahashi RU, Miyazaki H, Takeshita F, *et al.* Loss of microRNA-27b contributes to breast cancer stem cell generation by activating ENPP1. Nat Commun 2015; 6: 7318.
[http://dx.doi.org/10.1038/ncomms8318] [PMID: 26065921]

[82] Shimono Y, Mukohyama J, Nakamura S, Minami H. MicroRNA regulation of human breast cancer stem cells. J Clin Med 2015; 5(1): E2.
[http://dx.doi.org/10.3390/jcm5010002] [PMID: 26712794]

[83] Kang L, Mao J, Tao Y, *et al.* MicroRNA-34a suppresses the breast cancer stem cell-like characteristics by downregulating Notch1 pathway. Cancer Sci 2015; 106(6): 700-8.
[http://dx.doi.org/10.1111/cas.12656] [PMID: 25783790]

[84] Filipova A, Seifrtova M, Mokry J, *et al.* Breast cancer and cancer stem cells: a mini-review. Tumori 2014; 100(4): 363-9.
[http://dx.doi.org/10.1177/1636.17886] [PMID: 25296584]

[85] Yu F, Yao H, Zhu P, *et al.* let-7 regulates self renewal and tumorigenicity of breast cancer cells. Cell 2007; 131(6): 1109-23.
[http://dx.doi.org/10.1016/j.cell.2007.10.054] [PMID: 18083101]

[86] Blenkiron C, Goldstein LD, Thorne NP, *et al.* MicroRNA expression profiling of human breast cancer identifies new markers of tumor subtype. Genome Biol 2007; 8(10): R214.
[http://dx.doi.org/10.1186/gb-2007-8-10-r214] [PMID: 17922911]

[87] Enerly E, Steinfeld I, Kleivi K, *et al.* miRNA-mRNA integrated analysis reveals roles for miRNAs in primary breast tumors. PLoS One 2011; 6(2): e16915.
[http://dx.doi.org/10.1371/journal.pone.0016915] [PMID: 21364938]

[88] Okuda H, Xing F, Pandey PR, *et al.* miR-7 suppresses brain metastasis of breast cancer stem-like cells by modulating KLF4. Cancer Res 2013; 73(4): 1434-44.
[http://dx.doi.org/10.1158/0008-5472.CAN-12-2037] [PMID: 23384942]

[89] Liu S, Patel SH, Ginestier C, *et al.* MicroRNA93 regulates proliferation and differentiation of normal and malignant breast stem cells. PLoS Genet 2012; 8(6): e1002751.
[http://dx.doi.org/10.1371/journal.pgen.1002751] [PMID: 22685420]

[90]   Castilla MA, Díaz-Martín J, Sarrió D, *et al.* MicroRNA-200 family modulation in distinct breast cancer phenotypes. PLoS One 2012; 7(10): e47709.
[http://dx.doi.org/10.1371/journal.pone.0047709] [PMID: 23112837]

[91]   D'Ippolito E, Iorio MV. MicroRNAs and triple negative breast cancer. Int J Mol Sci 2013; 14(11): 22202-20.
[http://dx.doi.org/10.3390/ijms141122202] [PMID: 24284394]

[92]   Korpal M, Kang Y. The emerging role of miR-200 family of microRNAs in epithelial-mesenchymal transition and cancer metastasis. RNA Biol 2008; 5(3): 115-9.
[http://dx.doi.org/10.4161/rna.5.3.6558] [PMID: 19182522]

[93]   Hilmarsdottir B, Briem E, Bergthorsson JT, Magnusson MK, Gudjonsson T. Functional role of the microRNA-200 family in breast morphogenesis and neoplasia. Genes (Basel) 2014; 5(3): 804-20.
[http://dx.doi.org/10.3390/genes5030804] [PMID: 25216122]

[94]   Gregory PA, Bert AG, Paterson EL, *et al.* The miR-200 family and miR-205 regulate epithelial to mesenchymal transition by targeting ZEB1 and SIP1. Nat Cell Biol 2008; 10(5): 593-601.
[http://dx.doi.org/10.1038/ncb1722] [PMID: 18376396]

[95]   Shimono Y, Zabala M, Cho RW, *et al.* Downregulation of miRNA-200c links breast cancer stem cells with normal stem cells. Cell 2009; 138(3): 592-603.
[http://dx.doi.org/10.1016/j.cell.2009.07.011] [PMID: 19665978]

[96]   Wang Y, Yu Y, Tsuyada A, *et al.* Transforming growth factor-β regulates the sphere-initiating stem cell-like feature in breast cancer through miRNA-181 and ATM. Oncogene 2011; 30(12): 1470-80.
[http://dx.doi.org/10.1038/onc.2010.531] [PMID: 21102523]

[97]   Schwarzenbacher D, Balic M, Pichler M. The role of microRNAs in breast cancer stem cells. Int J Mol Sci 2013; 14(7): 14712-23.
[http://dx.doi.org/10.3390/ijms140714712] [PMID: 23860207]

[98]   Park EY, Chang E, Lee EJ, *et al.* Targeting of miR34a-NOTCH1 axis reduced breast cancer stemness and chemoresistance. Cancer Res 2014; 74(24): 7573-82.
[http://dx.doi.org/10.1158/0008-5472.CAN-14-1140] [PMID: 25368020]

[99]   Li X, Zhao J, Tang J. miR-34a may regulate sensitivity of breast cancer cells to adriamycin *via* targeting Notch1. Zhonghua Zhong Liu Za Zhi 2014; 36(12): 892-6.
[PMID: 25623761]

[100] Boo L, Ho WY, Ali NM, *et al.* MiRNA transcriptome profiling of spheroid-enriched cells with cancer stem cell properties in human breastMCF-7 Cell Line. Int J Biol Sci 2016; 12(4): 427-45.
[http://dx.doi.org/10.7150/ijbs.12777] [PMID: 27019627]

[101] Mandujano-Tinoco EA, Garcia-Venzor A, Muñoz-Galindo L, *et al.* miRNA expression profile in multicellular breast cancer spheroids. Biochim Biophys Acta Mol Cell Res 2017; 1864(10): 1642-55.
[http://dx.doi.org/10.1016/j.bbamcr.2017.05.023] [PMID: 28576513]

[102] Vahidian F, Mohammadi H, Ali-Hasanzadeh M, *et al.* MicroRNAs and breast cancer stem cells: Potential role in breast cancer therapy. J Cell Physiol 2019; 234(4): 3294-306.
[http://dx.doi.org/10.1002/jcp.27246] [PMID: 30362508]

[103] Liang R, Li Y, Wang M, *et al.* MiR-146a promotes the asymmetric division and inhibits the self-renewal ability of breast cancer stem-like cells *via* indirect upregulation of Let-7. Cell Cycle 2018; 17(12): 1445-56.
[http://dx.doi.org/10.1080/15384101.2018.1489176] [PMID: 29954239]

[104] Isobe T, Hisamori S, Hogan DJ, *et al.* miR-142 regulates the tumorigenicity of human breast cancer stem cells through the canonical WNT signaling pathway. eLife 2014; 3: 3.
[http://dx.doi.org/10.7554/eLife.01977] [PMID: 25406066]

[105] Abedi N, Mohammadi-Yeganeh S, Koochaki A, Karami F, Paryan M. miR-141 as potential suppressor

of β-catenin in breast cancer. Tumour Biol 2015; 36(12): 9895-901.
[http://dx.doi.org/10.1007/s13277-015-3738-y] [PMID: 26164002]

[106] Bonetti P, Climent M, Panebianco F, *et al.* Dual role for miR-34a in the control of early progenitor proliferation and commitment in the mammary gland and in breast cancer. Oncogene 2019; 38(3): 360-74.
[http://dx.doi.org/10.1038/s41388-018-0445-3] [PMID: 30093634]

[107] Kim NH, Kim HS, Kim NG, *et al.* p53 and microRNA-34 are suppressors of canonical Wnt signaling. Sci Signal 2011; 4(197): ra71.
[http://dx.doi.org/10.1126/scisignal.2001744] [PMID: 22045851]

[108] Burk U, Schubert J, Wellner U, *et al.* A reciprocal repression between ZEB1 and members of the miR-200 family promotes EMT and invasion in cancer cells. EMBO Rep 2008; 9(6): 582-9.
[http://dx.doi.org/10.1038/embor.2008.74] [PMID: 18483486]

[109] Chao CH, Chang CC, Wu MJ, *et al.* MicroRNA-205 signaling regulates mammary stem cell fate and tumorigenesis. J Clin Invest 2014; 124(7): 3093-106.
[http://dx.doi.org/10.1172/JCI73351] [PMID: 24911147]

[110] Smith AL, Iwanaga R, Drasin DJ, *et al.* The miR-106b-25 cluster targets Smad7, activates TGF-β signaling, and induces EMT and tumor initiating cell characteristics downstream of Six1 in human breast cancer. Oncogene 2012; 31(50): 5162-71.
[http://dx.doi.org/10.1038/onc.2012.11] [PMID: 22286770]

[111] Dai X, Fang M, Li S, Yan Y, Zhong Y, Du B. miR-21 is involved in transforming growth factor β1-induced chemoresistance and invasion by targeting PTEN in breast cancer. Oncol Lett 2017; 14(6): 6929-36.
[http://dx.doi.org/10.3892/ol.2017.7007] [PMID: 29151919]

[112] Wang X, Hang Y, Liu J, Hou Y, Wang N, Wang M. Anticancer effect of curcumin inhibits cell growth through miR-21/PTEN/Akt pathway in breast cancer cell. Oncol Lett 2017; 13(6): 4825-31.
[http://dx.doi.org/10.3892/ol.2017.6053] [PMID: 28599484]

[113] Li Q, Yao Y, Eades G, Liu Z, Zhang Y, Zhou Q. Downregulation of miR-140 promotes cancer stem cell formation in basal-like early stage breast cancer. Oncogene 2014; 33(20): 2589-600.
[http://dx.doi.org/10.1038/onc.2013.226] [PMID: 23752191]

[114] Ke J, Zhao Z, Hong SH, *et al.* Role of microRNA221 in regulating normal mammary epithelial hierarchy and breast cancer stem-like cells. Oncotarget 2015; 6(6): 3709-21.
[http://dx.doi.org/10.18632/oncotarget.2888] [PMID: 25686829]

[115] Lin Y, Liu AY, Fan C, *et al.* MicroRNA-33b inhibits breast cancer metastasis by targeting HMGA2, SALL4 and twist1. Sci Rep 2015; 5: 9995.
[http://dx.doi.org/10.1038/srep09995] [PMID: 25919570]

[116] Hwang-Verslues WW, Chang PH, Wei PC, *et al.* miR-495 is upregulated by E12/E47 in breast cancer stem cells, and promotes oncogenesis and hypoxia resistance *via* downregulation of E-cadherin and REDD1. Oncogene 2011; 30(21): 2463-74.
[http://dx.doi.org/10.1038/onc.2010.618] [PMID: 21258409]

[117] Song SJ, Poliseno L, Song MS, *et al.* MicroRNA-antagonism regulates breast cancer stemness and metastasis *via* TET-family-dependent chromatin remodeling. Cell 2013; 154(2): 311-24.
[http://dx.doi.org/10.1016/j.cell.2013.06.026] [PMID: 23830207]

[118] Huang S, Cai M, Zheng Y, Zhou L, Wang Q, Chen L. miR-888 in MCF-7 side population sphere cells directly targets E-cadherin. J Genet Genomics 2014; 41(1): 35-42.
[http://dx.doi.org/10.1016/j.jgg.2013.12.002] [PMID: 24480745]

[119] Zhang X, Wan G, Mlotshwa S, *et al.* Oncogenic Wip1 phosphatase is inhibited by miR-16 in the DNA damage signaling pathway. Cancer Res 2010; 70(18): 7176-86.
[http://dx.doi.org/10.1158/0008-5472.CAN-10-0697] [PMID: 20668064]

[120] Guo L, Cheng X, Chen H, *et al.* Induction of breast cancer stem cells by M1 macrophages through Lin-28B-let-7-HMGA2 axis. Cancer Lett 2019; 452: 213-25.
[http://dx.doi.org/10.1016/j.canlet.2019.03.032] [PMID: 30917918]

[121] Körner C, Keklikoglou I, Bender C, Wörner A, Münstermann E, Wiemann S. MicroRNA-31 sensitizes human breast cells to apoptosis by direct targeting of protein kinase C epsilon (PKCepsilon). J Biol Chem 2013; 288(12): 8750-61.
[http://dx.doi.org/10.1074/jbc.M112.414128] [PMID: 23364795]

[122] Zhang S, Kim K, Jin UH, *et al.* Aryl hydrocarbon receptor agonists induce microRNA-335 expression and inhibit lung metastasis of estrogen receptor negative breast cancer cells. Mol Cancer Ther 2012; 11(1): 108-18.
[http://dx.doi.org/10.1158/1535-7163.MCT-11-0548] [PMID: 22034498]

[123] Png KJ, Yoshida M, Zhang XH, *et al.* MicroRNA-335 inhibits tumor reinitiation and is silenced through genetic and epigenetic mechanisms in human breast cancer. Genes Dev 2011; 25(3): 226-31.
[http://dx.doi.org/10.1101/gad.1974211] [PMID: 21289068]

[124] Han ML, Wang F, Gu YT, *et al.* MicroR-760 suppresses cancer stem cell subpopulation and breast cancer cell proliferation and metastasis: By down-regulating NANOG. Biomed Pharmacother 2016; 80: 304-10.
[http://dx.doi.org/10.1016/j.biopha.2016.03.024] [PMID: 27133070]

[125] Martin G, Schouest K, Kovvuru P, Spillane C. Prediction and validation of microRNA targets in animal genomes. J Biosci 2007; 32(6): 1049-52.
[http://dx.doi.org/10.1007/s12038-007-0106-0] [PMID: 17954966]

[126] Yang Y, Chaerkady R, Beer MA, Mendell JT, Pandey A. Identification of miR-21 targets in breast cancer cells using a quantitative proteomic approach. Proteomics 2009; 9(5): 1374-84.
[http://dx.doi.org/10.1002/pmic.200800551] [PMID: 19253296]

[127] Mathonnet G, Fabian MR, Svitkin YV, *et al.* MicroRNA inhibition of translation initiation *in vitro* by targeting the cap-binding complex eIF4F. Science 2007; 317(5845): 1764-7.
[http://dx.doi.org/10.1126/science.1146067] [PMID: 17656684]

[128] Cheng J, Zhou L, Xie QF, *et al.* The impact of miR-34a on protein output in hepatocellular carcinoma HepG2 cells. Proteomics 2010; 10(8): 1557-72.
[http://dx.doi.org/10.1002/pmic.200900646] [PMID: 20186752]

[129] De Antonellis P, Carotenuto M, Vandenbussche J, *et al.* Early targets of miR-34a in neuroblastoma. Mol Cell Proteomics 2014; 13(8): 2114-31.
[http://dx.doi.org/10.1074/mcp.M113.035808] [PMID: 24912852]

[130] Kaller M, Liffers ST, Oeljeklaus S, *et al.* Genome-wide characterization of miR-34a induced changes in protein and mRNA expression by a combined pulsed SILAC and microarray analysis. Mol Cell Proteom 2011; 10(8): M111 010462.

[131] Ouchida M, Kanzaki H, Ito S, *et al.* Novel direct targets of miR-19a identified in breast cancer cells by a quantitative proteomic approach. PLoS One 2012; 7(8): e44095..
[http://dx.doi.org/10.1371/journal.pone.0044095] [PMID: 22952885]

[132] Ma Y, Zhang P, Wang F, Liu W, Yang J, Qin H. An integrated proteomics and metabolomics approach for defining oncofetal biomarkers in the colorectal cancer. Ann Surg 2012; 255(4): 720-30.
[http://dx.doi.org/10.1097/SLA.0b013e31824a9a8b] [PMID: 22395091]

[133] Eastlack SC, Dong S, Ivan C, Alahari SK. Suppression of PDHX by microRNA-27b deregulates cell metabolism and promotes growth in breast cancer. Mol Cancer 2018; 17(1): 100.
[http://dx.doi.org/10.1186/s12943-018-0851-8] [PMID: 30012170]

[134] Kim S, Lee E, Jung J, *et al.* microRNA-155 positively regulates glucose metabolism *via* PIK3R1-FOXO3a-cMYC axis in breast cancer. Oncogene 2018; 37(22): 2982-91.
[http://dx.doi.org/10.1038/s41388-018-0124-4] [PMID: 29527004]

[135] Gámez-Pozo A, Berges-Soria J, Arevalillo JM, *et al.* Combined label-free quantitative proteomics and microRNA expression analysis of breast cancer unravel molecular differences with clinical implications. Cancer Res 2015; 75(11): 2243-53.
[http://dx.doi.org/10.1158/0008-5472.CAN-14-1937] [PMID: 25883093]

[136] Yan GR, Xu SH, Tan ZL, Liu L, He QY. Global identification of miR-373-regulated genes in breast cancer by quantitative proteomics. Proteom 2011; 11(5): 912-20.
[http://dx.doi.org/10.1002/pmic.201000539] [PMID: 21271679]

[137] Ljepoja B, García-Roman J, Sommer AK, *et al.* A proteomic analysis of an *in vitro* knock-out of miR-200c. Sci Rep 2018; 8(1): 6927.
[http://dx.doi.org/10.1038/s41598-018-25240-y] [PMID: 29720730]

[138] Liu L, Xu Q, Hao S, Chen Y. A quasi-direct LC-MS/MS-based targeted proteomics approach for miRNA quantification *via* a covalently immobilized DNA-peptide probe. Sci Rep 2017; 7(1): 5669.
[http://dx.doi.org/10.1038/s41598-017-05495-7] [PMID: 28720752]

CHAPTER 11

Calcium Signaling in Breast Cancer: Current Perspective

Manuraj Pandey[1,*], Akanksha Nigam[2] and **Rajendra Mehta[3]**

[1]*Department of Biotechnology, Unique College, Jawahar Chowk, T.T. Nagar, Bhopal, M.P. India*
[2]*Department of Microbiology and Molecular genetics, IMRIC, The Hebrew University- Hadassah Medical School, Jerusalem, Israel*
[3]*Department of Rural Technology and Social Development, Guru Ghasidas Vishwavidhyalaya (Central University), Bilaspur, CG, India*

Abstract: Calcium (Ca^{2+}) signaling plays an important role in every aspect of cellular physiology, including cell proliferation, cell death, and cell motility. In the cellular environment, calcium signaling is tightly regulated to achieve a specific cellular response. Dysregulation in cell proliferation and cell death are crucial events in cancer evolution. There are several reports which have established the central role of calcium signaling in acquiring the hallmarks of cancer. Calcium signaling has been shown to be linked with several proteins and pathways, which are involved in the progression and advancement of breast cancer, including RANK/RANKL signaling pathway, EGFR and CAMK signaling, Rap2B, ERK1/2 signaling, Ca^{2+} influx pathways, MCU proteins, PTHrP, calmodulin, PARP1, NFAT, calpain, mitogen-activated protein kinase (MAPK), calmodulin-dependent protein kinase II (CaMKII), epithelial-mesenchymal transition (EMT), phospholipase C (PLC), inositol 1,4,5-trisphosphate (IP3), vascular endothelial growth factor (VEGF), estrogen, and estrogen receptor. In the recent past, several studies presented good enough pieces of evidence suggesting Ca^{2+} channels and transporters as a potential therapeutic target of breast cancer treatment. Therefore, in light of previous knowledge, in this chapter, we will discuss the role of Ca^{2+} signaling in breast cancer and its therapeutic implication as to the current perspective of breast cancer treatment.

Keywords: Breast cancer, Ca^{2+} homeostasis, Ca^{2+} channels, Cancer therapy, Ca^{2+} channel blockers, Mammary gland, ORAI, PMCA, Store-operated Ca^{2+} entry, TRP.

INTRODUCTION

In a cellular environment, calcium (Ca^{2+}) plays a crucial role in maintaining cellular homeostasis and signaling, where Ca^{2+} works as a secondary messenger

* **Corresponding author Manuraj Pandey:** Department of Biotechnology, Unique College, Jawahar Chowk, T.T. Nagar, Bhopal, M.P. India; E-mail: manuraj4b@gmail.com

Shankar Suman, Garima Suman and Sanjay Mishra (Eds.)

in the cellular signaling pathways [1, 2]. Cells maintain a 10,000 fold extracellular (1-2mM) to intracellular (100nM) Ca^{2+} gradient across plasma membrane in a resting state. Transporter proteins and ion channels [3] tightly maintain the Ca^{2+} gradient across the plasma membrane. Transient change in cytoplasmic Ca^{2+} concentration is achieved by the inflow of extracellular Ca^{2+} or the release of Ca^{2+} stored in the intracellular organelles. Change in Ca^{2+} gradient is exploited by the cell to initiate cascades of signaling, which trigger downstream signaling pathways [4-6]. Ca^{2+} binding proteins play important role in translating Ca^{2+} signal in cellular effect [3, 7] that play diverse role in fundamental cellular processes, including gene transcription, metabolism, cell growth, differentiation, apoptosis, autophagy, muscle contraction, neuronal plasticity, cell motility, phenotypic switching, and modulate the effector efficacy of immune cells [1, 2]. Cellular Ca^{2+} signaling has not only been implicated in the diverse physiological process but also varied pathological conditions, including cancers. It has been shown that calcium signaling plays an important role in many of the hallmarks of cancer. Proliferation, angiogenesis, invasion, and metastasis are the critical processes of cancer progression that are calcium-dependent [8].

Ca^{2+} flux has an important role in regulating the concentration of Ca^{2+} in breast epithelia, as it is one of the key components of milk. Specific Ca^{2+} pumps and channels are involved in transporting Ca^{2+} into milk, including plasma membrane Ca^{2+}ATPase (PMCA2), secretory pathway Ca^{2+}ATPase (SPCA), and store-operated Ca^{2+} channel (ORAI1) [4, 9]. Calcium homeostasis is tightly maintained in the breast from lactation to involution. Disruption in calcium homeostasis has been shown to involve in breast cancer progression and metastasis. Calcium transporters and pumps that are involved in Ca^{2+} transport into milk are shown to have an aberrant expression in some of the breast cancers and their subtypes [10]. This aberrant expression is not confined only to Ca^{2+} transporters involved in lactation but also to other Ca^{2+} transporter involved in diverse physiological processes and showed a specific pattern of expression to particular molecular subtypes of breast cancer [11].

Ca^{2+}CHANNELS, PUMPS, AND EXCHANGERS

The entry of Ca^{2+} is inevitable to initiate the specific signal, but at the same time, the elevated and prolonged intracellular Ca^{2+} could be toxic to the cell and trigger cell death [12]. Therefore, in the intracellular environment, Ca^{2+} homeostasis is tightly regulated by a complex network of diverse Ca^{2+} pumps, channels, and exchangers [7]. The elevation of intracellular Ca^{2+} is achieved by both extracellular calcium entry and release of Ca^{2+} from intracellular stores. Extracellular calcium entry is facilitated by Ca^{2+} channels on plasma membrane which includes voltage-gated calcium-permeable ion channels, ligand-gated calcium channels, transient receptor potential (TRP) channels and store-operated Ca^{2+} entry pathway [4], whereas Ca^{2+} release from internal calcium stores is facilitated by ligand-gated calcium channels present on the surface of Sarco/endoplasmic reticulum [1]. After serving the signaling purpose, Ca^{2+} concentration in intracellular space is decreased to normal cellular levels for maintaining intracellular Ca^{2+} homeostasis [1, 13]. Ca^{2+} is either effluxed to the extracellular environment by the calcium pumps such as plasma membrane Ca^{2+}-ATPase [PMCA] or the Na^{+}/Ca^{2+} exchanger (NCX), or it is sequestered by the sarcoplasmic/endoplasmic reticulum Ca^{2+}-ATPase (SERCA) into intracellular organelles [1, 14]. Apart from ER, two other organelles, Mitochondria and Golgi apparatus, also play an important role in calcium homeostasis. Mitochondria sequester cytoplasmic Ca^{2+} through mitochondrial Ca^{2+} uniporter (MCU) [15], and Golgi apparatus maintains the intracellular Ca^{2+} concentration by Ca^{2+}sequestering action of SPCAs transporters to modulate Ca^{2+} signaling [16].

Types of Calcium-permeable Ion Channels and Pumps

1- Transient Receptor Potential (TRP) Channels

TRP channel is plasma membrane Ca^{2+} channels and first identified in Drosophila.Since then, several types of Ca^{2+} permeable TRP channels have been discovered in mammalian cells [17]. TRP channels work as universal biological sensors by detecting environmental changes and responding to myriad of stimuli including light, temperatures [hot or cold], natural chemical compounds [hot pepper, camphor, menthol], mechanical stimuli, or changes in the composition of the lipid bilayer [18, 19]. TRP channels family consists of 7 subfamilies and 30 members, which are expressed in human cells. The seven subfamilies of TRP channels are TRPA (ankyrin), TRPV (vanilloid), TRPC (canonical), TRPN (no mechanoreceptor potential C), TRPM (melastatin), TRPML (mucolipin) and TRPP (polycystic) channels [20, 21]. Mutations and overexpression of specific TRP channels have been implicated in human diseases and some cancers, including breast cancer [22, 23].

2- Voltage-gated Calcium Channels (VGCCs)

VGCCs (CaV) are also plasma membrane Ca^{2+} channels that respond to changes in membrane potential and mediate a rapid Ca^{2+}entry in the cytoplasm. Ca_V channels are members of voltage-gated ion channels superfamily and share homology with voltage-gated Na^{+} and K^{+} channels. These channels are classified according to their voltage of activation, including high or low voltage-activated channels [24, 25]. The Ca_V1 (L-type) channels and Ca_V2 (P/Q-, N^{-}, and R-type) belong to high voltage-activated channels group, while low voltage-activated Ca_V channels include Ca_V3 (T-type) channels. Extensive alternative splicing and the subtypes of α_1 subunit conferred functional diversity to Ca_V channels. VGCC subfamilies significantly differ in physiological, regulatory, and pharmacological characteristics [26, 27]. L-type VGCC initiates contraction of muscles and endocrine secretion, whereas the N, P/Q, and R-type VGCCs initialize fast transmission in neurons. T-type VGCC activates and deactivates rapidly by membrane depolarization [4, 28, 29]. Voltage-gated calcium channels play an important role in the excitable cells including neurons and muscle tissue. Some studies suggested crucial roles of VGCC in cells other than neurons or muscle cells, *e.g.*, T-lymphocytes [30, 31]. Recent studies revealed the critical role of VGCCs in the progression and development of different tumor types, including breast cancer [32, 33].

3- Ligand-gated Ca²⁺Channels

Ligand-gatedCa²⁺channels operate in response to endogenous ligands and allow entry of Ca^{2+} in the cytoplasm. Ligand-gatedCa²⁺ channels expressed on both the plasma membrane and endoplasmic reticulum. Ligand-gated channels of plasma membrane include purinergic signaling receptors (P1 and P2 receptors), which respond to extracellular nucleotides and expressed nearly in all mammalian tissues [34, 35], α-amino3-hydroxy-5-methyl-4-isoxazole propionic acid [AMPA] receptors and N-methyl-D-aspartate (NMDA) receptors, which respond to neurotransmitter glutamate and expressed specifically in neurons [36, 37]. The P2X and P2Y are two subgroups of P2 receptors, containing several family members in each group. P2X Ca²⁺ channel has seven family members, which play crucial roles in the different cellular process including blood coagulation and neuronal signaling [36, 38, 39].

IP3 receptors (IP3Rs) are also ligand-gated Ca²⁺ channels, predominantly express on the endoplasmic reticulum and release calcium from intracellular Ca²⁺ store. These are the major intracellular Ca²⁺ channels of non-excitable cells. There are some reports that IP3R is also expressed on the plasma membrane, *e.g.*, IP3R3 in ciliated cells [40, 41] and IP3R1 in B-lymphocytes [42]. The IP3Rs activation mediated by IP3 binding to the receptor on the ER and causes the release of Ca²⁺to the cytoplasm, resulting in increased Ca²⁺ for several seconds [43-45]. There are three subtypes of IP3R - IP3R1, IP3R2, IP3R3 and each subtype form a Ca²⁺ channel, which is co-regulated by IP3 and Ca²⁺ both [43]. IP3R subtypes differ in their affinities for IP3, where IP3R2 is more sensitive than IP3R1, and the IP3R3 is least sensitive [46, 47]. The expression patterns of IP3Rs and their modulation by additional signals also differ significantly among subtypes [48, 49].

Ryanodine receptors (RyRs) are Ca²⁺ channels present on the Sarco/endoplasmic reticulum that open in response to Ca²⁺. Although, in mammals, RyRs are present in a wide variety of cells, including exocrine cells, neurons, lymphocytes, epithelial cells, *etc*. [50] but are prominently expressed in cells that involve in excitation-contraction coupling, *e.g.* muscle cells [51]. There are three subtypes of RyRs, including RyR1 RyR2 and RyR3. The RyR1 is extensively expressed in skeletal muscle [52]. RyR2 is primarily expressed in the heart [51], and RyR3 expression widely observed in different tissues [53].

4- Store-operated Calcium Channels

It is one of the major Ca^{2+} entry channels in non-excitable cells, such as epithelial cells. The main components of this Ca^{2+} entry pathway include the ORAI (a store-operated Ca^{2+} channel pore-forming subunit) calcium influx channel and the stromal interaction molecule (STIM), a Ca^{2+} depletion sensor of the endoplasmic reticulum [54, 55]. There are three subtypes of ORAI channel in humans (ORAI1-3) and two subtypes of STIM (STIM 1-2) [56, 57]. The mechanism of store-operated Ca^{2+} entry involves the detection of depleted Ca^{2+} stores in the endoplasmic reticulum by STIM1 sensor protein, which then oligomerizes on the ER section proximal to the plasma membrane. Interaction of oligomerized STIM1 with N-terminal domains of ORAI1 promotes the entry of Ca^{2+} through an oligomerized ORAI1 channel [58, 59]. The store operated Ca^{2+} entry pathway is an important route of Ca^{2+} trafficking during lactation and has been implicated in breast cancer [54].

5- Mitochondrial Ca^{2+} Uniporter (MCU)

Mitochondria is an important player of Ca^{2+} homeostasis, which is capable of rapid Ca^{2+} uptake and balance cell survival/cell death by modulating Ca^{2+} signaling. MCU largely mediates mitochondrial Ca^{2+} uptake and regulated by mitochondrial Ca^{2+} uptake 1 (MICU1) protein. MCU sequester Ca^{2+} temporarily during intense signaling, and it releases back into the cytosol after cessation of signaling. Rapid lowering of Ca^{2+} is beneficial for the cell as it prevents cell death due to Ca^{2+} toxicity [1, 3, 15]. The transport rate of mitochondrial uniporter is much greater than other pumps, and it helps to limit Ca^{2+} concentration over a wider dynamic range [60]. The quick uptake of mitochondrial Ca^{2+} is pumped back rapidly to the cytoplasm by mitochondrial H^+/Ca^{2+} exchangers (HCX) and mitochondrial NCX [3, 61].

6- The Plasma Membrane Ca^{2+}-ATPases (PMCs)-

The plasma membrane calcium ATPase (PMCs) is a member of the P-type ATPase family of ion transporters. PMCA transporters have four isoforms (PMCA1–4); all isoforms of PMCA are encoded by four separate genes present on different chromosomes [62]. Alternative splicing adds further PMCA isoform diversity by splicing primary transcripts [63, 64]. At least 25 splice variants have been identified so far [65]. All PMCA isoforms have ten transmembranes (TM) domains, and TM domains no. 4 –5 have major catalytic subunit of protein that includes aspartate residue and the ATP binding site. Catalytic activation of PMCAs depends on phosphorylation of this highly conserved aspartate residue in N terminal domains of PMCA protein [66]. C-terminal has a regulatory function and contains a calmodulin-binding site, which regulates the PMCA affinity for Ca^{2+} by changing its conformation. Calmodulin act as the key activator of the PMCA pumping function [65, 67, 68]. All isoforms have different affinity for CaM binding. PMCA 2/3 has a greater affinity for CaM than PMCA1/4. Ca^{2+} can also activate PMCA in the absence of key activator CaM [65].

In terms of tissue occurrence, the PMCAs expressed in all mammalian cells, but their isoforms show specific distribution patterns in different tissues. PMCA1 is referred to as housekeeping isoform and present almost in all tissue types. PMCA2 and PMCA3 show a restricted tissue distribution and primarily expressed in excitable cells such as muscles and neurons. Like PMCA1, the PMCA4 also has a wide tissue distribution [63, 69].

7- The sarco[endo]plasmic Reticulum Ca^{2+}-ATPases (SERCAs)

SERCA is one of the best characterized molecular pumps among the Ca^{2+}-ATPases family members that actively transport Ca^{2+} from the cytosol into the ER for maintaining ER Ca^{2+} stores. SERCA isoforms are encoded by three genes, ATP2A1-3 in higher vertebrates. Human cells contain three different isoforms of SERCA, which further divided into 11 splice variants that are species, tissue, and developmental stage-specific [3, 70]. SERCA isoforms are differentially expressed in different tissues. SERCA1 is specifically expressed in adult or neonatal fast-twitch skeletal muscle. SERCA2 isoforms are mainly expressed in the heart, slow-twitch muscle, smooth muscle, and in all non-muscle tissues. Limited tissue distribution has been observed for SERCA3 isoforms, and their expression has been detected in various non-muscle cells [71, 72].

8- The Secretory Pathway Ca^{2+}ATPases (SPCAs)

SPCAs calcium pumps belong to the P-type family of Ca^{2+}ATPase and accumulate Ca^{2+} into the Golgi apparatus [73, 74]. In humans, two isoforms of SPCA have been identified SPCA1-2, which are encoded by gene ATP2C1-2 [75, 76]. Keratinocytes show the highest SPCA1 expression, but it is expressed ubiquitously in other tissues as well, including the lung, brain, aorta, testes, and mammary gland [76-78]. SPCA1 is regarded as the housekeeping SPCA isoform whereas tissue distribution of SPCA2 is more restricted and mostly expressed in the trachea, gastrointestinal tract, mammary gland, and prostate [75]. Unlike SERCA, SPCAs have the ability to transport ionized manganese (Mn^{2+}) in the Golgi apparatus and help the cell to reduce Mn^{2+} toxicity. SPCA1 has been shown to have a greater Ca^{2+} affinity than SPCA2 [13].

CALCIUM SIGNALING AND MAMMARY GLAND

Calcium transport has a close association with breast as it is a lactating organ, and calcium is one of the key components of milk [79, 80]. Regulation of Ca^{2+} homeostasis and signaling in the breast has diverse cellular and physiological outcomes, which is not only restricted to transfer Ca^{2+} into milk during lactation but also affects the glandular organization and post-lactational involution of the breast by affecting epithelial cell differentiation, proliferation, and apoptosis. It is evident that breast growth and lactation are tightly regulated by many local and systemic hormonal effectors, including estrogen, an important modulator of proliferation, and differentiation of breast cells [81, 82]. Estrogen mediates its effects on mammary cells through genomic and non-genomic pathways, where the non-genomic pathway works through Ca^{2+} signaling [83]. Recent studies revealed that Ca^{2+} channels, Ca^{2+} transporters, and Ca^{2+} binding proteins play a crucial role during the sequential development of breast and lactation.

PMCA isoforms play diverse physiological roles in the mammary gland besides the regulation of Ca^{2+} signaling and homeostasis [84-86]. The protein expression of PMCA2 has been shown to increase by 100-fold in lactating rat mammary glands, compared to pregnant rats [76]. The localization of PMCA2 protein, during lactation, on the apical surface of secretory mammary epithelial cells suggests that PMCA2 has a crucial role in maintaining Ca^{2+} homeostasis by refluxing Ca^{2+} in milk [76]. Studies with PMCA2-null mice showed a significant reduction in Ca^{2+} content of milk compared to either wild type or heterozygous mice [76]. Some studies showed the involvement of PMCA-mediated apoptosis in mammary gland involution. Experimentally it has been demonstrated in the mouse model that PMCA2 expression in mammary epithelial cells drastically reduces after weaning, which triggers apoptosis and, ultimately, mammary gland involution by increasing Ca^{2+} in the cytosol [87, 88].

The SPCAs and SERCAs isoforms functions in the mammary gland and lactation is less known. SPCAs and SERCAs both are responsible for sequestering Ca^{2+} in the lumen of the Golgi apparatus and ER, respectively. Although Ca^{2+} accumulation in the ER and Golgi cisternae of luminal cells play a crucial role in the secretory pathway by controlling protein synthesis, processing, secretion and stability [89]. However, the link between SERCA isoforms regulation and its effect on cell cycle progression or proliferation in mammary epithelial cells is not well characterized until date [10, 13]. However, SPCA1 has been suggested to play an important role in milk production and secretion. In the mammary gland of rat, a 3-fold increase in protein expression of SPCA1 has been detected one week before litter birth and a further increase by approximately 6-fold compared to early pregnancy levels, which continued to remain higher during the lactation [10, 76].

During pregnancy, the mammary epithelium expands dramatically, is accompanied by significant angiogenesis in a way that the capillaries network covers each alveolus, and provide luminal cells with an adequate supply of Ca^{2+} and other nutrients necessary for milk production [9, 90]. It has been demonstrated recently that the ORAI1is significantly up-regulated in lactating mammary tissue of mice. Later it was suggested that during lactation ORAI1 Ca^{2+} entry channel was responsible for the entry of Ca^{2+} into luminal epithelial cells [55]. Experimentally it has been also demonstrated that the ORAI1 is crucial for Ca^{2+} enrichment in milk and transport about half of the milk Ca^{2+}across the basolateral membrane. These studies also suggest an important role of ORAI1 in milk ejection process, which is mediated by oxytocin through induced contractility of basal epithelial cells [10, 91]. TRP family of calcium channels are involved in calcium homeostasis in mammary gland but haven't been observed to be involved directly in the lactation and involution [10].

Calcium buffers are important regulators of transcellular Ca^{2+} transport in some cell types, but this property has not been suggested to be essential for secretory mammary epithelial cells to regulate calcium homeostasis. Mammary glands, during lactation, showed an upregulated expression of intra-organelle Ca^{2+}transporters, which maintain cytoplasmic Ca^{2+} homeostasis by coupling Ca^{2+} entry to its sequestration into intra-organelle stores and exclude the essentiality of calcium buffers. Further studies are needed to determine the specific roles of calcium buffers in the mammary gland if they are essential to the mammary gland [13]. Several Ca^{2+} modulated proteins are also important players in mammary gland calcium homeostasis. Important Ca^{2+}modulated proteins include calmodulin, the Ca^{2+}sensing receptor (CasR) and S100 family proteins [1, 67, 92, 93]. Calmodulin bind to $Ca^{2+}$and undergoes a conformational change and then interacts with several effector proteins, including the PMCAs and the calcineurin, a serine/threonine protein phosphatase [67]. Calmodulin plays physiological roles in the mammary gland *via* its effector proteins and also implicated in the pathophysiology of breast cancer [94], whereas the physiological roles of S100 proteins are almost unknown in the mammary gland [13]. CaSR is another important protein in Ca^{2+} signaling and has been shown to regulate cellular differentiation, proliferation and ions flux in many different tissues [95-97]. CaSR expression peaks during lactation, but reduces to a normal level with the initiation of mammary gland involution. Some studies have demonstrated that the CaSR signaling modulates the concentration of milk Ca^{2+} in response to circulating Ca^{2+} levels in blood [98]. However, to date, alterations in the CaSR have not been linked to any defects in the development or differentiation of the mammary gland [93].

BREAST CANCER AND CALCIUM SIGNALING

The mammary gland is unique for handling Ca^{2+} homeostasis, as it simultaneously adjusts the extraordinary demand for maintaining macro Ca^{2+} homeostasis while lactation along with maintaining intracellular Ca^{2+} homeostasis for controlling intracellular signaling to regulate normal physiology of breast epithelia and preventing Ca^{2+} toxicity. Therefore, Ca^{2+} channels, pumps, and Ca^{2+} binding proteins, which are key components for maintaining Ca^{2+} homeostasis, are assumed as an important physiological mediator of the mammary gland [4, 99]. There are several reports showing that deregulation of intracellular Ca^{2+} homeostasis alters the downstream signaling pathways, which contribute to mammary gland pathophysiology in the form of breast cancer. However, concurrently, it is also apparent that the calcium signaling alterations are not the driving force for initiating breast tumorigenesis [4]. Even altered calcium signaling does not appear to be similar between subtypes of breast cancer. It could differ significantly and operate with very different mechanisms in subtypes, which could lead to a different outcome of disease [11]. For example, ORAI isoforms 1 and 3 have a discrete association in different breast cancer subtypes, where ORAI1 is tightly linked with the basal molecular subtype, but ORAI3 being more closely linked to ER-positive breast cancer subtype [55, 100]. SPCA1 and PMCA2 are reported to be overexpressed in basal-like breast cancers and ErbB2 receptor-positive breast cancers respectively [87, 101].

Identification of such alterations in breast cancer subtypes could be exploited pharmacologically to develop targeted therapies. It has been reported that selective inhibition of altered calcium pathway, *in vitro*, seems promising in reducing breast cancer proliferation, metastasis and promote cell death in breast cancer cell lines [102, 103] see Table **1**. Some studies reported that the silencing of overexpressed SPCA1 in MDA-MB-231 cells (basal-like breast cancer cell line) reduces its proliferation. The mechanism behind this inhibition attributed to inhibition of the production of active insulin-like growth factor 1 receptor *via* modulation of Ca^{2+} dependent proprotein convertases in the Golgi lumen [101]. PMCA2 overexpression has been reported to link with ErbB2 receptor-positive breast cancers [87] tightly. It has been shown that exogenous overexpression of PMCA2 in T-47D breast cancer cells, confers cell death resistance to these cells, and indicates its clinical implications [87]. It has also been shown experimentally that carcinogens like Dimethylbenz[a]anthracene and benzo[a]pyrene could elevate cytoplasmic calcium in primary cultures of human mammary gland epithelial cells [104] suggesting role of Ca^{2+} in transformation process but still conclusive evidence is needed for such assumptions. Hereafter, we will discuss, in-depth, altered calcium channels and pumps in breast cancer.

Alteration of Ca^{2+} Transports in Breast Cancer

As we have discussed in the previous section of this chapter that Ca^{2+}channels, pumps, and Ca^{2+} binding proteins play an important role in maintaining Ca^{2+} homeostasis in the mammary gland, and their altered expression contributes to progression and advancement of breast carcinogenesis. Altered calcium channels in breast cancer. Below is the list of some of the calcium ion channels that are mostly disused in the context of breast cancer. Table **1** summarises some of the key Ca^{2+} transporters altered in breast cancer.

Table 1. Calcium transporter involved in lactation and involution

Calcium Transporters	Isoforms	Expression Status in the Breast During - lactation/Involution	References
PMCA isoforms	PMCA2	~200fold (Up) / ~90% (Down)	[85, 86, 88]
	PMCA-1,3 and 4	Slight (Up) /?	[85, 86, 88]
SPCAs isoforms	SPCA2	luminal cells (Up) / (Down)	[10, 88, 105]
	SPCA1	Cells of mammary gland (Up) / (Down)	[10, 88, 105]
	SERCA-2 and 3	~2fold (Up)/?	[13, 86]
	SERCA1	?	[13, 86]
ORAI-STIM isoforms	Orai1	(Up) / (Down)	[55, 106]
CaSR		basolateral membrane of the lactating alveolus (Up) / (Down)	[93, 107]

(Note: Up- up-regulated; Down- Downregulated?- not known)

1- Voltage-gated Calcium Channels

This Calcium channel includes T-type, R-type, P-type, Q-type, and N-type. The role of T-type calcium channels was strongly investigated in many breast cancer studies. This channel is mainly consisting of $\alpha 1$ subunit, which involved in the formation of pores on the cell membrane specifically for calcium ions. The expression of the $\alpha 1$ subunit was found in some of the breast cancer studies [108]. CACNA1G, CACNA1H, CACNA1I are the genes that encode for the $\alpha 1$ subunit for T-types calcium channels [109]. In T-type calcium channels, Cav3.1 was found to be very important to inhibit the proliferation in MCF-7 breast cancer cells [33]. On the other hand, NNC55-0396, a known calcium channel blocker demonstrated a potential inhibition in MCF-7 breast cancer cell proliferation [103]. One more calcium channel blocker, mibefradil, also found very effective in the growth inhibition of MCF-7 cells [110]. Microarray analysis of clinical cancer samples indicated the overexpression of the Ca^{++} channel subunit encoded by the gene CACNA1G and CACNA1I in breast cancer [111]. The upregulation of these genes is also known for the involvement in cancer progression, which could lead to the enhanced result of migration and invasion.

2- TRP Channel in Breast Cancer

TRP channels have been reported widely in some cancers, as they play an essential role in the growth as well as the progression of cancers. These channels were found to be highly overexpressed in breast cancer tissue [112]. TRPC1 was detected with a 30-fold increase in the mRNA level of human breast cancer samples when compared with its non-cancerous sample [112]. TRPC3 was also reported as highly overexpressed in its mRNA level in breast cancer cells [113]. The role of the TRP channel was also reported *in vitro* studies with breast cancer cell lines. Another TRP channel, that is very well known in breast cancer, is TRPM7. It is calcium as well as Magnesium ion-permeable channel [114, 115]. The role of TRPM7 was reported in the invasion and migration of breast cancer cells MDA-MB-435 [116]. Overexpression of TMPM7 levels was also reported in MCF-7 breast cancer cells, which may play a role in the proliferation of these cells [117]. Recently, TRPM7 levels reported being very high in tumors, which may have a role in metastasis [118]. Overexpression of TRPM8 was reported in two breast cancer cells MDA-MB-231 and BT-474 [119]. Its overexpression was also reported in estrogen receptor-positive breast cancer [120]. TRPV6 is the most studied TRPV channel in breast cancer. Bolanz *et al*. [121] reported the up-regulation of TRPV6 for the first time in 2008 and described its upregulation in breast adenocarcinoma tissue [122]. Furthermore, many research studies have noted the elevated levels of TRPV6 in breast tumors [112, 123]. In another study by Pla *et al*. 2012, demonstrated the higher level of TRPV4 expression in epithelial cells derived from breast cancers when compared to normal breast tissue [124]. He reported an increase in the migration of breast cancer-derived epithelial cells.

TRPV1 is one of the TRP channels, which were described to be highly expressed in triple negative breast cancer cells called SUM149PT breast cancer cells [125].

3- Calcium-activated K⁺ and Cl⁻ Channels in Breast Cancer

Many calcium-activated K^+ channels have been reported to be highly expressed in so many breast cancer cell lines. hIKCa1, calcium activated K^+ channel, was found to be involved in cell proliferation and activation of the JaK2 pathway in MCF-7 breast cancer cells [126]. Another calcium-activated K^+ channel [hIK1] was also noted to be highly expressed in MCF-7 cells. BKCa, this calcium-activated channel, was expressed in MDA-MB-231cancer cell lines [127]. hEag1, known as Ether agogo K^+ channel, was evident to be involved in breast cancer cell invasion [128]. ANO1, called anoctamin1, is a calcium-activated chloride channel. It was found to be expressed in breast cancer tumors and cell lines. Its higher expression may lead to cell proliferation and metastasis [129, 130].

4- ORAI Calcium Channels in Breast Cancer

Recently, two protein families were identified regarding the Ca^{2+} signaling in breast cancer. These proteins are known as STIM (Stromal interaction molecules) and ORAI. STIM proteins have been described to be involved in Ca^{2+} storage in the endoplasmic reticulum (ER), while Orai proteins have been involved in regulating the flow of Ca^{2+} inside the cells through the plasma membrane (PM) [131]. STIM allows the Ca^{2+} influx through the plasma membrane inside the cells when it is necessary for mammary epithelial cells to increase the concentration of milk with Ca^{2+} [55]. So many studies demonstrated the involvement of STIM proteins and ORAI channels in breast cancer. During lactation, ORAI is upregulated, and STIM1 is downregulated [55]. It is already known that ORAI is directly involved in the breast cancer cell and reported to be highly expressed in many breast cancer cells (MCF-7, ZR751, T-47D, BT474, HVV1500) when compared with non-breast cancer cell lines. Orai1 does not activate the STIM1/Orai1 pathway, while Orai3 functionally involved in the STIM1 and STIM2 pathway [100]. Generally, breast cancers are more likely to have higher expression of STIM1 and lower level of STIM2, which suggest that entry of Ca^{2+} ions inside the cells, could be responsible for the metastasis in breast cancer tissue [55]. Studies demonstrated that after the silencing of ORAI1, there was a reduction in cell proliferation in breast cancer cells both *in vitro* and *in vivo*. ORAI1 silencing with Orai1-siRNA reported in the reduction of cell migration in MDA-MB-231 cells, while overexpression of STIM1 and Orai1 was found to be involved in cell invasion process in non-tumorigenic epithelial MCF-10A cell line.

Recently Hammadi *et al.*, 2012 reported that reduced ether a-go-go K^+ channel shows a reduction in the cell migration process of MDA-MB-231 breast cancer cells, which happened due to the reduction of ORAI 1 mediated Ca^{2+} influx into the cells [128].

Another isoform of ORAI is ORAI3, which has recently been identified to be associated with estrogen-positive breast cancer [100]. The higher level of expression of Orai3 was found in MCF-7 breast cancer cells [estrogen receptor positive] compared with other breast cancer cells MDA-MB-231 (estrogen receptor-negative).

In Orai3 siRNA-treated MCF-7 cells inhibits cell proliferation and also the arrest cell cycle in the G1 phase by downregulation of cyclins E, D1 and low expression of p53 gene, when compared with non-breast cancer-derived MCF-10A cells. This study reported that ORAI3 could be used as a therapeutic target for breast cancer [132]. ORAI3 silencing demonstrated a reduction in cell proliferation in MCF-7 cancer cells *via* a c-Myc pathway, which was mediated through the MAPK pathway due to lower expression of pERK and cell cycle arrest in the G1 phase [133].

5- Muscarinic Acetylcholine Receptors in Breast Cancer

Acetylcholine (ACh), known as a neurotransmitter, is involved in the function of the central and peripheral nervous system. This receptor is also expressed in so many other types of cells, which includes smooth muscle, cells, endothelial cells, gastrointestinal tract, *etc*. Recently, emerging evidence revealed that Ach also participates in tumorigenesis which includes lung, stomach, colon, uterus, prostate, skin, pancreas, brain and breast cancer. This receptor participates in cell proliferation, invasion, migration, and metastasis [134-139].

Metabotropic cholinergic receptors are known for their ability to bind with agonist muscarine, which is the reason they called the muscarinic receptors (mAChRs). These receptors belong to the G-protein family, which consist of 7 transmembrane domains. Five different subtypes of muscarinic receptors have been identified M1-M5 [140]. Muscarinic receptor M1, M3, and M5 coupled with G protein and activate phospholipase C (PLC) to determine the release of Ca^{2+} from cells. The role of muscarinic acetylcholine receptors was detected in different mammary adenocarcinomas named LM2, LM3, and LMM3 cell lines that were developed in Balb/C mice. In LM2 cells, carbachol promoted proliferation *via* M2 and M1 receptor activation with arginase catabolism, while in LM3 cells, carbachol-induced proliferation *via* M3 receptor activation by a mechanism involving the activation of nitric oxide production [141, 142]. In LMM3 cells, the action of carbachol on cell proliferation was observed due to the involvement of M3 receptor activation [143]. Another study on MCF-7 showed that these cancer cells promoted cell proliferation mainly by the involvement of M3 receptor through the activation of MAPK kinase (MAPKK). One more study on MCF-7 cells reported the induction of angiogenesis and invasion by the higher expression of VEGF-A (Vascular endothelial growth factor-A [144]. These studies establish the role of the muscarinic receptor in tumor cell proliferation, growth, and angiogenesis.

CALCIUM SIGNALING AS A THERAPEUTIC TARGET IN BREAST CANCER

The involvement of Ca^{2+} signaling pathways in breast cancer pathogenesis also unfolds its strong potential to be used in breast cancer pharmacotherapy. These pathways have been used as a novel drug target in many breast cancer studies. Numerous inhibitors of Ca^{2+} ions channels are known for their pharmacological use in breast cancer. Table **2** enlists most of the studies conducted on malignant breast tumors and cell lines, which described specific Ca^{2+} signaling channels identified as potential therapeutic targets in *in vivo* and *in vitro* studies using inhibitors, siRNA, receptor modulators, and receptor antagonist. The use of inhibitors clearly shows a reduction in breast cancer proliferation, invasion, and migration. Another clear role of inhibitors as a pharmacological treatment is through the promotion of cancer cell death. Several studies have demonstrated the role of the TRPV1 channel as a therapeutic target of some regulators, which were involved in triggering apoptosis in breast cancer cells, *e.g.*, SUM149PT and MCF-7 [125, 145-147]. Capsaicin, a bioactive phytochemical, increases apoptosis in the breast cancer cell. Another study demonstrated that capsaicin when co applied with MRS1477 (a positive allosteric modulator of TRPV1), triggers apoptosis in MCF-7 cells [145].

Several other studies have shown the pharmacological potential of the muscarinic antagonist (*e.g.*, Atropine) to inhibit the cancer cell growth by targeting Muscarinic acetylcholine receptors (M3 and M4), which leads to reduce cell migration in MCF-7 breast cancer cells [148]. Another estrogen receptor modulator, Tamoxifen, is used as an anti-proliferative agent in MCF-7 breast cancer cells [122]. Blocking of Ca^{2+} influx in STIM1 and Orai1 channels also has been used as a pharmacological treatment in breast cancer [149]. 2-APB (2-aminoethoxydiphenyl borate), is another regulator known to decrease cell growth in MCF-7 and MDA-MB-231 cells [55]. Blockers like Astemizole (block hEAG1 channels) demonstrated a reduction in cell migration in MDA-MB-231 cells [128], while TRAM-34 and Clotrimazole (block hIKCa1 channel), showed inhibition in cell growth in MCF-7 breast cancer cells [126]. Another blocker, Iberiotoxin (block BKCa channels), showed a reduction in anchorage-independent growth in different breast cancer cell lines (UASS893, SK-BR-3, and MDA-M--231) [127]. CaCCinh-AO1, which blocks ANO1 channels, reduces the cell viability in breast cancer cells [130].

Carbachol, an agonist that acts on M1 and M3 receptors, leads to tumor progression in MCF-7 cells through the phosphorylation of the MAPK/ERK pathway in MCF-7 breast cancer cells [150]. When Wortmannin or LY294002 (both are inhibitors) applied with genistein reduced the carbachol-induced

MAPK/ERK phosphorylation. In one study, the treatment of paclitaxel with carbachol demonstrated the induction of tumor death in MCF-7 cells [151].

In conclusion, several Ca^{2+} ion channels, namely, TRP channels, STIM/Orai protein, hEAG1, Ca^{2+} activated $K^{+,}$ and Cl^- channels, muscarinic acetylcholine receptors reported their role as an important pharmacological target for the treatment of breast cancer.

Table 2. Pharmacological role of some of the Ca^{2+} permeable channels regulators in breast cancer.

Different Ca^{2+} Channels	Regulator	Studies in Breast Cancer Cells	References
TRPV1	Capsaicin	Triggers apoptosis in SUM149PT cells	[125]
	MRS1477 applied with capsaicin	Triggers pronounced apoptosis in MCF7 cells	[145]
	5-Fluorouracil	Induces apoptosis in MCF-7 cells	[146]
	cisplatin applied with selenium or alpha-lipoic acid	Increases cell death in MCF breast cancer cells	[147]
TRPC1/TRPV2	Fasudil, which is a Rho-kinase inhibitor	Increases the expression of TRPC1 and TRPC2 in MCF and MDA-MB-231 cells	[152]
TRPM6	Y-27632 (Rho-kinase inhibitor)	Downregulates TRPM6 in both the MCF and MDA-MB-231 cells	[152]
TRPV6	Tamoxifen, which is an estrogen receptor modulator	It has been reported as an anti-proliferative effect in MCF7 breast cancer cells.	[122]
TRPM8	AMTB (inhibitor)	Reduces proliferation and migration of SK-BR-3 and MDA-MB-231 breast cancer cells	[154]
TRPC3	PUFA (polyunsaturated fatty acids)	Reduces cell proliferation and migration by inhibiting TRPC-mediated calcium entry in MCF-7 breast cancer cells	[108]
TRPM7	Waixenicin	Inhibits cell growth in human Jurkat T-cells. It also reported to inhibits cell growth of human MCF-7 breast cancer cells	[155] [153]
TRPC6	Hyperforin	It decreases the growth and induces apoptosis in MCF-7 and MDA-MB-231 cells.	[113]
T-type Ca^{2+} channels	Mibefradil and pimozide	Inhibits cell proliferation in MCF-7 breast cancer cells.	[110]
	NNC55-0396	Inhibits cell proliferation in MCF-7 breast cancer cells	[103]

(Table 2) cont.....

Different Ca^{2+} Channels	Regulator	Studies in Breast Cancer Cells	References
STIM1/Orai	SKF9636 or Ni^{2+} or EGTA	A decrease in the number of invasive tumor cells in STIM1 siRNA or Orai1 si-RNA treated MDA-MB-231 cancer cells.	[149]
	2-APB (2-aminoethoxy diphenyl borate)	It decreases the cell growth of MCF-7 and MDA-MB-231 cells	[55]
hEAG1	Astemizole	Decrease cell migration in MDA-MB-231 breast cancer cells.	[128]
Ca^{2+} activated K$^+$ channels	TRAM-34 and clotrimazole	These hIKCa1 blockers inhibit cell growth in the MCF-7 cells.	[126]
	Iberiotoxin	Decrease the anchorage-independent growth of SK-BR-3, UACC893, and MDA-MB-231 breast cancer cell lines.	[127]
Ca^{2+} activated Cl$^-$ channels	CaCCinh-AO1	Inhibit ANO1 channel and helps in decreasing cell viability and cell colony formation in breast cancer cells	[130]
Muscarinic acetylcholine receptor	Atropine and Tropicamide (M$_3$ and M$_4$ receptor antagonist respectively)	They reduced cell migration in MCF-7 cells.	[148]
	Wortmanin or LY294002 with genistein	Reduced the MAPK/ERK phosphorylation in MCF-7 cells.	[150]
	Carbachol with paclitaxel	Induced apoptosis of breast tumor in MCF-7 cells	[151]

CONCLUDING REMARKS AND PERSPECTIVES

Calcium ion transporters play crucial roles virtually in every aspect of cellular physiology. These are intrinsically linked to breast development, lactation, and involution, as well. They are key regulators of calcium transport in milk. Studies in the past two decades reveal a tight link between altered expression of calcium transporters and breast cancer development and progression. Calcium transporters have been recognized as one of the important therapeutic targets, and several bioactive molecules, which work as inhibitors or antagonists of calcium transporters, have been identified and validated for their therapeutic potential. A better understanding of the calcium transporters' involvement in each of the hallmarks of breast cancer would help to develop potential measures for therapeutic intervention in breast cancer. Further, more studies are needed, specifically aimed toward exploring calcium transporter dependent biochemical pathways, improving selectivity and effectiveness of drug molecules, and assessing side effects to translate promising discoveries as a therapeutic approach against breast cancer and its subtypes.

CONSENT FOR PUBLICATION

Not applicable.

CONFLICT OF INTEREST

The authors confirm that the contents of this chapter have no conflict of interest.

ACKNOWLEDGEMENTS

Authors thank Mr. R. Choudhary, founder & chairman of Unique College, Bhopal, M.P. India, for his invaluable support. Thanks to Dr. Shivam Priya for his valuable suggestions and feedbacks.

REFERENCES

[1]   Berridge MJ, Bootman MD, Roderick HL. Calcium signalling: dynamics, homeostasis and remodelling. Nat Rev Mol Cell Biol 2003; 4(7): 517-29.
[http://dx.doi.org/10.1038/nrm1155] [PMID: 12838335]

[2]   Prevarskaya N, Ouadid-Ahidouch H, Skryma R, Shuba Y. Remodelling of Ca^{2+} transport in cancer: How it contributes to cancer hallmarks? Philos Trans R Soc B Biol Sci 2014; 369(1638)

[3]   Cui C, Merritt R, Fu L, Pan Z. Targeting calcium signaling in cancer therapy. Acta Pharm Sin B 2017; 7(1): 3-17.
[http://dx.doi.org/10.1016/j.apsb.2016.11.001] [PMID: 28119804]

[4]   Azimi I, Roberts-Thomson SJ, Monteith GR. Calcium influx pathways in breast cancer: opportunities for pharmacological intervention. Br J Pharmacol 2014; 171(4): 945-60.
[http://dx.doi.org/10.1111/bph.12486] [PMID: 24460676]

[5]   Carafoli E. Intracellular calcium homeostasis. Annu Rev Biochem 1987; 56(1): 395-433.
[http://dx.doi.org/10.1146/annurev.bi.56.070187.002143] [PMID: 3304139]

[6]   Clapham DE. Calcium signaling. Cell 2007; 131(6): 1047-58.
[http://dx.doi.org/10.1016/j.cell.2007.11.028] [PMID: 18083096]

[7]   Berridge MJ, Lipp P, Bootman MD. The versatility and universality of calcium signalling. Nat Rev Mol Cell Biol 2000; 1(1): 11-21.
[http://dx.doi.org/10.1038/35036035] [PMID: 11413485]

[8]   Monteith GR, Prevarskaya N, Roberts-Thomson SJ. The calcium-cancer signalling nexus. Nat Rev Cancer 2017; 17(6): 367-80.
[http://dx.doi.org/10.1038/nrc.2017.18] [PMID: 28386091]

[9]   Davis FM. The ins and outs of calcium signalling in lactation and involution: Implications for breast cancer treatment. Pharmacol Res 2017; 116: 100-4.
[http://dx.doi.org/10.1016/j.phrs.2016.12.007] [PMID: 27965034]

[10]   Cross BM, Breitwieser GE, Reinhardt TA, Rao R. Cellular calcium dynamics in lactation and breast cancer: from physiology to pathology. Am J Physiol Cell Physiol 2014; 306(6): C515-26.
[http://dx.doi.org/10.1152/ajpcell.00330.2013] [PMID: 24225884]

[11]   So CL, Saunus JM, Roberts-Thomson SJ, Monteith GR. Calcium signaling and breast cancer. Semin Cell Dev Biol 2019; 94: 74-83.
[PMID: 30439562]

[12]   Parkash J, Asotra K. Calcium wave signaling in cancer cells. Life Sci 2010; 87(19-22): 587-95.
[http://dx.doi.org/10.1016/j.lfs.2010.09.013] [PMID: 20875431]

[13]   Lee WJ, Monteith GR, Roberts-Thomson SJ. Calcium transport and signaling in the mammary gland: targets for breast cancer. Biochim Biophys Acta 2006; 1765(2): 235-55.
[PMID: 16410040]

[14]   Caride AJ, Filoteo AG, Penheiter AR, Pászty K, Enyedi A, Penniston JT. Delayed activation of the plasma membrane calcium pump by a sudden increase in Ca^{2+}: fast pumps reside in fast cells. Cell Calcium 2001; 30(1): 49-57.
[http://dx.doi.org/10.1054/ceca.2001.0212] [PMID: 11396987]

[15]   Kirichok Y, Krapivinsky G, Clapham DE. The mitochondrial calcium uniporter is a highly selective ion channel. Nature 2004; 427(6972): 360-4.
[http://dx.doi.org/10.1038/nature02246] [PMID: 14737170]

[16]   Wuytack F, Raeymaekers L, Missiaen L. PMR1/SPCA Ca^{2+} pumps and the role of the Golgi apparatus as a Ca^{2+} store. Pflugers Arch 2003; 446(2): 148-53.
[http://dx.doi.org/10.1007/s00424-003-1011-5] [PMID: 12739151]

[17]   Ramsey IS, Delling M, Clapham DE. An introduction to TRP channels. Annu Rev Physiol 2006; 68(1): 619-47.
[http://dx.doi.org/10.1146/annurev.physiol.68.040204.100431] [PMID: 16460286]

[18]   Minke B. TRP channels and Ca^{2+} signaling. Cell Calcium 2006; 40(3): 261-75.
[http://dx.doi.org/10.1016/j.ceca.2006.05.002] [PMID: 16806461]

[19]   Clapham DE. Hot and cold TRP ion channels 2002; 295(5563): 2228-9.

[20]   Gees M, Colsoul B, Nilius B. The role of transient receptor potential cation channels in Ca^{2+} signaling. Cold Spring Harb Perspect Biol 2010; 2(10): a003962.
[http://dx.doi.org/10.1101/cshperspect.a003962] [PMID: 20861159]

[21]   Benham CD, Gunthorpe MJ, Davis JB. TRPV channels as temperature sensors. Cell Calcium 2003; 33(5-6): 479-87.
[http://dx.doi.org/10.1016/S0143-4160(03)00063-0] [PMID: 12765693]

[22]   Prevarskaya N, Skryma R, Shuba Y. Calcium in tumour metastasis: new roles for known actors. Nat Rev Cancer 2011; 11(8): 609-18.
[http://dx.doi.org/10.1038/nrc3105] [PMID: 21779011]

[23]   Ouadid-Ahidouch H, Dhennin-Duthille I, Gautier M, Sevestre H, Ahidouch A. TRP channels: diagnostic markers and therapeutic targets for breast cancer? Trends Mol Med 2013; 19(2): 117-24.
[http://dx.doi.org/10.1016/j.molmed.2012.11.004] [PMID: 23253476]

[24]   Simms BA, Zamponi GW. Neuronal voltage-gated calcium channels: structure, function, and dysfunction. Neuron 2014; 82(1): 24-45.
[http://dx.doi.org/10.1016/j.neuron.2014.03.016] [PMID: 24698266]

[25]   Berridge MJ. Neuronal calcium signaling. Neuron 1998; 21(1): 13-26.
[http://dx.doi.org/10.1016/S0896-6273(00)80510-3] [PMID: 9697848]

[26]   Rao VR, Perez-Neut M, Kaja S, Gentile S. Voltage-gated ion channels in cancer cell proliferation. Cancers (Basel) 2015; 7(2): 849-75.
[http://dx.doi.org/10.3390/cancers7020813] [PMID: 26010603]

[27]   Catterall WA. Voltage-gated calcium channels. Cold Spring HarbPerspect Biol 2011; 3(8): a003947.
[http://dx.doi.org/10.1101/cshperspect.a003947]

[28]   Ertel EA, Campbell KP, Harpold MM, *et al.* Nomenclature of voltage-gated calcium channels. Neuron 2000; 25(3): 533-5.
[http://dx.doi.org/10.1016/S0896-6273(00)81057-0] [PMID: 10774722]

[29]   Cain SM, Snutch TP. Voltage-gated calcium channels and disease. Biofactors 2011; 37(3): 197-205.
[http://dx.doi.org/10.1002/biof.158] [PMID: 21698699]

[30]   Dolphin AC. Voltage-gated calcium channels and their auxiliary subunits: physiology and pathophysiology and pharmacology. J Physiol 2016; 594(19): 5369-90.
[http://dx.doi.org/10.1113/JP272262] [PMID: 27273705]

[31]   Robert V, Triffaux E, Savignac M, Pelletier L. Calcium signalling in T-lymphocytes. Biochimie 2011; 93(12): 2087-94.
[http://dx.doi.org/10.1016/j.biochi.2011.06.016] [PMID: 21712067]

[32]   Roberts-Thomson SJ, Chalmers SB, Monteith GR. The calcium-signaling toolkit in cancer: remodeling and targeting. Cold Spring Harb Perspect Biol 2019; 11(8) http://cshperspectives. cshlp.org/lookup/doi/10.1101/cshperspect.a035204 [Internet].
[http://dx.doi.org/10.1101/cshperspect.a035204] [PMID: 31088826]

[33]   Ohkubo T, Yamazaki J. T-type voltage-activated calcium channel Cav3.1, but not Cav3.2, is involved in the inhibition of proliferation and apoptosis in MCF-7 human breast cancer cells. Int J Oncol 2012; 41(1): 267-75.
[http://dx.doi.org/10.3892/ijo.2012.1422] [PMID: 22469755]

[34]   Burnstock G. Purine and purinergic receptors. Brain Neurosci Adv 2018; 2: 1-10.
[http://dx.doi.org/10.1177/2398212818817494]

[35]   Surprenant A, North RA. Signaling at purinergic P2X receptors. Annu Rev Physiol 2009; 71(1): 333-59.
[http://dx.doi.org/10.1146/annurev.physiol.70.113006.100630] [PMID: 18851707]

[36]   Li S, Wong AHC, Liu F. Ligand-gated ion channel interacting proteins and their role in neuroprotection. Front Cell Neurosci 2014; 8(125): 125.
[http://dx.doi.org/10.3389/fncel.2014.00125] [PMID: 24847210]

[37]   Watkins JC, Jane DE. The glutamate story 2006. http://www.ncbi.nlm.nih.gov/pubmed/16402093% 0Ahttp://www.pubmedcentral.nih.gov/articlerender.fcgi?artid=PMC1760733
[http://dx.doi.org/10.1038/sj.bjp.0706444]

[38]   Hechler B, Lenain N, Marchese P, *et al.* A role of the fast ATP-gated P2X1 cation channel in thrombosis of small arteries *in vivo*. J Exp Med 2003; 198(4): 661-7.
[http://dx.doi.org/10.1084/jem.20030144] [PMID: 12913094]

[39]   Pankratov Y, Castro E, Miras-Portugal MT, Krishtal O. A purinergic component of the excitatory postsynaptic current mediated by P2X receptors in the CA1 neurons of the rat hippocampus. Eur J Neurosci 1998; 10(12): 3898-902.
[http://dx.doi.org/10.1046/j.1460-9568.1998.00419.x] [PMID: 9875366]

[40]   Taylor CW, Tovey SC. IP(3) receptors: toward understanding their activation. Cold Spring Harb Perspect Biol 2010; 2(12): a004010.
[http://dx.doi.org/10.1101/cshperspect.a004010] [PMID: 20980441]

[41]   Barrera NP, Morales B, Villalón M. Plasma and intracellular membrane inositol 1,4,5-trisphosphate receptors mediate the $Ca^{(2+)}$ increase associated with the ATP-induced increase in ciliary beat frequency. Am J Physiol Cell Physiol 2004; 287(4): C1114-24.
[http://dx.doi.org/10.1152/ajpcell.00343.2003] [PMID: 15175223]

[42]   Dellis O, Rossi AM, Dedos SG, Taylor CW. Counting functional inositol 1,4,5-trisphosphate receptors into the plasma membrane. J Biol Chem 2008; 283(2): 751-5.
[http://dx.doi.org/10.1074/jbc.M706960200] [PMID: 17999955]

[43]   Mataragka S, Taylor CW. All three IP_3 receptor subtypes generate Ca^{2+} puffs, the universal building blocks of IP_3-evoked Ca^{2+} signals. J Cell Sci 2018; 131(16): jcs220848.
[http://dx.doi.org/10.1242/jcs.220848] [PMID: 30097556]

[44]   Berridge MJ. Inositol trisphosphate and calcium signalling mechanisms. Biochim Biophys Acta 2009; 1793(6): 933-40.
[http://dx.doi.org/10.1016/j.bbamcr.2008.10.005] [PMID: 19010359]

[45]   Mikoshiba K. IP3 receptor/Ca^{2+} channel: from discovery to new signaling concepts. J Neurochem 2007; 102(5): 1426-46.
[http://dx.doi.org/10.1111/j.1471-4159.2007.04825.x] [PMID: 17697045]

[46]   Berridge MJ. The inositol trisphosphate/calcium signaling pathway in health and disease. Physiol Rev 2016; 96(4): 1261-96.http://www.physiology.org/doi/10.1152/physrev.00006.2016 [Internet].
[http://dx.doi.org/10.1152/physrev.00006.2016] [PMID: 27512009]

[47]   Iwai M, Michikawa T, Bosanac I, Ikura M, Mikoshiba K. Molecular basis of the isoform-specific ligand-binding affinity of inositol 1,4,5-trisphosphate receptors. J Biol Chem 2007; 282(17): 12755-64.
[http://dx.doi.org/10.1074/jbc.M609833200] [PMID: 17327232]

[48]   Prole DL, Taylor CW. Inositol 1,4,5-trisphosphate receptors and their protein partners as signalling hubs. J Physiol 2016; 594(11): 2849-66.
[http://dx.doi.org/10.1113/JP271139] [PMID: 26830355]

[49]   Taylor CW, Genazzani AA, Morris SA. Expression of inositol trisphosphate receptors. Cell Calcium 1999; 26(6): 237-51.
[http://dx.doi.org/10.1054/ceca.1999.0090] [PMID: 10668562]

[50]   Lanner JT, Georgiou DK, Joshi AD, Hamilton SL. Ryanodine receptors: structure, expression, molecular details, and function in calcium release. Cold Spring Harb Perspect Biol 2010; 2(11): a003996.
[http://dx.doi.org/10.1101/cshperspect.a003996] [PMID: 20961976]

[51]   Van Petegem F. Ryanodine receptors: structure and function. J Biol Chem 2012; 287(38): 31624-32.
[http://dx.doi.org/10.1074/jbc.R112.349068] [PMID: 22822064]

[52]   Takeshima H, Nishimura S, Matsumoto T, *et al.* Primary structure and expression from complementary DNA of skeletal muscle ryanodine receptor. Nature 1989; 339(6224): 439-45.
[http://dx.doi.org/10.1038/339439a0] [PMID: 2725677]

[53]   Mishra J, Jhun BS, Hurst S, O-Uchi J, Csordás G, Sheu SS. The mitochondrial Ca^{2+} uniporter: Structure, function, and pharmacology Handb Exp Pharmacol 2017; 129-56.

[54]   Monteith GR, Davis FM, Roberts-Thomson SJ. Calcium channels and pumps in cancer: changes and consequences. J Biol Chem 2012; 287(38): 31666-73.
[http://dx.doi.org/10.1074/jbc.R112.343061] [PMID: 22822055]

[55]   McAndrew D, Grice DM, Peters AA, *et al.* ORAI1-mediated calcium influx in lactation and in breast cancer. Mol Cancer Ther 2011; 10(3): 448-60. http://mct.aacrjournals.org/ cgi/doi/10.1158/1535-7163.MCT-10-0923 [Internet].
[http://dx.doi.org/10.1158/1535-7163.MCT-10-0923] [PMID: 21224390]

[56]   Roberts-Thomson SJ, Peters AA, Grice DM, Monteith GR. ORAI-mediated calcium entry: mechanism and roles, diseases and pharmacology. Pharmacol Ther 2010; 127(2): 121-30.
[http://dx.doi.org/10.1016/j.pharmthera.2010.04.016] [PMID: 20546784]

[57]   Liou J, Kim ML, Heo WD, *et al.* STIM is a Ca^{2+} sensor essential for Ca^{2+}-store-depletion-triggered Ca^{2+} influx. Curr Biol 2005; 15(13): 1235-41.
[http://dx.doi.org/10.1016/j.cub.2005.05.055] [PMID: 16005298]

[58]   Lewis RS. Store-operated calcium channels: new perspectives on mechanism and function. Cold

Spring Harb Perspect Biol 2011; 3(12): a003970.
[http://dx.doi.org/10.1101/cshperspect.a003970] [PMID: 21791698]

[59] Mignen O, Thompson JL, Shuttleworth TJ. Orai1 subunit stoichiometry of the mammalian CRAC channel pore. J Physiol 2008; 586(2): 419-25.
[http://dx.doi.org/10.1113/jphysiol.2007.147249] [PMID: 18006576]

[60] Collins TJ, Lipp P, Berridge MJ, Bootman MD. Mitochondrial Ca(2+) uptake depends on the spatial and temporal profile of cytosolic Ca(2+) signals. J Biol Chem 2001; 276(28): 26411-20.
[http://dx.doi.org/10.1074/jbc.M101101200] [PMID: 11333261]

[61] Brookes PS, Yoon Y, Robotham JL, Anders MW, Sheu S-S. 2004.http://www.physiology.org/doi/10.1152/ajpcell.00139.2004

[62] Carafoli E. Biogenesis: plasma membrane calcium ATPase: 15 years of work on the purified enzyme. FASEB J 1994; 8(13): 993-1002.
[http://dx.doi.org/10.1096/fasebj.8.13.7926378] [PMID: 7926378]

[63] Strehler EE, Zacharias DA. Role of alternative splicing in generating isoform diversity among plasma membrane calcium pumps. Physiol Rev 2001; 81(1): 21-50.
[http://dx.doi.org/10.1152/physrev.2001.81.1.21] [PMID: 11152753]

[64] Stewart TA, Yapa KTDS, Monteith GR. Altered calcium signaling in cancer cells. Biochim Biophys Acta 2015; 1848(10 Pt B): 2502-11.
[http://dx.doi.org/10.1016/j.bbamem.2014.08.016] [PMID: 25150047]

[65] Stafford N, Wilson C, Oceandy D, Neyses L, Cartwright EJ. The Plasma Membrane Calcium ATPases and Their Role as Major New Players in Human Disease. Physiol Rev 2017; 97(3): 1089-125.
[http://dx.doi.org/10.1152/physrev.00028.2016] [PMID: 28566538]

[66] Pedersen PL, Carafoli E. Ion motive ATPases. I. Ubiquity, properties, and significance to cell function. Trends Biochem Sci 1987; 12(C): 146-50.
[http://dx.doi.org/10.1016/0968-0004(87)90071-5]

[67] Chin D, Means AR. Calmodulin: a prototypical calcium sensor. Trends Cell Biol 2000; 10(8): 322-8.
[http://dx.doi.org/10.1016/S0962-8924(00)01800-6] [PMID: 10884684]

[68] Falchetto R, Vorherr T, Carafoli E. The calmodulin-binding site of the plasma membrane Ca^{2+} pump interacts with the transduction domain of the enzyme. Protein Sci 1992; 1(12): 1613-21.
[http://dx.doi.org/10.1002/pro.5560011209] [PMID: 1339025]

[69] Monteith GR, Wanigasekara Y, Roufogalis BD. The plasma membrane calcium pump, its role and regulation: new complexities and possibilities. J Pharmacol Toxicol Methods 1998; 40(4): 183-90.
[http://dx.doi.org/10.1016/S1056-8719(99)00004-0] [PMID: 10465152]

[70] Altshuler I, Vaillant JJ, Xu S, Cristescu ME. The evolutionary history of sarco(endo)plasmic calcium ATPase (SERCA). PLoS One 2012; 7(12): e52617.
[http://dx.doi.org/10.1371/journal.pone.0052617] [PMID: 23285113]

[71] Dang D, Rao R. Calcium-ATPases: Gene disorders and dysregulation in cancer. Biochim Biophys Acta 2016; 1863(6 Pt B): 1344-50.
[http://dx.doi.org/10.1016/j.bbamcr.2015.11.016] [PMID: 26608610]

[72] Zwaal RR, Van Baelen K, Groenen JTM, et al. The sarco-endoplasmic reticulum Ca^{2+} ATPase is required for development and muscle function in Caenorhabditis elegans. J Biol Chem 2001; 276(47): 43557-63.
[http://dx.doi.org/10.1074/jbc.M104693200] [PMID: 11559701]

[73] Van Baelen K, Dode L, Vanoevelen J, Callewaert G, De Smedt H, Missiaen L, et al. The Ca^{2+}/Mn^{2+} pumps in the Golgi apparatus Biochimica et BiophysicaActa - Mol Cell Res. 2004; pp. 103-2.

[74] Wuytack F, Raeymaekers L, Missiaen L. Molecular physiology of the SERCA and SPCA pumps. Cell Calcium 2002; 32(5-6): 279-305.

[http://dx.doi.org/10.1016/S0143416002001847] [PMID: 12543090]

[75]   Vanoevelen J, Dode L, Van Baelen K, *et al.* The secretory pathway Ca^{2+}/Mn^{2+}-ATPase 2 is a Golgi-localized pump with high affinity for Ca^{2+} ions. J Biol Chem 2005; 280(24): 22800-8.
[http://dx.doi.org/10.1074/jbc.M501026200] [PMID: 15831496]

[76]   Reinhardt TA, Filoteo AG, Penniston JT, Horst RL. Ca(2+)-ATPase protein expression in mammary tissue. Am J Physiol Cell Physiol 2000; 279(5): C1595-602.
[http://dx.doi.org/10.1152/ajpcell.2000.279.5.C1595] [PMID: 11029307]

[77]   Hu Z, Bonifas JM, Beech J, *et al.* Mutations in ATP2C1, encoding a calcium pump, cause Hailey-Hailey disease. Nat Genet 2000; 24(1): 61-5.
[http://dx.doi.org/10.1038/71701] [PMID: 10615129]

[78]   Wootton LL, Argent CCH, Wheatley M, Michelangeli F. The expression, activity and localisation of the secretory pathway Ca^{2+}-ATPase (SPCA1) in different mammalian tissues. Biochim Biophys Acta 2004; 1664(2): 189-97.
[http://dx.doi.org/10.1016/j.bbamem.2004.05.009] [PMID: 15328051]

[79]   Shennan DBPM, Peaker M. Transport of milk constituents by the mammary gland. Physiol Rev 2000; 80(3): 925-51.
[http://dx.doi.org/10.1152/physrev.2000.80.3.925] [PMID: 10893427]

[80]   Neville MC. Calcium secretion into milk. J Mammary Gland Biol Neoplasia 2005; 10(2): 119-28.
[http://dx.doi.org/10.1007/s10911-005-5395-z] [PMID: 16025219]

[81]   Tajbakhsh A, Pasdar A, Rezaee M, *et al.* The current status and perspectives regarding the clinical implication of intracellular calcium in breast cancer. J Cell Physiol 2018; 233(8): 5623-41.
[http://dx.doi.org/10.1002/jcp.26277] [PMID: 29150934]

[82]   Oftedal OT. The evolution of milk secretion and its ancient origins. Animal 2012; pp. 355-68.

[83]   Nadal A, Ropero AB, Laribi O, Maillet M, Fuentes E, Soria B. Nongenomic actions of estrogens and xenoestrogens by binding at a plasma membrane receptor unrelated to estrogen receptor alpha and estrogen receptor beta. Proc Natl Acad Sci USA 2000; 97(21): 11603-8. [In Process Citation].
[http://dx.doi.org/10.1073/pnas.97.21.11603] [PMID: 11027358]

[84]   Guerini D. The significance of the isoforms of plasma membrane calcium ATPase. Cell Tissue Res 1998; 292(2): 191-7.
[http://dx.doi.org/10.1007/s004410051050] [PMID: 9560462]

[85]   Reinhardt TA, Lippolis JD, Shull GE, Horst RL. Null mutation in the gene encoding plasma membrane Ca^{2+}-ATPase isoform 2 impairs calcium transport into milk. J Biol Chem 2004; 279(41): 42369-73.
[http://dx.doi.org/10.1074/jbc.M407788200] [PMID: 15302868]

[86]   Reinhardt TA, Horst RL. Ca^{2+}-ATPases and their expression in the mammary gland of pregnant and lactating rats. Am J Physiol 1999; 276(4): C796-802.
[http://dx.doi.org/10.1152/ajpcell.1999.276.4.C796] [PMID: 10199809]

[87]   VanHouten J, Sullivan C, Bazinet C, *et al.* PMCA2 regulates apoptosis during mammary gland involution and predicts outcome in breast cancer. Proc Natl Acad Sci USA 2010; 107(25): 11405-10.
[http://dx.doi.org/10.1073/pnas.0911186107] [PMID: 20534448]

[88]   Reinhardt TA, Lippolis JD. Mammary gland involution is associated with rapid down regulation of major mammary Ca^{2+}-ATPases. Biochem Biophys Res Commun 2009; 378(1): 99-102.
[http://dx.doi.org/10.1016/j.bbrc.2008.11.004] [PMID: 19000904]

[89]   Burgoyne RD, Duncan JS, Sudlow AW. Role of calcium in the pathway for milk protein secretion and possible relevance for mammary gland physiology. Biochem Soc Symp 1998; 63: 91-100.
[PMID: 9513714]

[90]   Djonov V, Andres AC, Ziemiecki A. Vascular remodelling during the normal and malignant life cycle

of the mammary gland. Microsc Res Tech 2001; 52(2): 182-9.
[http://dx.doi.org/10.1002/1097-0029(20010115)52:2<182::AID-JEMT1004>3.0.CO;2-M] [PMID: 11169866]

[91] Davis FM, Janoshazi A, Janardhan KS, *et al.* Essential role of Orai1 store-operated calcium channels in lactation. Proc Natl Acad Sci USA 2015; 112(18): 5827-32.
[http://dx.doi.org/10.1073/pnas.1502264112] [PMID: 25902527]

[92] Donato R. S100: a multigenic family of calcium-modulated proteins of the EF-hand type with intracellular and extracellular functional roles. Int J Biochem Cell Biol 2001; 33(7): 637-68.
[http://dx.doi.org/10.1016/S1357-2725(01)00046-2] [PMID: 11390274]

[93] Vanhouten JN, Wysolmerski JJ. The calcium-sensing receptor in the breast. Best Pract Res Clin Endocrinol Metab 2013; 27(3): 403-14.
[http://dx.doi.org/10.1016/j.beem.2013.02.011] [PMID: 23856268]

[94] Berchtold MW, Villalobo A. The many faces of calmodulin in cell proliferation, programmed cell death, autophagy, and cancer. Biochim Biophys Acta 2014; 1843(2): 398-435.
[http://dx.doi.org/10.1016/j.bbamcr.2013.10.021] [PMID: 24188867]

[95] Brennan SC, Thiem U, Roth S, *et al.* Calcium sensing receptor signalling in physiology and cancer. Biochim Biophys Acta 2013; 1833(7): 1732-44.
[http://dx.doi.org/10.1016/j.bbamcr.2012.12.011] [PMID: 23267858]

[96] Quinn SJ, Kifor O, Kifor I, Butters RR Jr, Brown EM. Role of the cytoskeleton in extracellular calcium-regulated PTH release. Biochem Biophys Res Commun 2007; 354(1): 8-13.
[http://dx.doi.org/10.1016/j.bbrc.2006.12.160] [PMID: 17223073]

[97] Hofer AM, Brown EM. Extracellular calcium sensing and signalling. Nat Rev Mol Cell Biol 2003; 4(7): 530-8.
[http://dx.doi.org/10.1038/nrm1154] [PMID: 12838336]

[98] VanHouten J, Dann P, McGeoch G, *et al.* The calcium-sensing receptor regulates mammary gland parathyroid hormone-related protein production and calcium transport. J Clin Invest 2004; 113(4): 598-608.
[http://dx.doi.org/10.1172/JCI200418776] [PMID: 14966569]

[99] Roderick HL, Cook SJ. Ca^{2+} signalling checkpoints in cancer: remodelling Ca^{2+} for cancer cell proliferation and survival. Nat Rev Cancer 2008; 8(5): 361-75.
[http://dx.doi.org/10.1038/nrc2374] [PMID: 18432251]

[100] Motiani RK, Abdullaev IF, Trebak M. A novel native store-operated calcium channel encoded by Orai3: selective requirement of Orai3 *versus* Orai1 in estrogen receptor-positive *versus* estrogen receptor-negative breast cancer cells. J Biol Chem 2010; 285(25): 19173-83.
[http://dx.doi.org/10.1074/jbc.M110.102582] [PMID: 20395295]

[101] Grice DM, Vetter I, Faddy HM, Kenny PA, Roberts-Thomson SJ, Monteith GR. Golgi calcium pump secretory pathway calcium ATPase 1 (SPCA1) is a key regulator of insulin-like growth factor receptor (IGF1R) processing in the basal-like breast cancer cell line MDA-MB-231. J Biol Chem 2010; 285(48): 37458-66.
[http://dx.doi.org/10.1074/jbc.M110.163329] [PMID: 20837466]

[102] Motiani RK, Zhang X, Harmon KE, *et al.* Orai3 is an estrogen receptor α-regulated Ca^{2+} channel that promotes tumorigenesis. FASEB J 2013; 27(1): 63-75.
[http://dx.doi.org/10.1096/fj.12-213801] [PMID: 22993197]

[103] Taylor JT, Huang L, Pottle JE, *et al.* Selective blockade of T-type Ca^{2+} channels suppresses human breast cancer cell proliferation. Cancer Lett 2008; 267(1): 116-24.
[http://dx.doi.org/10.1016/j.canlet.2008.03.032] [PMID: 18455293]

[104] Tannheimer SL, Barton SL, Ethier SP, Burchiel SW. Carcinogenic polycyclic aromatic hydrocarbons increase intracellular Ca^{2+} and cell proliferation in primary human mammary epithelial cells.

Carcinogenesis 1997; 18(6): 1177-82.
[http://dx.doi.org/10.1093/carcin/18.6.1177] [PMID: 9214600]

[105] Faddy HM, Smart CE, Xu R, *et al.* Localization of plasma membrane and secretory calcium pumps in the mammary gland. Biochem Biophys Res Commun 2008; 369(3): 977-81.
[http://dx.doi.org/10.1016/j.bbrc.2008.03.003] [PMID: 18334228]

[106] Feng M, Grice DM, Faddy HM, *et al.* Store-independent activation of Orai1 by SPCA2 in mammary tumors. Cell 2010; 143(1): 84-98.
[http://dx.doi.org/10.1016/j.cell.2010.08.040] [PMID: 20887894]

[107] Ardeshirpour L, Dann P, Pollak M, Wysolmerski J, VanHouten J. The calcium-sensing receptor regulates PTHrP production and calcium transport in the lactating mammary gland. Bone 2006; 38(6): 787-93.
[http://dx.doi.org/10.1016/j.bone.2005.11.009] [PMID: 16377269]

[108] Zhang H, Zhou L, Shi W, Song N, Yu K, Gu Y. A mechanism underlying the effects of polyunsaturated fatty acids on breast cancer. Int J Mol Med 2012; 30(3): 487-94.
[http://dx.doi.org/10.3892/ijmm.2012.1022] [PMID: 22692672]

[109] Bidaud I, Mezghrani A, Swayne LA, Monteil A, Lory P. Voltage-gated calcium channels in genetic diseases. Biochim Biophys Acta 2006; 1763(11): 1169-74.
[http://dx.doi.org/10.1016/j.bbamcr.2006.08.049] [PMID: 17034879]

[110] Bertolesi GE, Shi C, Elbaum L, *et al.* The Ca(2+) channel antagonists mibefradil and pimozide inhibit cell growth *via* different cytotoxic mechanisms. Mol Pharmacol 2002; 62(2): 210-9.
[http://dx.doi.org/10.1124/mol.62.2.210] [PMID: 12130671]

[111] Wang CY, Lai MD, Phan NN, Sun Z, Lin YC. Meta-analysis of public microarray datasets reveals voltage-gated calcium gene signatures in clinical cancer patients. PLoS One 2015; 10(7): e0125766.
[http://dx.doi.org/10.1371/journal.pone.0125766] [PMID: 26147197]

[112] Dhennin-Duthille I, Gautier M, Faouzi M, *et al.* High expression of transient receptor potential channels in human breast cancer epithelial cells and tissues: correlation with pathological parameters. Cell Physiol Biochem 2011; 28(5): 813-22.
[http://dx.doi.org/10.1159/000335795] [PMID: 22178934]

[113] Aydar E, Yeo S, Djamgoz M, Palmer C. Abnormal expression, localization and interaction of canonical transient receptor potential ion channels in human breast cancer cell lines and tissues: a potential target for breast cancer diagnosis and therapy. Cancer Cell Int 2009; 9(23): 23.
[http://dx.doi.org/10.1186/1475-2867-9-23] [PMID: 19689790]

[114] Prevarskaya N, Zhang L, Barritt G. TRP channels in cancer. Biochim Biophys Acta 2007; 1772(8): 937-46.
[http://dx.doi.org/10.1016/j.bbadis.2007.05.006] [PMID: 17616360]

[115] Bates-Withers C, Sah R, Clapham DE. TRPM7, the Mg^{2+} inhibited channel and kinase Advances in Experimental Medicine and Biology. 2011; pp. 173-83.

[116] Meng X, Cai C, Wu J, *et al.* TRPM7 mediates breast cancer cell migration and invasion through the MAPK pathway. Cancer Lett 2013; 333(1): 96-102.
[http://dx.doi.org/10.1016/j.canlet.2013.01.031] [PMID: 23353055]

[117] Guilbert A, Gautier M, Dhennin-Duthille I, Haren N, Sevestre H, Ouadid-Ahidouch H. Evidence that TRPM7 is required for breast cancer cell proliferation. Am J Physiol Cell Physiol 2009; 297(3): C493-502.
[http://dx.doi.org/10.1152/ajpcell.00624.2008] [PMID: 19515901]

[118] Middelbeek J, Kuipers AJ, Henneman L, *et al.* TRPM7 is required for breast tumor cell metastasis. Cancer Res 2012; 72(16): 4250-61.
[http://dx.doi.org/10.1158/0008-5472.CAN-11-3863] [PMID: 22871386]

[119] Nazıroğlu M, Blum W, Jósvay K, *et al.* Menthol evokes Ca^{2+} signals and induces oxidative stress

independently of the presence of TRPM8 (menthol) receptor in cancer cells. Redox Biol 2018; 14: 439-49.
[http://dx.doi.org/10.1016/j.redox.2017.10.009] [PMID: 29078169]

[120]   Chodon D, Guilbert A, Dhennin-Duthille I, *et al.* Estrogen regulation of TRPM8 expression in breast cancer cells. BMC Cancer 2010; 10(212): 212.
[http://dx.doi.org/10.1186/1471-2407-10-212] [PMID: 20482834]

[121]   Bolanz KA, Hediger MA, Landowski CP. The role of TRPV6 in breast carcinogenesis. Mol Cancer Ther 2008; 7(2): 271-9.
[http://dx.doi.org/10.1158/1535-7163.MCT-07-0478] [PMID: 18245667]

[122]   Bolanz KA, Kovacs GG, Landowski CP, Hediger MA. Tamoxifen inhibits TRPV6 activity *via* estrogen receptor-independent pathways in TRPV6-expressing MCF-7 breast cancer cells. Mol Cancer Res 2009; 7(12): 2000-10.
[http://dx.doi.org/10.1158/1541-7786.MCR-09-0188] [PMID: 19996302]

[123]   Peters AA, Simpson PT, Bassett JJ, *et al.* Calcium channel TRPV6 as a potential therapeutic target in estrogen receptor-negative breast cancer. Mol Cancer Ther 2012; 11(10): 2158-68.
[http://dx.doi.org/10.1158/1535-7163.MCT-11-0965] [PMID: 22807578]

[124]   Fiorio Pla A, Ong HL, Cheng KT, *et al.* TRPV4 mediates tumor-derived endothelial cell migration *via* arachidonic acid-activated actin remodeling. Oncogene 2012; 31(2): 200-12.
[http://dx.doi.org/10.1038/onc.2011.231] [PMID: 21685934]

[125]   Weber LV, Al-Refae K, Wölk G, *et al.* Expression and functionality of TRPV1 in breast cancer cells. Breast Cancer (Dove Med Press) 2016; 8: 243-52.
[http://dx.doi.org/10.2147/BCTT.S121610] [PMID: 28008282]

[126]   Faouzi M, Chopin V, Ahidouch A, Ouadid-Ahidouch H. Intermediate Ca^{2+}-sensitive K^+ channels are necessary for prolactin-induced proliferation in breast cancer cells. J Membr Biol 2010; 234(1): 47-56.
[http://dx.doi.org/10.1007/s00232-010-9238-5] [PMID: 20177667]

[127]   Schickling BM, England SK, Aykin-Burns N, Norian LA, Leslie KK, Frieden-Korovkina VP. BKCa channel inhibitor modulates the tumorigenic ability of hormone-independent breast cancer cells *via* the Wnt pathway. Oncol Rep 2015; 33(2): 533-8.
[http://dx.doi.org/10.3892/or.2014.3617] [PMID: 25422049]

[128]   Hammadi M, Chopin V, Matifat F, *et al.* Human ether à-gogo K(+) channel 1 (hEag1) regulates MDA-MB-231 breast cancer cell migration through Orai1-dependent calcium entry. J Cell Physiol 2012; 227(12): 3837-46.
[http://dx.doi.org/10.1002/jcp.24095] [PMID: 22495877]

[129]   Du C, Chen L, Zhang H, *et al.* Caveolin-1 limits the contribution of BKCa channel to MCF-7 breast cancer cell proliferation and invasion. Int J Mol Sci 2014; 15(11): 20706-22.
[http://dx.doi.org/10.3390/ijms151120706] [PMID: 25397596]

[130]   Britschgi A, Bill A, Brinkhaus H, *et al.* Calcium-activated chloride channel ANO1 promotes breast cancer progression by activating EGFR and CAMK signaling. Proc Natl Acad Sci USA 2013; 110(11): E1026-34.http://www.pnas.org/lookup/doi/10.1073/pnas.1217072110 [Internet].
[http://dx.doi.org/10.1073/pnas.1217072110] [PMID: 23431153]

[131]   Wang Y, Deng X, Gill DL. Calcium signaling by STIM and Orai: intimate coupling details revealed. Sci Signal 2010; 3(148): pe42.
[http://dx.doi.org/10.1126/scisignal.3148pe42] [PMID: 21081752]

[132]   Faouzi M, Hague F, Potier M, Ahidouch A, Sevestre H, Ouadid-Ahidouch H. Down-regulation of Orai3 arrests cell-cycle progression and induces apoptosis in breast cancer cells but not in normal breast epithelial cells. J Cell Physiol 2011; 226(2): 542-51.
[http://dx.doi.org/10.1002/jcp.22363] [PMID: 20683915]

[133]   Faouzi M, Kischel P, Hague F, *et al.* ORAI3 silencing alters cell proliferation and cell cycle

progression *via* c-myc pathway in breast cancer cells. Biochim Biophys Acta 2013; 1833(3): 752-60.
[http://dx.doi.org/10.1016/j.bbamcr.2012.12.009] [PMID: 23266555]

[134] Castillo-González AC, Pelegrín-Hernández JP, Nieto-Cerón S, *et al.* Unbalanced acetylcholinesterase activity in larynx squamous cell carcinoma. Int Immunopharmacol 2015; 29(1): 81-6.
[http://dx.doi.org/10.1016/j.intimp.2015.05.011] [PMID: 26002584]

[135] Song P, Sekhon HS, Lu A, *et al.* M3 muscarinic receptor antagonists inhibit small cell lung carcinoma growth and mitogen-activated protein kinase phosphorylation induced by acetylcholine secretion. Cancer Res 2007; 67(8): 3936-44.
[http://dx.doi.org/10.1158/0008-5472.CAN-06-2484] [PMID: 17440109]

[136] Kodaira M, Kajimura M, Takeuchi K, Lin S, Hanai H, Kaneko E. Functional muscarinic m3 receptor expressed in gastric cancer cells stimulates tyrosine phosphorylation and MAP kinase. J Gastroenterol 1999; 34(2): 163-71.
[http://dx.doi.org/10.1007/s005350050238] [PMID: 10213113]

[137] Von Rosenvinge EC, Raufman JP. Muscarinic receptor signaling in colon cancer. Cancers (Basel) 2011; 3(1): 971-81.
[http://dx.doi.org/10.3390/cancers3010971] [PMID: 24212649]

[138] Boss A, Oppitz M, Lippert G, Drews U. Muscarinic cholinergic receptors in the human melanoma cell line SK-Mel 28: modulation of chemotaxis. Clin Exp Dermatol 2005; 30(5): 557-64.
[http://dx.doi.org/10.1111/j.1365-2230.2005.01865.x] [PMID: 16045692]

[139] Song W, Yuan M, Zhao S. Variation of M3 muscarinic receptor expression in different prostate tissues and its significance. Saudi Med J 2009; 30(8): 1010-6.
[PMID: 19668880]

[140] Eglen RM. Muscarinic receptor subtypes in neuronal and non-neuronal cholinergic function. Auton Autacoid Pharmacol 2006; 26(3): 219-33.
[http://dx.doi.org/10.1111/j.1474-8673.2006.00368.x] [PMID: 16879488]

[141] Español A, Eiján AM, Mazzoni E, *et al.* Nitric oxide synthase, arginase and cyclooxygenase are involved in muscarinic receptor activation in different murine mammary adenocarcinoma cell lines. Int J Mol Med 2002; 9(6): 651-7.
[http://dx.doi.org/10.3892/ijmm.9.6.651] [PMID: 12011984]

[142] Español AJ, Sales ME. Different muscarinc receptors are involved in the proliferation of murine mammary adenocarcinoma cell lines. Int J Mol Med 2004; 13(2): 311-7.
[http://dx.doi.org/10.3892/ijmm.13.2.311] [PMID: 14719140]

[143] Rimmaudo LE, de la Torre E, Sacerdote de Lustig E, Sales ME. Muscarinic receptors are involved in LMM3 tumor cells proliferation and angiogenesis. Biochem Biophys Res Commun 2005; 334(4): 1359-64.
[http://dx.doi.org/10.1016/j.bbrc.2005.07.031] [PMID: 16040004]

[144] Negroni MP, Fiszman GL, Azar ME, *et al.* Immunoglobulin G from breast cancer patients in stage I stimulates muscarinic acetylcholine receptors in MCF7 cells and induces proliferation. Participation of nitric oxide synthase-derived nitric oxide. J Clin Immunol 2010; 30(3): 474-84.
[http://dx.doi.org/10.1007/s10875-010-9370-0] [PMID: 20157846]

[145] Nazıroğlu M, Çiğ B, Blum W, *et al.* Targeting breast cancer cells by MRS1477, a positive allosteric modulator of TRPV1 channels. PLoS One 2017; 12(6): e0179950.
[http://dx.doi.org/10.1371/journal.pone.0179950] [PMID: 28640864]

[146] Deveci HA, Nazıroğlu M, Nur G. 5-Fluorouracil-induced mitochondrial oxidative cytotoxicity and apoptosis are increased in MCF-7 human breast cancer cells by TRPV1 channel activation but not Hypericum perforatum treatment. Mol Cell Biochem 2018; 439(1-2): 189-98.
[http://dx.doi.org/10.1007/s11010-017-3147-1] [PMID: 28795251]

[147] Nur G, Nazıroğlu M, Deveci HA. Synergic prooxidant, apoptotic and TRPV1 channel activator effects

of alpha-lipoic acid and cisplatin in MCF-7 breast cancer cells. J Recept Signal Transduct Res 2017; 37(6): 569-77.
[http://dx.doi.org/10.1080/10799893.2017.1369121] [PMID: 28849985]

[148] Pelegrina LT, Lombardi MG, Fiszman GL, Azar ME, Morgado CC, Sales ME. Immunoglobulin g from breast cancer patients regulates MCF-7 cells migration and MMP-9 activity by stimulating muscarinic acetylcholine receptors. J Clin Immunol 2013; 33(2): 427-35.
[http://dx.doi.org/10.1007/s10875-012-9804-y] [PMID: 23007238]

[149] Yang S, Zhang JJ, Huang XY. Orai1 and STIM1 are critical for breast tumor cell migration and metastasis. Cancer Cell 2009; 15(2): 124-34.
[http://dx.doi.org/10.1016/j.ccr.2008.12.019] [PMID: 19185847]

[150] Jiménez E, Montiel M. Activation of MAP kinase by muscarinic cholinergic receptors induces cell proliferation and protein synthesis in human breast cancer cells. J Cell Physiol 2005; 204(2): 678-86.
[http://dx.doi.org/10.1002/jcp.20326] [PMID: 15744749]

[151] Español AJ, Salem A, Rojo D, Sales ME. Participation of non-neuronal muscarinic receptors in the effect of carbachol with paclitaxel on human breast adenocarcinoma cells. Roles of nitric oxide synthase and arginase. Int Immunopharmacol 2015; 29(1): 87-92.
[http://dx.doi.org/10.1016/j.intimp.2015.03.018] [PMID: 25812766]

[152] Gogebakan B, Bayraktar R, Suner A, *et al.* Do fasudil and Y-27632 affect the level of transient receptor potential (TRP) gene expressions in breast cancer cell lines? Tumour Biol 2014; 35(8): 8033-41.
[http://dx.doi.org/10.1007/s13277-014-1752-0] [PMID: 24839003]

[153] Kim BJ, Nam JH, Kwon YK, So I, Kim SJ. The role of waixenicin A as transient receptor potential melastatin 7 blocker. Basic Clin Pharmacol Toxicol 2013; 112(2): 83-9.
[http://dx.doi.org/10.1111/j.1742-7843.2012.00929.x] [PMID: 22901271]

[154] Yapa KTDS, Deuis J, Peters AA, *et al.* Assessment of the TRPM8 inhibitor AMTB in breast cancer cells and its identification as an inhibitor of voltage gated sodium channels. Life Sci 2018; 198: 128-35.
[http://dx.doi.org/10.1016/j.lfs.2018.02.030] [PMID: 29496495]

[155] Zierler S, Yao G, Zhang Z, *et al.* Waixenicin A inhibits cell proliferation through magnesium-dependent block of transient receptor potential melastatin 7 (TRPM7) channels. J Biol Chem 2011; 286(45): 39328-35.
[http://dx.doi.org/10.1074/jbc.M111.264341] [PMID: 21926172]

CHAPTER 12

Role of Mitochondrial-mediated Pathways in Breast Cancer: An Overview

Nabanita Chatterjee*, **Debangshi Das, Ashna Jha** and **Sraddhya Roy**

Chittaranjan National Cancer Institute, 37, Shyama Prasad Mukherjee Road, Kolkata-700026, India

Abstract: The powerhouse of the cell, mitochondria play several cellular functions, and it also regulates the physiological adjustment of the body. The deregulation of any of the key factors in the regulation pathway of energy production or cellular metabolism leads to disease conditions and, sometimes even cancer. Several studies emphasize the fact that the alteration in metabolic pathways, generate or evoke cancer susceptibility including breast cancer. Among the several cancers, breast cancer is a major concern in the female population. Thus, the alteration of any mitochondrial factors or metabolites associated with the mitochondrial energy cycle, the changes in breast cancer development or progression of metastasis is high. Mitochondrial regulation could be a promising therapeutic approach in the treatment of breast cancer.

Keywords: Breast cancer, Metabolic pathway, Mitochondria, mtDNA, Reactive oxygen species, Warburg effect.

INTRODUCTION

The Powerful Cellular Organelle: Mitochondria

Mitochondria is a membrane-bound organelle found in the cytoplasm of almost all eukaryotic organisms [1]. The role of mitochondria is the production of the ATP which is known as the energy currency of the cell *via* respiration. It helps in the regulation of cellular metabolism. It is also known as the 'powerhouse' of the cell [2]. Citric acid cycle and Krebs's cycle are involved in the production of ATP molecules [3, 4]. Signaling, cell growth, maintaining cell cycle and cell death are several other functions performed by the mitochondria.

It is also involved in various human disorders such as cardiac dysfunction, mitochondrial disorders, autism, and heart failure [5 - 10].

---

* **Corresponding Author Dr. Nabanita Chatterjee**: Chittaranjan National Cancer Institute, 37, Shyama Prasad Mukherjee Road, Kolkata -700026, India; E-mails: nabanita.chatterje@yahoo.com/nabanitachatterjee@cnci.org.in

Shankar Suman, Garima Suman and Sanjay Mishra (Eds.)

The number of mitochondria varies in the cell, depending on the organism, cells, and type of tissues. For instance, the liver has around 2000 mitochondria whereas RBCs do not contain any mitochondria. These organelles consist of compartments that include the outer membrane, inner membrane, cristae, matrix and the intermembrane space that individually performs specialized functions [11]. The genome of mitochondria shows similarity to bacterial genomes. In addition, mitochondrial proteins differ widely based on tissues and species type.

Mitochondrial Energy

The primary function of mitochondria is ATP production. The oxidization mainly does energy conversion. In the cytosol, the main compound is glucose, which gets converted to pyruvate, NADH and this process is known as aerobic respiration, which is an oxygen-dependent process during oxidation. Sometimes, the process is oxygen-independent when the oxygen supply is limited, and it starts anaerobic fermentation [12]. In this process, the ATP production is 13-times higher in aerobic respiration than fermentation [13]. The release of ATP occurs through the outer membrane channel porin from the inner membrane with the help of several other proteins.

The Process of ATP Production: Pyruvate and Citric Acid Cycle

In the process of glycolysis, the out product is pyruvate, which is actively transported to the matrix. After that, it gets oxidized and followed by the combination with co-enzyme A and its associates, leading to form acetyl CoA or decarboxylated to oxaloacetate. The second reaction, denoted with it, is the citric acid cycle, where all the intermediates like citrate, alpha-keto-glutarate, and succinate oxaloacetate again turn into the cycle whenever it needs the regeneration of cycles. That cycle could produce citric acid in a combination of excess or low mount of oxaloacetate with reacting acetyl-CoA that might be referred to as anaplerotic or cataplerotic effect. Thus, the amount of ATP production is directly or indirectly regulated by mitochondria. After this reaction of oxidative reaction, the acetate portion of acetyl-CoA gets oxidized to carbon dioxide, water, and ATP. More importantly, acetyl-CoA is the only compound that enters the TCA cycle either from pyruvate oxidation or β-oxidation of fatty acids. This also affects several disease conditions including cancer [14]. Few more parameters of oxidation also influence the interaction process like the gluconeogenic pathway [15].

Pyruvate and the TCA Cycle

Pyruvate molecules produced *via* the glycolysis pathway are carried across the inner membrane of mitochondria and into the matrix where pyruvate molecules get oxidized and combine with coenzyme-A forming CO_2, acetyl-CoA, and NADH. It can be carboxylated by pyruvate carboxylase that forms oxaloacetate [16]. This results in an increase in the amount of oxaloacetate in the TCA cycle which in [17] turn increases the cycle's capacity to metabolize acetyl Co-A to form citric acid. Thus, the increase or decrease in the rate of ATP production is regulated by the mitochondria. All the intermediates (*e.g.*, citrate, iso-citrate, alpha-ketoglutarate, succinate, fumarate, *etc.*) are generated during each turn of the TCA cycle. Acetyl CoA is the only combustible fuel that enters the citric acid or TCA cycle derived from pyruvate oxidation or β-oxidation of the fatty acids [18], and it is consumed for each of the molecules of oxaloacetate which is present in the mitochondrial matrix. CO_2, water, and energy are produced by the oxidation of acetate protein of acetyl CoA captured in the form of ATP [14, 19].

In the liver, the cytosolic pyruvate is carboxylated into oxaloacetate in gluconeogenic pathway, which under the influence of an increased level of glucan in the blood converts lactate and as well as de-aminated alanine into the glucose. Most of the enzymes of the TCA cycle are located in the mitochondrial matrix, but succinate dehydrogenase is bound to the inner mitochondrial membrane as a part of complex II [20]. Oxidization of acetyl-CoA to CO_2 by the citric acid cycle or TCA cycle produces reduced cofactors that include three molecules of NADH and one molecule of FADH2. These reduced cofactors are a source of electrons for electron transport chain [21].

Electron Transport Chain [NADH and FADH2]

Through the electron transport chain, redox energy from NADH and FADH2 is transferred to oxygen [22]. NADH and FADH2 molecules are produced *via* the TCA cycle within the matrix and through the process of glycolysis in the cytoplasm. Using the glycerol phosphate shuttle or the malate-aspartate shuttle system, the reducing equivalents from the cytoplasm can be imported. NADH dehydrogenase, cytochrome c reductase, cytochrome c oxidase in the inner membrane performs the transfer process, and the energy released is used for pumping protons into the intermembrane space. This process can lead to mitochondrial dysfunction associated with aging and oxidative stress [23, 24].

Heat Production

The process by which protons can enter the mitochondrial matrix without the synthesis of ATP is known as Proton leak or mitochondrial uncoupling [11]. This process takes place due to the facilitated diffusion of protons resulting in the release of electrochemical gradient energy in the form of heat mediated by a proton channel called thermogenin or UCP1 [25].

Storage of Calcium Ions

Many reactions can be regulated by the concentration of free calcium in the cell which is significant for signal transduction in the cell. Calcium is stored in mitochondria that contribute to the cell's homeostasis of calcium. Mitochondria can also help in the take-up and release of calcium ions [26].

A series of second messenger system proteins are activated by the release of calcium, which coordinates the process such as the release of hormones in endocrine cells and release of neurotransmitters in nerve cells [27]. Mitochondria play a central role in many other metabolic tasks, such as signaling through mitochondrial reactive oxygen species, regulating membrane potential, apoptosis, calcium signaling (including calcium-evoked apoptosis), regulating of cellular metabolism, certain heme synthesis reactions, steroid synthesis, and hormonal imbalance *etc.* [28, 29].

Cancer: Breast Cancer

Cancer that specifically develops from breast and its associate ductal parts occurs mainly in females. Lack of physical exercise, obesity, early age at first menstruation, having children late, family history of breast cancer, drinking alcohol, *etc.*, are the risk factors concerned with developing breast cancer. Around 5-10% of breast cancer occurs due to genes inherited from parents, including BRCA1 and BRCA2 [30]. It commonly occurs in the lining of milk ducts and the lobules. Cancers developed from the lining of duct are called ductal carcinomas, whereas ones developed from lobules known as lobular carcinomas. Ductal carcinomas are developed from pre-invasive lesions. Breast cancer is determined by performing a biopsy of concerning lump [31]. After the diagnosis, more tests are performed in order to determine if carcinoma cells have spread beyond the breast [32].

Triple-negative Breast Cancer

Triple-negative breast cancer (TNBC) is a type of breast cancer that tests negative for estrogen receptors, progesterone receptors and excess HER2 protein. The hormone receptors inside and on the surface of the healthy breast cells receive a message from estrogen and progesterone. The hormones attach to these receptors thereby provide instructions to the cells to grow and function properly. However, triple-negative breast cancer does not have these receptors. On the other hand, TNBC has about 20% of the excess HER2 protein. When the breast cancer cells have an excessive amount of HER2 protein, they grow, divide quickly and develop metastasis. Among others, about 10-20% of cancer of breast cancers are found as TNBC [33, 34]. They are unlikely to respond to medicines that target

HER2 protein, such as Herceptin [chemical name: Trastuzumab], Kadcyla (chemical name: T-DMA or ado-Trastuzumabemtansine), Nerlynx (chemical name: neratinib), Perjeta (chemical name: Pertuzumab), or Tykerb (chemical name: Lapatinib) [35].

Common Features of TNBC [36]:

• TNBC is considered aggressive, having a poorer prognosis than any other breast cancer types.

• It tends to be higher in grade.

• It is the "basal-like" cell type.

TNBC is commonly found in younger people, African-American and Hispanic women, and people with BRCA1 mutation [37].

Treatment for TNBC: Triple-negative breast cancer is treated with a combination of surgery, radiation therapy, and chemotherapy [38].

Some of them are listed below:

• Neo-adjuvant chemotherapy- Triple negative breast cancer treated with chemotherapy before surgery is called neo-adjuvant chemotherapy. This type of treatment makes disease-free survival and other survival better [39].

• PARP inhibitor- PARP inhibitor, such as Lynparza (chemical name: olaparib), Talzenna (chemical name: talazoparib) are used to treat advanced-stage HER2-negative breast cancer in people with BRCA1 or BRCA2 mutation. This helps in preventing poly ADP-ribose polymerase (PARP) enzyme from fixing DNA damage in breast cancer cells [40].

• Immunotherapy- The immunotherapy medicines, Tecentriq and Abraxane, is used for treating unresectable locally advanced or metastatic triple-negative, PD-L1 positive breast cancer. Tecentriq is an immune checkpoint inhibitor medicine that targets a specific protein inhibiting PD-L1 protein expression. By doing so, it allows the immune system cells to recognize cancer cells and kill them [41].

Alterations in Cancer Cells

Normal cell growth and development requires the optimal function of regulatory signaling pathways, which resist or tolerate in response to external or internal stimuli. Deregulation of these signaling pathways can lead to the occurrence of various diseases, such as diabetes, a neurodegenerative disorder, developmental defects and cancer [42]. Defects in the cellular growth and apoptotic pathway can lead to carcinogenesis and metastatic tumor progression. However, defects in apoptosis are observed as the primary cellular malfunction in tumor growth and metastatic progression. Cancer cells exhibit strong metabolic faults in the mitochondrial apoptotic process which includes increased fatty acid synthesis, boosting glutamine metabolism and dependence on aerobic glycolysis for gaining energy. All these metabolic adaptations take place due to the defects in normal mitochondria function, thereby developing resistance towards cancer treatments and apoptotic evasion, which leads to an increase in cancer growth and progression [43, 44].

Therefore, targeting and restoring mitochondrial steady state is considered to be a useful strategy for cancer control and management. Metabolic inhibitors, such as 2-deoxy-D-glucose (2DG), dichloroacetate (DCA), hexokinase inhibitors, and lactate dehydrogenase inhibitors, have commonly been used to inhibit aerobic glycolysis pathway and restore steady-state oxidative phosphorylation in mitochondria [45]. These have been effective against various cancer cells [46].

MITOCHONDRIAL INVOLVEMENT: BETWEEN NORMAL AND CANCER CELLS IN RESPECT OF METABOLISM

Cancer cells vary from normal cells in separate metabolic aspects. Differential cellular metabolisms of cells are a fully dependent anaerobic glycolytic pathway, glutaminolysis and fatty acid synthesis that helps in cellular proliferation, development, survival, and growth. Oxidization of glucose by normal cells through the TCA cycle generates 30 ATP per molecule of glucose in the mitochondria to fulfill their cellular requirements [47]. Cancer cells also depend on glycolysis for generating 2 ATP per glucose molecule in the cytoplasm. Therefore, cancer cells help in the up-regulation of glucose transporter extending the uptake of glucose to meet their energy needs [47, 48]. Glucose oxidation through TCA in the mitochondrial cell prevents respiratory dysfunction in cancer cells. An increase in glycolysis provides substance for gluconeogenesis, lipid metabolism and the pentose phosphate pathway for macromolecules required in anabolic reaction and to generate NADH. This distinguished alteration in the bioenergetics metabolic process stipulates a new era of cancer research in the therapy of cancer treatment [49].

Metabolic Pathway and its Resistance in Cancer

Apoptosis resistance in cancer cells develops due to altered metabolism and active glycolytic processes. Upregulation and activation of hexokinase in cancer cells, translocates it into the mitochondria and inhibits mitochondria-mediated apoptosis. Phosphate and tensin homolog (PTEN), oncogenic activation and hypoxic conditions are the events that help in the modulation of glycolytic factors and act as resistant to carcinoma cells. Inhibition of cellular respiration is due to hexokinase 2 expression and PDH inactivation by PDK. PDK-PDH circuit plays a very significant role in the regulation of energy metabolism between oxidative phosphorylation and glucose. The role of PDK is to phosphorylate and inhibits PDH activity with the help of ATP. PDH Phosphatase causes dephosphorylation of PDH thus restoring its activity. This PDH activation helps in the conversion of pyruvate to acetyl CoA leading to the entry of pyruvate molecules in mitochondria. Glucose is converted into lactate through the glycolysis pathway when PDH is deactivated and PDK activity is enhanced.

Similarly, in the presence of activated PDH and inhibited PDK, glucose oxidation through the TCA cycle occurs in the mitochondria. In cancer cells, overexpression of PDK3 enhances glycolysis which in turn increases the chances of cancer recurrence and drug resistance. Hence, a hyperactive glycolytic pathway leads to the inhibition of the apoptotic pathway in cancer cells. Thus, the PDK–PDH signaling circuit is considered a very significant target in cancer therapy, expecting better treatments in cancer patients [50, 51].

Regulation of Tumorigenesis in Mitochondria

The formation of a mass of cells is known as a tumor and the process involved is called tumorigenesis. It may not be cancerous, the mass of cells can be either malignant or benign [52]. Mitochondria has a central role in most eukaryotic cells, ranging from regulation of apoptosis to energy production. Energy metabolism plays a vital role in carcinogenesis. Mitochondria modulate Reactive Oxygen Species (ROS) production, Ca^{+2} homeostasis and apoptosis, which are necessary for normal cellular homeostasis. Mitochondria possess the capability of sensing the overall level of cellular physiological stress and synchronize the liberation of various apoptosis initiating factors, that lead to caspase activation and cell death [53]. The flaw in the mitochondrial system including mtDNA mutations, deletions and alternations in nuclear-coded proteins are pivotal for mitochondrial function leading to the formation of cancer cells. mtDNA mutations are found to affect the functions of mitochondrial physiology, also considering oxidative phosphorylation complexes, ROS-producing potential, Ca^{+2} homeostasis and apoptosis-initiating potential, that gets serious by a high rate of glycolytic pathway or by the oxidative phosphorylation activity [54].

Mitochondria metabolism varies from their normal counterparts in cancer cells. ROS accumulation, aerobic glycolysis, hypoxia, anti-apoptotic signals are the important characteristics of mitochondria in cancer cells. Mutations in mtDNA lead to the deregulation of enzymes. This trait is interlinked which in turn accelerates tumorigenesis in cancer cells by reductive carboxylation of glutamine. Behind the activation of hypoxia-inducible factors (HIFs), mutations in TCA cycle enzymes encoding genes have a vital role [55].

As we know, mitochondria regulate programmed cell death, and apoptotic inducing factors are generally preserved inside mitochondria, which upon the opening of the MTP (mito-transition pores) are released into the cytosol to initiate cell death. Increased ROS and mitochondrial depolarization modulate the opening of MTPs, ROS production and redox state which are determined by the flux of electrons in ETC (electron transport chain). Production of NADH and FADH2 electron donors from the TCA cycle decide the redox state [56].

The accession of a glycolytic phenotype and halting of pyruvate entry into the mitochondria suppresses acetyl-CoA formation, thus reducing the effect both Krebs's cycle and ETC, which leads to MTP closure and reduction in apoptosis [57]. Mitochondria are also involved in programmed cell death *via* other mechanisms, which include intracellular Ca^{+2} uptake and H_2O_2 production by dismutation of mitochondrial superoxide by manganese superoxide dismutase. Reversing signaling from mitochondria to the nucleus modulates cell death initiation and energy metabolism. Retrograde signaling of mitochondria and Ca^{+2} signaling regulates genetic and epigenetic changes that assist cellular metabolism favoring tumorigenesis [58].

The altered regulation in mitochondrial functions could promote transformational changes, which leads to malignancies [59]. There are few important factors moderate the consequences of healthy cells including (i) alteration in reactive oxygen species, (ii) abundance of metabolic factors (succinate, fumarate, 2-hydrxyglutarate), denoted as oncometabolite, (iii) mitochondrial outer membrane potential permeabilization/mitochondrial permeability transition increases resistances due to oncogenic driven [60].

The pivotal metabolic process glycolysis regulates energy production in mitochondria and anabolic growth in cancer cells. Cancer cells mainly required an amount of ATP, which induces the growth of malignant cells. According to the 'Warburg phenotype' high amount of glucose uptake during the high-level glycolytic activity, the pyruvate is produced by mitochondrial metabolism (Fig. 1). MAPK pathway is the oncogenic signaling pathway, which increases the glucose uptake and reroutes the mitochondrial metabolism into glycolysis and provides the cell the energy for proliferation. The cancer cell mitochondria are involved in ATP biosynthesis and macromolecular biosynthesis mitochondrial metabolism plays a key role in cancer cell development and growth [61].

Warburg Effect on Cancer Cells

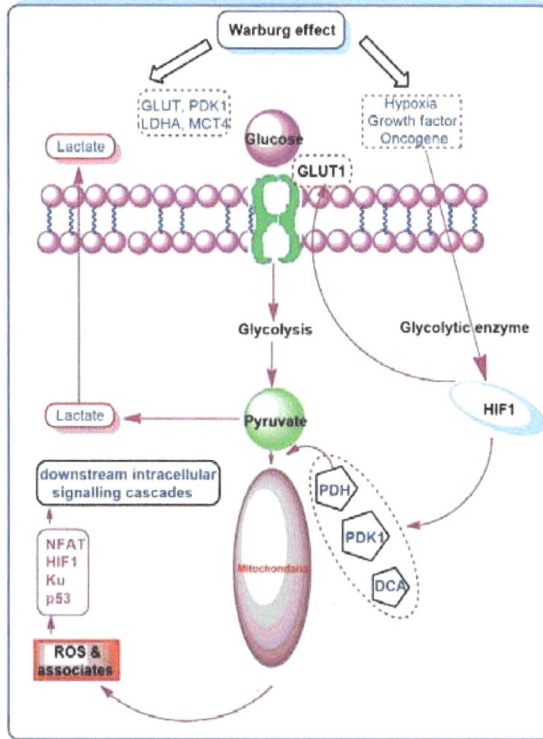

Fig. (1). As per the Warburg effect, hypoxia-inducible factor 1 alpha is upregulated during aerobic glycolysis that regulates glucose metabolism. H1F1-alpha also regulated the glucose transporter GLUT1 that increases the demand for glucose by cancer cells. The process glycolysis is upregulated *via* glycolytic enzymes whereas PDK inhibits several conversations. HIF1alpha induces the lactate production and simultaneously, ROS and αKG regulate several cellular functions in cellular physiology.

MITOCHONDRIAL METABOLISM IN BREAST CANCER PROGRESSION

The key features altered in tumor progression due to the involvement of mitochondria are:

I. Building blocks for anabolism.

II. Generation of ROS.

III. Regulation in RCD signaling.

Proliferation

During glycolysis, cancer cells can obtain enough ATP under optimal growth conditions. Mitochondria acts in the proliferation process while enough amounts of pyruvate and uridine are provided exogenously to compensate for aspartate and pyrimidine biosynthesis. In response to fluctuating conditions regarding the microenvironment, they can use glycolysis, oxidative phosphorylation and fatty acid oxidation interchangeably as the source of energy. For proliferation at optimal rates, cancer cells require an enzyme that can convert citrate into acetyl-Co A, such as ATP citrate lyase. In breast cancers, which are highly proliferating, cytosolic malic enzyme 1 induces a function that leads to the production of NADPH from glutamate. Aceto-acetate is derived from Acetyl-CoA which can support the cancer cells to proliferate by activating and boosting the BRAF-kinase and MAPK signaling consequently. By stabilizing HIF1A or by inactivating the tumor suppressors like phosphate and tensin homolog, minutely increased level of ROS can stimulate proliferation [62].

Alteration in RCD

Some tumors are specified by an increased level of mitochondrial transmembrane potential which is linked to the high rates of glycolysis and gained resistance towards RCD. Unfavorable micro-environmental conditions (such as low nutrient availability, hypoxia, GF withdrawal, *etc.*) are encountered with the progressing neoplasms, for which mitochondrial RCD is derived normally *via* MPT or MOMP. However, for irreversible permeabilization (beyond overexpression of BCL2 family members), several alterations are acquired by the malignant cells which increase the mitochondrial threshold. So, with the help of the chemical PDK1 inhibitors, the restoration of pyruvate generation is sufficient for causing RCD and as well as inhibiting tumor growth *in vivo*. Similarly, in malignant cells, the detachment of hexokinase 2 or hexokinase 1 from mitochondria causes MOMP [63].

Metastatic Modification

Metastatic modification occurs by dissemination, a multistep process where the malignant cells can acquire the ability for colonization and at distant sites macroscopic lesions are formed. This process requires oxidative phosphorylation and optimal mitochondrial biogenesis. By favoring the overproduction of mild ROS, metastatic dissemination is also promoted by mitophagy defects. There are many signal transduction cascades like SRC and protein tyrosine kinase 2 beta, which are associated with this process and ROS activates these signal transduction cascades. If there is an imbalance in mitochondrial dynamics, a little bit overproduction of ROS and as well as consequent metastatic dissemination can occur as a result [64]. Conversely, ROS can inhibit metastatic dissemination in the presence of high oxidative stress, probably as a direct consequence of RCD and reduced fitness or cellular senescence [65].

Mitochondrial Metabolism in Breast Cancer and its Therapeutic Approaches

Mitochondrial metabolism in response to the treatments and the several metabolic characteristics are involved in the therapeutic responses. All forms of treatments such as chemotherapy, radiation therapy and immune therapy inactivate malignant cells *via* cellular senescence and regulating cell death. Mitochondria control the therapy driven RCD in cancer cells, which alters the molecular mechanism in mitochondria. As a result, MOMP (mitochondrial outer membrane permeabilization) and MPT (Mitochondrial permeability transition) as a major resistance source. The mitochondrial metabolic enzyme, IDH2, is used for the development of anticancer agents. FDA approved agent venetoclax for killing the transform cells or can be used for treatment by MOMP or MPT. BRAF^{V600E} inhibits this FDA approved agent. As a result, the malignant cells can switch from glycolysis to OXPHOS (oxidative phosphorylation), which is required for melanoma cells to resist the treatments. Malignant cells utilize the OXPHOS for the ATP production which resists the treatment *via* cancer cell-intrinsic and extrinsic pathways. Mitochondrial ATP has several pumps that activate the various transporter of ATP binding cassettes family hence support the chemoresistance. Finally, malignant cells can switch between glycolysis and OXPHOS plays a major role in the resistance of oncogenic development [66].

Mitochondrial Metabolism in Breast Cancer and Immunosurveillance

In breast cancer, both intrinsic and extrinsic cancer cells have influenced the mitochondria, and it produces the dangerous signals which are released from cancer cells and the consequence of activating the tumor-targeting immune response. Mitochondrial products such as ATP, operate the extracellularly dangerous signals and intracellularly signals operate from ROS and mtDNA. Mitochondrial components are participating in immune functions *via* metabolic pathways such as the TCA cycle, OXPHOS, and fatty acid oxidation are important for T cell differentiation. ROS is required not only for TCR signaling but also for activating various transcription factors necessary for T cell activation. OXPHOS gives metabolic support to the memory T cell, as a result, it involves mitochondrial elongation and inhibits the mTOR (mechanistic target of rapamycin complex 1) for autophagy activation. Mitochondrial metabolism influences macrophage polarization. M1 macrophage activity is inhibited by the ETC to promote the tumoricidal and pro-inflammatory state, which displays the predominantly glycolytic metabolism in mitochondria. OXPHOS is a source of

ATP and it is the differentiation of immunosuppressive cells, including M2 macrophages, $CD4^+$, $CD25^+$, FOX, $P3^+$ regulatory T (Treg) cells and myeloid-derived suppressor cells (MDSCs), CTL (cytotoxic T lymphocyte) [67, 68]. Mitochondria acts as a target for the development of noble anticancer agents because they underlie their phenotypic and metabolic plasticity and resist the malignant cells by RCD induction treatments [69].

Role of the Mitochondrial Metabolism in Malignant Transformation

Malignant transformation is the process by which the cells acquire the properties of cancer in the case of breast cancer, specially. Mitochondria are involved in the malignant transformation by three key mechanisms:

1. The reactive oxygen species or ROS support to increase the potentially oncogenic DNA defects.

2. The abnormal accumulation of specific mitochondrial metabolites such as fumarate, succinate, 2-hydroxyglutarate (2-HG), has significant transforming effects.

3. Functional deficits in mitochondrial permeable transitions (MPT) are generally required for the endurance of neo-formed malignant transformed malignant transformation [70].

The mitophagy should maintain mitochondrial fitness and it also removes the ROS (Reactive Oxygen Species). The different group has shown the knockout and knockdown of the autophagy-related gene Atg7 and Atg5 which are essential for which promotes the oncogenesis. ROS are genotoxins, mtDNA mutations that affect various components of Electron Transport Chain (ETC) and they increase the ROS production to form breast associated tumors. ROS activates many signaling cascades that are Mitogen-activated protein kinase (MAPK), Hypoxia Inducible Factor 1α (HIF-1) and Epidermal Growth Factor Receptor (EGFR) signaling. The produced ROS activate MAPK for breast cancer and increased the cytotoxic level for breast cancer by using GSH inhibitors [71]. The role of the ROS in cancer progression by alteration in redox balance deregulated the redox signaling [72].

What are the Potential Mitochondrial Targets on Breast Cancer?

Mitochondria are the membrane-bound organelles that are found in eukaryotic cells. They are responsible for mobilizing cellular energy production. They have a central role in the maintenance of life and they also serve as the gatekeepers of cell death, as per Fig. (**2**) [73, 74].

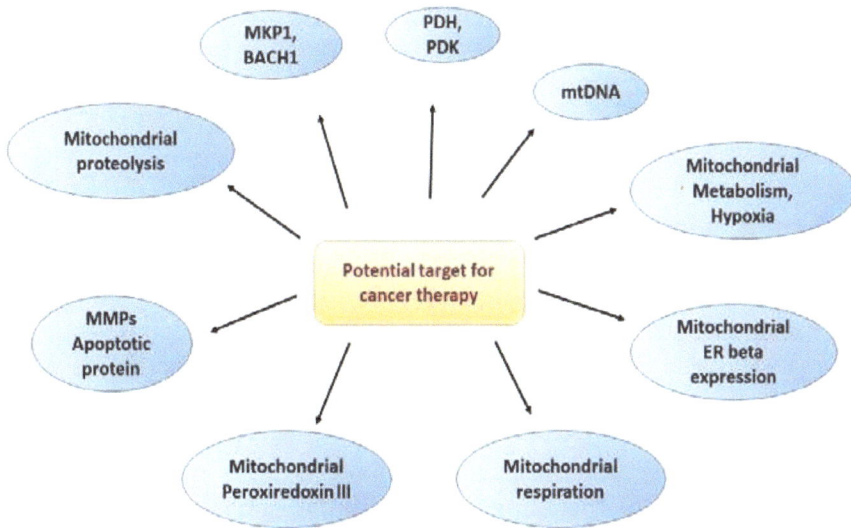

Fig. (2).   Different mitochondrial targets for breast cancer therapy.

Targeting the Apoptotic Proteins

Mitochondria are having a normal homeostasis and cell death initiation when the cell experiences stress responses [73]. Induction of apoptosis cell death necessitates Mitochondrial Membrane Permeabilization (MMP). Agents are responsible for regulating MMP affect the outer MMP, the inner MMP or both of them. Evolutionarily conserved B-cell lymphoma 2 (Bcl-2) family proteins are responsible for the modulation of the coherence of the outer mitochondrial membrane [75].

In humans, BCL-2 is encoded by the BCL-2 gene, which is the initiating member of the BCL-2 family of regulator proteins that are responsible for modulating cell death [apoptosis], by either inhibiting (anti-apoptotic) or inducing (pro-apoptotic) apoptosis [76].

Proteins like BCL-2 and BCL-XL block the emancipation of apoptogenic factors from mitochondria. On the other hand, BCL-2 associated x protein (Bax) and BCL-2 antagonist (Bak), which are proapoptotic BCL-2 members induce outer MMP, allowing the liberation of proapoptotic factors from MMP [60]. Therefore a balance competition between these two processes decides the death and the survival of the cell.

Targeting mtDNA Regulation

mtDNA encodes crucial oxidative phosphorylation proteins, the modulation of mtDNA copy number can be embarked for cancer therapy and mtDNA has a significant role in diagnosing the sensitivity of cancer cells in reciprocation to multiple chemotherapeutic agents. In mammalian cells, many agents are accountable for causing depletion of mtDNA like 4-quinolone drugs such as ciprofloxacin which inhibits TOP2β in mtDNA, resulting in the accumulation of positively supercoiled mtDNA, along with the cessation of mitochondrial transcription and the initiation of replication that leads to the depletion of mtDNA copy number. This leads to the disruption of the function of mitochondria. There are also other agents such as cisplatin, resveratrol, *etc*. So, it can be suggested that mtDNA is involved in regulating cancer cell death as it is observed that cancer agents have the ability to bind with mtDNA. On the other hand, anti-cancer agents can also deplete DNA. Oxidative phosphorylation can be another mitochondrial target in the treatment of cancer. In cancer cells, cell death is generally initiated by the activation of oxidative phosphorylation with the initiation of apoptosis *via* the production of ROS [74]. By subduing the activity of oxidative phosphorylation and inhibiting the glycolytic pathway results in reduction of cell death in the extremely proliferative tumor cells [77]. On low-level glucose conditions, the activity of mitochondria is stimulated by forskolin, generally growing cancer cells are comparatively more sensitive to the very low level of oxidative phosphorylation inhibitors and cell death. Due to defective mitochondrial functions, cancer cells have the ability to resist treatment strategies. DCA can restore the oxidative phosphorylation function which in turn initiates the ROS production with apoptotic cell death [78].

Targeting Pyruvate Dehydrogenase and Pyruvate Dehydrogenase Kinase (PDH-PDK) and Associates in Breast Cancer

Managing and controlling cancer cells are essential by restoring mitochondrial function in the therapy of breast cancer. Mitochondria are hyperpolarized in breast cancer cells, causing an increase in intracellular calcium ion, activation of the nuclear factor activated T cells, increase in aerobic glycolysis, reduction of ROS level, upregulation of antiapoptotic Bcl-2 [67]. The rate of glycolysis increases in the cancer cell formation, and as a result of the hexokinase level also increases, for which mitochondria are translocated, and it leads to apoptosis inhibition & hyperpolarization of mitochondria. In cancer cells, all these events lead towards apoptosis and induce cell proliferation, enhance the survival rate, terminate cell senescence. So, if the mitochondrial functions are reactivated, then it will reverse these events and lead to suppressing the aerobic glycolysis process & apoptosis. The decision either to undergo glucose oxidation or to follow aerobic glycolysis, depends on the overall LBH and PDH-PDK regulatory circuit interactions. Both suppress LDH and activates PDH by inhibiting PDK that can increase the pumping of pyruvate into mitochondria. Thus in oxidative phosphorylation, ETC is reactivated, leading to ROS production, calcium ions flux into the mitochondria as well as induction of apoptosis [79, 80].

Agents such as DCA can increase the rate of oxidation of glucose by pumping pyruvate to the citric acid cycle reactive oxidative phosphorylation and it can induce the ROS production, which leads to apoptotic cell death of the tumor cells. Against the metastatic cells of breast cancer, potential anticancer effects are offered by DCA. Against the T cell lymphoma, the antitumor effects of DCA are associated with the alterations in pH homeostasis and the metabolism of glucose, which leads to suppression in the survival rate of the tumor cells in breast cancer.

There is an increased rate of delivery of pyruvate into the mitochondria due to PDH is activated by DCA, which is followed by an increased level of glucose oxidation, which will lead to the restoration of the mitochondrial function [81]. By producing ROS and activating NFAT, the apoptosis inducing effects are mediated by DCA which leads to the release of Cytochrome C and apoptosis-inducing factors into the cytosol from mitochondria. DCA disrupts HIF-1α dependent adaptive response in tumors under hypoxia. For killing the hypoxic tumor cells, the effectiveness of chemotherapy is gradually increasing [82] (Table **1**).

Table 1. Signalling pathways involved in the activation and regulation of HIF in breast cancer [82].

Increase In HIFs Regulation		
Hypoxia	Increase in reactive oxygen species (ROS) formation	NF-kB
RTK	Notch	IL6/IL6R
TGF-â/ TGF-âR	TNF-á	PI3K
Akt/mTOR	STAT3	MAPK

CONCLUDING REMARKS AND FUTURE PERSPECTIVES

Mitochondria have been considered as the target for developing novel anti-cancer agents in breast cancer. It has a major impact on processes linked to oncogenesis, encompassing malignant transformation, tumor progression, response to treatment and anticancer immune-surveillance, dying of cancer cell, metastatic cancer cell, MOMP, MPT, reactive oxygen species, and tumor microenvironment [83, 84] (Table **2**). Regulation of aerobic glycolysis and mitochondrial dysfunction are linked to cancer survival, apoptotic invasion and resistance to cancer therapies.

All these may be associated with the sequestration of proapoptotic proteins or the nonapoptotic function of various proapoptotic proteins in mitochondria leading to the inhibition of cancer cell apoptosis. Hexokinase and PDK activation inhibits the function of proapoptotic Bax and Bak. Thus the PDK inhibition may activate these pro-apoptotic proteins, causing cytochrome c release and enhancing cancer cell apoptosis.

Table. 2 Signalling factors and factors promoted by an increase in HIFs regulation in breast cancer [83,84]:

Increase in HIFs regulation causing to				
Oct-3/4, Nanog, SOX-2 increase	GLUT-1/2 hexokinase 2, aldolase A, PGK1, PKM, CAIX, MCT4 increase	TGF-á, EGFR, CXCL4, snail, twist, lox, lox2, MMPs increase	VEGF increase	BCL-2, survivin, BCL-xl, MUG-1, Pgp, ABCG2 increase
Stemnessself-renewal	Glycolysis pH regulation	EMT metastatic spread	Angiogenesis	Resistance to CT/RT survival Antiapoptotic effect
Causing tumor growth, metastasizing, resistance to therapy				

On the other hand, HSP folding machinery plays an important role in proper mitochondrial function. A defect in this machinery causes cells to grow and divide uncontrollably, forming tumors. Thus, targeting the downregulation of pre-cancerous HSPs or upregulation of anti-cancerous HSPs can be an important approach in controlling tumorigenesis. Also, restoration of mitochondrial OXPHOS and inhibition of the glycolytic pathway can be another approach in treating cancer patients.

Besides, there are various challenges to establish potent anticancer agents. DCA regulation contains strong anticancer agents. Its higher dose may be essential in therapeutic approaches, but it can be toxic to normal tissues. Thus, the synthesis of DCA analogs proved to have a better efficacy that selectively targets tumor cells. Hence, future researchers are focusing on DCA analog synthesis alone or with nanoparticle encapsulation or in combination with other anticancer agents to develop more efficient anticancer agents that can effectively kill the cancer cells. Thus, the function of mitochondria provides building blocks for tumor anabolism, controlling of redox and calcium signaling, participate in transcriptional regulation and cell death. The promising contribution of this powerful cellular organelle develops constant focus as the novel target in regards to anti-metastatic drug development. By altering cellular metabolism, it also regulates the drug resistance, especially in the tumor micro-environment. The altered strategies in mitochondrial regulation allow the selected cell populations to devise for the therapeutic potential of mitochondria-targeting agents in clinics. More preclinical and clinical approaches are required to achieve this ambitious and useful objective.

ABBREVIATIONS

AIF:	Apoptosis inducing factor
BCL-2:	B cell lymphoma-2
BCL-XL:	B cell lymphoma-extra-large
BCRPs:	Breast cancer resistance proteins
CAFs:	Cancer associated fibroblast
CAIX:	Carbonic Anhydrase
CT:	Chemotherapy
CXCL 4:	Chemokine ligands 4
EGFR:	Epidermal Growth factor Receptor
EMT:	Epithelial to mesenchymal transition
GLUT:	Glucose Transporter
HIFs:	Hypoxia Inducible Factors
IL-6/IL-6R:	Interleukin 6/ Interleukin 6 Receptor
MAPK:	Mitogen-activated Protein kinase
MCT-4:	Monocarboxylate transporter 4
MIC-1:	Macrophage inhibitory cytokine-1
MMPs:	Metalloproteinases
MOMP:	Mitochondrial Outer Membrane Permeabilization
MPT:	Mitochondrial Permeability Transition
mTOR:	Molecular target of rapamycin
MUC-1:	Mucin-1
NF-KB:	Nuclear Factor KB
Oct-3/4:	Octamer binding transcriptional Factor 3/4
P13K:	Phosphatidyl inositol-3-kinase
PGK-1:	Phosphogylcerate kinase-1
Pgp:	P Glycoprotein
PKM:	Pyruvate kinase M
RCD:	Regulated cell death Signaling
ROS:	Reactive Oxygen Species
RT:	Radiotherapy
RTK:	Receptor tyrosine kinase
SOX-2:	Sex Determining Region Y
STAT 3:	Signal transducer activator of transcription 3
TGF-β/TGFR:	Transforming growth factor-β/Transforming growth factor-β Receptor
TNF-α:	Tumor necrosis factor-α

VEGF:　　Vascular endothelial growth factor

CONSENT FOR PUBLICATION

Not applicable.

CONFLICT OF INTEREST

The authors confirm that the contents of this chapter have no conflict of interest.

ACKNOWLEDGEMENT

We acknowledge the Director of CNCI, Kolkata, for providing the research environment and continuous support.

REFERENCES

[1]　Henze K, Martin W. Evolutionary biology: essence of mitochondria. Nature 2003; 426(6963): 127-8.
[http://dx.doi.org/10.1038/426127a] [PMID: 14614484]

[2]　Birceanu O. Mitochondria are too hot to handle! J Exp Biol. 2018; 221(9): 1-4.
[http://dx.doi.org/10.1242/jeb.170027]

[3]　Campbell NA, Williamson B, Heyden RJ. Pearson/Prentice Hallexploring life. 0--13--250882-6 Boston, Massachusetts: Pearson Prentice Hall 2006.

[4]　McBride HM, Neuspiel M, Wasiak S. Mitochondria: more than just a powerhouse. Curr Biol 2006; 16(14): R551-60.
[http://dx.doi.org/10.1016/j.cub.2006.06.054] [PMID: 16860735]

[5]　Valero T. Mitochondrial biogenesis: pharmacological approaches. Curr Pharm Des 2014; 20(35): 5507-9.
[http://dx.doi.org/10.2174/13816128203514091114218] [PMID: 24606795]

[6]　Sanchis-Gomar F, Garcia-Gimenez J, Gomez-Cabrera M, Pallardo F. Mitochondrial biogenesis in health and disease. Molecular and therapeutic approaches. Curr Pharm Des 2014; 20(35): 5619-33.

[7]　Gardner A, Boles R. Is a "mitochondrial psychiatry" in the future? A review. Curr Psychiatry Rev 2005.
[http://dx.doi.org/10.2174/157340005774575064]

[8]　Lesnefsky EJ, Moghaddas S, Tandler B, Kerner J, Hoppel CL. Mitochondrial dysfunction in cardiac disease: ischemia--reperfusion, aging, and heart failure. J Mol Cell Cardiol 2001; 33(6): 1065-89.
[http://dx.doi.org/10.1006/jmcc.2001.1378] [PMID: 11444914]

[9]　Dorn GW II, Vega RB, Kelly DP. Mitochondrial biogenesis and dynamics in the developing and diseased heart. Genes Dev 2015; 29(19): 1981-91.
[http://dx.doi.org/10.1101/gad.269894.115] [PMID: 26443844]

[10]　Griffiths KK, Levy RJ. Evidence of mitochondrial dysfunction in autism: Biochemical links, genetic-based associations, and non-energy-related mechanisms. Oxid Med Cell Longev 2017; 2017: 4314025.
[http://dx.doi.org/10.1155/2017/4314025] [PMID: 28630658]

[11]　Andersson SGE, Karlberg O, Kurland CG. On the origin of mitochondria : a genomics perspective. 2003; (December 2002): 165-79.
[http://dx.doi.org/10.1098/rstb.2002.1193]

[12]　Rich PR. The molecular machinery of Keilin's respiratory chain. Biochem Soc Trans 2003; 31(Pt 6):

1095-105.
[http://dx.doi.org/10.1042/bst0311095] [PMID: 14641005]

[13] Stoimenova M, Igamberdiev AU, Gupta KJ, Hill RD. Nitrite-driven anaerobic ATP synthesis in barley and rice root mitochondria. Planta 2007; 226(2): 465-74.
[http://dx.doi.org/10.1007/s00425-007-0496-0] [PMID: 17333252]

[14] King A, Selak MA, Gottlieb E. Succinate dehydrogenase and fumarate hydratase: linking mitochondrial dysfunction and cancer. Oncogene 2006; 25(34): 4675-82.
[http://dx.doi.org/10.1038/sj.onc.1209594] [PMID: 16892081]

[15] Berg J, Tymoczko J, Stryer L. Biochemistry. 5th edition. New York: W H Freeman; 2002. Section 24.2, Amino Acids Are Made from Intermediates of the Citric Acid Cycle and Other Major Pathways. Available from: https://www.ncbi.nlm.nih.gov/books/NBK22459/.

[16] Akram M. Citric acid cycle and role of its intermediates in metabolism. Cell Biochem Biophys 2014; 68(3): 475-8.
[http://dx.doi.org/10.1007/s12013-013-9750-1] [PMID: 24068518]

[17] Mailloux RJ, Bériault R, Lemire J, *et al.* The tricarboxylic acid cycle, an ancient metabolic network with a novel twist. PLoS One 2007; 2(8): e690.
[http://dx.doi.org/10.1371/journal.pone.0000690] [PMID: 17668068]

[18] Hui S, Ghergurovich JM, Morscher RJ, *et al.* Glucose feeds the TCA cycle *via* circulating lactate. Nature 2017; 551(7678): 115-8.
[http://dx.doi.org/10.1038/nature24057] [PMID: 29045397]

[19] Ramakrishna R, Edwards JS, McCulloch A, Palsson BO. Flux-balance analysis of mitochondrial energy metabolism: Consequences of systemic stoichiometric constraints. Am J Physiol - Regul Integr Comp Physiol 2001; 280(349-3): 695-704.
[http://dx.doi.org/10.1152/ajpregu.2001.280.3.r695]

[20] Cortassa S, Aon MA, O'Rourke B, Winslow RL. Metabolic control analysis applied to mitochondrial networks. Proc Annu Int Conf IEEE Eng Med Biol Soc EMBS 2011; 4673-6.
[http://dx.doi.org/10.1109/IEMBS.2011.6091157]

[21] Nazaret C, Heiske M, Thurley K, Mazat JP. Mitochondrial energetic metabolism: a simplified model of TCA cycle with ATP production. J Theor Biol 2009; 258(3): 455-64.
[http://dx.doi.org/10.1016/j.jtbi.2008.09.037] [PMID: 19007794]

[22] Silverstein TP. An exploration of how the thermodynamic efficiency of bioenergetic membrane systems varies with c-subunit stoichiometry of F_1F_0 ATP synthases. J Bioenerg Biomembr 2014; 46(3): 229-41.
[http://dx.doi.org/10.1007/s10863-014-9547-y] [PMID: 24706236]

[23] Durieux J, Wolff S, Dillin A. The cell-non-autonomous nature of electron transport chain-mediated longevity. Cell 2011; 144(1): 79-91.
[http://dx.doi.org/10.1016/j.cell.2010.12.016] [PMID: 21215371]

[24] Huang H, Manton KG. The role of oxidative damage in mitochondria during aging: a review. Front Biosci 2004; 9: 1100-17.
[http://dx.doi.org/10.2741/1298] [PMID: 14977532]

[25] Mozo J, Emre Y, Bouillaud F, Ricquier D, Criscuolo F. Thermoregulation: what role for UCPs in mammals and birds? Biosci Rep 2005; 25(3-4): 227-49.
[http://dx.doi.org/10.1007/s10540-005-2887-4] [PMID: 16283555]

[26] Denton RM. Regulation of mitochondrial dehydrogenases by calcium ions. Biochim Biophys Acta - Bioenerg 2009; 1787(11): 1309-16.
[http://dx.doi.org/10.1016/j.bbabio.2009.01.005]

[27] Kirichok Y, Krapivinsky G, Clapham DE. The mitochondrial calcium uniporter is a highly selective ion channel. Nature 2004; 427(6972): 360-4.

[http://dx.doi.org/10.1038/nature02246] [PMID: 14737170]

[28]   Pinto MCX, Kihara AH, Goulart VAM, *et al.* Calcium signaling and cell proliferation. Cell Signal 2015; 27(11): 2139-49.
[http://dx.doi.org/10.1016/j.cellsig.2015.08.006] [PMID: 26275497]

[29]   Collins S, Meyer T. Cell biology: A sensor for calcium uptake. Nature 2010; 467(7313): 283.
[http://dx.doi.org/10.1038/467283a] [PMID: 20844529]

[30]   Carriers M. Cancer Risks in BRCA2 Mutation Carriers. 1999; 91 (15).

[31]   Stephens PJ, Tarpey PS, Davies H, *et al.* Oslo Breast Cancer Consortium (OSBREAC). The landscape of cancer genes and mutational processes in breast cancer. Nature 2012; 486(7403): 400-4.
[http://dx.doi.org/10.1038/nature11017] [PMID: 22722201]

[32]   Marcom PK. Breast Cancer. Elsevier Inc.; 2017.
[http://dx.doi.org/10.1016/B978-0-12-800685-6.00010-2]

[33]   Dent R, Trudeau M, Pritchard KI, *et al.* Triple-negative breast cancer: clinical features and patterns of recurrence. Clin Cancer Res 2007; 13(15 Pt 1): 4429-34.
[http://dx.doi.org/10.1158/1078-0432.CCR-06-3045] [PMID: 17671126]

[34]   Schneider BP, Winer EP, Foulkes WD, *et al.* Triple-negative breast cancer: risk factors to potential targets. Clin Cancer Res 2008; 14(24): 8010-8.
[http://dx.doi.org/10.1158/1078-0432.CCR-08-1208] [PMID: 19088017]

[35]   Oakman C, Viale G, Di Leo A. Management of triple negative breast cancer. Breast 2010; 19(5): 312-21.
[http://dx.doi.org/10.1016/j.breast.2010.03.026] [PMID: 20382530]

[36]   Chavez KJ, Garimella SV, Lipkowitz S. Triple negative breast cancer cell lines: one tool in the search for better treatment of triple negative breast cancer. Breast Dis 2010; 32(1-2): 35-48.
[http://dx.doi.org/10.3233/BD-2010-0307] [PMID: 21778573]

[37]   Atchley DP, Albarracin CT, Lopez A, *et al.* Clinical and pathologic characteristics of patients with BRCA-positive and BRCA-negative breast cancer. J Clin Oncol 2008; 26(26): 4282-8.
[http://dx.doi.org/10.1200/JCO.2008.16.6231] [PMID: 18779615]

[38]   Telli ML. Triple-negative breast cancer In: Badve S., Gökmen-Polar Y. (eds). Mol Path of Breast Cancer. Springer, Cham 2016; pp 71-80.
[http://dx.doi.org/10.1007/978-3-319-41761-5_6]

[39]   Liu SV, Melstrom L, Yao K, Russell CA, Sener SF. Neoadjuvant therapy for breast cancer. J Surg Oncol 2010; 101(4): 283-91.
[http://dx.doi.org/10.1002/jso.21446] [PMID: 20187061]

[40]   Lin KY, Kraus WL. PARP Inhibitors for Cancer Therapy. Cell 2017; 169(2): 183.
[http://dx.doi.org/10.1016/j.cell.2017.03.034] [PMID: 28388401]

[41]   Nathan MR, Schmid P. The emerging world of breast cancer immunotherapy. Breast 2018; 37: 200-6.
[http://dx.doi.org/10.1016/j.breast.2017.05.013] [PMID: 28583398]

[42]   Hanahan D, Weinberg RA. The hallmarks of cancer. Cell 2000; 100(1): 57-70.
[http://dx.doi.org/10.1016/S0092-8674(00)81683-9] [PMID: 10647931]

[43]   Cairns RA, Harris IS, Mak TW. Regulation of cancer cell metabolism. Nat Rev Cancer 2011; 11(2): 85-95.
[http://dx.doi.org/10.1038/nrc2981] [PMID: 21258394]

[44]   DeBerardinis RJ, Chandel NS. Fundamentals of cancer metabolism. Sci Adv 2016; 2(5): e1600200.
[http://dx.doi.org/10.1126/sciadv.1600200] [PMID: 27386546]

[45]   Pelicano H, Martin DS, Xu RH, Huang P. Glycolysis inhibition for anticancer treatment. Oncogene 2006; 25(34): 4633-46.

[http://dx.doi.org/10.1038/sj.onc.1209597] [PMID: 16892078]

[46] Muñoz-Pinedo C, El Mjiyad N, Ricci JE. Cancer metabolism: current perspectives and future directions. Cell Death Dis 2012; 3: e248.
[http://dx.doi.org/10.1038/cddis.2011.123] [PMID: 22237205]

[47] Szent-Gyorgyi A. Metabolism and cancer. *Int J Quantum Chem.* 1985;28(12 S):257-261.
[http://dx.doi.org/10.1002/qua.560280725]

[48] Seyfried TN, Shelton LM. Cancer as a metabolic disease. Nutr Metab (Lond) 2010; 7: 7.
[http://dx.doi.org/10.1186/1743-7075-7-7] [PMID: 20181022]

[49] Cantor JR, Sabatini DM. Cancer cell metabolism: one hallmark, many faces. Cancer Discov 2012; 2(10): 881-98.
[http://dx.doi.org/10.1158/2159-8290.CD-12-0345] [PMID: 23009760]

[50] Jain M, Nilsson R, Sharma S, *et al.* Metabolite profiling identifies a key role for glycine in rapid cancer cell proliferation. Science (80-) 2012; 336(6084): 1040-4.
[http://dx.doi.org/10.1126/science.1218595]

[51] Dagogo-Jack I, Shaw AT. Tumour heterogeneity and resistance to cancer therapies. Nat Rev Clin Oncol 2018; 15(2): 81-94.
[http://dx.doi.org/10.1038/nrclinonc.2017.166] [PMID: 29115304]

[52] Vyas S, Zaganjor E, Haigis MC. Mitochondria and cancer. Cell 2016; 166(3): 555-66.
[http://dx.doi.org/10.1016/j.cell.2016.07.002] [PMID: 27471965]

[53] Idelchik MDPS, Begley U, Begley TJ, Melendez JA. Mitochondrial ROS control of cancer. Semin Cancer Biol 2017; 47: 57-66.
[http://dx.doi.org/10.1016/j.semcancer.2017.04.005] [PMID: 28445781]

[54] Tubbs A, Nussenzweig A. Endogenous DNA damage as a source of genomic instability in cancer. Cell 2017; 168(4): 644-56.
[http://dx.doi.org/10.1016/j.cell.2017.01.002] [PMID: 28187286]

[55] Calabrese C, Iommarini L, Kurelac I, *et al.* Respiratory complex I is essential to induce a Warburg profile in mitochondria-defective tumor cells. Cancer Metab 2013; 1(1): 11.
[http://dx.doi.org/10.1186/2049-3002-1-11] [PMID: 24280190]

[56] Cherian MG, Jayasurya A, Bay BH. Metallothioneins in human tumors and potential roles in carcinogenesis. Mutat Res 2003; 533(1-2): 201-9.
[http://dx.doi.org/10.1016/j.mrfmmm.2003.07.013] [PMID: 14643421]

[57] Lapuente-Brun E, Moreno-Loshuertos R, Aciń-Pérez R, *et al.* Supercomplex assembly determines electron flux in the mitochondrial electron transport chain. Science (80-) 2013; 340(6140): 1567-70.
[http://dx.doi.org/10.1126/science.1230381]

[58] Turrens JF. Mitochondrial formation of reactive oxygen species. J Physiol 2003; 552(Pt 2): 335-44.
[http://dx.doi.org/10.1113/jphysiol.2003.049478] [PMID: 14561818]

[59] Schmitt S, Zischka H, Hygiene E. Targeting Mitochondria for Cancer Therapy The Role of Mitochondria in Programmed Cell Death Apoptosis as Cancer Therapy. 2018. German Journal of Oncology 2018; 50: 124-130.
[http://dx.doi.org/10.1055/a-0657-4437]

[60] Yang M, Brackenbury WJ. Membrane potential and cancer progression. Front Physiol 2013; 4: 185.
[http://dx.doi.org/10.3389/fphys.2013.00185] [PMID: 23882223]

[61] Xie J, Wu H, Dai C, *et al.* Beyond Warburg effect--dual metabolic nature of cancer cells. Sci Rep 2014; 4: 4927.
[http://dx.doi.org/10.1038/srep04927] [PMID: 24820099]

[62] Shaw RJ. Glucose metabolism and cancer. Curr Opin Cell Biol 2006; 18(6): 598-608.
[http://dx.doi.org/10.1016/j.ceb.2006.10.005] [PMID: 17046224]

[63]   Zhong H, De Marzo AM, Laughner E, *et al.* Overexpression of hypoxia-inducible factor 1α in common human cancers and their metastases. Cancer Res 1999; 59(22): 5830-5.
[PMID: 10582706]

[64]   Liou GY, Storz P. Reactive oxygen species in cancer. Free Radic Res 2010; 44(5): 479-96.
[http://dx.doi.org/10.3109/10715761003667554] [PMID: 20370557]

[65]   Kim JW, Tchernyshyov I, Semenza GL, Dang CV. HIF-1-mediated expression of pyruvate dehydrogenase kinase: a metabolic switch required for cellular adaptation to hypoxia. Cell Metab 2006; 3(3): 177-85.
[http://dx.doi.org/10.1016/j.cmet.2006.02.002] [PMID: 16517405]

[66]   Weinberg SE, Chandel NS. Targeting mitochondria metabolism for cancer therapy. Nat Chem Biol 2015; 11(1): 9-15.
[http://dx.doi.org/10.1038/nchembio.1712] [PMID: 25517383]

[67]   Scharping NE, Menk AV, Moreci RS, *et al.* The tumor microenvironment represses T cell mitochondrial biogenesis to drive intratumoral T Cell metabolic insufficiency and dysfunction. Immunity 2017; 45(2): 374-88.
[http://dx.doi.org/10.1016/j.immuni.2016.08.009]

[68]   Wang JB, Erickson JW, Fuji R, *et al.* Targeting mitochondrial glutaminase activity inhibits oncogenic transformation. Cancer Cell 2010; 18(3): 207-19.
[http://dx.doi.org/10.1016/j.ccr.2010.08.009] [PMID: 20832749]

[69]   Sotgia F, Whitaker-Menezes D, Martinez-Outschoorn UE, *et al.* Mitochondria "fuel" breast cancer metabolism: fifteen markers of mitochondrial biogenesis label epithelial cancer cells, but are excluded from adjacent stromal cells. Cell Cycle 2012; 11(23): 4390-401.
[http://dx.doi.org/10.4161/cc.22777] [PMID: 23172368]

[70]   Glunde K, Bhujwalla ZM, Ronen SM. Choline metabolism in malignant transformation. Nat Rev Cancer 2011; 11(12): 835-48.
[http://dx.doi.org/10.1038/nrc3162] [PMID: 22089420]

[71]   Sabharwal SS, Schumacker PT. Mitochondrial ROS in cancer: initiators, amplifiers or an Achilles' heel? Nat Rev Cancer 2014; 14(11): 709-21.
[http://dx.doi.org/10.1038/nrc3803] [PMID: 25342630]

[72]   Frezza C, Gottlieb E. Mitochondria in cancer: not just innocent bystanders. Semin Cancer Biol 2009; 19(1): 4-11.
[http://dx.doi.org/10.1016/j.semcancer.2008.11.008] [PMID: 19101633]

[73]   Galluzzi L, Kepp O, Vander Heiden MG, Kroemer G. Metabolic targets for cancer therapy. Nat Rev Drug Discov 2013; 12(11): 829-46.
[http://dx.doi.org/10.1038/nrd4145] [PMID: 24113830]

[74]   Gogvadze V, Orrenius S, Zhivotovsky B. Mitochondria in cancer cells: what is so special about them? Trends Cell Biol 2008; 18(4): 165-73.
[http://dx.doi.org/10.1016/j.tcb.2008.01.006] [PMID: 18296052]

[75]   Panieri E, Santoro MM. ROS homeostasis and metabolism: a dangerous liason in cancer cells. Cell Death Dis 2016; 7(6): e2253.
[http://dx.doi.org/10.1038/cddis.2016.105] [PMID: 27277675]

[76]   Jin Z, El-Deiry WS. Overview of cell death signaling pathways. Cancer Biol Ther 2005; 4(2): 139-63.
[http://dx.doi.org/10.4161/cbt.4.2.1508] [PMID: 15725726]

[77]   Vander Heiden MG, Locasale JW, Swanson KD, *et al.* Evidence for an alternative glycolytic pathway in rapidly proliferating cells. Science 2010; 329(5998): 1492-9.
[http://dx.doi.org/10.1126/science.1188015]

[78]   Harrison H, Farnie G, Howell SJ, *et al.* Regulation of breast cancer stem cell activity by signaling

through the Notch4 receptor. Cancer Res 2010; 70(2): 709-18.
[http://dx.doi.org/10.1158/0008-5472.CAN-09-1681] [PMID: 20068161]

[79]　Liu AM, Wang W, Luk JM. Liu A.M., Wang W., Luk J.M. (2013) Targeting Cancer Metabolisms. In: Lee N., Cheng C., Luk J. (eds) New Advances on Disease Biomarkers and Molecular Targets in Biomedicine. Humana Press, Totowa,NJ.
[http://dx.doi.org/10.1007/978-1-62703-456-2_9]

[80]　Zhao Y, Butler EB, Tan M. Targeting cellular metabolism to improve cancer therapeutics. Cell Death Dis 2013; 4: e532.
[http://dx.doi.org/10.1038/cddis.2013.60] [PMID: 23470539]

[81]　Hitosugi T, Fan J, Chung TW, *et al.* Tyrosine phosphorylation of mitochondrial pyruvate dehydrogenase kinase 1 is important for cancer metabolism. Mol Cell 2011; 44(6): 864-77.
[http://dx.doi.org/10.1016/j.molcel.2011.10.015] [PMID: 22195962]

[82]　Kim JW, Gao P, Liu Y-C, Semenza GL, Dang CV. Hypoxia-inducible factor 1 and dysregulated c-Myc cooperatively induce vascular endothelial growth factor and metabolic switches hexokinase 2 and pyruvate dehydrogenase kinase 1. Mol Cell Biol 2007; 27(21): 7381-93.
[http://dx.doi.org/10.1128/MCB.00440-07] [PMID: 17785433]

CHAPTER 13

Advances of the Current Therapeutic Approach for the Management of Breast Cancer

Saroj Kumar Amar[1,2,*], **Ajeet Kumar Srivastav**[3] and **Swayam Prakash Srivastava**[4,*]

[1]*Department of Forensic Science, School of Bioengineering and Biosciences, Lovely Professional University, Punjab, India*
[2]*Department of Therapeutic Radiology, School of Medicine, Yale University, New Haven, CT, USA*
[3]*Universal Corporation Limited (LuvLap), 4/1 Middleton Street, Sikkim Commerce House Kolkata, India-700071*
[4] *Department of Pediatrics, Yale University School of Medicine, New Haven, CT, 06511, USA*

Abstract: Breast cancer is the most common type of malignancy in women worldwide. There are several factors associated with breast cancer for manifesting a heterogeneous disease in nature. Chemotherapeutic drugs significantly reduce the mortality rate of breast cancer. The recent development of chemotherapeutic drugs is targeting heterogeneity by including hormone receptors, expression of genes, epidermal growth factors, *etc*. The therapeutic response is dependent on a variety of factors, including stages, subtypes, metastasis, *etc*. For example,- endocrine therapy is preferred for positive hormone response in luminal breast cancer. In the recent therapeutic regimens, CDK4/6 quenchers are emerged, which regulate cell cycle by interacting with cyclin D1. It is also because, in the case of resistant hormonal therapy, tumors still showed its dependency on CDK4/6- cyclin D1 for proliferation. Apart from chemotherapy, immunotherapy is one of the emerging therapeutical regimens for breast cancer. There are also a number of vaccination approaches against breast cancer, including Nelipepimut–S, derived from the extracellular domain of the human epidermal factor receptor, which is used as a vaccine to prevent the reoccurrence of refractory breast cancer. Epithelial-to-mesenchymal transition (EMT) is a crucial mechanism for breast cancer progression. Currently, EMT inhibitor is used for preclinical testing to further used as a drug molecule to treat breast cancer. Thus, the advancement of chemo- or immunotherapy can substitute over invasive treatment strategies such as the surgical method for the treatment of breast cancer.

Keywords: Breast cancer, Cyclin-dependent kinases 4 and 6 inhibitors, Chemotherapy, Human epidermal growth factor receptor, Immunotherapy.

* **Corresponding Authors Saroj Kumar Amar and Swayam Prakash Srivastava:** Department of Forensic Science, School of Bioengineering and Biosciences, Lovely Professional University, Punjab, India; E-mail: sarojkumaramar@gmail.com and Department of Pediatrics, Yale University School of Medicine, New Haven CT USA 06511; E-mail: swayam.srivastava@yale.edu

INTRODUCTION

Breast cancer is the most common malignancy among women, but there is still lack of clarity in origin and preventions despite in-depth research in breast cancer biology. Moreover, the inheritance of oncogenes, obesity, aging, and hormonal imbalances are the key factors for the progression of breast cancer. The advanced treatment approaches have reduced the mortality rate of breast cancer patients in the last few years. Cancer susceptibility gene types 1 and 2, BRCA-1 and BRCA-2, expression of human epidermal growth factor receptors 1 and 2, and activation of vascular endothelial growth factor receptors are considered as efficient markers of breast cancer. Based on these markers, new strategies have evolved as targeted therapies in breast cancer [1]. In chemotherapy, drugs may be given to the patients intravenously or orally. In some severe cases, it can be given directly into the spinal fluid. Chemotherapies reduce the tumor burden induced by the cytotoxic effects of chemicals on cancer cells. These "anti-cancer" drugs stop the growth of tumor cells by discontinuing their duplication and cell growth. However, normal healthy cells are also affected by these chemicals, thus cause the side effects of chemotherapy. The normal cells have a planned structure and renewal mechanisms in place. Thus the daughter cell produced after chemotherapy is a new normal cell [2]. In the current therapeutic regimen, the use of more than one drug is preferred over just a single drug alone. The effect of drugs in combination is much better than the same drugs treated alone. In order to minimize the side effect of chemotherapy drugs on healthy tissues, adjuvant endocrine therapy is preferred [3]. Depending upon the stage of cancer and side effects of the drug used, chemotherapy can be administered as part of adjuvant or neoadjuvant with a period of six months or less [4].

Chemotherapy plays an important role in the prevention of cancer, and clinical data show that it can precisely block mutations carrying tumors burden. Poly-ADP ribose polymerase (PARP) inhibitors can be used as a novel effective therapeutic strategy [5]. One can classify the chemotherapy drug based on the chemical structure of the drug, working method, and association with other drugs. Drugs with known mechanisms of action are combined for better therapeutic efficacy, which can be termed as combinational chemotherapy. Based on the working mechanism, chemotherapy might incorporate alkylating agents, which can directly damage the DNA of tumor cells. Another drug, cyclophosphamide, induces apoptosis of target tumor cells [6].

Drugs, such as methotrexate and 5- fluorouracil, act as anti-metabolites in the S phase of the cell cycle. In the S phase of the cell cycle, genetic material replicates for cell division. Methotrexate and 5- fluorouracil induce apoptosis in tumor cells by decreasing the level of thymidine triphosphate, a nucleotide that participates in

DNA replication via blocking N5, N10-methylenetetrahydrofolate synthesis [5]. An anti-tumor agent, such as Anthracyclins, causes DNA damage, facilitated by topoisomerase II isoform, which finally leads to cell death [6]. Mitotic inhibitors are used as chemotherapeutic drugs, such as paclitaxel, taxanes, and docetaxel interfere M phase of the cell cycle by interrupting spindle formation through binding with β tubulin [6].

The objectives of chemotherapy are:

• To reduce the tumor burden.

• To regulate the propagation of tumor.

• To recover disease-associated symptoms such as discomfort in cancer.

Current regimens of breast cancer therapy include chemotherapy, surgical methods, and radiotherapy, which may be used in combination also for enhancing the efficacy of the treatment [2]. Apart from these therapies, gene therapy, hormonal therapy, targeted therapy, and immunotherapy are the new treatment regimes of breast cancer, which have shown a very high potency to eliminate breast cancer cells.

CHEMOTHERAPY

Chemotherapy is the main regimen of cancer treatment if the tumors cells growth extends outside of the breast, especially in locally advanced breast cancer. There are different kinds of chemotherapy, which depend upon heterogeneity of breast cancer. A number of drug doses are dependent on the physiological mechanism and degree of tolerance of each and every individual patient. Oncotype DX and mammoprint are common techniques used to reduce the side effects of chemotherapy post tumor surgery. The details of the different chemotherapy used in clinics are as follows:

Adjuvant Chemotherapy

After surgery, the remaining tumor cells can form tumors in other parts of the body that cannot be visualized by imaging easily. Thus, adjuvant chemotherapy is given to destroy those cells. This adjuvant chemotherapy technique minimizes the chances of the breast tumor for recurring.

Neoadjuvant Chemotherapy

This technique is helpful if the tumor is big in size, which cannot be removed by surgery properly. This technique is used to narrow down the broad tumor area before surgery. Hence, tumor cells can be removed without extensive surgery. Thus, if cancer is locally advanced, there are high chances that tumor cells remain after surgery. Therefore, this pre-surgery treatment is preferred. Apart from this, the next step of this technique is to get the exact response of chemotherapy before the removal of a tumor so that the doctor can decide the number of chemo sessions required.

Chemotherapy: Drugs that are Used for the Treatment of Breast Tumor

The common drugs are recommended for chemotherapy either in single or in a combination of two or more for adjuvant or neoadjuvant chemotherapy. Some of the common drugs are eribulin, gemcitabine, ixabepilone, capecitabine, vinorelbine, platinum agents, anthracyclines, taxanes, paclitaxel, docetaxel, cyclophosphamide, carboplatin, 5-fluorouracil, adriamycin, anthracyclines, epirubicin, *etc.* Generally, the combination therapies are more preferred over the single chemotherapeutic drug for the early stage as well as advanced-stage breast cancer cases.

Chemotherapy: Mode of Administration

The most preferred mode for chemotherapy drugs is intravenous, by either injection or diffusion over the period.

The ideal model of diffusion over periods of administration through a device, called a central line access device, is used for administering not only medicine but also nutrients or fluids directly into the bloodstream. These systems are also useful for drawing blood from the vein for diagnostic purposes. The most common types of central line access devices are venous access ports, and the central lines are located opposite to the side of the breast underwent surgery.

Chemotherapy is given at certain intervals. The gap periods followed by each cycle of chemotherapy are given to recover from the side effect of drugs administered. The interval between two cycles is 10 – 15 days, dependent on the drug used.

Dose-interval Chemotherapy

It has been observed that the minimum interval of the chemotherapy cycle has decreased the chance of reoccurrence of breast cancer and hence, this helps in increasing the life expectancy of breast cancer patients. In chemotherapy, one can reduce the time interval of the next dose by 20 to 30% and this can be applicable for both adjuvant and neoadjuvant therapies. However, the chances of side effects from chemotherapy always remain with breast cancer patients. Sometimes the side effects are very severe; in such cases, it has recommended to reduce the time intervals of the drug in use [7].

Side Effects of Chemotherapy in Breast Cancer

The side effects of chemotherapy are dependent on types of drugs, the dose of drugs, physiology, stage of the tumor, *etc*. The common side effects of chemotherapy include loss of hair, inflammation in the mouth, loss of weight, loss of appetite, nausea, vomiting, diarrhea, *etc*. Apart from these, there are also several known changes in the physiology of patients reported so far.

Effect on the Premature Blood Cells of the Bone Marrow

The side effects of chemotherapy are based on the type of drugs, frequencies, and individual physiology of the patient. Chemotherapy can reduce the total count of red blood cells (RBC), white blood cells (WBC), and blood platelets. Chemotherapy can also weaken the blood clotting factors resulting in the low counts of blood platelets. There are several ways by which we can reduce these side effects [8].

Impact on Fertility and Menstrual Cycle

Fertility and changes in the mensural cycle are common side effects observed. Young women undergoing chemotherapy can have early menopause, irregular menstrual cycle, and difficulties in conceiving, which may result in premature menopause and permanent infertility [9]. The common side effects of chemotherapy in older women are osteoporosis and poor bone density [10]. In such patients, more calcium intake is advised to enhance bone density.

Effect on the Heart Muscle

Chemotherapeutic drugs are responsible for heart problems like cardiomyopathy. Certain drugs, such as doxorubicin and epirubicin, are more preferred for chemotherapy if there is an existing risk of heart damage in breast cancer patients. The risk of damaging cardiac muscle is increased when a high dose of drugs is used for an extended time [11].

Effect on the Nervous System

Nerves of the brain and spinal cord are more susceptible to damage by chemo-therapy, but it is dependent on the kind of drug used. Common drugs used to treat breast cancer are taxanes, cisplatin, vinorelbine, eribulin, and ixabepilone, which may enhance the chances of nerve damage. The common symptoms include weakness, sensitivity towards heat and cold, numbness, burning, and pain [12].

Inflammation in Limbs

Few drugs used for chemotherapy promotes irritation in hands and feet, including numbness, redness, swelling, and pain, called hand and foot syndrome. Usually, for the treatment of breast cancer, anti-inflammatory drugs or steroids in the form of cream are used [13].

Menace of Leukemia

Although it is a rare report, it cannot be ignored that few chemotherapeutic drugs can lead to blood cancer and other bone marrow diseases such as myeloid leukemia [14, 15].

HORMONAL THERAPY

Hormonal therapy works on the principle of lowering the level of hormones to neutralize its proliferating role in breast cancer. Tamoxifen, raloxifene, and toremifene work as anti-estrogen agents that block the activity of estrogen receptors. Palbociclib works by blocking CDK4 & 6 in hormone receptor-positive cells and some other drugs that support hormone therapy to be more effective [5]. Aromatase inhibitors stop the biosynthesis of estrogen by binding to enzyme aromatase [16, 17].

TARGETED THERAPY

Apart from chemotherapy and hormonal therapy, targeted therapy is new and specific approaches, which have shown comparatively lesser side effects. Targeted therapy is patient specific, personalized, and not a generalized treatment. The toxicity report of target-oriented therapy is comparatively low. The beauty of this effective therapy is that it attacks tumor cells only, and the normal cells remain unaffected. Thus targeted therapy will be more effective when used as combination therapy with conventional chemotherapeutic drugs. The study shows that drugs used in targeted therapy have a lesser side effect than traditional chemotherapy. For example, for HER2 positive breast cancer patients, it is useful to find a drug that can block the translational effect on HER2 mediated cell proliferation. Trastuzumab, a recombinant antibody, can be used for HER2 positive patients. If tumors are expressing a high level of HER2, then the recommended medicines are trastuzumab, lapatinib, T-DM1, pertuzumab and MM-111. HER2 expression can be opposed by tamoxifen, fulvestrant, and cabozantinib. For BRCA1 and BRCA2 mutant breast tumor PARP is preferred. In the case of PI3K mutant and HER2 positive tumor, anti- PI3K and anti-AKT therapies are used respectively [18, 19]. In the case of estrogen-positive cases of breast cancer, estrogen receptor modulators are used to suppress tumor growth by inhibiting the estrogen-signaling pathway. Since estrogen receptors play a critical role in the proliferation of breast tumors. Tamoxifen was the first-line drug used for the inhibition of estrogen signaling pathways. The report also suggests that aromatase inhibitors like anastrozole can also achieve a reduction in estrogen levels in breast tumors.

IMMUNOTHERAPY

The activation of the immune system is important to eradicate the cancer cells from the BC patients completely. Immunotherapy plays an important role, which can easily mark, recognize and neutralize the cancer cells. The immunogenicity of tumors is important for therapeutic efficacy in the case of breast cancer [20, 21]. The development of vaccines for breast cancer is dependent on associated antigens only [20]. The significant tumor linked antigens are human epithelial growth factor receptor (HER2), hTERT (carbohydrate antigens, telomerase reverse transcriptase) and mucin-1 [20]. Monoclonal antibodies, such as trastuzumab, prevent additional signal transduction that activates cell cycle progression.

The cancer cell-specific vaccine is developed from cell extracts or entire cancer cells based on the use of peptides or protein subunits [21]. A vaccine based on DNA and dendritic cell-specific vaccines are in the process of development. For clinical trials, the utmost consideration is given to HER2-derived peptide after the extracellular domain of HER2 and categorized by HLA-A2 restriction. HER2 derived peptide from provoking a joint response from CD4+ T and CD8+ T cell. MUC-1, a membrane-based glycoprotein cancer antigen, has been reported to aberrantly glycosylated by altered cells, comprising the breast epithelium. MUC-1 epitope, in combination with limpet hemocyanin, is reported to work well [21]. The amalgamation of immunotherapeutic tactics with other innovative approaches, such as radiotherapy, chemotherapy, vaccination, and immunomodulating instruments, improves the healing process in breast cancer [21].

RESEARCH DEVELOPMENT FOR NEW THERAPEUTIC APPROACH

Ligand-based Approach

Toll-like receptor (TLR) agonists have been confirmed to show anticancer properties [22]. TLR 7 agonist displays a relapse in a tumor in a transgenic mouse and a model of human HER-2/neu positive breast tumor [23]. TLR2 agonist inhibits breast tumor progress in transgenic mice [22]. The contribution of TLRs toward cancer-cell resistance to cell death is appreciable [24]. A consequence of TLR agonists is well studied in human breast tumor cell lines. The knockdown of

TLR4 in cells demonstrated an enormous decrease in breast tumor cell proliferation [25, 26].

Nanotechnology-based Drug Delivery in Tumor Cells

Nano based drug delivery is selective and more effective over chemotherapeutic treatment. Especially in the case of metastatic breast tumors, it is effective to control the release of the drug on a particular site. Magnetic polymers are used as an external magnet to direct the path of drug delivery for chemotherapeutic drugs in the body. This approach-enhanced cytotoxicity towards cancerous cells has simultaneously reduced the toxicity to normal cells and decreased the resistance capacity towards multi drugs.

Targeting Epithelial-to-mesenchymal Transition

Invasion and metastasis are the final common pathways in the progression of any human malignancy [27]. Breast cancer is the most commonly diagnosed cancer in women worldwide [28]. Most of the breast cancer deaths are caused by metastasis rather than the primary tumor itself [28, 29]. The major parallels between cell elasticity during the process of embryonic development and carcinoma progression, have eased to understand the significance of the epithelial-t--mesenchymal transition (EMT) in several human diseases [30, 31].

EMT is a cell-to-cell transition program in which epithelial cells transform into a polarized, differentiated phenotype with numerous cell-cell junctions to a mesenchymal phenotype [32, 33]. EMTs are classified into three biological types that carry different functional significances [34]. 1. Type 1 EMT-The EMT that is associated with embryo formation, and organ development, is organized to generate diverse cell types that share a common mesenchymal phenotype. Type 1 EMT can generate mesenchymal cells (primary mesenchyme) that have the ability to subsequently undergo a mesenchymal-to-epithelial transition (MET) processes to generate secondary epithelia [34]. 2. Type 2 EMT- This form of EMT is linked with wound healing, tissue regeneration, and organ fibrosis. Type 2 EMT, normally generates fibroblasts and other related cells to repair tissues following trauma and inflammatory injury. However, in contrast to type 1 EMT, the type 2 EMT is linked with inflammation. Tissue fibrosis is, in essence, an aberrant form of wound healing due to persistent inflammation [34]. 3. Type 3 EMT- it occurs in neoplastic cells that have undergone genetic and epigenetic changes in genes that favor the clonal outgrowth and development of localized tumors. Type 3 EMT, remarkably affects oncogenes and tumor suppressor genes. Carcinoma cells undergoing type 3 EMT can invade, metastasize, and generate the final, life-threatening manifestations of cancer progression [34]. EMT is associated with increased cancer cell motility, metastasis, and chemotherapy resistance [35].

The reverse of the EMT process is the mesenchymal-epithelial transition (MET) that is linked with a loss of the migratory ability, with cells adopting an apicobasal polarization and expressing the junctional complexes that are features of epithelial tissues [34 - 36]. The EMT is performed in response to pleiotropic factors that induce the expression of specific transcription factors, *e.g.*, Snail, Zeb, Twist, *etc.* and microRNAs together with epigenetic and post-translational modulators, many of which are involved in embryonic development, wound healing, fibrosis, and cancer metastasis [30]. EMT and its intermediate phenotypes have recently been identified as critical modulators of organ fibrosis and tumor progression [30, 37 - 41]. Here, the current state-of-the-art and latest findings regarding the concept of cellular plasticity and heterogeneity in EMT have been discussed [42, 43]. The chief function of fibroblasts, which are pro-typical mesenchymal cells, is to maintain structural integrity by secreting extracellular matrix (ECM) [41]. Fibroblast-specific protein 1 (FSP-1), alpha-smooth muscle actin (αSMA), fibronectin, and collagen I have proved to be key markers to describe the mesenchymal products generated by EMT that occurs during the development of fibrosis in various organs and breast cancer [31, 34, 41, 44, 45].

Inflammatory injury can result in the recruitment of a diverse array of cells that trigger EMT through their release of growth factors, such as transforming growth factor-β (TGF-β), platelet-derived growth factor (PDGF), epidermal growth factor (EGF), and fibroblast growth factor-2 (FGF-2) [34, 44 - 46]. Targeting EMT could be beneficial for the treatment of breast cancer [45]. Fig. (**1**) represents the contribution of type 3 EMT processes in the generation of cancer-associated fibroblasts. Accumulation and metastasis of cancer-associated fibroblasts lead to advancement in breast cancer [47].

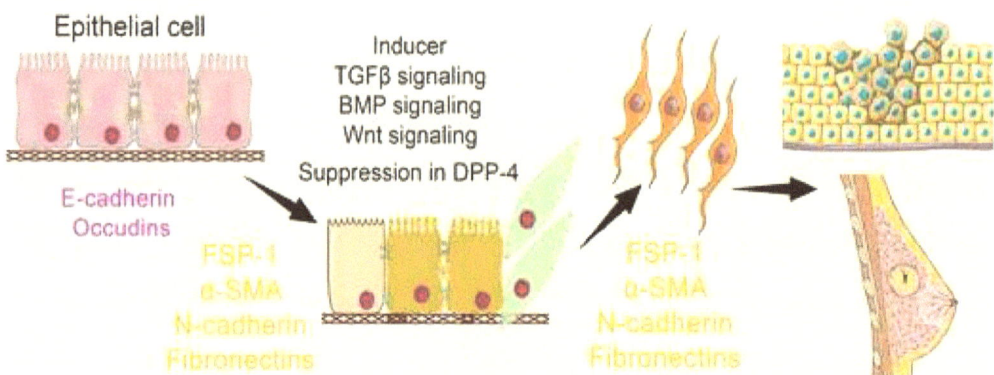

Fig. (1). Epithelial-to-mesenchymal transition is critical in the generation of cancer-associated fibroblasts. *(Note: Figures were created using the Servier medical art illustration resources).*

EMT Inhibitors

Small chemical molecules that inhibit TGF-β signaling and EMT are now under development [48]. Silmitasertib (CX-4945) is an inhibitor of protein kinase CK2, inhibits TGF-β-induced EMT, and is currently in phase II clinical trials for cholangiocarcinoma, and in preclinical development for hematological and lymphoid cancer [49, 50]. Silmitasertib was an orphan drug approved by the U.S. Food and Drug Administration for cholangiocarcinoma and is currently in phase II clinical trials. Another chemical molecule Galunisertib (LY2157299), is a TGF-β type I receptor kinase inhibitor that decreased the tumor size and tumor growth, in triple-negative breast cancer cell lines using mouse xenografts [51]. Inhibitors of EMT are suggested to not work as a replacement for traditional chemotherapeutic agents but are likely to show the best efficacy in treating malignancies when used in conjunction with known drugs.

MicroRNAs Antagonist

MicroRNA (miRNA) is a small non-coding RNA molecule (about 22 nucleotides) found in plants, animals, and some viruses, which functions in RNA silencing and post-transcriptional regulation of gene expression. MicroRNAs are involved in the regulation of several disease processes, including diabetes and cancer [52 - 56]. Antagomirs (inhibitors of microRNAs) and microRNA mimics have shown a potential source of therapeutics to target EMT-induced carcinogenesis in breast cancer as well as treating many other diseases [57]. A microRNA mimic of miR-655 mitigates EMT through the targeting transcription factor ZEB1 and TGFβR2 in a pancreatic cancer cell line [58]. However, microRNA mimics and antagomirs experience a lack of stability *in vivo* and lack of an accurate delivery system to target these molecules to the cancer cells [59]. Chemical modifications such as locked nucleic acid (LNA), oligonucleotides, or peptide nucleic acids (PNA) can prevent the fast clearing of these mimics and antagomirs by RNases [57, 59]. Delivery of antagomirs and microRNA mimics into the cells by liposome-nanoparticles has gained attention, however; liposome structures suffer from their drawbacks that need to be overcome for their effective use as a drug delivery mechanism [59]. These drawbacks of liposome-mediated-nanoparticles include non-specific uptake by the cells [60]. The role of microRNAs in tumor advancement is under examination, and it is yet to be verified whether microRNA mimics or antagomirs may use as clinical treatments to suppress EMT and associated complications or to suppress oncogenic microRNAs in breast cancer.

DPP-4 Biology in Breast Cancer

Dipeptidyl peptidase (DPP)-4, a membrane glycoprotein, has been shown to affect several biological processes, such as cell differentiation, cell adhesion, immunomodulation, and apoptosis [61]. Accumulating evidence specifies that DPP-4 plays a significant role in several disease processes including cancer progression [62 - 64] and diabetic kidney disease [65 - 67]. A recent study displayed that a DPP-4 inhibitor may promote the metastasis of multiple cancer cell lines [45]. DPP-4 regulates the activity of peptides by proteolytically cleaving several peptides, cytokines, and chemokines [68, 69]. C-X-C motif chemokine 12 (CXCL12), also known as stromal cell-derived factor 1 (SDF1), is a known substrate of DPP-4 [70]. CXCL12 binds to C-X-C receptor 4 (CXCR4) and CXCR7 and thus regulates tumor growth and metastasis [71]. In breast cancer, the CXCL12/CXCR4 axis plays a significant role in directing the metastasis of CXCR4 positive cancer cells to organs that express elevated CXCL12 levels, such as the lungs, bone marrow, and lymph nodes [72]. Therefore, an increase in CXCL12 levels in response to DPP-4 inhibitor treatment can be relevant to the metastasis of CXCR4-positive cancer [73].

Mammalian target of rapamycin (mTOR), a major regulator of the PI3K/AKT pathway, is associated with mRNA translation, metabolism, and autophagy and is linked with malignant transformation [74]. mTOR exists in two complexes: mTORC1 (containing mTOR, Raptor, *etc.*) and mTORC2 (containing mTOR, Rictor, *etc.*). mTORC1 is sensitive to rapamycin treatment, whereas mTORC2 is rapamycin-insensitive [75]. A recent finding connected mTORC1 and mTORC2 as key regulators of EMT. Knockdown of mTORC1 and mTORC2 induced mesenchymal-epithelial transition (MET), and suppression of mTOR signaling inhibited cancer cell invasion [76, 77]. Activation of the CXCL12/CXCR4-mTOR signaling pathway in response to DPP-4 inhibition regulates EMT and metastasis in breast cancer [57]. DPP-4 inhibition stimulates breast cancer metastasis by inducing EMT through CXCL12/CXCR4-linked mTOR activation. DPP-4 inhibitors, thought to be safe, can be harmful in a selective population of patients with CXCR4-positive cancer [45].

SUMMARY AND FUTURE DIRECTION

The present chapter describes the recent advancement in the therapeutics of breast cancer. The major risk factors for breast cancer are aging, hormonal imbalance of reproductive hormone, alcoholism, genetic predisposition, and breast tissue disposition. Alteration in the expression level of certain genes, such as BRCA 1, BRCA 2, phosphoinositide 3-kinase (PIK3), retinoblastoma gene (RB), mouse double minute 2 homolog (MDM2), TPK53, HER2, and different oncogenic microRNAs, is the key factor in the development of breast cancer [1]. Physicians appreciate the individual approach and personalized medicine for the treatment of breast cancer. The patient-centric approach should be preferred over the one common approach for all patients due to the heterogeneity of cancer cells. Thus, to confirm clear clinical benefits, an individual approach is dominating the general methodology of breast cancer management. Immunotherapy and the use of natural drugs are also recommended as targeted therapy. Targeted therapy alone or in combination with chemotherapy is effective but still is a matter of ongoing research [19, 20]. Furthermore, therapeutic potentials of microRNAs mimics and antagomiR can be utilized for future drug development for breast cancer. In addition, targeting EMT could be helpful, and hence, EMT inhibitors can be safely utilized in the treatment of breast cancer. Such cellular transition processes are linked with alterations in the DPP-4 level, which has a crucial role in the pathobiology of diabetes. However, the effect of DPP-4 is diverse in several cell types like in the endothelial cells, it promotes mesenchymal activations, party involve in the development of endothelial derive-fibroblasts formation, which is critical for understanding of diabetes, organ fibrosis and cancer [41, 78]. As a part, the current chapter reveals the novel approaches that connect the key modulators in type II diabetes and breast cancer. Moreover, further study is necessary to analyze the effects of DPP-4 inhibitors on human tumorigenesis. DPP-4 shows a connecting link between type 2 diabetes and cancer; it needs further attention by the researchers. Several plant-derived or synthetic antidiabetic molecules, which are in preclinical settings, can be tested for DPP-4 activity and their association with breast cancer [79 - 88]. Moreover, these biological characteristics of DPP-4 in cancer cells could lead to the identification of novel therapeutic targets for cancer.

CONSENT FOR PUBLICATION

Not applicable.

CONFLICT OF INTEREST

The authors confirm that the contents of this chapter have no conflict of interest.

ACKNOWLEDGEMENTS

The author would like to thank the editors for providing the opportunity to write on women's imperative issues in the current world scenario.

REFERENCES

[1]   Bhinder A, Carothers S, Ramaswamy B. Antiangiogenesis therapy in breast cancer. Curr Breast Cancer Rep 2010; 2: 4-15.
[http://dx.doi.org/10.1007/s12609-010-0005-5]

[2]   Lee A, Mavaddat N, Wilcox AN, *et al.* Correction: BOADICEA: a comprehensive breast cancer risk prediction model incorporating genetic and nongenetic risk factors. Genet Med 2019; 21(6): 1462.
[http://dx.doi.org/10.1038/s41436-019-0459-4] [PMID: 30787466]

[3]   Matthews A, Stanway S, Farmer RE, *et al.* Long term adjuvant endocrine therapy and risk of

cardiovascular disease in female breast cancer survivors: systematic review. BMJ 2018; 363: k3845.
[http://dx.doi.org/10.1136/bmj.k3845] [PMID: 30297439]

[4]   Zerah L, Bun RS, Guillo S, Collet JP, Bonnet-Zamponi D, Tubach F. A prescription support-tool for chronic management of oral antithrombotic combinations in adults based on a systematic review of international guidelines. PLoS One 2019; 14(2): e0211695.
[http://dx.doi.org/10.1371/journal.pone.0211695] [PMID: 30763325]

[5]   Nathanson KL, Domchek SM. Therapeutic approaches for women predisposed to breast cancer. Annu Rev Med 2011; 62: 295-306.
[http://dx.doi.org/10.1146/annurev-med-010910-110221] [PMID: 21034216]

[6]   Navolanic PM, McCubrey JA. Pharmacological breast cancer therapy (review). Int J Oncol 2005; 27(5): 1341-4. [review].
[PMID: 16211230]

[7]   Bast RC Jr, Ravdin P, Hayes DF, *et al.* 2000 update of recommendations for the use of tumor markers in breast and colorectal cancer: clinical practice guidelines of the American Society of Clinical Oncology. J Clin Oncol 2001; 19(6): 1865-78.
[http://dx.doi.org/10.1200/JCO.2001.19.6.1865] [PMID: 11251019]

[8]   Sparmann A, Bar-Sagi D. Ras-induced interleukin-8 expression plays a critical role in tumor growth and angiogenesis. Cancer Cell 2004; 6(5): 447-58.
[http://dx.doi.org/10.1016/j.ccr.2004.09.028] [PMID: 15542429]

[9]   Stern RS. Prevalence of a history of skin cancer in 2007: results of an incidence-based model. Arch Dermatol 2010; 146(3): 279-82.
[http://dx.doi.org/10.1001/archdermatol.2010.4] [PMID: 20231498]

[10]   Badowski ME, Burton B, Shaeer KM, Dicristofano J. Oral oncolytic and antiretroviral therapy administration: dose adjustments, drug interactions, and other considerations for clinical use. Drugs Context 2019; 8: 212550.
[http://dx.doi.org/10.7573/dic.212550] [PMID: 30815023]

[11]   Lam F, Pro G, Agrawal S, *et al.* Effect of enhanced detailing and mass media on community use of oral rehydration salts and zinc during a scale-up program in Gujarat and Uttar Pradesh. J Glob Health 2019; 9(1): 010501.
[http://dx.doi.org/10.7189/jogh.09.010501] [PMID: 30546870]

[12]   Classe JM, Bordes V, Campion L, *et al.* Sentinel lymph node biopsy after neoadjuvant chemotherapy for advanced breast cancer: results of ganglion sentinelle et chimiotherapie neoadjuvante, a French prospective multicentric study. J Clin Oncol 2009; 27(5): 726-32.
[http://dx.doi.org/10.1200/JCO.2008.18.3228] [PMID: 19114697]

[13]   Mauri D, Pavlidis N, Ioannidis JP. Neoadjuvant versus adjuvant systemic treatment in breast cancer: a meta-analysis. J Natl Cancer Inst 2005; 97(3): 188-94.
[http://dx.doi.org/10.1093/jnci/dji021] [PMID: 15687361]

[14]   Houghton J, George WD, Cuzick J, Duggan C, Fentiman IS, Spittle M. Radiotherapy and tamoxifen in women with completely excised ductal carcinoma in situ of the breast in the UK, Australia, and New Zealand: randomised controlled trial. Lancet 2003; 362(9378): 95-102.
[http://dx.doi.org/10.1016/S0140-6736(03)13859-7] [PMID: 12867108]

[15]   Kurtz JM, Jacquemier J, Amalric R, *et al.* Risk factors for breast recurrence in premenopausal and postmenopausal patients with ductal cancers treated by conservation therapy. Cancer 1990; 65(8): 1867-78.
[http://dx.doi.org/10.1002/1097-0142(19900415)65:8<1867::AID-CNCR2820650833>3.0.CO;2-I] [PMID: 2156607]

[16]   Chumsri S, Howes T, Bao T, Sabnis G, Brodie A. Aromatase, aromatase inhibitors, and breast cancer. J Steroid Biochem Mol Biol 2011; 125(1-2): 13-22.
[http://dx.doi.org/10.1016/j.jsbmb.2011.02.001] [PMID: 21335088]

[17] Zhao M, Ramaswamy B. Mechanisms and therapeutic advances in the management of endocrine-resistant breast cancer. World J Clin Oncol 2014; 5(3): 248-62.
[http://dx.doi.org/10.5306/wjco.v5.i3.248] [PMID: 25114842]

[18] Higgins MJ, Baselga J. Targeted therapies for breast cancer. J Clin Invest 2011; 121(10): 3797-803.
[http://dx.doi.org/10.1172/JCI57152] [PMID: 21965336]

[19] Mohamed A, Krajewski K, Cakar B, Ma CX. Targeted therapy for breast cancer. Am J Pathol 2013; 183(4): 1096-112.
[http://dx.doi.org/10.1016/j.ajpath.2013.07.005] [PMID: 23988612]

[20] Emens LA. Breast cancer immunobiology driving immunotherapy: vaccines and immune checkpoint blockade. Expert Rev Anticancer Ther 2012; 12(12): 1597-611.
[http://dx.doi.org/10.1586/era.12.147] [PMID: 23253225]

[21] Soliman H. Immunotherapy strategies in the treatment of breast cancer. Cancer Contr 2013; 20(1): 17-21.
[http://dx.doi.org/10.1177/107327481302000104] [PMID: 23302903]

[22] Yusuf N. Toll like receptors and breast cancer. Front Immunol 2014; 5: 84.

[23] Lu H, Wagner WM, Gad E, et al. Treatment failure of a TLR-7 agonist occurs due to self-regulation of acute inflammation and can be overcome by IL-10 blockade. J Immunol 2010; 184(9): 5360-7.
[http://dx.doi.org/10.4049/jimmunol.0902997] [PMID: 20308630]

[24] Yang H, Zhou H, Feng P, et al. Reduced expression of Toll-like receptor 4 inhibits human breast cancer cells proliferation and inflammatory cytokines secretion. J Exp Clin Cancer Res 2010; 29: 92.
[http://dx.doi.org/10.1186/1756-9966-29-92] [PMID: 20618976]

[25] Allavena P, Sica A, Garlanda C, Mantovani A. The Yin-Yang of tumor-associated macrophages in neoplastic progression and immune surveillance. Immunol Rev 2008; 222: 155-61.
[http://dx.doi.org/10.1111/j.1600-065X.2008.00607.x] [PMID: 18364000]

[26] Merrell MA, Ilvesaro JM, Lehtonen N, et al. Toll-like receptor 9 agonists promote cellular invasion by increasing matrix metalloproteinase activity. Mol Cancer Res 2006; 4(7): 437-47.
[http://dx.doi.org/10.1158/1541-7786.MCR-06-0007] [PMID: 16849519]

[27] Heerboth S, Housman G, Leary M, et al. EMT and tumor metastasis. Clin Transl Med 2015; 4: 6.
[http://dx.doi.org/10.1186/s40169-015-0048-3] [PMID: 25852822]

[28] Ghoncheh M, Pournamdar Z, Salehiniya H. Incidence and mortality and epidemiology of breast cancer in the world. Asian Pac J Cancer Prev 2016; 17(S3): 43-6.
[http://dx.doi.org/10.7314/APJCP.2016.17.S3.43] [PMID: 27165206]

[29] Tohme S, Simmons RL, Tsung A. Surgery for cancer: A trigger for metastases. Cancer Res 2017; 77(7): 1548-52.
[http://dx.doi.org/10.1158/0008-5472.CAN-16-1536] [PMID: 28330928]

[30] Nieto MA, Huang RY, Jackson RA, Thiery JP. Emt: 2016. Cell 2016; 166(1): 21-45.
[http://dx.doi.org/10.1016/j.cell.2016.06.028] [PMID: 27368099]

[31] Srivastava SP, Koya D, Kanasaki K. MicroRNAs in kidney fibrosis and diabetic nephropathy: roles on EMT and EndMT. BioMed Res Int 2013; 2013: 125469.
[http://dx.doi.org/10.1155/2013/125469] [PMID: 24089659]

[32] Wu Y, Zhou BP. New insights of epithelial-mesenchymal transition in cancer metastasis. Acta Biochim Biophys Sin (Shanghai) 2008; 40(7): 643-50.
[http://dx.doi.org/10.1111/j.1745-7270.2008.00443.x] [PMID: 18604456]

[33] Lamouille S, Xu J, Derynck R. Molecular mechanisms of epithelial-mesenchymal transition. Nat Rev Mol Cell Biol 2014; 15(3): 178-96.
[http://dx.doi.org/10.1038/nrm3758] [PMID: 24556840]

[34]   Kalluri R, Weinberg RA. The basics of epithelial-mesenchymal transition. J Clin Invest 2009; 119(6): 1420-8.
[http://dx.doi.org/10.1172/JCI39104] [PMID: 19487818]

[35]   Tomaskovic-Crook E, Thompson EW, Thiery JP. Epithelial to mesenchymal transition and breast cancer. Breast Cancer Res 2009; 11(6): 213.
[http://dx.doi.org/10.1186/bcr2416] [PMID: 19909494]

[36]   Thiery JP, Acloque H, Huang RYJ, Nieto MA. Epithelial-mesenchymal transitions in development and disease. Cell 2009; 139(5): 871-90.
[http://dx.doi.org/10.1016/j.cell.2009.11.007] [PMID: 19945376]

[37]   Srivastava SP, Li J, Kitada M, *et al.* SIRT3 deficiency leads to induction of abnormal glycolysis in diabetic kidney with fibrosis. Cell Death Dis 2018; 9(10): 997.
[http://dx.doi.org/10.1038/s41419-018-1057-0] [PMID: 30250024]

[38]   Nagai T, Kanasaki M, Srivastava SP, *et al.* N-acetyl-seryl-aspartyl-lysyl-proline inhibits diabetes-associated kidney fibrosis and endothelial-mesenchymal transition. BioMed Res Int 2014; 2014: 696475.
[http://dx.doi.org/10.1155/2014/696475] [PMID: 24783220]

[39]   Nitta K, Shi S, Nagai T, *et al.* Oral administration of N-acetyl-seryl-aspartyl-lysyl-proline ameliorates kidney disease in both type 1 and type 2 diabetic mice *via* a therapeutic regimen. BioMed Res Int 2016; 2016: 9172157.
[http://dx.doi.org/10.1155/2016/9172157] [PMID: 27088094]

[40]   Li J, Shi S, Srivastava SP, *et al.* FGFR1 is critical for the anti-endothelial mesenchymal transition effect of N-acetyl-seryl-aspartyl-lysyl-proline *via* induction of the MAP4K4 pathway. Cell Death Dis 2017; 8(8): e2965.
[http://dx.doi.org/10.1038/cddis.2017.353] [PMID: 28771231]

[41]   Srivastava SP, Hedayat AF, Kanasaki K, Goodwin JE. microRNA crosstalk influences epithelial-t--mesenchymal, endothelial-to-mesenchymal, and macrophage-to-mesenchymal transitions in the Kidney. Front Pharmacol 2019; 10: 904.
[http://dx.doi.org/10.3389/fphar.2019.00904] [PMID: 31474862]

[42]   Gould R, Bassen DM, Chakrabarti A, Varner JD, Butcher J. Population heterogeneity in the epithelial to mesenchymal transition is controlled by NFAT and phosphorylated Sp1. PLOS Comput Biol 2016; 12(12): e1005251.
[http://dx.doi.org/10.1371/journal.pcbi.1005251] [PMID: 28027307]

[43]   Wendt MK, Allington TM, Schiemann WP. Mechanisms of the epithelial-mesenchymal transition by TGF-beta. Future Oncol 2009; 5(8): 1145-68.
[http://dx.doi.org/10.2217/fon.09.90] [PMID: 19852727]

[44]   Alidadiani N, Ghaderi S, Dilaver N, Bakhshamin S, Bayat M. Epithelial mesenchymal transition Transcription Factor (TF): The structure, function and microRNA feedback loop. Gene 2018; 674: 115-20.
[http://dx.doi.org/10.1016/j.gene.2018.06.049] [PMID: 29936265]

[45]   Yang F, Takagaki Y, Yoshitomi Y, *et al.* Inhibition of dipeptidyl peptidase-4 accelerates epithelial-mesenchymal transition and breast cancer metastasis *via* the CXCL12/CXCR4/mTOR axis. Cancer Res 2019; 79(4): 735-46.
[http://dx.doi.org/10.1158/0008-5472.CAN-18-0620] [PMID: 30584072]

[46]   Liu X, Sun N, Mo N, *et al.* Quercetin inhibits kidney fibrosis and the epithelial to mesenchymal transition of the renal tubular system involving suppression of the Sonic Hedgehog signaling pathway. Food Funct 2019; 10(6): 3782-97.
[http://dx.doi.org/10.1039/C9FO00373H] [PMID: 31180394]

[47]   Fiori ME, Di Franco S, Villanova L, Bianca P, Stassi G, De Maria R. Cancer-associated fibroblasts as

abettors of tumor progression at the crossroads of EMT and therapy resistance. Mol Cancer 2019; 18(1): 70.
[http://dx.doi.org/10.1186/s12943-019-0994-2] [PMID: 30927908]

[48]   Yingling JM, Blanchard KL, Sawyer JS. Development of TGF-beta signalling inhibitors for cancer therapy. Nat Rev Drug Discov 2004; 3(12): 1011-22.
[http://dx.doi.org/10.1038/nrd1580] [PMID: 15573100]

[49]   Zou J, Luo H, Zeng Q, Dong Z, Wu D, Liu L. Protein kinase CK2α is overexpressed in colorectal cancer and modulates cell proliferation and invasion *via* regulating EMT-related genes. J Transl Med 2011; 9: 97.
[http://dx.doi.org/10.1186/1479-5876-9-97] [PMID: 21702981]

[50]   Gowda C, Sachdev M, Muthusami S, *et al.* Casein kinase II (CK2) as a therapeutic target for hematological malignancies. Curr Pharm Des 2017; 23(1): 95-107.
[PMID: 27719640]

[51]   Bhola NE, Balko JM, Dugger TC, *et al.* TGF-β inhibition enhances chemotherapy action against triple-negative breast cancer. J Clin Invest 2013; 123(3): 1348-58.
[http://dx.doi.org/10.1172/JCI65416] [PMID: 23391723]

[52]   Pandey AK, Verma G, Vig S, Srivastava S, Srivastava AK, Datta M. miR-29a levels are elevated in the db/db mice liver and its overexpression leads to attenuation of insulin action on PEPCK gene expression in HepG2 cells. Mol Cell Endocrinol 2011; 332(1-2): 125-33.
[http://dx.doi.org/10.1016/j.mce.2010.10.004] [PMID: 20943204]

[53]   Kaur K, Pandey AK, Srivastava S, Srivastava AK, Datta M. Comprehensive miRNome and in silico analyses identify the Wnt signaling pathway to be altered in the diabetic liver. Mol Biosyst 2011; 7(12): 3234-44.
[http://dx.doi.org/10.1039/c1mb05041a] [PMID: 21968817]

[54]   McDonald AC, Vira M, Walter V, *et al.* Circulating microRNAs in plasma among men with low-grade and high-grade prostate cancer at prostate biopsy. Prostate 2019; 79(9): 961-8.
[http://dx.doi.org/10.1002/pros.23803] [PMID: 30958910]

[55]   Chen G, Ye B. The key microRNAs regulated the development of non-small cell lung cancer by targeting TGF-beta-induced epithelial-mesenchymal transition. Comb Chem High Throughput Screen 2019; 22(4): 238-44.
[http://dx.doi.org/10.2174/1386207322666190410151945] [PMID: 30968775]

[56]   Srivastava SP, Shi S, Koya D, Kanasaki K. Lipid mediators in diabetic nephropathy. Fibrogenesis Tissue Repair 2014; 7: 12.
[http://dx.doi.org/10.1186/1755-1536-7-12] [PMID: 25206927]

[57]   Rupaimoole R, Slack FJ. MicroRNA therapeutics: towards a new era for the management of cancer and other diseases. Nat Rev Drug Discov 2017; 16(3): 203-22.
[http://dx.doi.org/10.1038/nrd.2016.246] [PMID: 28209991]

[58]   Rupaimoole R, Han HD, Lopez-Berestein G, Sood AK. MicroRNA therapeutics: principles, expectations, and challenges. Chin J Cancer 2011; 30(6): 368-70.
[http://dx.doi.org/10.5732/cjc.011.10186] [PMID: 21627858]

[59]   Rothschild SI. microRNA therapies in cancer. Mol Cell Ther 2014; 2: 7.
[http://dx.doi.org/10.1186/2052-8426-2-7] [PMID: 26056576]

[60]   Lv H, Zhang S, Wang B, Cui S, Yan J. Toxicity of cationic lipids and cationic polymers in gene delivery. J Control Release 2006; 114(1): 100-9.
[http://dx.doi.org/10.1016/j.jconrel.2006.04.014] [PMID: 16831482]

[61]   Bae EJ. DPP-4 inhibitors in diabetic complications: role of DPP-4 beyond glucose control. Arch Pharm Res 2016; 39(8): 1114-28.
[http://dx.doi.org/10.1007/s12272-016-0813-x] [PMID: 27502601]

[62]   Gokhale M, Buse JB, Gray CL, Pate V, Marquis MA, Stürmer T. Dipeptidyl-peptidase-4 inhibitors and pancreatic cancer: a cohort study. Diabetes Obes Metab 2014; 16(12): 1247-56.
[http://dx.doi.org/10.1111/dom.12379] [PMID: 25109825]

[63]   Amritha CA, Kumaravelu P, Chellathai DD. Evaluation of anti cancer effects of DPP-4 inhibitors in colon cancer- an *in vitro* study. J Clin Diagn Res 2015; 9(12): FC14-6.
[PMID: 26816911]

[64]   Nagel AK, Ahmed-Sarwar N, Werner PM, Cipriano GC, Van Manen RP, Brown JE. Dipeptidyl peptidase-4 inhibitor-associated pancreatic carcinoma: a review of the FAERS database. Ann Pharmacother 2016; 50(1): 27-31.
[http://dx.doi.org/10.1177/1060028015610123] [PMID: 26497885]

[65]   Kanasaki K, Shi S, Kanasaki M, *et al.* Linagliptin-mediated DPP-4 inhibition ameliorates kidney fibrosis in streptozotocin-induced diabetic mice by inhibiting endothelial-to-mesenchymal transition in a therapeutic regimen. Diabetes 2014; 63(6): 2120-31.
[http://dx.doi.org/10.2337/db13-1029] [PMID: 24574044]

[66]   Shi S, Srivastava SP, Kanasaki M, *et al.* Interactions of DPP-4 and integrin β1 influences endothelial-to-mesenchymal transition. Kidney Int 2015; 88(3): 479-89.
[http://dx.doi.org/10.1038/ki.2015.103] [PMID: 25830763]

[67]   Srivastava SP, Shi S, Kanasaki M, *et al.* Effect of antifibrotic MicroRNAs crosstalk on the action of n-acetyl-seryl-aspartyl-lysyl-proline in diabetes-related kidney fibrosis. Sci Rep 2016; 6: 29884.
[http://dx.doi.org/10.1038/srep29884] [PMID: 27425816]

[68]   Amin S, Boffetta P, Lucas AL. The role of common pharmaceutical agents on the prevention and treatment of pancreatic cancer. Gut Liver 2016; 10(5): 665-71.
[http://dx.doi.org/10.5009/gnl15451] [PMID: 27563018]

[69]   Metzemaekers M, Van Damme J, Mortier A, Proost P. Regulation of chemokine activity - a focus on the role of dipeptidyl peptidase IV/CD26. Front Immunol 2016; 7: 483.
[http://dx.doi.org/10.3389/fimmu.2016.00483] [PMID: 27891127]

[70]   Christopherson KW II, Frank RR, Jagan S, Paganessi LA, Gregory SA, Fung HC. CD26 protease inhibition improves functional response of unfractionated cord blood, bone marrow, and mobilized peripheral blood cells to CXCL12/SDF-1. Exp Hematol 2012; 40(11): 945-52.
[http://dx.doi.org/10.1016/j.exphem.2012.07.009] [PMID: 22846168]

[71]   Mego M, Cholujova D, Minarik G, *et al.* CXCR4-SDF-1 interaction potentially mediates trafficking of circulating tumor cells in primary breast cancer. BMC Cancer 2016; 16: 127.
[http://dx.doi.org/10.1186/s12885-016-2143-2] [PMID: 26896000]

[72]   Hernandez L, Magalhaes MA, Coniglio SJ, Condeelis JS, Segall JE. Opposing roles of CXCR4 and CXCR7 in breast cancer metastasis. Breast Cancer Res 2011; 13(6): R128.
[http://dx.doi.org/10.1186/bcr3074] [PMID: 22152016]

[73]   Mortier A, Gouwy M, Van Damme J, Proost P, Struyf S. CD26/dipeptidylpeptidase IV-chemokine interactions: double-edged regulation of inflammation and tumor biology. J Leukoc Biol 2016; 99(6): 955-69.
[http://dx.doi.org/10.1189/jlb.3MR0915-401R] [PMID: 26744452]

[74]   Engelman JA. Targeting PI3K signalling in cancer: opportunities, challenges and limitations. Nat Rev Cancer 2009; 9(8): 550-62.
[http://dx.doi.org/10.1038/nrc2664] [PMID: 19629070]

[75]   Bracho-Valdés I, Moreno-Alvarez P, Valencia-Martínez I, Robles-Molina E, Chávez-Vargas L, Vázquez-Prado J. mTORC1- and mTORC2-interacting proteins keep their multifunctional partners focused. IUBMB Life 2011; 63(10): 896-914.
[http://dx.doi.org/10.1002/iub.558] [PMID: 21905202]

[76]   Chang LH, Chen CH, Huang DY, Pai HC, Pan SL, Teng CM. Thrombin induces expression of twist

and cell motility *via* the hypoxia-inducible factor-1α translational pathway in colorectal cancer cells. J Cell Physiol 2011; 226(4): 1060-8.
[http://dx.doi.org/10.1002/jcp.22428] [PMID: 20857420]

[77]   Chen G, Chen SM, Wang X, Ding XF, Ding J, Meng LH. Inhibition of chemokine (CXC motif) ligand 12/chemokine (CXC motif) receptor 4 axis (CXCL12/CXCR4)-mediated cell migration by targeting mammalian target of rapamycin (mTOR) pathway in human gastric carcinoma cells. J Biol Chem 2012; 287(15): 12132-41.
[http://dx.doi.org/10.1074/jbc.M111.302299] [PMID: 22337890]

[78]   Srivastava SP, Goodwin JE, Kanasaki K, Koya D. Inhibition of Angiotensin-Converting Enzyme Ameliorates Renal Fibrosis by Mitigating DPP-4 Level and Restoring Antifibrotic MicroRNAs. Genes (Basel) 2020; 11(2): 211.
[http://dx.doi.org/10.3390/genes11020211] [PMID: 32085655]

[79]   Kumar A, Sharma S, Tripathi VD, *et al.* Design and synthesis of 2,4-disubstituted polyhydroquinolines as prospective antihyperglycemic and lipid modulating agents. Bioorg Med Chem 2010; 18(11): 4138-48.
[http://dx.doi.org/10.1016/j.bmc.2009.11.061] [PMID: 20471838]

[80]   Jaiswal N, Bhatia V, Srivastava SP, Srivastava AK, Tamrakar AK. Antidiabetic effect of Eclipta alba associated with the inhibition of alpha-glucosidase and aldose reductase. Nat Prod Res 2012; 26(24): 2363-7.
[http://dx.doi.org/10.1080/14786419.2012.662648] [PMID: 22348789]

[81]   Kumar A, Sharma S, Gupta LP, *et al.* Synthesis of propiophenone derivatives as new class of antidiabetic agents reducing body weight in db/db mice. Bioorg Med Chem 2012; 20(6): 2172-9.
[http://dx.doi.org/10.1016/j.bmc.2011.12.027] [PMID: 22341243]

[82]   Balaramnavar VM, Srivastava R, Rahuja N, *et al.* Identification of novel PTP1B inhibitors by pharmacophore based virtual screening, scaffold hopping and docking. Eur J Med Chem 2014; 87: 578-94.
[http://dx.doi.org/10.1016/j.ejmech.2014.09.097] [PMID: 25299681]

[83]   Kanasaki M, Srivastava SP, Yang F, *et al.* Deficiency in catechol-o-methyltransferase is linked to a disruption of glucose homeostasis in mice. Sci Rep 2017; 7(1): 7927.
[http://dx.doi.org/10.1038/s41598-017-08513-w] [PMID: 28801594]

[84]   Arha D, Pandeti S, Mishra A, *et al.* Deoxyandrographolide promotes glucose uptake through glucose transporter-4 translocation to plasma membrane in L6 myotubes and exerts antihyperglycemic effect *in vivo*. Eur J Pharmacol 2015; 768: 207-16.
[http://dx.doi.org/10.1016/j.ejphar.2015.10.055] [PMID: 26528798]

[85]   Shukla P, Srivastava SP, Srivastava R, Rawat AK, Srivastava AK, Pratap R. Synthesis and antidyslipidemic activity of chalcone fibrates. Bioorg Med Chem Lett 2011; 21(11): 3475-8.
[http://dx.doi.org/10.1016/j.bmcl.2011.03.057] [PMID: 21515043]

[86]   Verma AK, Singh H, Satyanarayana M, *et al.* Flavone-based novel antidiabetic and antidyslipidemic agents. J Med Chem 2012; 55(10): 4551-67.
[http://dx.doi.org/10.1021/jm201107g] [PMID: 22524508]

[87]   Mishra A, Srivastava R, Srivastava SP, *et al.* Antidiabetic activity of heart wood of Pterocarpus marsupium Roxb. and analysis of phytoconstituents. Indian J Exp Biol 2013; 51(5): 363-74.
[PMID: 23821824]

[88]   Raza S, Srivastava SP, Srivastava DS, Srivastava AK, Haq W, Katti SB. Thiazolidin-4-one and thiazinan-4-one derivatives analogous to rosiglitazone as potential antihyperglycemic and antidyslipidemic agents. Eur J Med Chem 2013; 63: 611-20.
[http://dx.doi.org/10.1016/j.ejmech.2013.01.054] [PMID: 23567949]

CHAPTER 14

Micro and Nano-scale Technologies for Breast Cancer Detection and Destruction

Pranay Agarwal*

Department of Orthopaedic Surgery, Stanford University, 450 Broadway, Redwood City, CA94063, California, USA

Abstract: In this chapter, we thoroughly review the current developments and challenges in the field of tissue engineering of normal and breast cancer cells. We also briefly describe the current advances in cell culture techniques and common biomaterials, which are useful in the field of tissue engineering. Further, the need for a new microencapsulation technology of cells utilizing the microfluidic method is illustrated. Moreover, the most recent applications of cell-laden microcapsules in tissue engineering are summarized. Lastly, the chapter is concluded with an outline of the future prospective.

Keywords: Breast cancer, Extracellular matrix, Nanodevice, Tissue engineering, Two and three-dimensional culture.

INTRODUCTION

Tissue engineering utilizes cells in a variety of ways to restore, maintain, and improve the function of tissues and organs [1, 2]. Tissue engineering envisions building organs from a tissue scratch in the laboratory, ready to be transplanted into the patients. The potential impacts of tissue engineering are immense: (1) engineered tissues can reduce the need for organ replacement; (2) engineered tissues can accelerate the development of novel drugs and evaluate the cytotoxicity of available drugs, thus eliminating the need for an organ transplant [3 - 5]. However, engineering a living tissue *in vitro* is a complex process because cells are typically cultured on a bioactive degradable scaffold, which provides biochemical clues to guide them to become functional 3D tissues [3 - 5]. Furthermore, the time scale of these events can range from seconds to several weeks [6]. Inducing cells to form functional tissues is currently a major biological challenge, and it requires extensive engineering design, which must be accom-

* **Corresponding author Dr. Pranay Agarwal:** Department of Orthopaedic Surgery, Stanford University, 450 Broadway, Redwood City, CA94063, California, USA; E-mail: agpranay@stanford.edu

Shankar Suman, Garima Suman and Sanjay Mishra (Eds.)

plished with high fidelity and low cost [7]. The other technical challenges that are needed to be overcome to create "off-the-shelf" tissues include (1) the availability of adequate source of healthy expandable cells, (2) optimization of scaffolds, (3) creation of large-scale bioreactors that mimic the native microenvironment of tissues, and (4) long-term preservation of engineered tissues [7].

Additional key aspects of tissue engineering and its challenges are provided in Table **1** [3, 7 - 14].

Table 1. Key aspects of tissue engineering.

Cell source	• **Unlimited availability of embryonic stem cells, adult stem cells or differentiated cells.**
Scaffold design requirement	• Injectability. • Ability to encapsulate cells. • Ability to mimic the biomechanical microenvironment of the native tissue. • Degradation at a rate fast enough to allow the growth of surrounding tissues.
Cell surface interactions	• Ability to manipulate the interaction of cells with the surface.
Growth factor and cellular delivery	• Increased efficiency of loading physiological amounts of growth factors. • Controlled release of the growth factors. • High survival and viability of transplanted cells.
Assessment	• Development of clinically relevant models to assess the functionality of tissue-engineered products.
Scale up or tissue vascularization	• Ability to use large tissue-engineered products where diffusion limitation may limit the viability of encapsulated cells.

Sources of Cells For Tissue Engineering

The production of successful tissue engineering products utilizes the cells to proliferate within the scaffolds. Recently, more attention has been given to stem cells, including embryonic stem (ES) cells and bone marrow-derived stem cells (BM-MSCs). Stem cells are pluripotent cells and can be differentiated into all different cell types. However, there are two critical steps for the use of stem cells in tissue engineering applications, (1) maintenance of pluripotency for extending the culture period in the laboratory and (2) the ability to control the differentiation of these cells to the desired tissue lineage [15 - 17]. It is also equally important to be able to engineer cells in order to express or secrete small biological molecules or desired functions for therapeutic purposes. Controlling the cell aggregation (stem or non-stem cells) and stiffness of the supporting matrix is known to modulate the functional capabilities of cells. Moreover, in the case of stem cell-based therapies, well-planned strategies are required to deliver cells *in vivo* that ensure high retention and better survival post-transplantation [15 - 17]. Other applications of controlled cell aggregation are drug discovery and cytotoxicity screening. Therefore, this chapter focuses on the application of different biomaterial systems that may affect the proliferation, development, and survival of various types of cells including breast cancer cells.

Native Tissue Microenvironment

The function and regeneration of any tissue are a result of intricate coordination between numerous individual cellular processes, which are induced by different signals originating from extracellular matrices. For example, complex biochemical and biophysical signals, communicated from outside microenvironments, are combined *via* intracellular signaling, ultimately converging to regulate gene and protein expression, which establishes cell/tissue function and phenotype. The extracellular microenvironment surrounding the cells consists of insoluble macromolecules (fibrillary protein such as collagen, laminin, fibronectin), soluble molecules (growth factors, cytokines, chemokines), and proteins on the surface of the adjacent cells [18].

Current Techniques For Culturing Cells (2D *vs.* 3D culture system)

Typically, in *in vitro* experiments, cells are cultured on a stiff plastic surface, which does not capture the properties of *in vivo* biology. Monolayer culture allows all the cells to receive a homogeneous amount of nutrients and growth factors. They mostly consist of proliferating cells since necrotic cells are detached from the surface. Furthermore, the morphology of cells in 2D is flatter and stretched compared to *in vivo* settings [19, 20]. This abnormal growth condition influences cell proliferation, differentiation, and gene/protein expression. In contrast to 2D cultures, cells in the 3D system are either grown into aggregates on the matrix or embedded within the scaffold/matrix. The cells in 3D can also be grown in a scaffold-free microenvironment. The cells in these 3D conditions more closely mimic the natural microenvironment. They have cell-matrix and cell-cell interactions [19, 20]. In addition, the cells in 3D culture coexist in different stages, such as outer proliferative, hypoxic, and necrotic cells. They have nutrient and oxygen gradient as present *in vivo*. Furthermore, the proliferation of cells in 2D and 3D cell cultures is different as it is dependent on ECM. This 3D culture system has also been utilized for the co-culture of different types of cells as well to gain invaluable information. For example, tumor stromal cells have been co-cultured with mammary cancer cells and have been shown to regulate tumor growth, metastasis, and even drug response [19, 20].

In addition to the morphological differences between 2D and 3D culture systems, it has been shown that 3D cell cultures differ in gene and protein expression profiles compared to 2D cultured cells. For example, mouse embryonic stem cells cultured in 3D scaffolds (Cytomatrix) have a significantly higher expression of ECM related genes, as well as genes that regulate cell growth, proliferation and differentiation [21]. Various cancer cells grown in 2D and 3D cultures often display differential gene expression of genes involved in proliferation, angiogenesis, migration, invasion, and chemosensitivity. In a study, it was shown that cell-ECM interactions in 3D culture (on matrigel) of prostate cancer cells could modulate overall tumor morphology and upregulate CXCR4 and CXCR7 expression [22]. Loessner *et al.* reported that ovarian cancer cells grown in the 3D culture system showed increased expression of integrin, metalloprotease and MMP9 compared to traditional 2D culture systems [23]. Altogether, these observations suggest that the 3D microenvironment of the cell is important to maintain the gene and protein expressions similar to *in vivo* like systems.

Cell-based assays are critical for drug and cytotoxicity screening. Most of the drug screening assays utilize 2D cell culture tests, followed by animal model tests and clinical trials [19]. However, the information obtained from 2D experiments sometimes provides misleading or non-predictive data in drug screening. For example, numerous studies have shown that cells cultured in 3D models are more resistant to anticancer drugs compared to 2D cultures. Karlsson *et al.*, investigated the drug sensitivity of colorectal cancer cells, HCT-116, in 3D spheroids and 2D monolayer cultures to melphalan, 5-FU, oxaliplatin and irinotecan, and the results showed that all the drugs were less active on 3D spheroids in contrast to 2D monolayer cells [24]. It has been shown that high drug resistance in 3D cultured cells is due to increased cell-cell interactions between neighboring cells, limited diffusion, and hypoxic condition [19]. Another possible explanation could be an altered gene and protein expression in 3D cultured cells as compared to 2D cells [19]. This phenomenon observed in 3D spheroids is similar to what was observed *in vivo*. Key differences between 2D and 3D culture systems are provided in Table **2**.

Table 2. Key differences between two-dimensional and three-dimensional culture systems.

Property	Two dimensional (2D)	Three-dimensional (3D)
Morphology	Flat and stretched	Natural shape in spheroids and aggregates
Proliferation	Very proliferative compared to *in vivo*	Proliferation depends on cell type and matrix
Gradients	Cells are exposed to an equal concentration of medium and growth factors	Spheroids have concentration gradients. High concentration on the outer surface
Cell Stage	Typically, cells are in a similar stage	Contains proliferative, quiescent, apoptotic, and necrotic zones

(Table 2) cont.....

Property	Two dimensional (2D)	Three-dimensional (3D)
Gene/Protein expression	Different compared to *in vivo*	More similar to *in vivo* conditions
Drug sensitivity	Cells are typically more sensitive	Cells are more resistant to drugs compared to 2D cultured cells

Altogether, it is evident that 3D cell culture models are better than 2D culture systems since they closely resemble the *in vivo* architecture. They hold great promise in the application in drug discovery, breast cancer cell biology, and cancer stem cell research. However, there are still many hurdles that must be overcome before they can be widely utilized. (1) Currently, they are more expensive for large-scale studies and high throughput assays. (2) Some methods generate spheroids that differ greatly in size, which results in high variability in results. (3) 3D models still lack vasculature, which plays a vital role in tissue proliferation, survival, and drug delivery [12].

BIOMATERIALS FOR 3D CELL CULTURE

Definition of Biomaterials

According to the National Institutes of Health Consensus Development symposium, biomaterial may be defined as "any substance (other than a drug) or combination of substances, synthetic or natural in origin, which can be used for any period of time, as a whole or as a part of a system which treats, augments, or replaces any tissue, organ, or function of the body".

BIOMATERIALS AND TISSUE ENGINEERING

Biomaterials in the form of grafts (sutures, joint replacements, bone plates, *etc.*) and medical devices (pacemakers, artificial organs, blood tubes, *etc.*) are broadly used to replace and/or restore the function of damaged organs and thus, improve the patient outcomes. The most important requirement for the selection of the biomaterial is its acceptability/compatibility by the human body. A biomaterial used for transplantation should have some important qualities for long-term usage in the body without any immunological rejection [25]. Initially, various types of natural products such as wood, resin, rubber, and tissues from living organisms, and synthetic materials such as iron, gold, silver, and glass were used as biomaterials. The host immunological responses to these materials/natural products tremendously vary. Polymers are suitable candidates as scaffold materials for tissue engineering since they can be tailored to have desired sizes, shape, and properties (*e.g.,* mechanical properties, geometrical shapes, biocompatibility, and least toxicity, *etc.*) and can be degraded at the same rate as new tissues are formed [26]. Here, some commonly used natural and synthetic biopolymers are discussed for their application as biomaterials in 3D culture, as well as the biochemical functions.

Types of Biomaterials

Natural Polymers

Natural products-based biomaterials possess perfect bioactivity and biodegradability *in vivo*. Proteins, peptides and other molecules of these biopolymers can be very similar to native ones, so cells can attach, recognize, and respond. Biopolymers derived from natural materials such as collagen type-I, fibrin, alginate, chitosan, chondroitin sulfate, and HA have been used to fabricate hydrogel scaffolds [27 - 30]. Hydrogels of naturally derived biopolymers have the benefit of rapid biodegradability and resemble the natural ECM. However, some of them also have their disadvantages. Collagen hydrogels can be immune responsive while fibrin hydrogels can produce insoluble fibrin peptide aggregates and can be linked with a certain degree of shrinkage when used as matrices for cell encapsulation [31].

Collagen

Collagen is considered a perfect choice as biomaterials for tissue engineering because it is the main fibrous protein in the extracellular matrix (ECM) and offers strength and structural integrity to various types of connective tissues, including bone, skin, cartilage, blood vessels, tendons, and ligaments. Collagen biopolymers show biocompatibility, high porosity and permeability, hydrophilicity, biodegradability, but less mechanical strength for bone tissue engineering in weight-bearing applications [32]. Various physical and chemical cross-linking methods can increase the decomposition rate and compressive and tensile strength.

Chitosan

Chitosan, derived from chitin, is a linear polysaccharide biopolymer comprising copolymers of β (1-4)-glucosamine and N-acetyl-D-glucosamine moiety. Chitin occurs in the exoskeleton of crustaceans (such as scorpion, crabs, and shrimps), cuticles of insects, and cell walls of bacteria (bacilli). Chitosan has attained much attention from scientists because of its biocompatibility, less toxicity, biodegradability, controllable mechanical and structural features, and capability of being managed in several forms, sizes, and shapes. However, pure chitosan as a biopolymeric tissue engineering scaffold is inadequate because of its weak mechanical properties and inconsistent behavior with seeded cells. Chitosan can be physically and chemically altered and produce materials with a broad range of properties [33].

Alginate

Alginate is a brown sea algae-derived linear polysaccharide. It belongs to a family of linear block polyanionic copolymers containing (1-4)-linked β-D-mannuronic acid and (1-4)-linked α-L-Guluronic acid residues. Alginate can produce stable and well-categorized hydrogels in the presence of divalent cations (*e.g.*, Ca^{2+}, Sr^{2+}, Ba^{2+}). In order to prevent immunological responses after implantation, alginate must undergo extensive purification. Alginate shows various properties like biocompatibility, hydrophilicity, less-toxicity, biodegradability, and is relatively less expensive. However, some limitations have restricted its use in tissue engineering such as weak mechanical properties, less cell adhesion (for highly hydrophilic nature), and uncontrollable decomposition [30].

Hyaluronic Acid

HA is a naturally derived polysaccharide, which is present in the ECM of delicate connective tissues and body fluids. Concerning its mechanism of synthesis, size, and physiochemical properties, HA is exclusive among other glycosaminoglycans. In addition, HA can interact with other molecules (*e.g.*, proteins) in order to participate in regulating cell behavior during various morphogenic, restorative and pathological developments in the human body. The role of HA in diseases, such as several types of malignancies, arthritis, and osteoporosis, is leading to new research. Although, the fabrication of the safest and well-organized HA-based biomaterials for theranostic medicine for any type of damage, regardless of their surface, remains a challenge [34].

Synthetic Polymers

Many synthetic polymers have been used to produce biomaterials because of their several benefits as a scaffold material and also due to their availability. Synthetic polymers can be biodegradable and non-biodegradable. Synthetic polymeric materials can be synthesized with personalized architecture and properties (*e.g.* porosity, degradability, and mechanical features), as per their applications. Polymers, such as Poly (lactic-co-glycolic) acid (PLGA), PEG, and poly(ethylene glycol) (PEG), have been broadly used because of their relatively simple way to fabricate gels with required mechanical and physical properties [35].

Poly (lactic-co-glycolic) acid (PLGA)

PLGA is fabricated by random ring-opening copolymerization of glycolic acid and lactic acid monomers. PLGA possesses unique features, including extraordinary mechanical strength, excellent biocompatibility, less toxicity and immunogenicity, and adaptable degradation kinetics [36]. The properties of PLGA are tailored by altering the monomer ratios and molecular weight [36].

Poly (ethylene glycol) (PEG)

PEG, the most commercially used polyether, also known as polyethylene oxide (PEO) or polyoxyethylene (POE) based on its molecular weight, refers to an oligomer or polymer of ethylene oxide. PEG has some important properties, including good biocompatibility, hypoimmunogenicity, and resistance to protein adsorption and cell adhesion, for which it has been a central hydrophilic polymer in biomedical applications, including bioconjugation, surface alteration, drug delivery, and tissue engineering [36].

Properties of Ideal Biomaterials

Ideal biomaterials must be non-toxic, non-carcinogenic, hypo-immunogenic, chemically inert, stable, and mechanically durable to withstand repeated forces [37]. Irrespective of the tissue type, a number of key factors are important when designing or determining the appropriateness of a biomaterial for use in tissue engineering:

Biocompatibility

The first criteria of any biomaterial to be used for tissue engineering are as follows 1). It must be biocompatible; 2). Cells must adhere and drift onto the surface and eventually through the scaffold and begin to multiply before laying down the new matrix. After implantation, the biomaterial or tissue-engineered construct must induce a negligible immunological response to prevent it, causing such a severe inflammatory response that it might decrease healing or cause rejection by the body [37, 38].

Biodegradability

The main goal of tissue engineering is to allow the body's own cells/tissues, over time, to ultimately replace the grafted biomaterial or tissue-engineered construct. Biomaterials and tissue engineering constructs are not envisioned as permanent implants. The biomaterial must, therefore, be biodegradable to allow cells to produce their own ECM. The by-products of this degradation should also be non-toxic and able to exit the body without interference in other organs [37, 38].

Mechanical Properties

Ideally, the biomaterial should possess mechanical properties consistent with the anatomical site into which it is to be grafted, and, from a practical viewpoint, it must be strong enough to permit surgical handling during implantation [37, 38].

Biomaterial Architecture

The architecture of biomaterials applied for tissue engineering is of crucial importance. Biomaterials must possess an interconnected pore architecture and high porous structure to ensure cellular penetration and suitable diffusion of nutrients to cells within the construct and to the ECM made by these cells. Moreover, a porous interconnected structure is required to allow the diffusion of waste products/toxic agents out of the biomaterial, and the products of scaffold degradation should be able to exit the body without interfering with the surrounding tissues [37, 38]. The issue of core degradation, arising from less vascularization and waste removal from the center of tissue-engineered constructs, is of major concern in the field of tissue engineering [37, 38].

Manufacturing Technology

For a particular biomaterial or tissue-engineered construct to become clinically and commercially applicable, it should be less expensive and promising to scale-up from manufacturing one at a time in a research laboratory to significant batch production in the industry. The progress of ascendable manufacturing procedures to good manufacturing practice standards is crucially important in ensuring effective translation of tissue engineering methods to clinical applicability. `This will determine how either the biomaterial or the tissue-engineered construct will be stored.

Cell Encapsulation in Micro-Hydrogels for Tissue Engineering

The encapsulation of cells in tiny hydrogels offers numerous advantages for tissue engineering. It is easy to handle and provides a 3D microenvironment of cell and tissue growth. Furthermore, many features of micro-hydrogels, such as swelling, mechanical properties, degradation, biochemical properties, and diffusion, can be modulated through a myriad of processing conditions [39 - 41]. The encapsulation of cells can be performed using macro-platforms, micro-molding techniques, and microfluidic-based technologies [42]. Among these technologies, the encapsulation of cells in small size microbeads/microcapsules is very attractive. The encapsulation of cells in microcapsules composed of a semi-permeable membrane can prevent direct contact of encapsulated cells and immune cells after *in vivo* implantation in the host system [43]. Furthermore, the small size of microcapsules allows facile diffusion of nutrients, oxygen, metabolic waste, and therapeutic agents secreted by the encapsulated cells. Since the free diffusion limit is ~200 μm [12], and the ideal size of microcapsules to encapsulate cells is ~400 μm, it ensures that cells buried in the core of microcapsules will obtain sufficient nutrients and oxygen. Cell encapsulation is advantageous for 3D *in vitro* cell culture. Single or multiple cells can be encapsulated to proliferate in microcapsules, which serve as a micro-bioreactor. Furthermore, microcapsules can also be used as a carrier to deliver bioactive agents or growth factors. Depending on the application, microcapsules can be fabricated using poly (ethylene glycol), polysaccharides (alginate and hyaluronic acid), and proteins (collagen, fibrinogen, and gelatin). In addition, various crosslinking mechanisms of biomaterials to form hydrogels must be considered. Generally, photo-cross linkers, ions, and heat are utilized to form the particles [39 - 41].

Core-Shell Microcapsules for Cell Encapsulation and their Advantages

Alginate beads are generally used for the encapsulation of cells owing to their excellent biocompatibility and biodegradability, low toxicity, and rapid gelation in the presence of divalent cations such as Ca^{2+} and Ba^{2+} [44, 45]. Even though the solid alginate beads have been shown to encapsulate cells for the culture, the homogenous mixing of cells with alginate is not ideal (Fig. **1**) [45]. This is because alginate does not adhere to the mammalian cells. Furthermore, solid beads are ineffective in forming spherical aggregates of cells. Another disadvantage of solid beads is that cell or cell aggregate can grow near the edge of the beads, which may lead to inadequate immune protection. In order to effectively use the microencapsulation of cell culture and related applications, it is desirable to use tissue-specific ECM with desired biomechanical and biochemical properties. The present methods generate microcapsules that do not effectively solve the abovementioned problems.

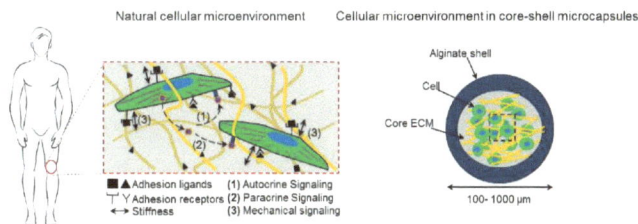

Fig. (1). Schematic of the two types of microfluidic device generally used to form droplets. (**A**) Shows the T-shaped junction device and (**B**) shows the flow-focusing (FF) device.

Cell Encapsulation via Droplet Microfluidics

Droplet microfluidics has emerged as an important approach to fabricate microcapsules [46 - 50]. Using the microfluidic device, the high-throughput production of microcapsules with low polydispersity can be achieved. Furthermore, a microfluidic system for droplet formation provides more control over the droplet size. For example, other methods for preparing microparticles such as electrospray and emulsification using sonification generate particles with broad size distribution. In order to generate microparticles *via* microfluidics, two or more immiscible liquids are used, which are independently controlled using syringe pumps (either pressure control or volumetric flow rate control). Various microfluidic geometries to produce microcapsules have been introduced over the years [51, 52]. For example, T-shaped junctions and flow focusing (FF) devices are the most common, as shown in Fig. (**2**). The two liquid phases meet at a junction at which the dispersed phase liquid forms a droplet. The geometry of the microfluidic device determines the flow or velocity field during the experiments. Ultimately, the droplet pinches off from the dispersed phase due to the interfacial tension between the two phases [51, 52]. Continuous and uniform generation of droplets is dependent on the steadiness of the flow rates. The wettability of the microfluidic channels is also important for the successful generation of droplets [52]. For example, if the dispersed and continuous phase is in aqueous and oil solutions, the channels of the microfluidic device must be hydrophobic. In other words, the continuous phase liquid must preferentially wet the walls of the microfluidic channels. Therefore, the selection of material for fabricating a microfluidic device is also important. To make oil-in-water droplets, microfluidic channels in polydimethylsiloxane (PDMS) are fabricated using soft lithography since PDMS is hydrophobic. However, the surface properties of PDMS can be readily changed by chemical modifications in order to make oil-in-water droplets [53]. Otherwise, materials like silicon can be used, which is hydrophilic. In addition, the choice of fabricating material also depends on its strength and compatibility with fluids [52].

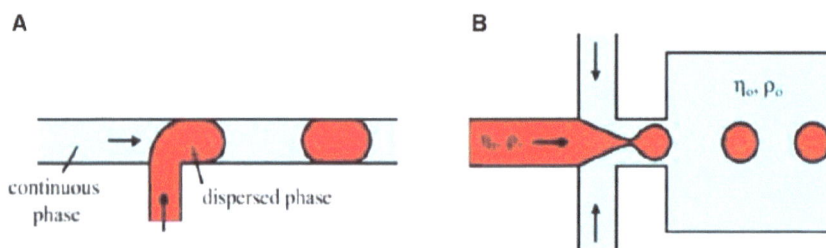

Fig. (2). Schematic of the two types of microfluidic device generally used to form droplets. (**A**) Shows the T-shaped junction device and (**B**) shows the flow-focusing (FF) device.

The size of continuous and dispersed phase channels, height and width, are important parameters that determine the flow field and, ultimately, the size of the droplets. Several important fluid properties that need to be considered are the viscosities (η) and densities (ρ) of dispersed (d) and continuous (c) phase, and the interfacial tension between the two (σ) [52]. Key dimensionless parameters are used to analyze the important forces acting in the microfluidic system. Capillary number (*Ca*) represents the relative effect of viscous force and the surface tension [52]. The capillary number for the droplet formation process is defined in terms of continuous/dispersed phase flow field as:

$$Ca = \frac{\mu V}{\eta} \tag{1}$$

Where ρ is the dynamic viscosity of the continuous/dispersed phase, V is the characteristic velocity, and σ is the surface tension. The typical values of *Ca* range from 10^{-3} to 10^{1}. Another important parameter is the ratio of volumetric flow rate φ, given by

$$\varphi = \frac{Q_d}{Q_c} \tag{2}$$

The Reynold number *Re* is also another dimensionless quantity that is used to predict the flow pattern in the microfluidic device and is defined as the ratio of inertial forces to viscous forces,

$$Re = \frac{\rho V D}{\eta} \tag{3}$$

Where D is the hydraulic diameter of the channel. Typically, for microfluidic experiments, *Re*<< 1.

In a typical flow-focusing device, as shown in Fig. (**2B**), continuous and dispersed phase flow coaxially in separate channels in a planar microfluidic device. Also, continuous flow channels flank dispersed phase channels on both sides, and they meet at the flow-focusing junction. As a result of the velocity field of the continuous phase at the junction, the dispersed phase liquid breaks into droplets. Droplets in this device can be generated in dripping and jetting regimes, which are based on the flow rates of flown liquids as well as on the capillary number [51, 52]. In the dripping regime, the dispersed phase immediately forms a droplet at the FF junction, whereas in jetting elongation of the dispersed phase, droplets are formed downstream of the FF junction. In both the regimes, the frequency of droplet formation and the droplet sizes are different. Furthermore, as the capillary number increases or the flow rates of liquids increase, the transition of dripping to jetting is observed.

In order to form hydrogel particles for cell culture in an FF microfluidic device, a suitable gelling/solidification mechanism should be included in the downstream channels. The solidification can occur by various chemical reactions. Mostly, chemical crosslinking (use of photoinitiators and UV light) or physical crosslinking (in the presence of ions) is utilized [54]. For the cell encapsulation purposes, it is always desirable to have a gentle crosslinking mechanism to ensure high viability of encapsulated cells. Kim *et al.* demonstrated the use of microfluidic FF devices to encapsulate embryonic carcinoma cells to form aggregates in microcapsules with a liquid core and alginate hydrogel shell. In addition, they compared the aggregate formation of cells in core-shell microcapsules and microbeads. They reported the formation of several clusters of cells in microbeads whereas uniform size aggregates were formed in core-shell microcapsules [55]. In this study, however, they utilized oleic acid with infused calcium chloride to gel the alginate, which could be harmful to cells. Furthermore, the inclusion of glycerol in the core of microcapsules could also compromise the viability of the encapsulated cells. In another study by Leong and co-workers, a microfluidic device was utilized to encapsulate hepatocyte cells alginate-collagen and alginate microcapsules [56]. The study showed that the encapsulation of hepatocyte enhanced its long-term performance.

MODULAR TISSUE ENGINEERING FOR FABRICATING COMPLEX TISSUES

There is still less number of *in vitro* engineered tissues due to the current inability to mimic the tissue vasculature. *In vivo,* all the tissues get nutrients and oxygen from blood vessels (larger blood vessels and microcapillaries). Since the free diffusion limit is ~200 μm, currently, it is not possible to efficiently fabricate tissue-engineered products larger than this without creating a vascular architecture [12].

There are two broad strategies which can be used to create hierarchical tissue structures: top-down and bottom-up approaches. In the top-down approach, cells are seeded on a biodegradable polymeric scaffold such as PLGA (synthetically manufactured vascularized scaffolds) and are expected to secrete ECM and recreate microarchitecture similar to the *in vivo* conditions. Typically, perfusion systems, growth factors, and mechanical stimulation are provided that aid cellular growth. However, such a top-down system is often limited to mimic the intricate microstructural details of the desired tissue [57]. In bottom-up approaches, modular structures are first micro-engineered, which can be used as building blocks to create larger tissues. These modules can be prepared using different ways: encapsulation of cells, cell sheet formation, or bioprinting. Since most of the tissues are made up of repeating units, bottom-up approaches are preferred to create more biomimetic engineered tissues [57].

As an example of the bottom-up approach, Takeuchi *et al.* seeded 3T3 fibroblast cells on the surface of collagen gels [58]. Later, they assembled a large number of beads to generate a 3D hierarchical system. They formed an arbitrary shape macroscopic object by using a molding approach to form a dense tissue. Such a system could be used to form vascularized complex tissues because different micro-tissues can be easily prepared with tissue relevant cells. Furthermore, using core-shell microcapsules composed of tissue-specific biomaterials as an ECM can be utilized as a building block. This would potentially enable us to replicate more intricate *in vivo* like structures needed for tissue engineering applications.

APPLICATION OF NANO DEVICE IN STUDYING BREAST TUMOR MICROENVIRONMENT

The role of the 3D microenvironment in tumor development has been extensively studied in recent years [6, 13, 59 - 63]. It has been reported that the surrounding extracellular matrix (ECM), mesenchymal cells (fibroblasts and adult stem cells), and supporting blood vessels play a vital role in tumor growth, invasion, and metastasis [64, 65]. For example, the ECM (collagen, laminin, and fibronectin) provides structural support to the resident cells and acts as a reservoir of growth factors and cytokines [13, 60, 61]. Moreover, communications between cancer cells and stromal cells in the microenvironment enable tumor proliferation and distant colony formation [61]. Importantly, the tumor microenvironment has received growing attention due to its role in chemoresistance, relapse, and metastasis [61]. Therefore, an *in vitro* 3D biomimetic model is essential that takes into account the complex interplay between different types of cells and their microenvironment for investigating tumor biology and drug screening applications.

Several methods have been proposed lately to mimic the native microenvironment of the tumor. They include suspension culture to form multicellular tumor spheroids and encapsulation of cells in porous scaffolds [13, 59, 61, 64, 66]. The former is simple and inexpensive. However, it is difficult to achieve high-throughput production and obtain aggregates of uniform size [61, 64]. 3D tumor models have also been developed by introducing cells into porous synthetic scaffolds (*e.g.*, polylactide or PLA, polyglycolide or PGA, and copolymers of PLA and PGA (PLGA)) and hydrogels (*e.g.*, polyethylene glycol or PEG) [61,

64]. Although studies on these models have made significant contributions to tumor biology, the synthetic ECM does not accurately mimic the natural tumor microenvironment. The lack of vascularization is another fundamental limitation of most contemporary 3D tumor models where the diffusional restrictions of nutrients and oxygen in highly cellularized tissues (typically less than ~200 μm [61, 67 - 69]) may result in viable cells only in the surface layer of less than ~200 μm thick. Vascularization is also required for tumor metastasis. The differences between normal vasculature and vasculature in solid tumors [70 - 72] (immature, tortuous, and hyperpermeable vessels) offer a unique target for anticancer therapies [73 - 75]. Moreover, the abnormal vasculature greatly affects the transport of anti-cancer drugs within the tumor tissues. Therefore, tumor vasculature is an important component of the tumor microenvironment that must be incorporated in the 3D tumor models. However, contemporary work on vascularization *in vitro* is focused on either the random assembly of endothelial cells in a homogeneous system (*e.g.*, hydrogel or medium) to form new blood vessels (*i.e.*, vasculogenesis) with no control on their distribution [76 - 81], or the sprouting of existing or microfabricated vessels to produce new capillaries (*i.e.*, angiogenesis) [70, 71, 76, 82, 83].

To mimic the vasculature of *in vivo* tissues, "bottom-up" tissue engineering principles can be utilized. Bottom-up approaches have the potential to construct vascularized tissues with defined properties, including spatial and temporal control, at the cellular level [6, 57]. Recent progress in encapsulating and culturing cells in core-shell microcapsules with a tumor relevant ECM core and an alginate hydrogel shell using a high-throughput microfluidic device is one of the ways to create these microscale modules [45, 84, 85]. To develop an avascular network, the cell-laden modules may be packaged with tumor-relevant ECM and supporting vascular and stromal cells for them to self-assemble and form a vascularized tumor. Moreover, the microscale modules may provide geometric guidance to the vascular cells [81], enabling the formation of a complex 3D vascular network around the cancer cells in the modules to mimic the vasculature in the tumor *in vivo*.

Agarwal *et al*. also described the fabrication of 3D vascularized human mammary tumors (Fig. **3**) [86]. In this study, authors first encapsulated and cultured MCF-7 cells in core-shell microcapsules (< ~200 μm in radius) composed of type 1 collagen-rich ECM enclosed in a semipermeable alginate hydrogel shell using a high-throughput non-planar microfluidic device. Then, they characterized the proliferation and gene expression of the encapsulated MCF-7 cells in different core ECMs with different biophysical properties. Next, these engineered individual micro-tumors (μtumor) in core-shell microcapsules were assembled in a microfluidic device with endothelial and stromal cells to form a millimeter-sized

3D vascularized breast tumor. The endothelial cells were guided by the microcapsules to form complex tortuous 3D vascular beds around the encapsulated µtumours, mimicking the vasculature of an *in vivo* tumor. Lastly, to illustrate the capability of their model for high-throughput drug screening, they investigated the effect of the tumor microenvironment on cancer drug resistance and demonstrated the use of nanotechnology to overcome cancer drug resistance. Therefore, this biomimetic 3D model may be valuable for studying the effect of microenvironment on tumor progression, invasion, and metastasis, and for developing an effective therapeutic strategy to combat cancer.

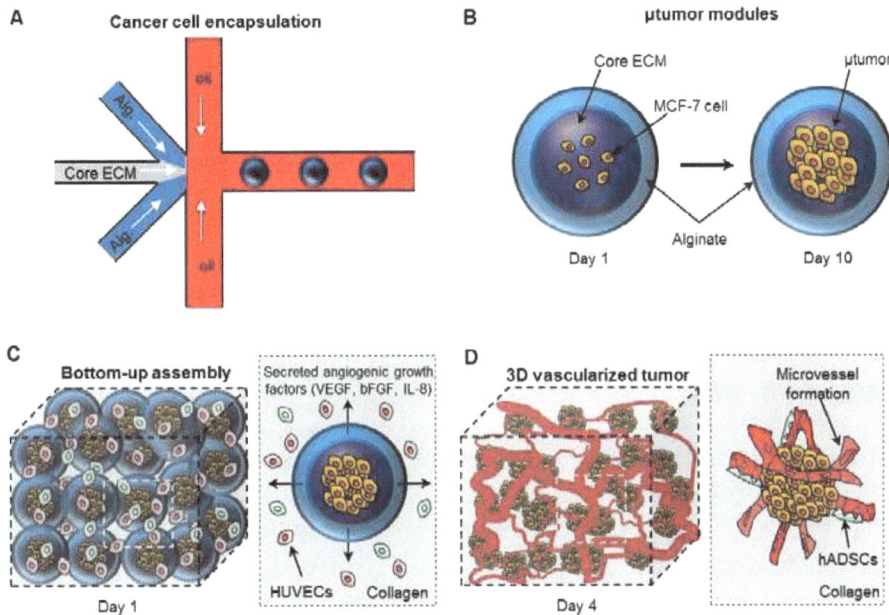

Fig. (3). Schematic of the bottom up tissue engineering method to prepare 3D vascularized breast tumor. (**A**) Non-planar microfluidic device is utilized to encapsulate cancer cells in core-shell microcapsules. (**B**) Encapsulated cancer cells are cultured in microcapsules for 10 days to form cancer cell aggregates. (**C**) Encapsulated micro aggregates are assembled together with stromal cells and collagen hydrogel to form 3D vascularized tumor (**D**).

CONCLUSION

The main objective of tissue engineering is to construct living tissues that can be used to replace or repair damaged tissue or organs. This is designed to address the critical gap between the growing number of patients and the available organs for transplantation. However, since the last decade or so, only a few products have been approved by the US Food and Drug Administration (FDA). As discussed in this book chapter, scalable/high-throughput 3D biomimetic culture systems, ability to control cellular proliferation and differentiation, sustainable delivery of growth factors and cells after transplantation can contribute to solving many present challenges.

Employing stem cells as a cell source is an important aspect of tissue engineering/regenerative medicine since they can be programmed to differentiate into any cell type. However, large quantities of cells with high pluripotency are essential for any tissue engineering application. In addition to using core-shell microcapsules in regenerative medicine, the application of micro and nano devices has also been used in investigating breast tumor biology. In summary, this chapter discussed the novel biomaterial systems involving microencapsulation of cells and explored their applications in stem cell-based tissue regeneration and breast cancer biology with promising results. This chapter provides a brief overview of the studies conducted in the field of tissue engineering. Building on these findings, this chapter can help biomedical engineers to develop more advanced biomaterial systems and seek potential therapies/diagnosis for other diseases in the near future.

CONSENT FOR PUBLICATION

Not applicable.

CONFLICT OF INTEREST

I want to declare that most of the content of this chapter has been taken from my graduate thesis (Ph.D.), submitted to the Ohio State University (OSU). However, being a student at OSU, I own the copyrights to my dissertation (library.osu.edu/document-registry/docs/774/stream).

ACKNOWLEDGEMENT

I want to thank my Ph.D. advisor and the Ohio State University for all the support.

REFERENCES

[1]   Atala A, Kasper FK, Mikos AG. Engineering complex tissues. Sci Transl Med 2012; 4(160): 160rv12.
[http://dx.doi.org/10.1126/scitranslmed.3004890] [PMID: 23152327]

[2]   Mikos AG, Herring SW, Ochareon P, *et al.* Engineering complex tissues. Tissue Eng 2006; 12(12): 3307-39.
[http://dx.doi.org/10.1089/ten.2006.12.3307] [PMID: 17518671]

[3]   Langer R, Vacanti JP. Tissue engineering. Science 1993; 260(5110): 920-6.
[http://dx.doi.org/10.1126/science.8493529] [PMID: 8493529]

[4]   Lee KY, Mooney DJ. Hydrogels for tissue engineering. Chem Rev 2001; 101(7): 1869-79.
[http://dx.doi.org/10.1021/cr000108x] [PMID: 11710233]

[5]   Vunjak-Novakovic G, Tandon N, Godier A, *et al.* Challenges in cardiac tissue engineering. Tissue Eng Part B Rev 2010; 16(2): 169-87.
[http://dx.doi.org/10.1089/ten.teb.2009.0352] [PMID: 19698068]

[6]   Guven S, Chen P, Inci F, Tasoglu S, Erkmen B, Demirci U. Multiscale assembly for tissue engineering and regenerative medicine. Trends Biotechnol 2015; 33(5): 269-79.
[http://dx.doi.org/10.1016/j.tibtech.2015.02.003] [PMID: 25796488]

[7]   Griffith LG, Naughton G. Tissue engineering--current challenges and expanding opportunities. Science 2002; 295(5557): 1009-14.
[http://dx.doi.org/10.1126/science.1069210] [PMID: 11834815]

[8]   Dhandayuthapani B, Yoshida Y, Maekawa T, Kumar DS. Polymeric scaffolds in tissue engineering application: A review. Int J Polym Sci 2011.
[http://dx.doi.org/10.1155/2011/290602]

[9]   Griffith LG, Swartz MA. Capturing complex 3D tissue physiology *in vitro*. Nat Rev Mol Cell Biol 2006; 7(3): 211-24.
[http://dx.doi.org/10.1038/nrm1858] [PMID: 16496023]

[10]   Kang HW, Lee SJ, Ko IK, Kengla C, Yoo JJ, Atala A. A 3D bioprinting system to produce human-scale tissue constructs with structural integrity. Nat Biotechnol 2016; 34(3): 312-9.
[http://dx.doi.org/10.1038/nbt.3413] [PMID: 26878319]

[11]   Luttun A, Tjwa M, Moons L, *et al.* Revascularization of ischemic tissues by PlGF treatment, and inhibition of tumor angiogenesis, arthritis and atherosclerosis by anti-Flt1. Nat Med 2002; 8(8): 831-40.
[http://dx.doi.org/10.1038/nm731] [PMID: 12091877]

[12]   Novosel EC, Kleinhans C, Kluger PJ. Vascularization is the key challenge in tissue engineering. Adv Drug Deliv Rev 2011; 63(4-5): 300-11.
[http://dx.doi.org/10.1016/j.addr.2011.03.004] [PMID: 21396416]

[13]   Yamada KM, Cukierman E. Modeling tissue morphogenesis and cancer in 3D. Cell 2007; 130(4): 601-10.
[http://dx.doi.org/10.1016/j.cell.2007.08.006] [PMID: 17719539]

[14]   Amini AR, Laurencin CT, Nukavarapu SP. Bone tissue engineering: recent advances and challenges. Crit Rev Biomed Eng 2012; 40(5): 363-408.
[http://dx.doi.org/10.1615/CritRevBiomedEng.v40.i5.10] [PMID: 23339648]

[15]   Lutolf MP, Gilbert PM, Blau HM. Designing materials to direct stem-cell fate. Nature 2009; 462(7272): 433-41.
[http://dx.doi.org/10.1038/nature08602] [PMID: 19940913]

[16]   Bianco P, Cao X, Frenette PS, *et al.* The meaning, the sense and the significance: translating the science of mesenchymal stem cells into medicine. Nat Med 2013; 19(1): 35-42.
[http://dx.doi.org/10.1038/nm.3028] [PMID: 23296015]

[17]   Bianco P, Robey PG. Stem cells in tissue engineering. Nature 2001; 414(6859): 118-21.
[http://dx.doi.org/10.1038/35102181] [PMID: 11689957]

[18]   Lutolf MP, Hubbell JA. Synthetic biomaterials as instructive extracellular microenvironments for morphogenesis in tissue engineering. Nat Biotechnol 2005; 23(1): 47-55.
[http://dx.doi.org/10.1038/nbt1055] [PMID: 15637621]

[19]   Edmondson R, Broglie JJ, Adcock AF, Yang L. Three-dimensional cell culture systems and their applications in drug discovery and cell-based biosensors. Assay Drug Dev Technol 2014; 12(4): 207-18.
[http://dx.doi.org/10.1089/adt.2014.573] [PMID: 24831787]

[20]   Haycock JW. 3D cell culture: a review of current approaches and techniques. Methods Mol Biol 2011;

695: 1-15.
[http://dx.doi.org/10.1007/978-1-60761-984-0_1] [PMID: 21042962]

[21]   Liu H, Lin J, Roy K. Effect of 3D scaffold and dynamic culture condition on the global gene expression profile of mouse embryonic stem cells. Biomaterials 2006; 27(36): 5978-89.
[http://dx.doi.org/10.1016/j.biomaterials.2006.05.053] [PMID: 16824594]

[22]   Kiss DL, Windus LC, Avery VM. Chemokine receptor expression on integrin-mediated stellate projections of prostate cancer cells in 3D culture. Cytokine 2013; 64(1): 122-30.
[http://dx.doi.org/10.1016/j.cyto.2013.07.012] [PMID: 23921147]

[23]   Loessner D, Stok KS, Lutolf MP, Hutmacher DW, Clements JA, Rizzi SC. Bioengineered 3D platform to explore cell-ECM interactions and drug resistance of epithelial ovarian cancer cells. Biomaterials 2010; 31(32): 8494-506.
[http://dx.doi.org/10.1016/j.biomaterials.2010.07.064] [PMID: 20709389]

[24]   Karlsson H, Fryknäs M, Larsson R, Nygren P. Loss of cancer drug activity in colon cancer HCT-116 cells during spheroid formation in a new 3-D spheroid cell culture system. Exp Cell Res 2012; 318(13): 1577-85.
[http://dx.doi.org/10.1016/j.yexcr.2012.03.026] [PMID: 22487097]

[25]   Qi C, Yan X, Huang C, Melerzanov A, Du Y. Biomaterials as carrier, barrier and reactor for cell-based regenerative medicine. Protein Cell 2015; 6(9): 638-53.
[http://dx.doi.org/10.1007/s13238-015-0179-8] [PMID: 26088192]

[26]   Levenberg S, Langer R. Advances in tissue engineering. Curr Top Dev Biol 2004; 61: 113-34.
[http://dx.doi.org/10.1016/S0070-2153(04)61005-2] [PMID: 15350399]

[27]   Augst AD, Kong HJ, Mooney DJ. Alginate hydrogels as biomaterials. Macromol Biosci 2006; 6(8): 623-33.
[http://dx.doi.org/10.1002/mabi.200600069] [PMID: 16881042]

[28]   Hoffman AS. Hydrogels for biomedical applications. Ann N Y Acad Sci 2001; 944: 62-73.
[http://dx.doi.org/10.1111/j.1749-6632.2001.tb03823.x] [PMID: 11797696]

[29]   Khademhosseini A, Langer R. Microengineered hydrogels for tissue engineering. Biomaterials 2007; 28(34): 5087-92.
[http://dx.doi.org/10.1016/j.biomaterials.2007.07.021] [PMID: 17707502]

[30]   Lee KY, Mooney DJ. Alginate: properties and biomedical applications. Prog Polym Sci 2012; 37(1): 106-26.
[http://dx.doi.org/10.1016/j.progpolymsci.2011.06.003] [PMID: 22125349]

[31]   Rowe SL, Lee S, Stegemann JP. Influence of thrombin concentration on the mechanical and morphological properties of cell-seeded fibrin hydrogels. Acta Biomater 2007; 3(1): 59-67.
[http://dx.doi.org/10.1016/j.actbio.2006.08.006] [PMID: 17085089]

[32]   Glowacki J, Mizuno S. Collagen scaffolds for tissue engineering. Biopolymers 2008; 89(5): 338-44.
[http://dx.doi.org/10.1002/bip.20871] [PMID: 17941007]

[33]   Chandy T, Sharma CP. Chitosan--as a biomaterial. Biomater Artif Cells Artif Organs 1990; 18(1): 1-24.
[http://dx.doi.org/10.3109/10731199009117286] [PMID: 2185854]

[34]   Collins MN, Birkinshaw C. Hyaluronic acid based scaffolds for tissue engineering--a review. Carbohydr Polym 2013; 92(2): 1262-79.
[http://dx.doi.org/10.1016/j.carbpol.2012.10.028] [PMID: 23399155]

[35]   Gunatillake P, Mayadunne R, Adhikari R. Recent developments in biodegradable synthetic polymers. Biotechnol Annu Rev 2006; 12: 301-47.
[http://dx.doi.org/10.1016/S1387-2656(06)12009-8] [PMID: 17045198]

[36]   Gentile P, Chiono V, Carmagnola I, Hatton PV. An overview of poly(lactic-co-glycolic) acid (PLGA)-

based biomaterials for bone tissue engineering. Int J Mol Sci 2014; 15(3): 3640-59.
[http://dx.doi.org/10.3390/ijms15033640] [PMID: 24590126]

[37]   Buddy D Ratner ASH, Frederick J Schoen, Jack E Lemons. Biomaterials Science: An introduction to materials in medicine. Academic Press 2004.

[38]   O'Brien FJ. Biomaterials & scaffolds for tissue engineering. Mater Today 2011; 14(3): 88-95.
[http://dx.doi.org/10.1016/S1369-7021(11)70058-X]

[39]   Nicodemus GD, Bryant SJ. Cell encapsulation in biodegradable hydrogels for tissue engineering applications. Tissue Eng Part B Rev 2008; 14(2): 149-65.
[http://dx.doi.org/10.1089/ten.teb.2007.0332] [PMID: 18498217]

[40]   Overhauser J. Encapsulation of cells in agarose beads. Methods Mol Biol 1992; 12: 129-34.
[PMID: 21409630]

[41]   Serra M, Correia C, Malpique R, *et al.* Microencapsulation technology: a powerful tool for integrating expansion and cryopreservation of human embryonic stem cells. PLoS One 2011; 6(8): e23212.
[http://dx.doi.org/10.1371/journal.pone.0023212] [PMID: 21850261]

[42]   Kang A, Park J, Ju J, Jeong GS, Lee SH. Cell encapsulation *via* microtechnologies. Biomaterials 2014; 35(9): 2651-63.
[http://dx.doi.org/10.1016/j.biomaterials.2013.12.073] [PMID: 24439405]

[43]   Orive G, Hernández RM, Rodríguez Gascón A, *et al.* History, challenges and perspectives of cell microencapsulation. Trends Biotechnol 2004; 22(2): 87-92.
[http://dx.doi.org/10.1016/j.tibtech.2003.11.004] [PMID: 14757043]

[44]   Agarwal P, Choi JK, Huang H, *et al.* A Biomimetic Core-Shell Platform for Miniaturized 3D Cell and Tissue Engineering. Part Part Syst Charact 2015; 32(8): 809-16.
[http://dx.doi.org/10.1002/ppsc.201500025] [PMID: 26457002]

[45]   Agarwal P, Zhao S, Bielecki P, *et al.* One-step microfluidic generation of pre-hatching embryo-like core-shell microcapsules for miniaturized 3D culture of pluripotent stem cells. Lab Chip 2013; 13(23): 4525-33.
[http://dx.doi.org/10.1039/c3lc50678a] [PMID: 24113543]

[46]   Arriaga LR, Amstad E, Weitz DA. Scalable single-step microfluidic production of single-core double emulsions with ultra-thin shells. Lab Chip 2015; 15(16): 3335-40.
[http://dx.doi.org/10.1039/C5LC00631G] [PMID: 26152396]

[47]   Fischer AE, Wu SK, Proescher JBG, *et al.* A high-throughput drop microfluidic system for virus culture and analysis. J Virol Methods 2015; 213: 111-7.
[http://dx.doi.org/10.1016/j.jviromet.2014.12.003] [PMID: 25522923]

[48]   Lee H, Choi CH, Abbaspourrad A, *et al.* Encapsulation and enhanced retention of fragrance in polymer microcapsules. ACS Appl Mater Interfaces 2016; 8(6): 4007-13.
[http://dx.doi.org/10.1021/acsami.5b11351] [PMID: 26799189]

[49]   Mazutis L, Vasiliauskas R, Weitz DA. Microfluidic production of alginate hydrogel particles for antibody encapsulation and release. Macromol Biosci 2015; 15(12): 1641-6.
[http://dx.doi.org/10.1002/mabi.201500226] [PMID: 26198619]

[50]   Pessi J, Santos HA, Miroshnyk I, Yliruusi J, Weitz DA, Mirza S. Microfluidics-assisted engineering of polymeric microcapsules with high encapsulation efficiency for protein drug delivery. Int J Pharm 2014; 472(1-2): 82-7.
[http://dx.doi.org/10.1016/j.ijpharm.2014.06.012] [PMID: 24928131]

[51]   Anna SL, Bontoux N, Stone HA. Formation of dispersions using "flow focusing" in microchannels. Appl Phys Lett 2003; 82(3): 364-6.
[http://dx.doi.org/10.1063/1.1537519]

[52]   Christopher GF, Anna SL. Microfluidic methods for generating continuous droplet streams. J Phys D

Appl Phys 2007; 40(19): R319-6.
[http://dx.doi.org/10.1088/0022-3727/40/19/R01]

[53]   Zhou J, Khodakov DA, Ellis AV, Voelcker NH. Surface modification for PDMS-based microfluidic devices. Electrophoresis 2012; 33(1): 89-104.
[http://dx.doi.org/10.1002/elps.201100482] [PMID: 22128067]

[54]   Shah RK, Shum HC, Rowat AC, *et al.* Designer emulsions using microfluidics. Mater Today 2008; 11(4): 18-27.
[http://dx.doi.org/10.1016/S1369-7021(08)70053-1]

[55]   Kim C, Chung S, Kim YE, *et al.* Generation of core-shell microcapsules with three-dimensional focusing device for efficient formation of cell spheroid. Lab Chip 2011; 11(2): 246-52.
[http://dx.doi.org/10.1039/C0LC00036A] [PMID: 20967338]

[56]   Chan HF, Zhang Y, Leong KW. Efficient One-Step Production of Microencapsulated Hepatocyte Spheroids with Enhanced Functions. Small 2016; 12(20): 2720-30.
[http://dx.doi.org/10.1002/smll.201502932] [PMID: 27038291]

[57]   Nichol JW, Khademhosseini A. Modular Tissue Engineering: Engineering Biological Tissues from the Bottom Up. Soft Matter 2009; 5(7): 1312-9.
[http://dx.doi.org/10.1039/b814285h] [PMID: 20179781]

[58]   Matsunaga YT, Morimoto Y, Takeuchi S. Molding cell beads for rapid construction of macroscopic 3D tissue architecture. Adv Mater 2011; 23(12): H90-4.
[http://dx.doi.org/10.1002/adma.201004375] [PMID: 21360782]

[59]   Xu X, Farach-Carson MC, Jia X. Three-dimensional *in vitro* tumor models for cancer research and drug evaluation. Biotechnol Adv 2014; 32(7): 1256-68.
[http://dx.doi.org/10.1016/j.biotechadv.2014.07.009] [PMID: 25116894]

[60]   Villasante A, Marturano-Kruik A, Vunjak-Novakovic G. Bioengineered human tumor within a bone niche. Biomaterials 2014; 35(22): 5785-94.
[http://dx.doi.org/10.1016/j.biomaterials.2014.03.081] [PMID: 24746967]

[61]   Villasante A, Vunjak-Novakovic G. Tissue-engineered models of human tumors for cancer research. Expert Opin Drug Discov 2015; 10(3): 257-68.
[http://dx.doi.org/10.1517/17460441.2015.1009442] [PMID: 25662589]

[62]   Fischbach C, Chen R, Matsumoto T, *et al.* Engineering tumors with 3D scaffolds. Nat Methods 2007; 4(10): 855-60.
[http://dx.doi.org/10.1038/nmeth1085] [PMID: 17767164]

[63]   Weaver VM, Petersen OW, Wang F, *et al.* Reversion of the malignant phenotype of human breast cells in three-dimensional culture and *in vivo* by integrin blocking antibodies. J Cell Biol 1997; 137(1): 231-45.
[http://dx.doi.org/10.1083/jcb.137.1.231] [PMID: 9105051]

[64]   Asghar W, El Assal R, Shafiee H, Pitteri S, Paulmurugan R, Demirci U. Engineering cancer microenvironments for *in vitro* 3-D tumor models. Mater Today (Kidlington) 2015; 18(10): 539-53.
[http://dx.doi.org/10.1016/j.mattod.2015.05.002] [PMID: 28458612]

[65]   Barcellos-de-Souza P, Gori V, Bambi F, Chiarugi P. Tumor microenvironment: bone marrow-mesenchymal stem cells as key players. Biochim Biophys Acta 2013; 1836(2): 321-35.
[PMID: 24183942]

[66]   Yip D, Cho CH. A multicellular 3D heterospheroid model of liver tumor and stromal cells in collagen gel for anti-cancer drug testing. Biochem Biophys Res Commun 2013; 433(3): 327-32.
[http://dx.doi.org/10.1016/j.bbrc.2013.03.008] [PMID: 23501105]

[67]   Jain RK. Normalization of tumor vasculature: an emerging concept in antiangiogenic therapy. Science 2005; 307(5706): 58-62.
[http://dx.doi.org/10.1126/science.1104819] [PMID: 15637262]

[68]   Ruoslahti E. Specialization of tumour vasculature. Nat Rev Cancer 2002; 2(2): 83-90.
[http://dx.doi.org/10.1038/nrc724] [PMID: 12635171]

[69]   Chung AS, Lee J, Ferrara N. Targeting the tumour vasculature: insights from physiological angiogenesis. Nat Rev Cancer 2010; 10(7): 505-14.
[http://dx.doi.org/10.1038/nrc2868] [PMID: 20574450]

[70]   Song JW, Bazou D, Munn LL. Anastomosis of endothelial sprouts forms new vessels in a tissue analogue of angiogenesis. Integr Biol 2012; 4(8): 857-62.
[http://dx.doi.org/10.1039/c2ib20061a] [PMID: 22673771]

[71]   Song JW, Munn LL. Fluid forces control endothelial sprouting. Proc Natl Acad Sci USA 2011; 108(37): 15342-7.
[http://dx.doi.org/10.1073/pnas.1105316108] [PMID: 21876168]

[72]   Zheng Y, Chen J, Craven M, *et al. In vitro* microvessels for the study of angiogenesis and thrombosis. Proc Natl Acad Sci USA 2012; 109(24): 9342-7.
[http://dx.doi.org/10.1073/pnas.1201240109] [PMID: 22645376]

[73]   Farokhzad OC, Langer R. Impact of nanotechnology on drug delivery. ACS Nano 2009; 3(1): 16-20.
[http://dx.doi.org/10.1021/nn900002m] [PMID: 19206243]

[74]   Sykes EA, Chen J, Zheng G, Chan WC. Investigating the impact of nanoparticle size on active and passive tumor targeting efficiency. ACS Nano 2014; 8(6): 5696-706.
[http://dx.doi.org/10.1021/nn500299p] [PMID: 24821383]

[75]   Wang H, Yu J, Lu X, He X. Nanoparticle systems reduce systemic toxicity in cancer treatment. Nanomedicine (Lond) 2016; 11(2): 103-6.
[http://dx.doi.org/10.2217/nnm.15.166] [PMID: 26653177]

[76]   Chan JM, Zervantonakis IK, Rimchala T, Polacheck WJ, Whisler J, Kamm RD. Engineering of *in vitro* 3D capillary beds by self-directed angiogenic sprouting. PLoS One 2012; 7(12): e50582.
[http://dx.doi.org/10.1371/journal.pone.0050582] [PMID: 23226527]

[77]   Ma M, Chiu A, Sahay G, Doloff JC, Dholakia N, Thakrar R, *et al.* Core-Shell Hydrogel Microcapsules for Improved Islets Encapsulation. Adv Healthc Mater 2013; 2(4): 10.
[PMID: 23208618]

[78]   Ehsan SM, Welch-Reardon KM, Waterman ML, Hughes CC, George SC. A three-dimensional *in vitro* model of tumor cell intravasation. Integr Biol 2014; 6(6): 603-10.
[http://dx.doi.org/10.1039/c3ib40170g] [PMID: 24763498]

[79]   Hsu YH, Moya ML, Abiri P, Hughes CC, George SC, Lee AP. Full range physiological mass transport control in 3D tissue cultures. Lab Chip 2013; 13(1): 81-9.
[http://dx.doi.org/10.1039/C2LC40787F] [PMID: 23090158]

[80]   Moya ML, Hsu YH, Lee AP, Hughes CC, George SC. *In vitro* perfused human capillary networks. Tissue Eng Part C Methods 2013; 19(9): 730-7.
[http://dx.doi.org/10.1089/ten.tec.2012.0430] [PMID: 23320912]

[81]   Baranski JD, Chaturvedi RR, Stevens KR, *et al.* Geometric control of vascular networks to enhance engineered tissue integration and function. Proc Natl Acad Sci USA 2013; 110(19): 7586-91.
[http://dx.doi.org/10.1073/pnas.1217796110] [PMID: 23610423]

[82]   Bischel LL, Young EW, Mader BR, Beebe DJ. Tubeless microfluidic angiogenesis assay with three-dimensional endothelial-lined microvessels. Biomaterials 2013; 34(5): 1471-7.
[http://dx.doi.org/10.1016/j.biomaterials.2012.11.005] [PMID: 23191982]

[83]   Kim C, Kasuya J, Jeon J, Chung S, Kamm RD. A quantitative microfluidic angiogenesis screen for studying anti-angiogenic therapeutic drugs. Lab Chip 2015; 15(1): 301-10.
[http://dx.doi.org/10.1039/C4LC00866A] [PMID: 25370780]

[84]   Agarwal P, Choi JK, Huang H, *et al.* A biomimetic core–shell platform for miniaturized 3D cell and

tissue engineering. Part Part Syst Charact 2015; 32(8): 809-16.
[http://dx.doi.org/10.1002/ppsc.201500025] [PMID: 26457002]

[85]   Rao W, Zhao S, Yu J, Lu X, Zynger DL, He X. Enhanced enrichment of prostate cancer stem-like cells with miniaturized 3D culture in liquid core-hydrogel shell microcapsules. Biomaterials 2014; 35(27): 7762-73.
[http://dx.doi.org/10.1016/j.biomaterials.2014.06.011] [PMID: 24952981]

[86]   Agarwal P, Wang H, Sun M, *et al.* Microfluidics Enabled Bottom-Up Engineering of 3D Vascularized Tumor for Drug Discovery. ACS Nano 2017; 11(7): 6691-702.
[http://dx.doi.org/10.1021/acsnano.7b00824] [PMID: 28614653]

SUBJECT INDEX

A

Accelerated partial breast irradiation (APBI) 19
Acids 65, 95, 110, 124, 131, 189, 191, 193, 352, 355, 358
  benzoic 110
  glucuronic 124
  glycolic 352
  hyaluronic 352, 355
  indoleacetic 95
  ketoglutaric 193
  lactic 191
  nicotinuric 95
  nitric 131
  nucleic ribose 189
  ribonucleic 65
  utilized oleic 358
Actin 108, 126, 183
  crosslinking protein transgelin 108
  filament 183
  polymerization 126
Activating gene expression 245
Activation 144, 147, 151, 154, 179, 180, 190, 193, 209, 213, 243, 245, 289, 290, 310, 311, 312, 318, 319
  caspase 311
  estrogen-independent 147
  oncogene 209
  oncogenic 190, 213, 310
Adenocarcinomas 3, 88
Adenosine Diphosphate (ADP) 67, 130
  -ribose 67
Adherens junctions component 243
Aerobic glycolysis 179, 190, 191, 193, 310, 311, 313, 318, 319
  process 318
Agents 95, 185, 317, 318, 319, 321, 329, 331, 333, 355
  alkylating 329
  anti-estrogen 333
  antitumor candidate 95
  bioactive 355

  mitochondria-targeting 321
  platinum 331
  therapeutic 185, 355
Aggregates 348, 349, 351, 359
  insoluble fibrin peptide 351
Amino acid 128, 131, 187, 188
  metabolism 187, 188
  residues 128, 131
Aminotransferase 194
Androgen receptor (AR) 143, 148, 149
Angiosarcoma 5
Antagomirs experience 337
Apolipoprotein 116
Apoptosis 150, 155, 157, 258, 267, 284, 291, 292, 308, 310, 311, 312, 317, 318, 319, 329
  calcium-evoked 308
  cell death 317
  inhibition 155, 318
  mitochondria-mediated 310
  resistance in cancer cells 310
  triggering 291
Apoptotic 310, 317
  evasion 310
  proteins 317
Aromatase inhibitors (AIs) 70, 147, 333, 334
Arteriovenous malformations 46
Aspartate transcarbamylase 189
Ataxia telangiectasia mutated (ATM) 10, 76, 141, 143, 263
Atomic bomb 11, 218
  explosion 218
  survivors 11
ATP-binding 152, 283
  cassette (ABC) 152
  site 283
ATP citrate lyase 186, 314
Avidin affinity chromatography 113

B

Biopolymers 93, 351
  derived 351

www.ingramcontent.com/pod-product-compliance
Lightning Source LLC
Chambersburg PA
CBHW050800220326
41598CB00006B/77